CW01475931

TO THE THREE WOMEN IN MY LIFE—
MY MOTHER AND TWO GRANDMOTHERS:
CLAUDETTE, LEA, AND GINETTE
– FRANÇOIS NARS

FRANÇOIS NARS

To Lucy,
With Lots of
Love.

RIZZOLI
NEW YORK

New York · Paris · London · Milan

Franco

London 2018

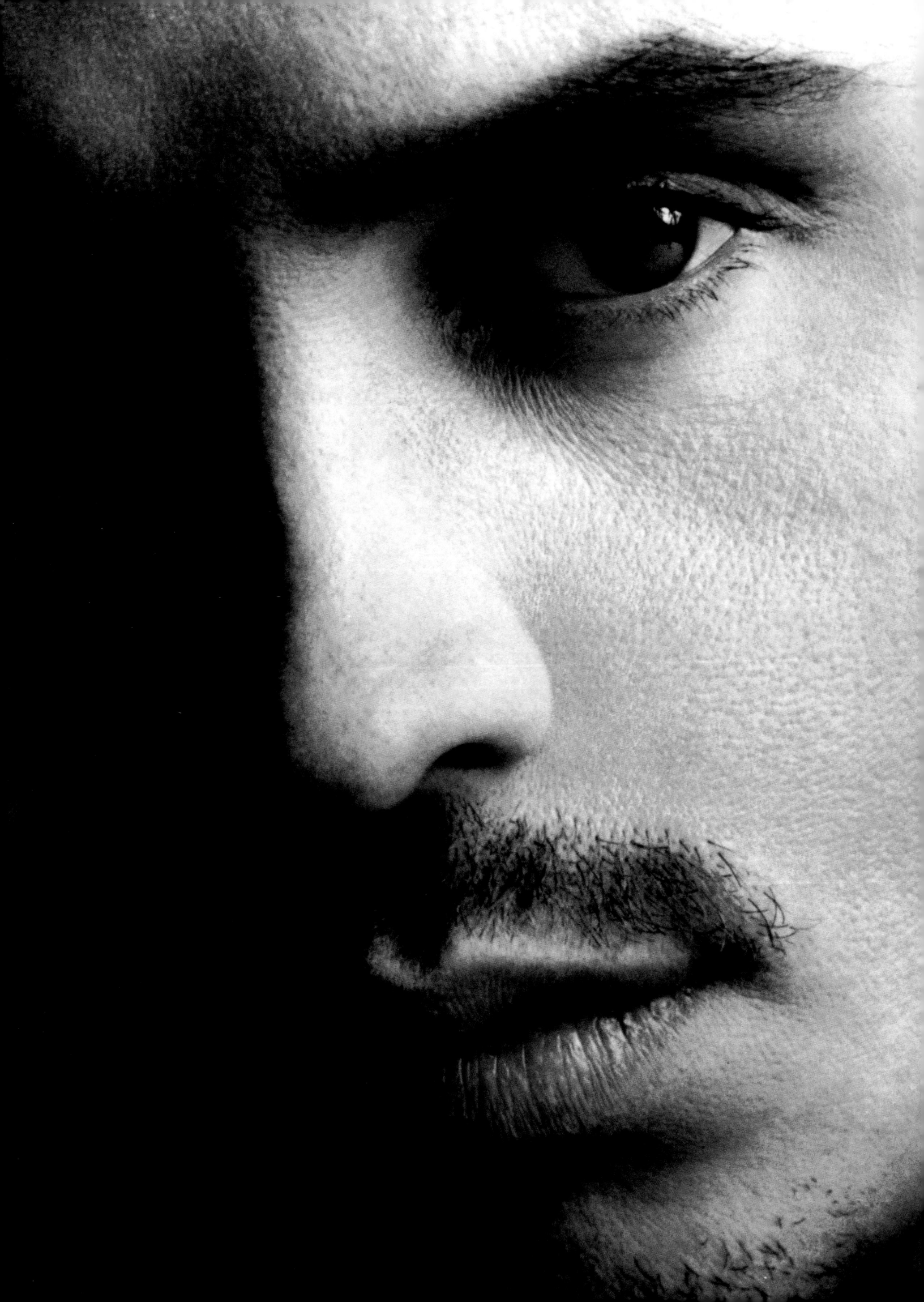

"I DON'T BELIEVE
IN BLANK BEAUTY.
I NEED CHARACTER
AND PERSONALITY."
– FRANÇOIS NARS

NEW YORK, 1984. ENTER THE TURN OF A NEW CREATIVE GUARD, WHERE FASHION WAS REBORN AND STARS ROSE TO LEGENDS—OFTEN AT THE HAND OF FRANÇOIS NARS. THRIVING IN MANHATTAN'S CREATIVE CIRCLE, HE PAINTED A DECADE OF BEAUTY THAT NOT ONLY CHALLENGED CONVENTION, BUT GAVE IT A NEW FACE: THE SUPERMODEL. BACKSTAGE, ON SET, IN PRINT: FRANÇOIS'S WORK WAS EVERYWHERE, ELECTRIFYING NEW AESTHETIC DIMENSIONS WITH HIS REVOLUTIONARY APPROACH TO TEXTURE AND TECHNIQUE.

SHORTLY AFTER MOVING FROM PARIS TO NEW YORK AT THE INSISTENCE OF EDITOR POLLY MELLEN, FRANÇOIS BEGAN SHAPING NEW STANDARDS OF BEAUTY FOR THE PAGES OF *VOGUE*, *ELLE*, *HARPER'S BAZAAR*, AND BEYOND. "POLLY CAME FROM AN ERA THAT WAS FASCINATING TO ME BECAUSE SHE WORKED WITH AVEDON IN THE 60s. IT WAS A DREAM," HE SAYS. "THAT'S WHY I MOVED: I WANTED TO WORK WITH THOSE PEOPLE, THOSE LEGENDS."

HIS NAME WOULD JOIN THEIRS WITHIN THE YEAR. EVOCATIVE AND ARRESTING, FRANÇOIS'S ARTISTRY FOR EDITORIALS SHOT BY RICHARD AVEDON, IRVING PENN, PATRICK DEMARCHELIER, STEVEN MEISEL, BRUCE WEBER, AND BILL KING, AMONG OTHERS, INSPIRED A SWELL OF DEMAND FROM LEADING DESIGNERS, CATAPULTING HIM INTO A RARIFIED STRATA WITHIN THE FASHION INDUSTRY. FRANÇOIS'S SIGNATURE TOUCH OF ELEGANT, ECLECTIC, STARTLINGLY MODERN BEAUTY SOON LAUNCHED A THOUSAND RUNWAY LOOKS FOR LIKE-MINDED IMAGE-MAKERS SUCH AS KARL LAGERFELD, MARC JACOBS, DOLCE & GABBANA, AND ANNA SUI. BUT IT WASN'T UNTIL HE TOOK ON THE WORLD OF ADVERTISING THAT HIS INFLUENCE CHANGED THE FACE OF BEAUTY ON A GLOBAL SCALE.

WITH VERSACE, FRANÇOIS USHERED IN A BOLD NEW ERA. AS THE MAISON'S EXCLUSIVE MAKEUP ARTIST FOR ALL CAMPAIGNS BETWEEN 1994 AND 1996, HE HELPED INTRODUCE A NEW GLAMOUR OF HIGH STYLE AND OUTSIZED PERSONALITY. ICONIC CAMPAIGNS FOR CALVIN KLEIN, RALPH LAUREN, PRADA, AND BARNEYS NEW YORK DEFINED THE SHIFT. BEHIND THE DECADE'S FAÇADE—KATE, LINDA, NAOMI, CLAUDIA—STOOD FRANÇOIS, VISION IN HAND.

"I LIKE TO SHOCK—I TRY NOT TO BE BORING." — FRANÇOIS NARS

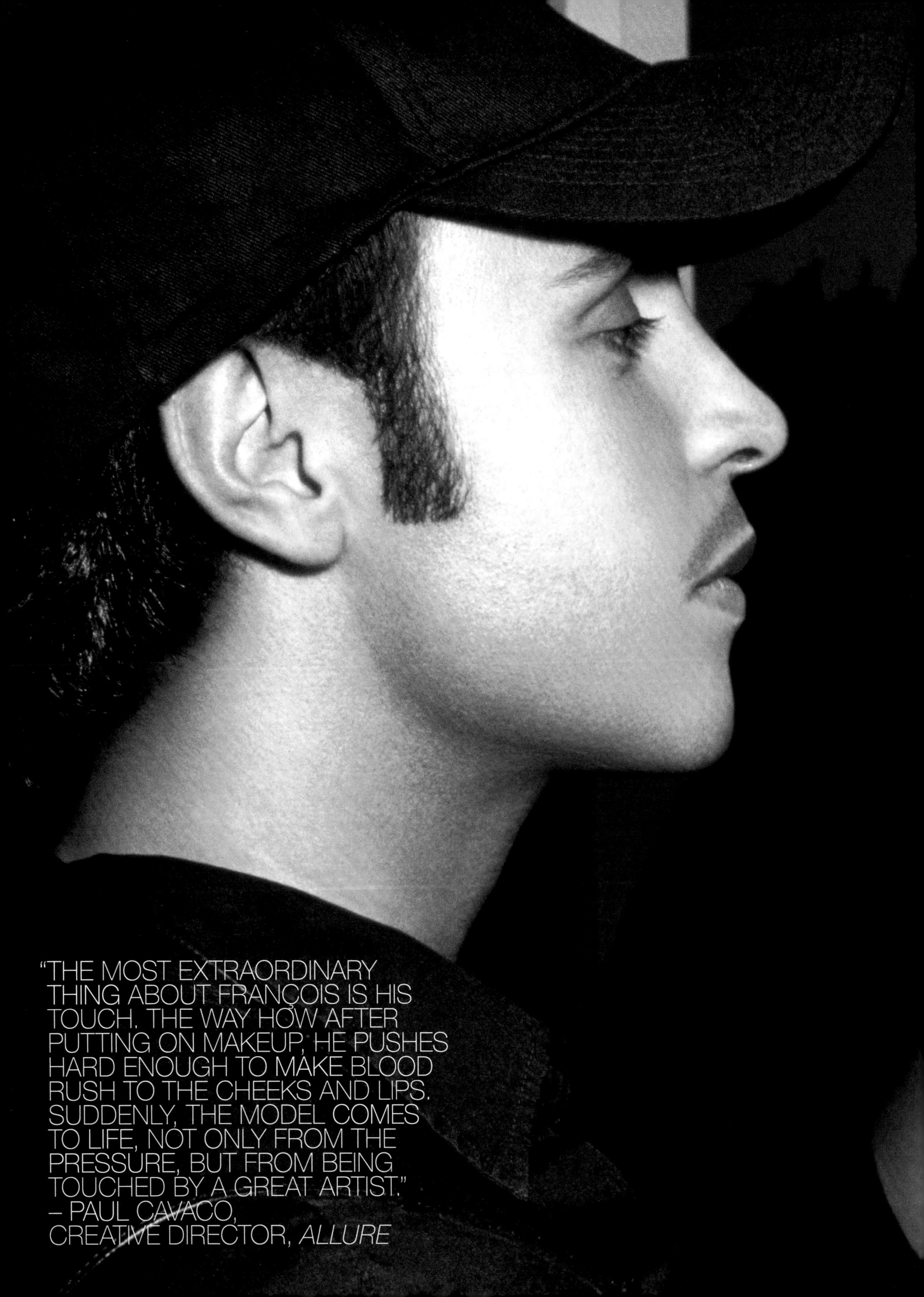

"THE MOST EXTRAORDINARY
THING ABOUT FRANÇOIS IS HIS
TOUCH. THE WAY HOW AFTER
PUTTING ON MAKEUP, HE PUSHES
HARD ENOUGH TO MAKE BLOOD
RUSH TO THE CHEEKS AND LIPS.
SUDDENLY, THE MODEL COMES
TO LIFE, NOT ONLY FROM THE
PRESSURE, BUT FROM BEING
TOUCHED BY A GREAT ARTIST."
– PAUL CAVACO,
CREATIVE DIRECTOR, *ALLURE*

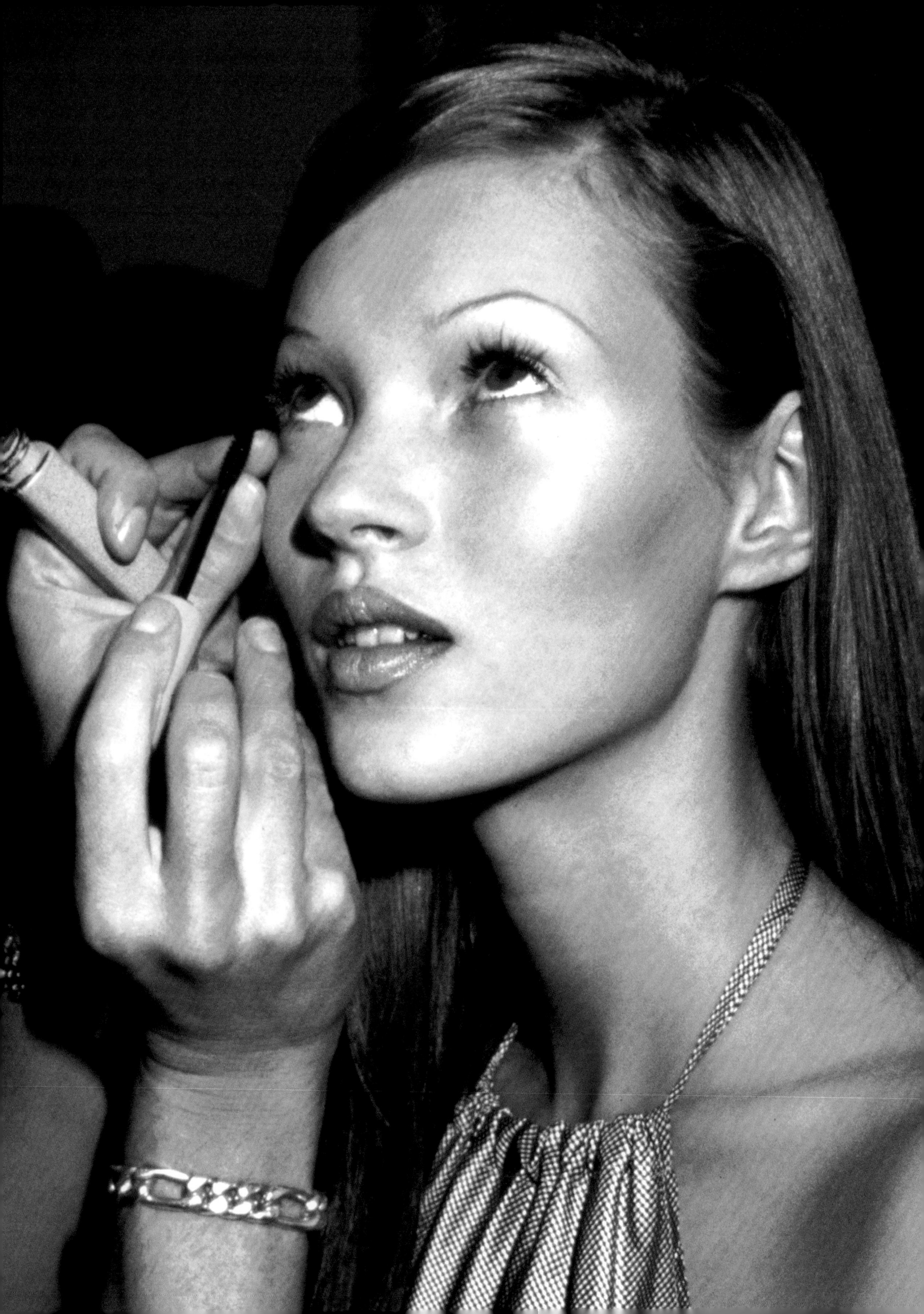

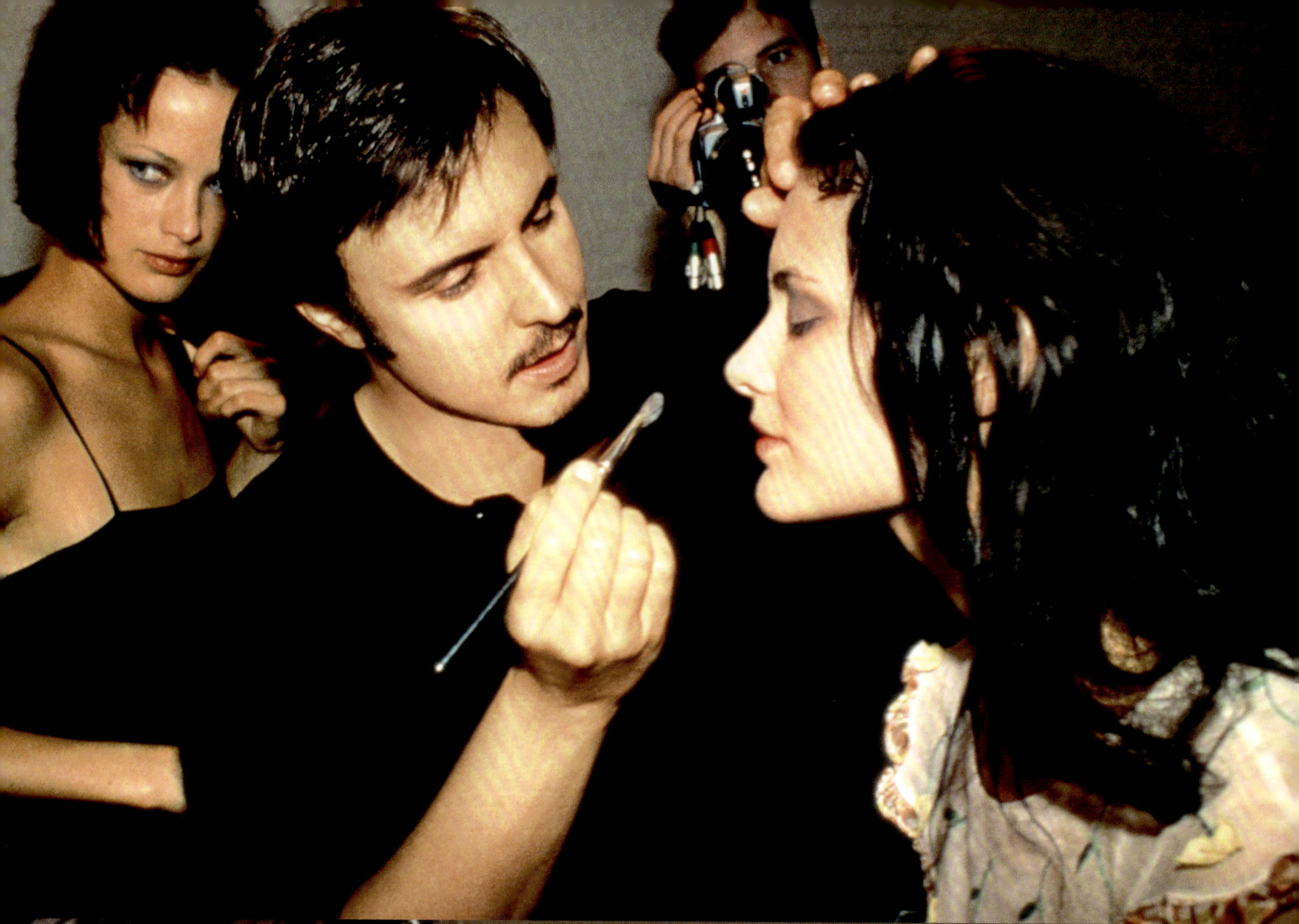

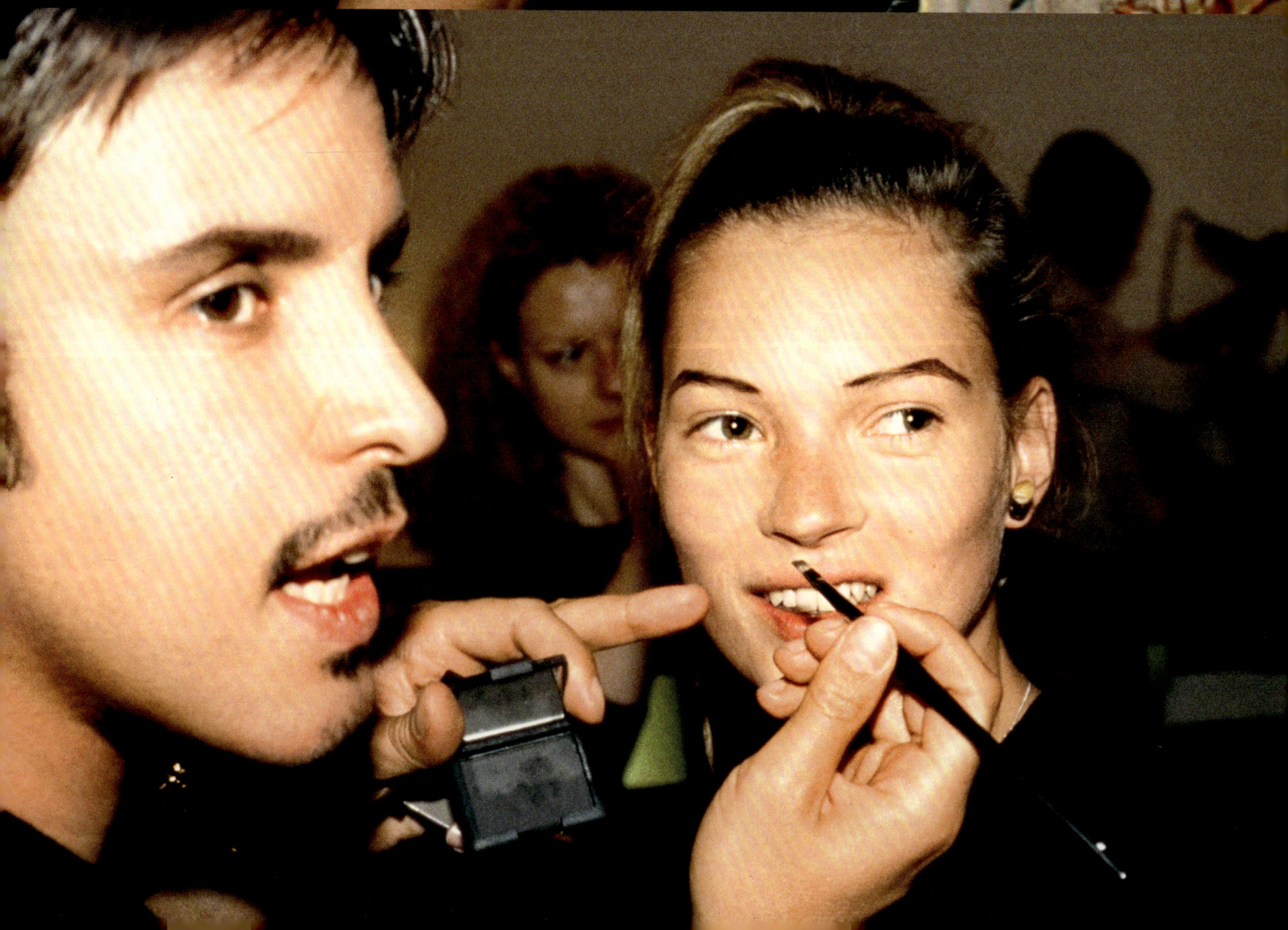

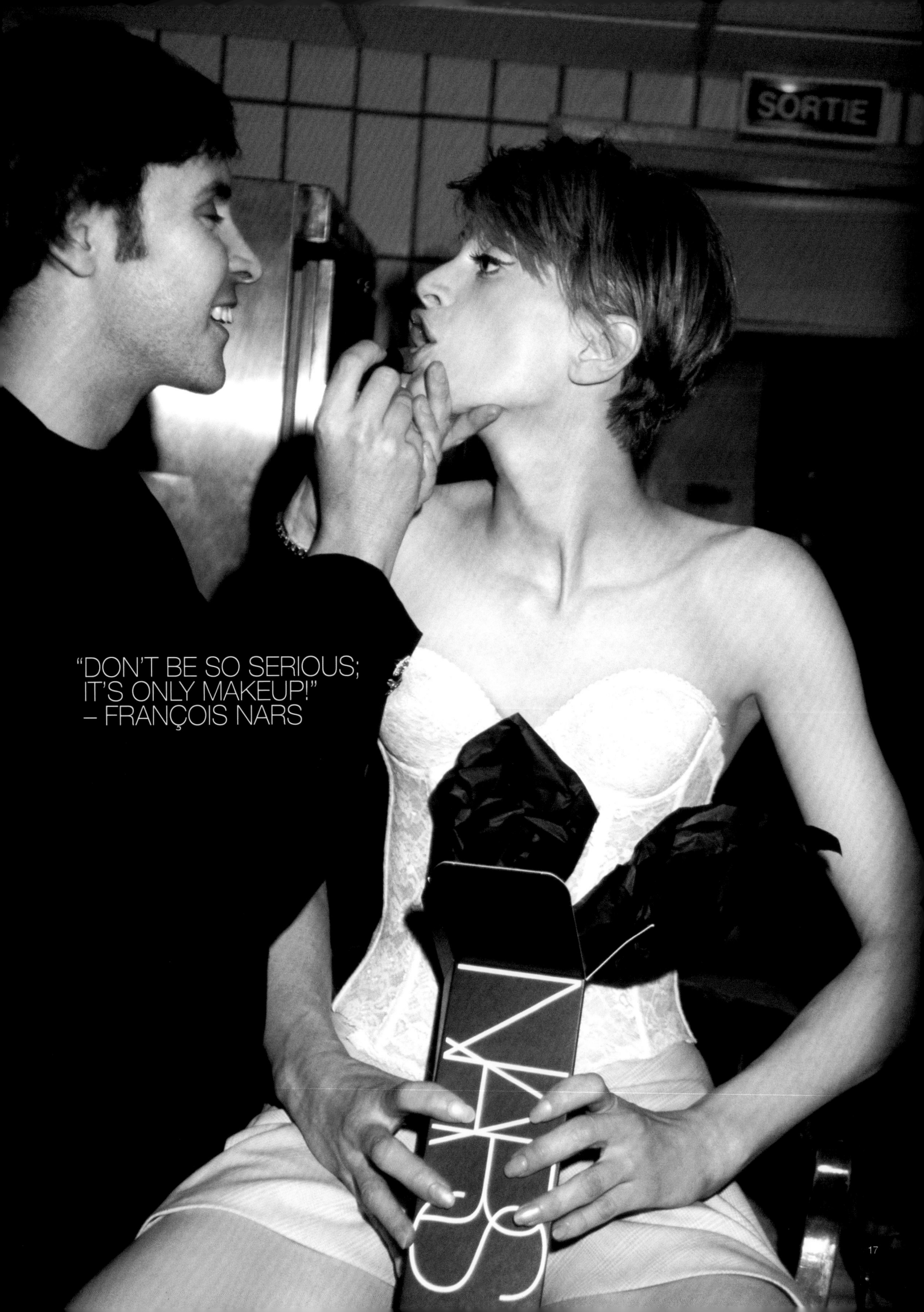

"DON'T BE SO SERIOUS; IT'S ONLY MAKEUP!"
– FRANÇOIS NARS

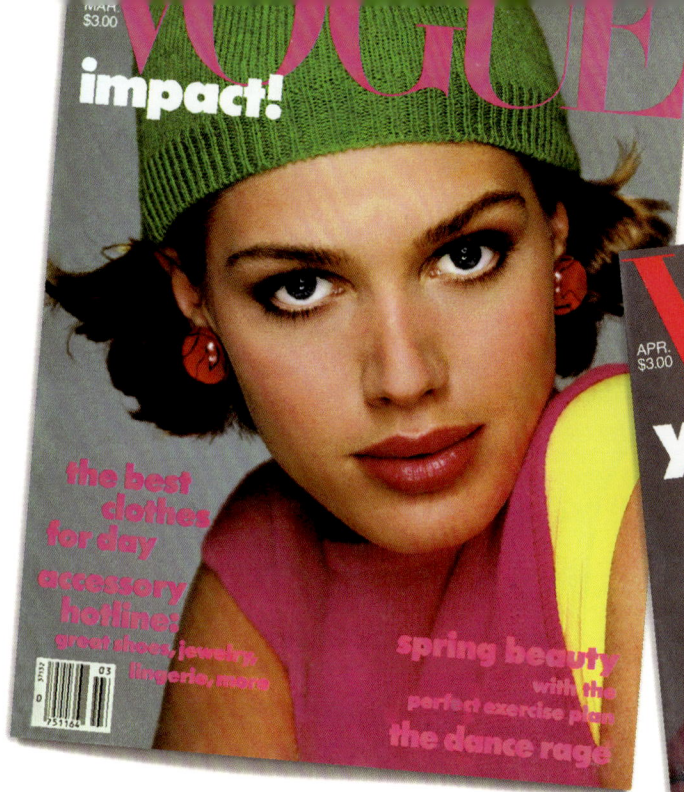

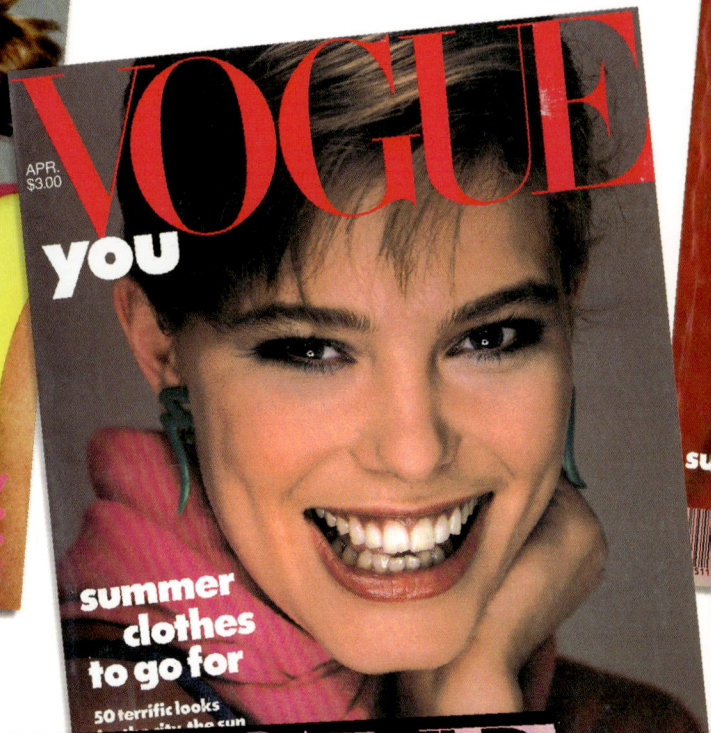

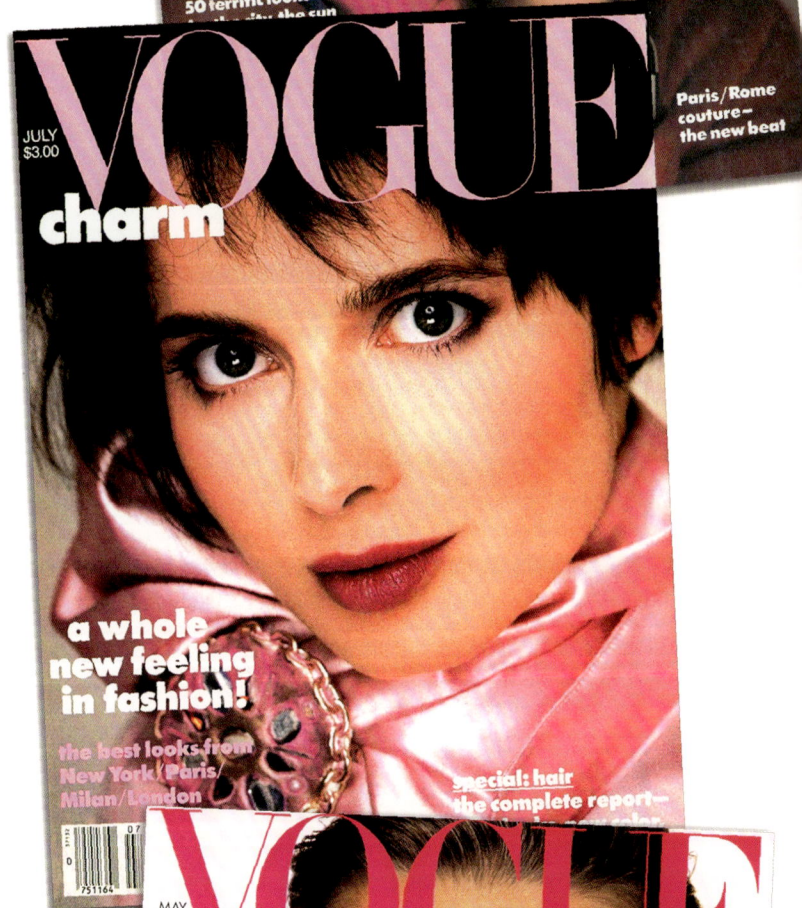

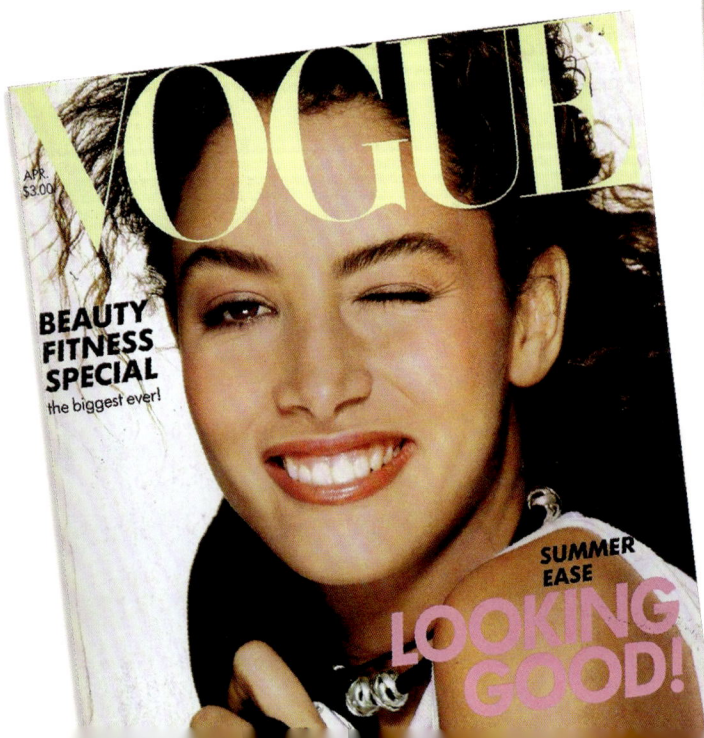

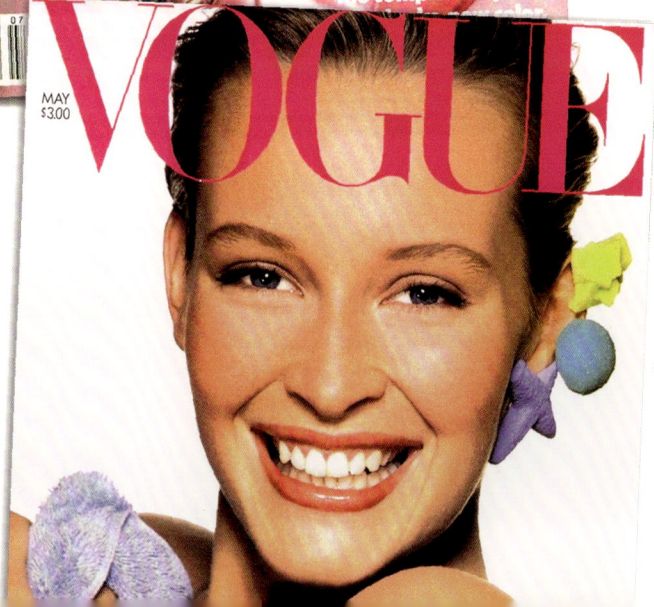

"WE MAY BE PHOTOGRAPHING THE MOST BEAUTIFUL DRESS OR EXTRAORDINARY MODEL, BUT IT'S THE MAKEUP AND HAIR THAT DEFINES A PHOTO AND EITHER MAKES IT GREAT, INSTANTLY DATES IT, OR EVEN RUINS IT. WHEN WE WORKED TOGETHER, FRANÇOIS'S EYE MADE IT SO EXCITING BECAUSE HE DIDN'T JUST DO MAKEUP: HE WAS A COLLABORATOR WHO HELPED MAKE THE PHOTO BETTER."
– PHYLLIS POSNICK, FASHION EDITOR, *VOGUE*

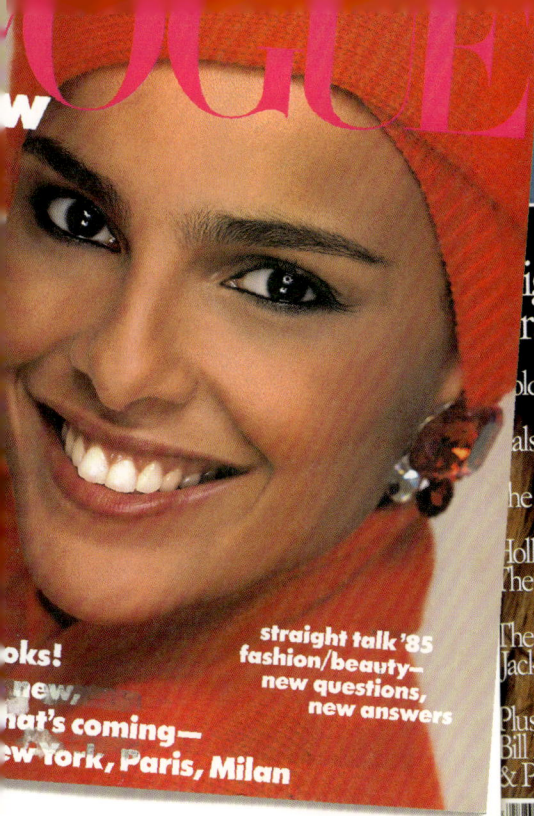

VOGUE

straight talk '85
fashion/beauty—
new questions,
new answers

...oks!
...new,
...hat's coming—
...ew York, Paris, Milan

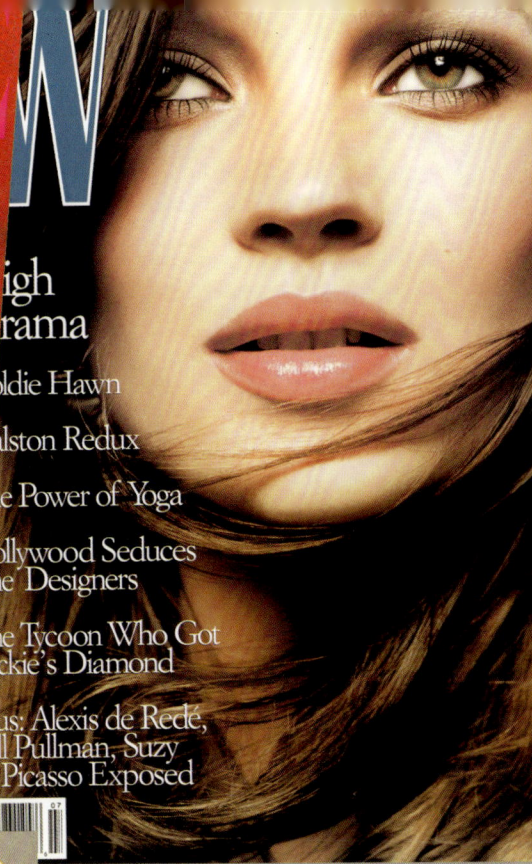

igh
rama

oldie Hawn

alston Redux

he Power of Yoga

Hollywood Seduces
The Designers

The Tycoon Who Got
Jackie's Diamond

Plus: Alexis de Redé,
Bill Pullman, Suzy
& Picasso Exposed

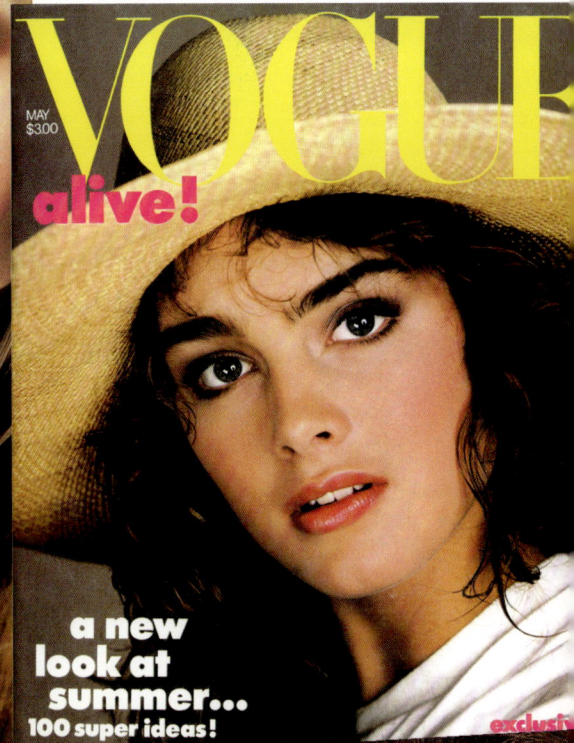

VOGUE

MAY
$3.00

alive!

a new
look at
summer...
100 super ideas!

exclusiv

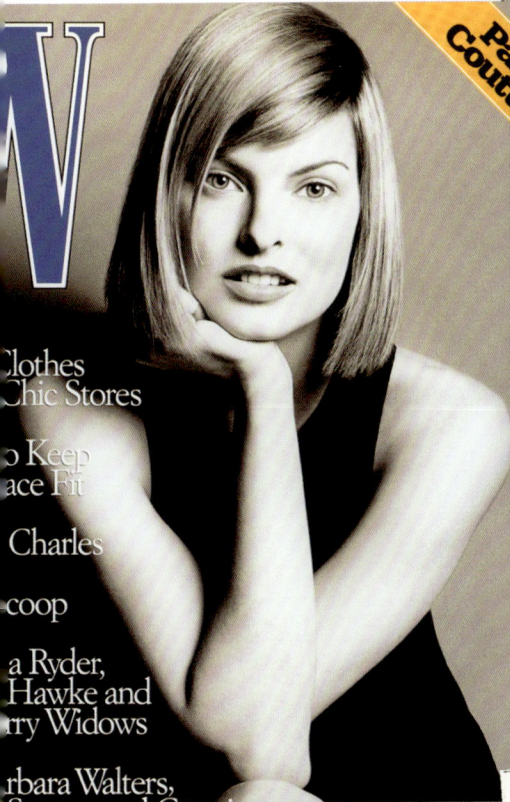

W

Clothes
Chic Stores

o Keep
ace Fit

Charles

coop

a Ryder,
Hawke and
rry Widows

rbara Walters,

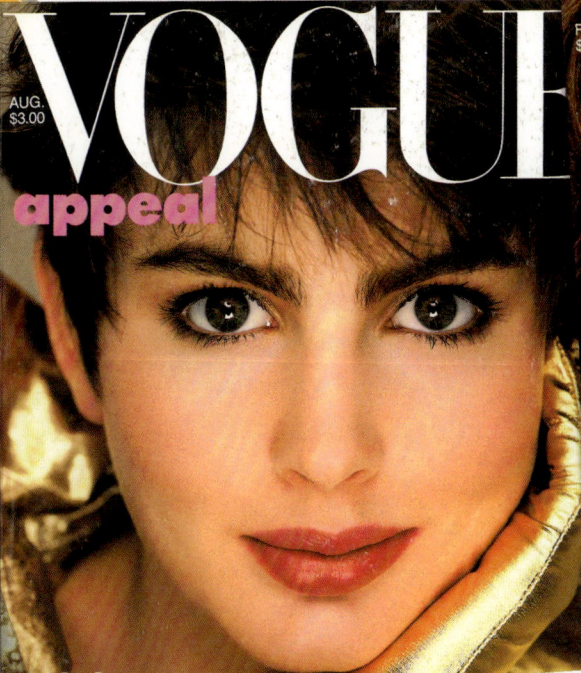

AUG.
$3.00

VOGUE

appeal

a whole new

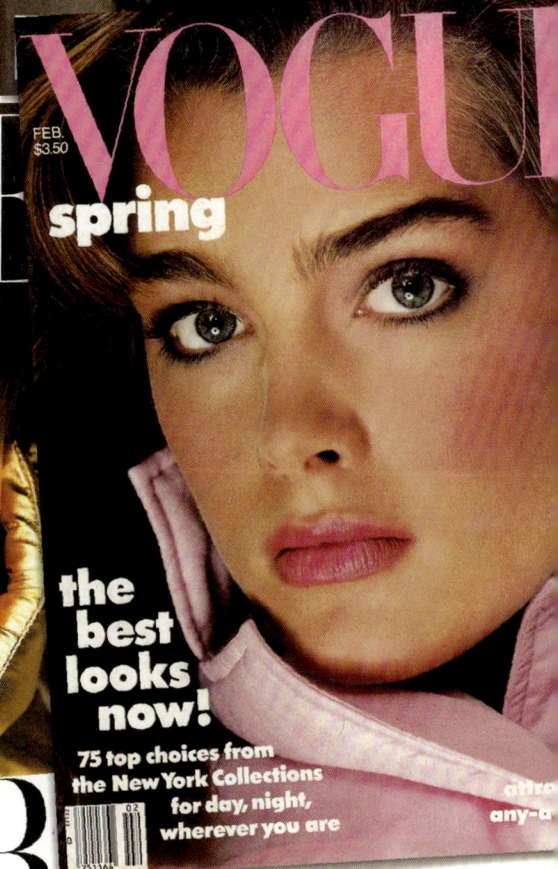

FEB.
$3.50

VOGUE

spring

the
best
looks
now!

75 top choices from
the New York Collections
for day, night,
wherever you are

attire
any-a

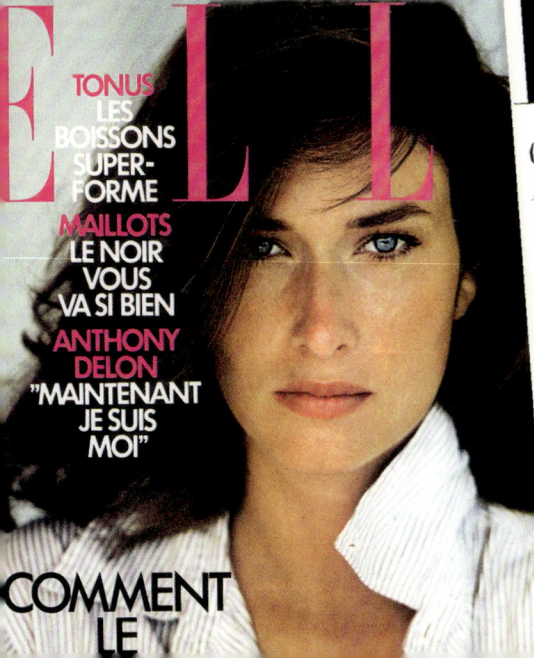

ELLE

TONUS:
LES
BOISSONS
SUPER-
FORME

MAILLOTS
LE NOIR
VOUS
VA SI BIEN

ANTHONY
DELON
"MAINTENANT
JE SUIS
MOI"

COMMENT
LE

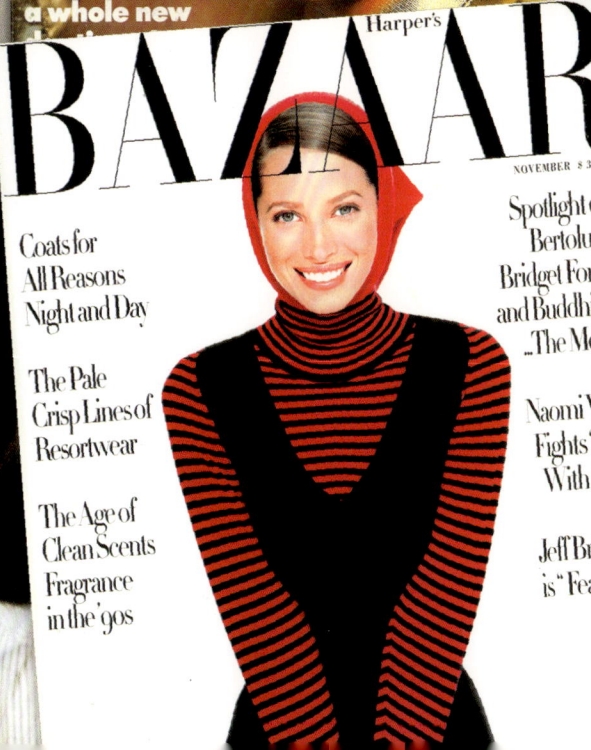

Harper's
BAZAAR

NOVEMBER $ 3.00

Coats for
All Reasons
Night and Day

The Pale
Crisp Lines of
Resortwear

The Age of
Clean Scents
Fragrance
in the '90s

Spotlight on:
Bertolucci
Bridget Fonda
and Buddhism
...The Movie

Naomi Wolf
Fights "Fire
With Fire"

Jeff Bridges
is "Fearless"

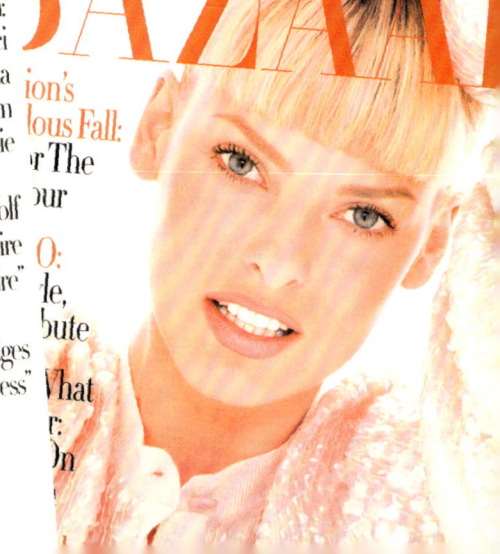

Harper's
BAZAAR

ion's
lous Fall:
r The
ur

O:
le,
bute

What
r: On

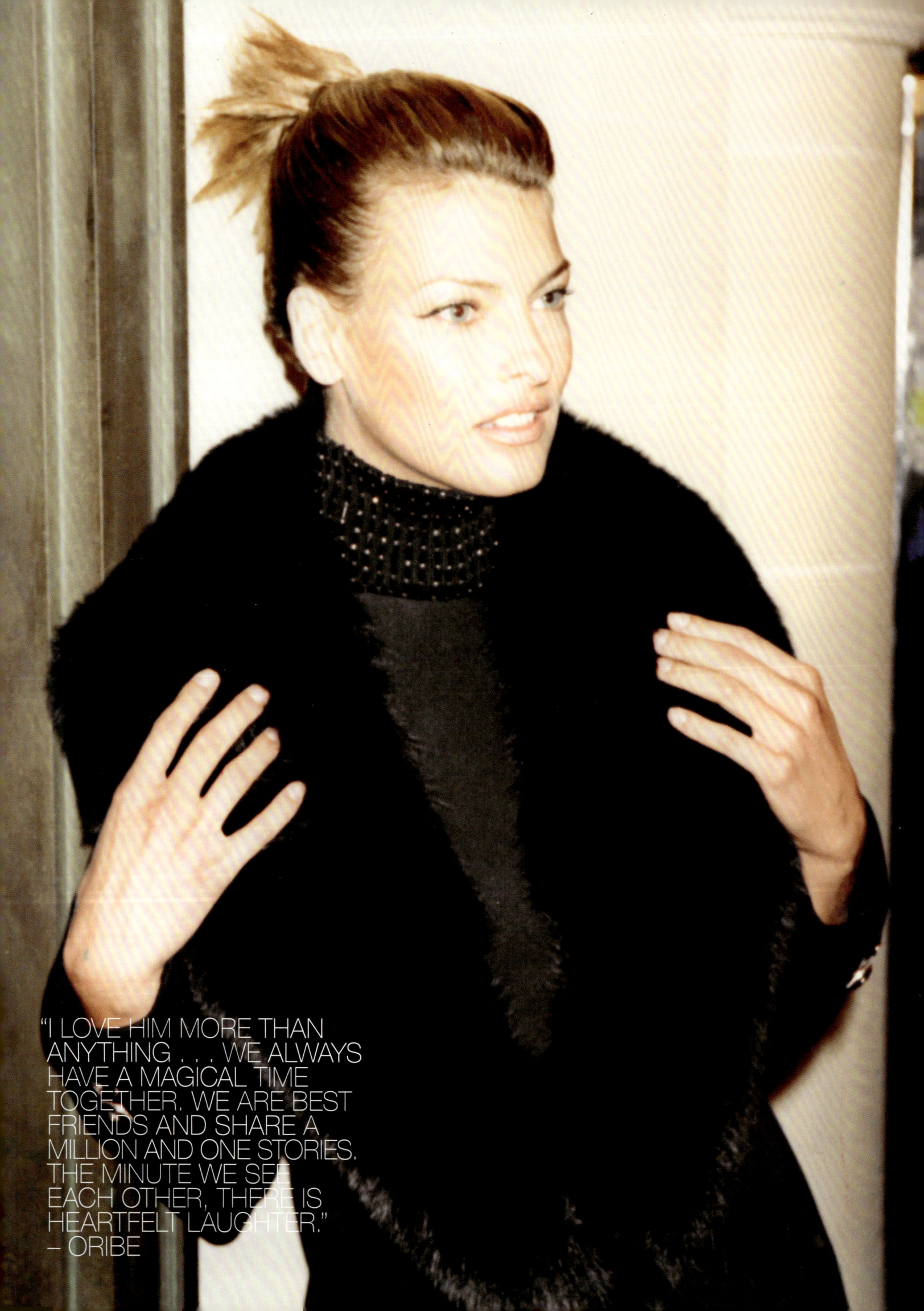

"I LOVE HIM MORE THAN ANYTHING . . . WE ALWAYS HAVE A MAGICAL TIME TOGETHER. WE ARE BEST FRIENDS AND SHARE A MILLION AND ONE STORIES. THE MINUTE WE SEE EACH OTHER, THERE IS HEARTFELT LAUGHTER."
– ORIBE

"ORIBE AND I WERE PARTNERS IN CRIME, ALWAYS LAUGHING, MAKING JOKES AND GIGGLING LIKE FIVE-YEAR-OLD KIDS, BUT ALWAYS DELIVERING. I ADORE HIM." – FRANÇOIS NARS

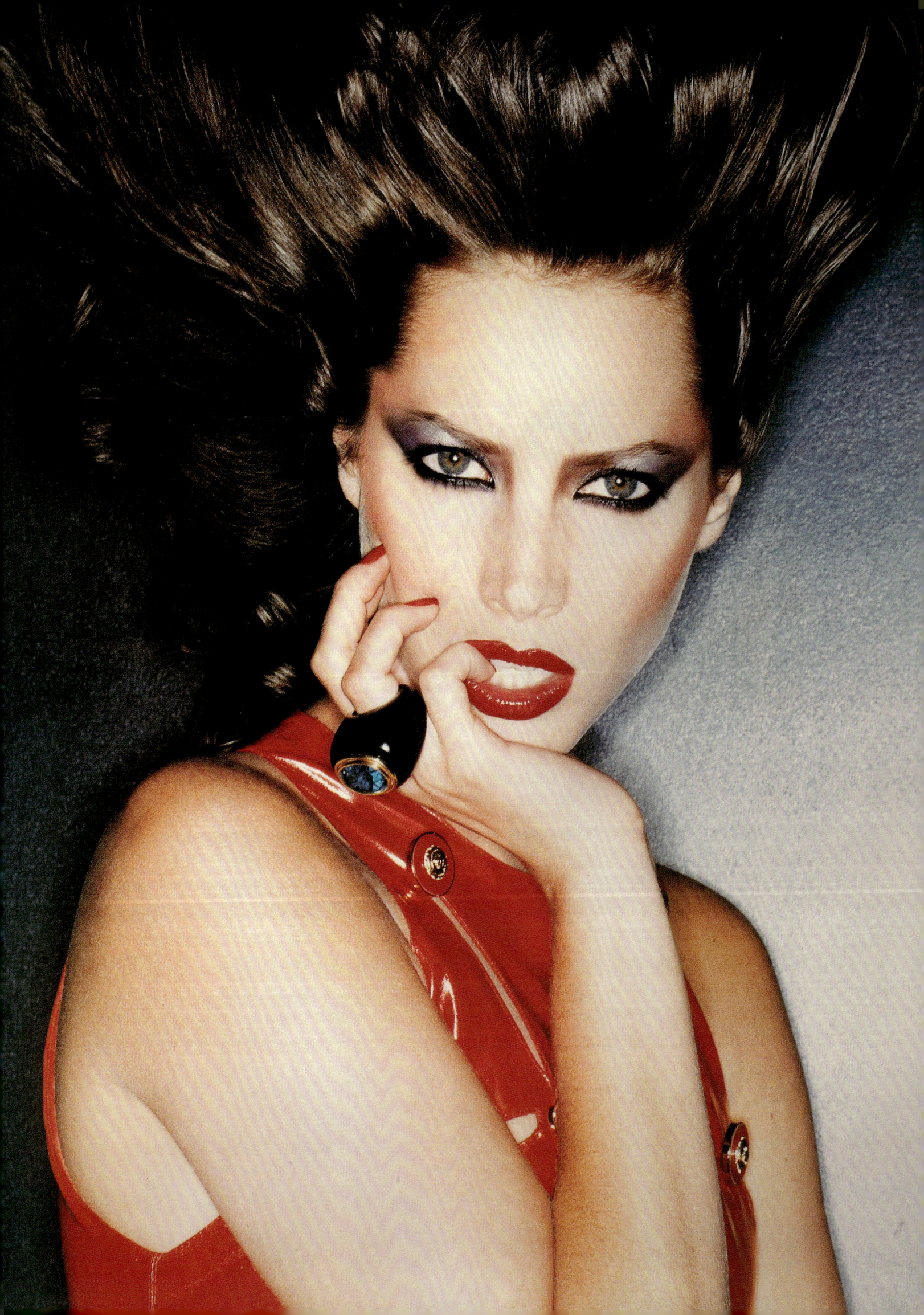

"FRANÇOIS IS AN AMAZING MAKEUP ARTIST WHOM I'VE WORKED WITH A LOT. WE'VE SHOT TOGETHER MANY TIMES, INCLUDING FOR *VOGUE* YEARS AGO. HE IS A GREAT TALENT WITH A GREAT PERSONALITY. THE GUY IS FANTASTIC!" — PATRICK DEMARCHELIER

"PATRICK IS SO WONDERFUL, I LOVE HIS ENERGY! HE MAKES EVERYBODY ON THE SET FEEL COMFORTABLE. THIS IS ONE OF HIS SECRETS TO GET THOSE AMAZING IMAGES."
– FRANÇOIS NARS

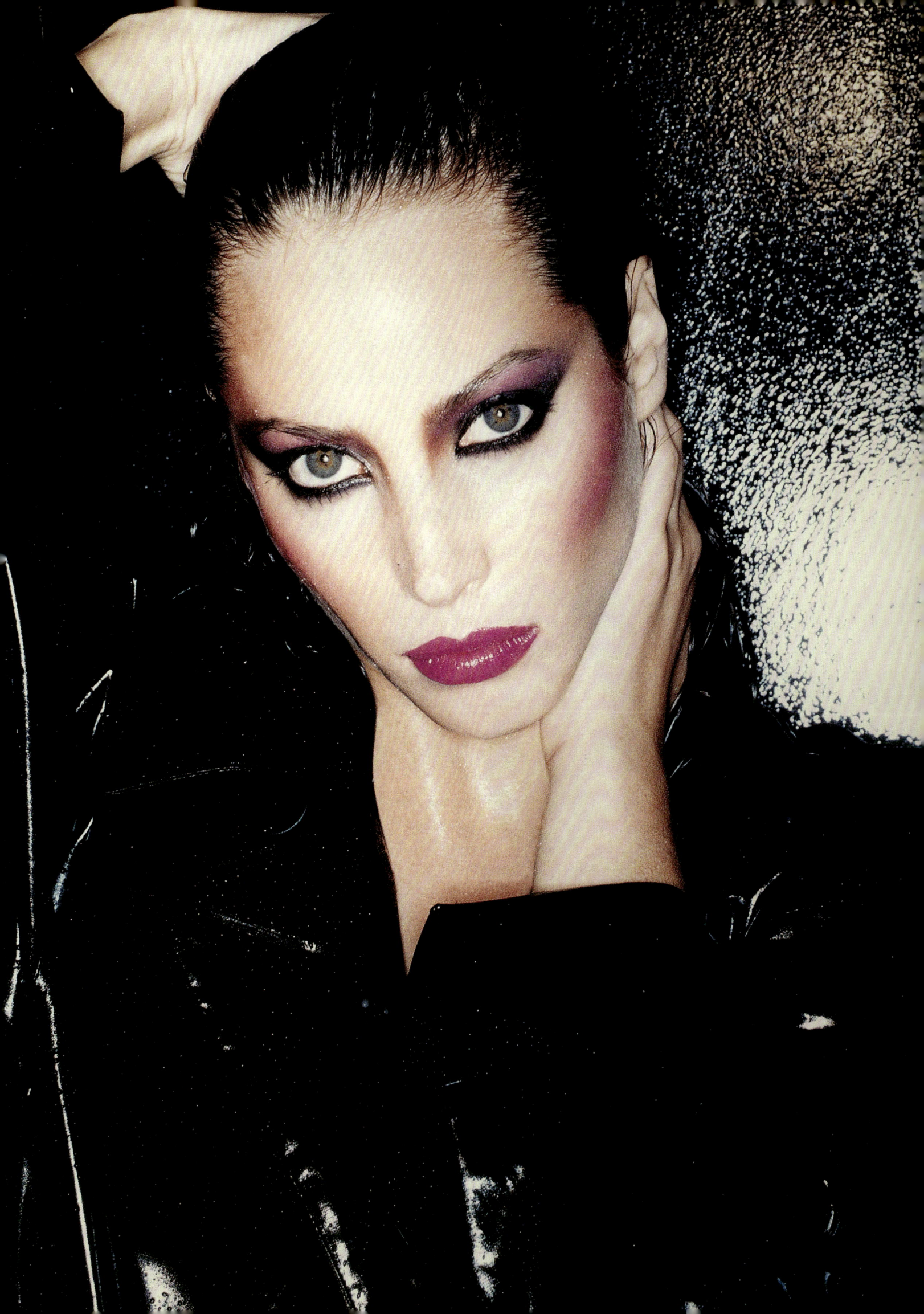

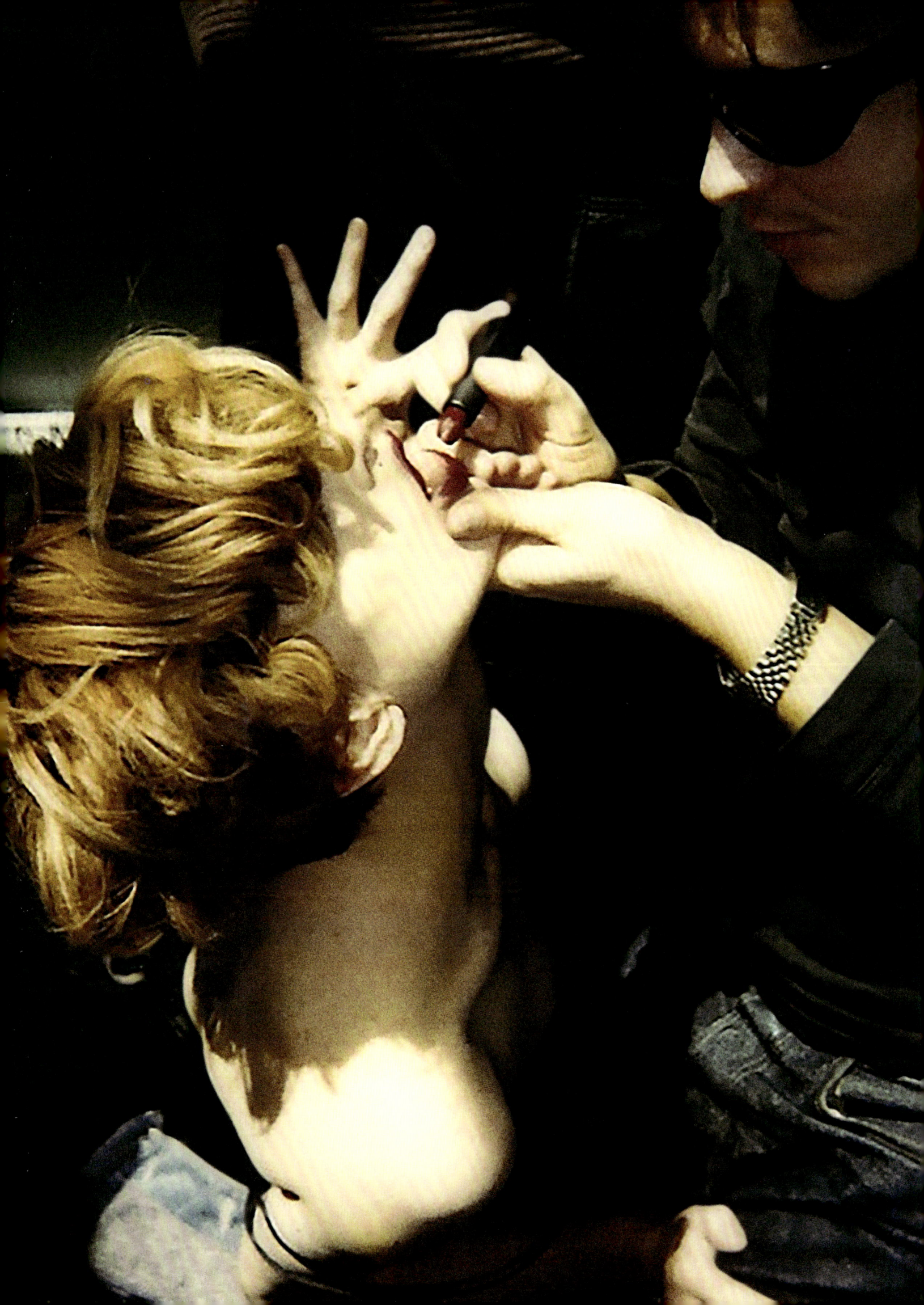

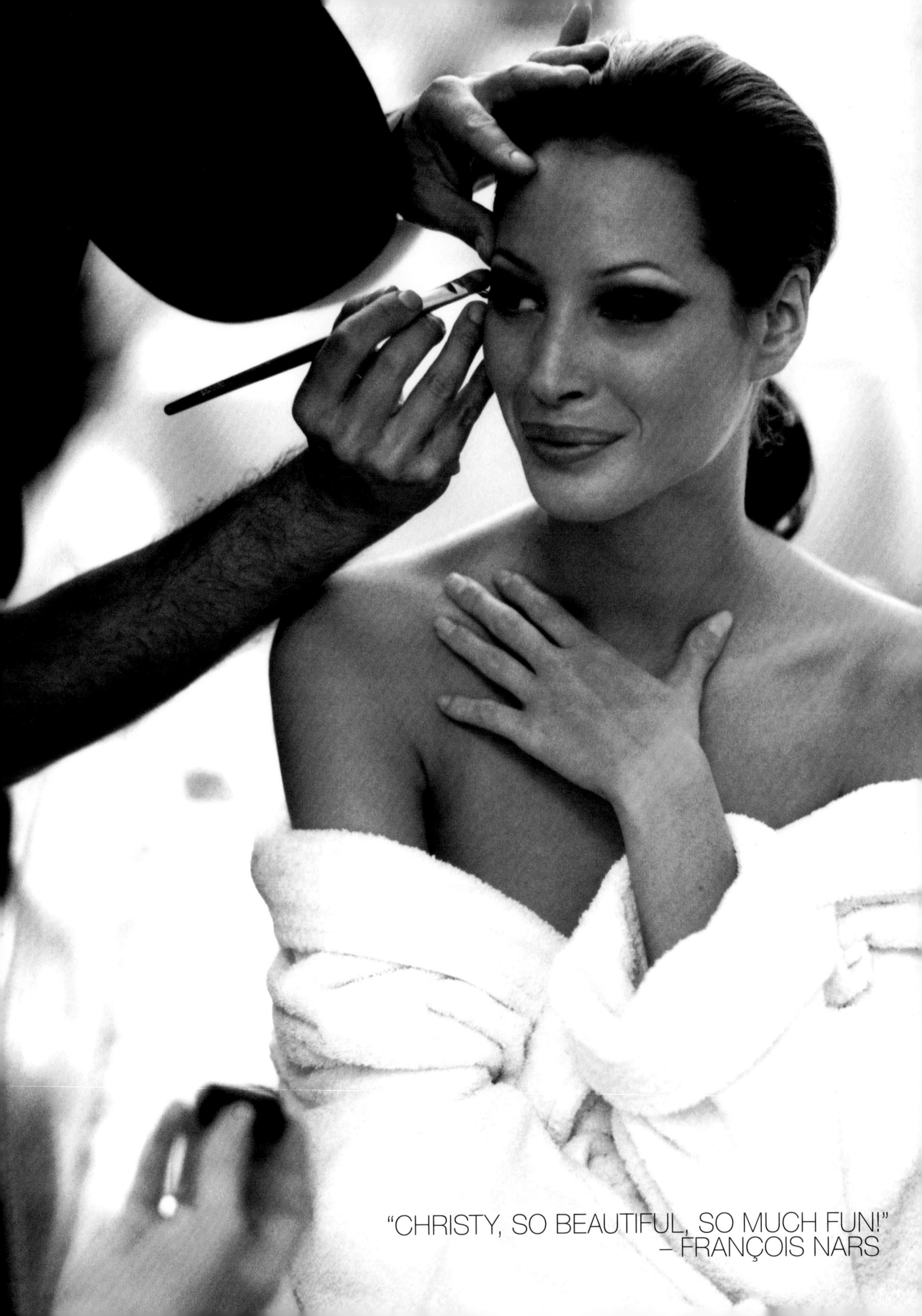

"CHRISTY, SO BEAUTIFUL, SO MUCH FUN!"
– FRANÇOIS NARS

"MAKEUP IS A GREAT
TOOL FOR SEDUCTION.
IT SHOULD EMPOWER
WOMEN AND HELP
THEM FACE THE
WORLD GRACEFULLY."
– FRANÇOIS NARS

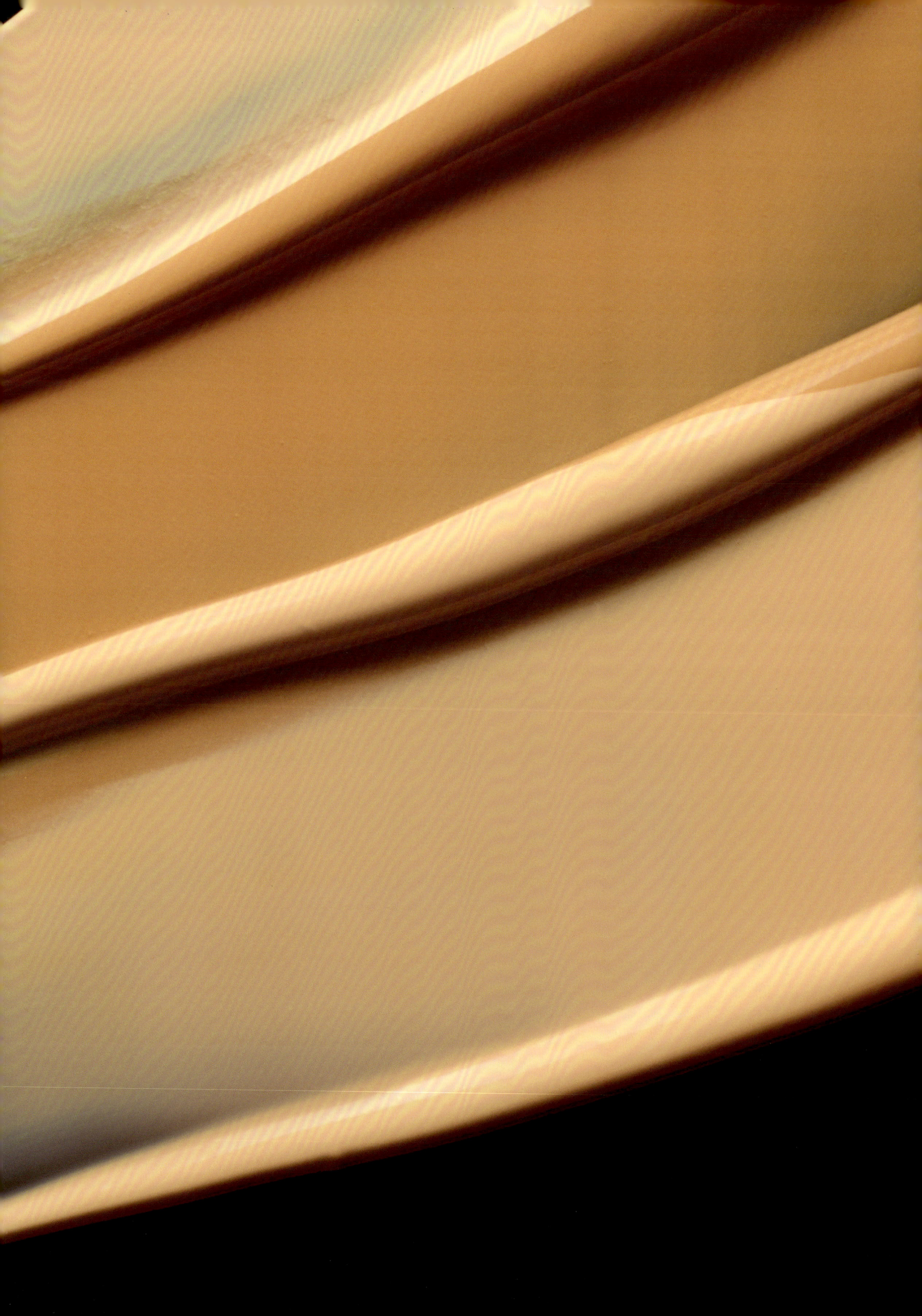

"ONE OF THE MOST MEMORABLE *VOGUE* COVERS I DID WAS WITH RICHARD AVEDON, POLLY MELLEN, AND PAULINA PORIZKOVA. THEY HAD TRIED TO PUT PAULINA ON THE COVER A COUPLE OF TIMES, BUT SHE NEVER MADE IT, AS DICK NEVER GOT A PICTURE HE WAS REALLY HAPPY WITH. SO THEY BOOKED ME FOR ONE LAST COVER TRY. I DECIDED TO MAKE HER EXTREMELY SOFT—NO OBVIOUS MAKEUP, NO DARK EYESHADOW—JUST VERY CLEAN, VERY FRESH. DICK LOVED IT, POLLY LOVED IT, GRACE MIRABELLA LOVED IT. THE REST IS HISTORY."
– FRANÇOIS NARS

VOGUE

MAY
$3.00

cool!

free & easy
fashion
CITY, SUN
DAY, NIGHT

diet bliss
eat healthy,
lose weight,
and win!

IN/OUT/HOT/NOT
celebrities on celebrity

"DICK AVEDON WAS NOT JUST A FASHION PHOTOGRAPHER, HE WAS SO MUCH MORE THAN THAT, HE WAS A COMPLETE ARTIST WITH AN AMAZING EYE FOR HIS TIME. HIS INFLUENCE TODAY MAKES HIM ONE OF THE MOST COPIED ARTISTS EVER." — FRANÇOIS NARS

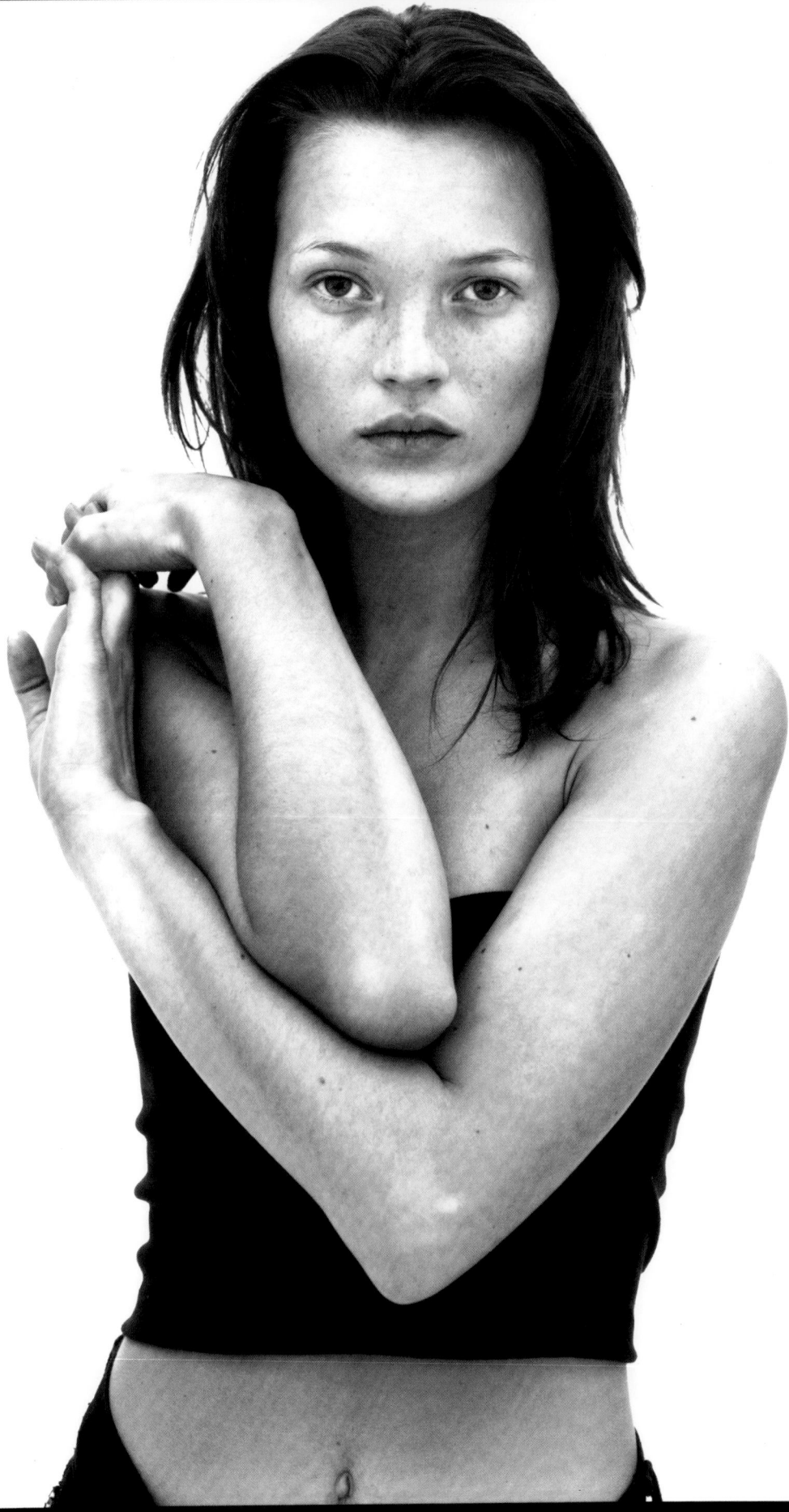

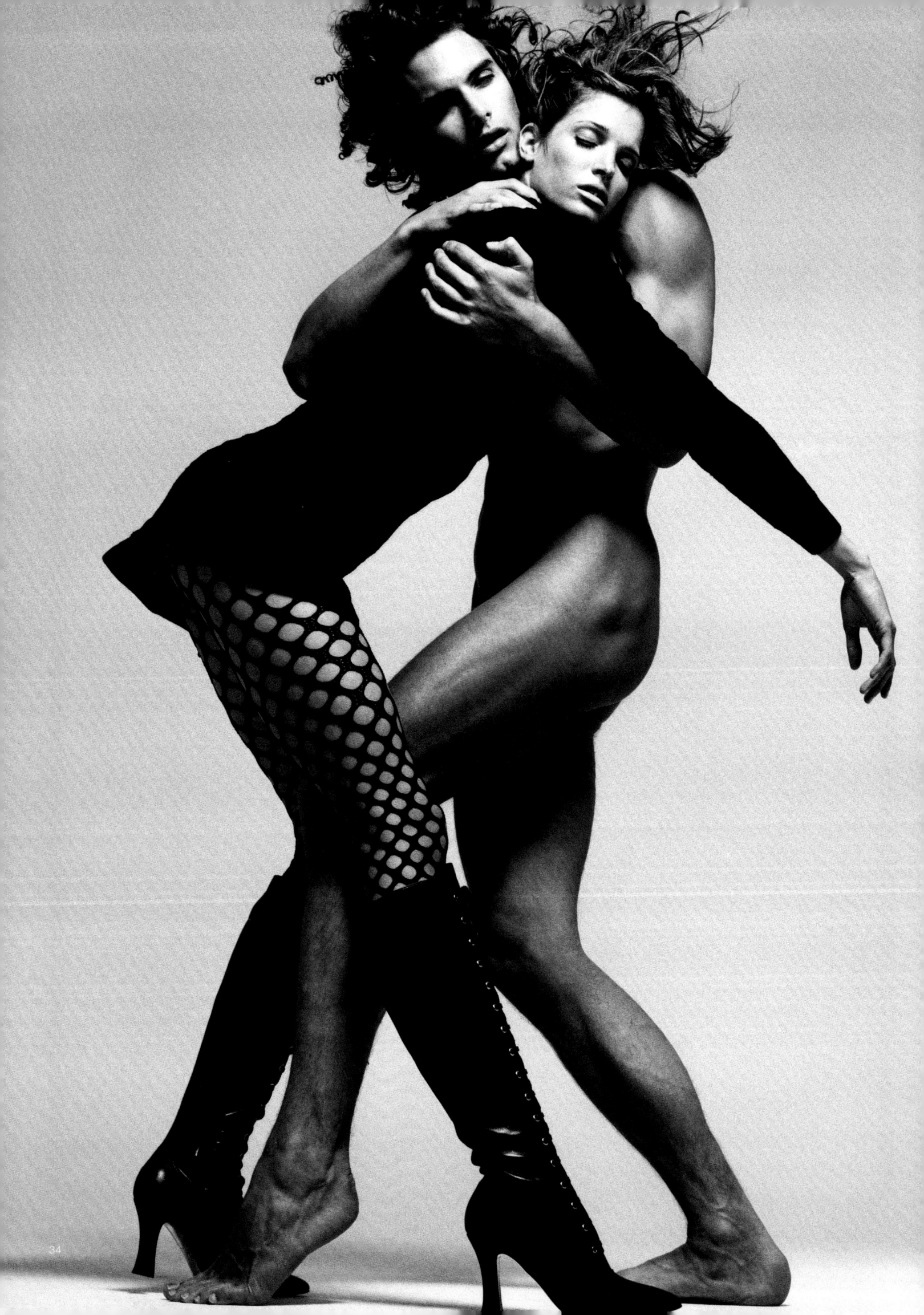

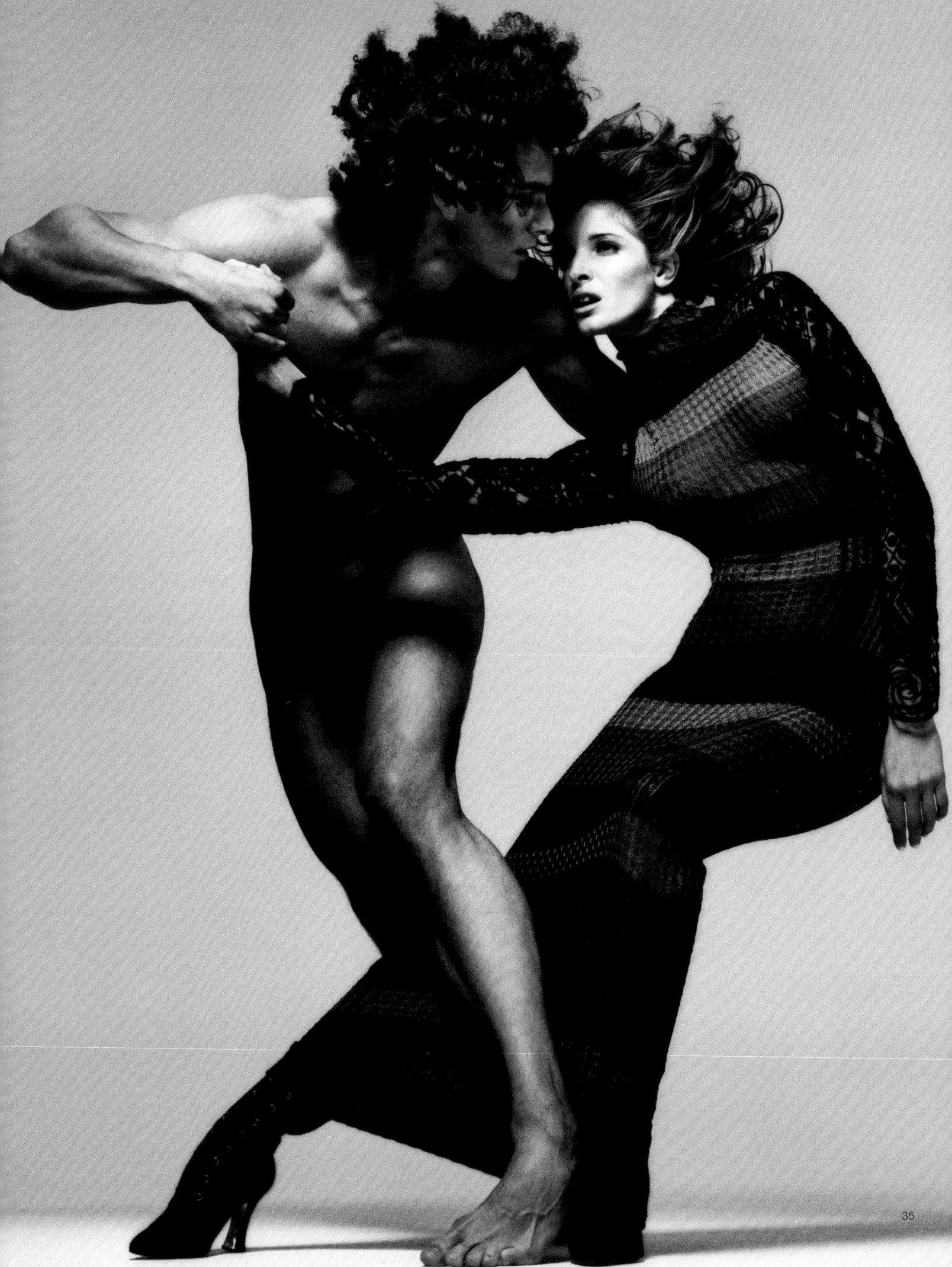

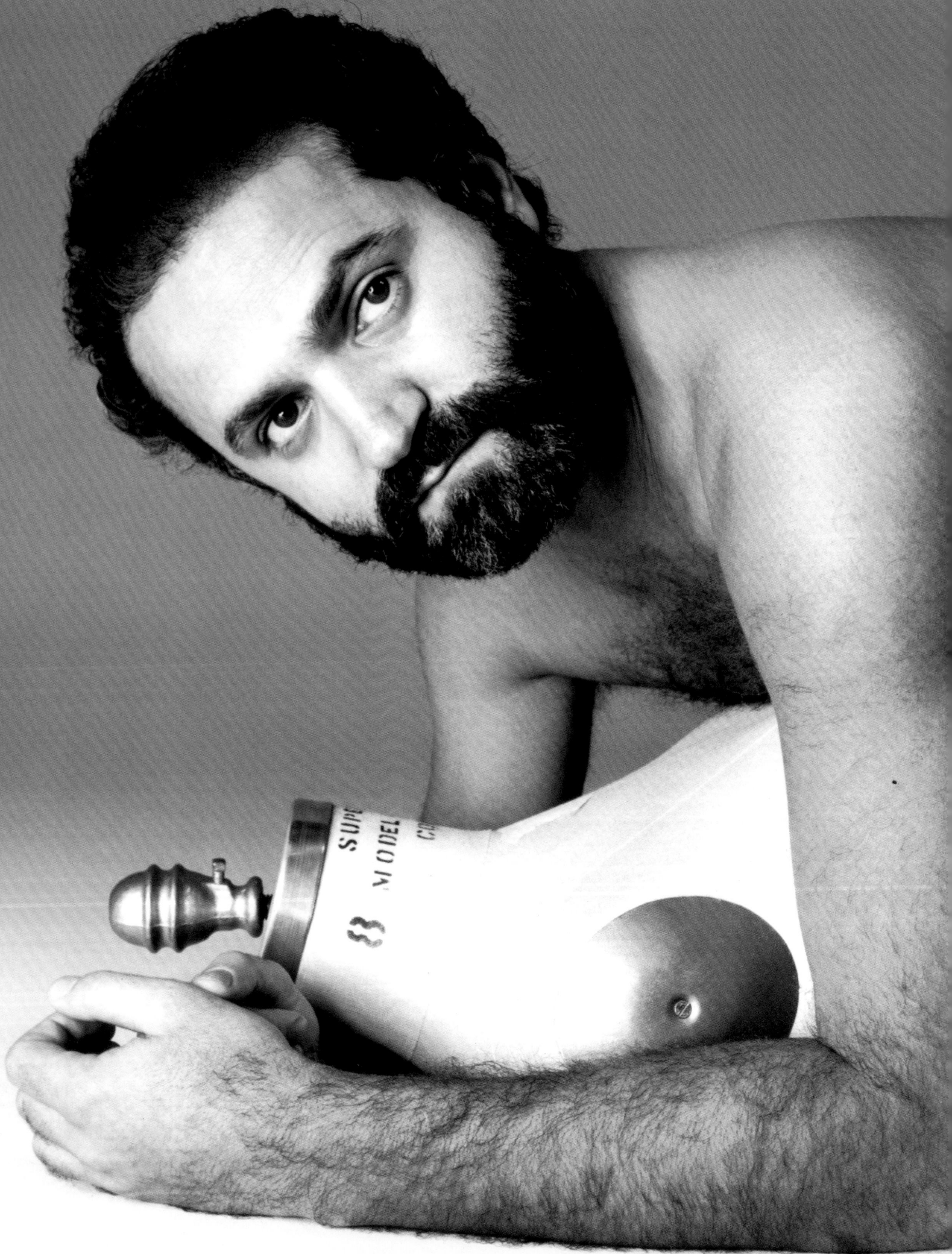

"GIANNI WAS WONDERFUL, SO ITALIAN. HE NEEDED BEAUTY IN HIS LIFE AND YOU WANTED TO MAKE THOSE MODELS LOOK LARGER-THAN-LIFE FOR HIM. I MISS HIM."
– FRANÇOIS NARS

"I'VE HAD THE GREAT
OPPORTUNITY TO WORK
WITH FRANÇOIS MANY
TIMES OVER THE YEARS,
AND I NEVER ONCE
HEARD HIM COMPLAIN
ABOUT BEING TOO WET,
SANDY, DIRTY, FREEZING,
OR SWEATY IN THE
PURSUIT OF BEAUTY."
– BRUCE WEBER

"WHEN I FIRST ARRIVED IN NEW YORK
IN THE EARLY 80s, I HAD A MISSION
TO WORK WITH SOME VERY SPECIFIC
PHOTOGRAPHERS; BRUCE WAS THE
FIRST ONE ON MY LIST WITH AVEDON
AND PENN. HELMUT NEWTON ONCE
SAID ABOUT BRUCE THAT HE WAS
'THE BEST PHOTOGRAPHER IN
AMERICA.' WORKING WITH BRUCE ALL
THOSE YEARS HAS ALWAYS BEEN
AN ADVENTURE FOR ME. WHEREVER
BRUCE TOOK US, YOU ALWAYS FELT
LIKE YOU WERE PART OF THE STORY
HE WAS TELLING THROUGH HIS
PHOTOGRAPHS. HIS VERY SPECIFIC,
DIFFERENT EYE ON FASHION, AND HIS
AMAZING CULTURE AND AESTHETICS
ALWAYS MADE IT A GREAT AND VERY
SPECIAL EXPERIENCE."
– FRANÇOIS NARS

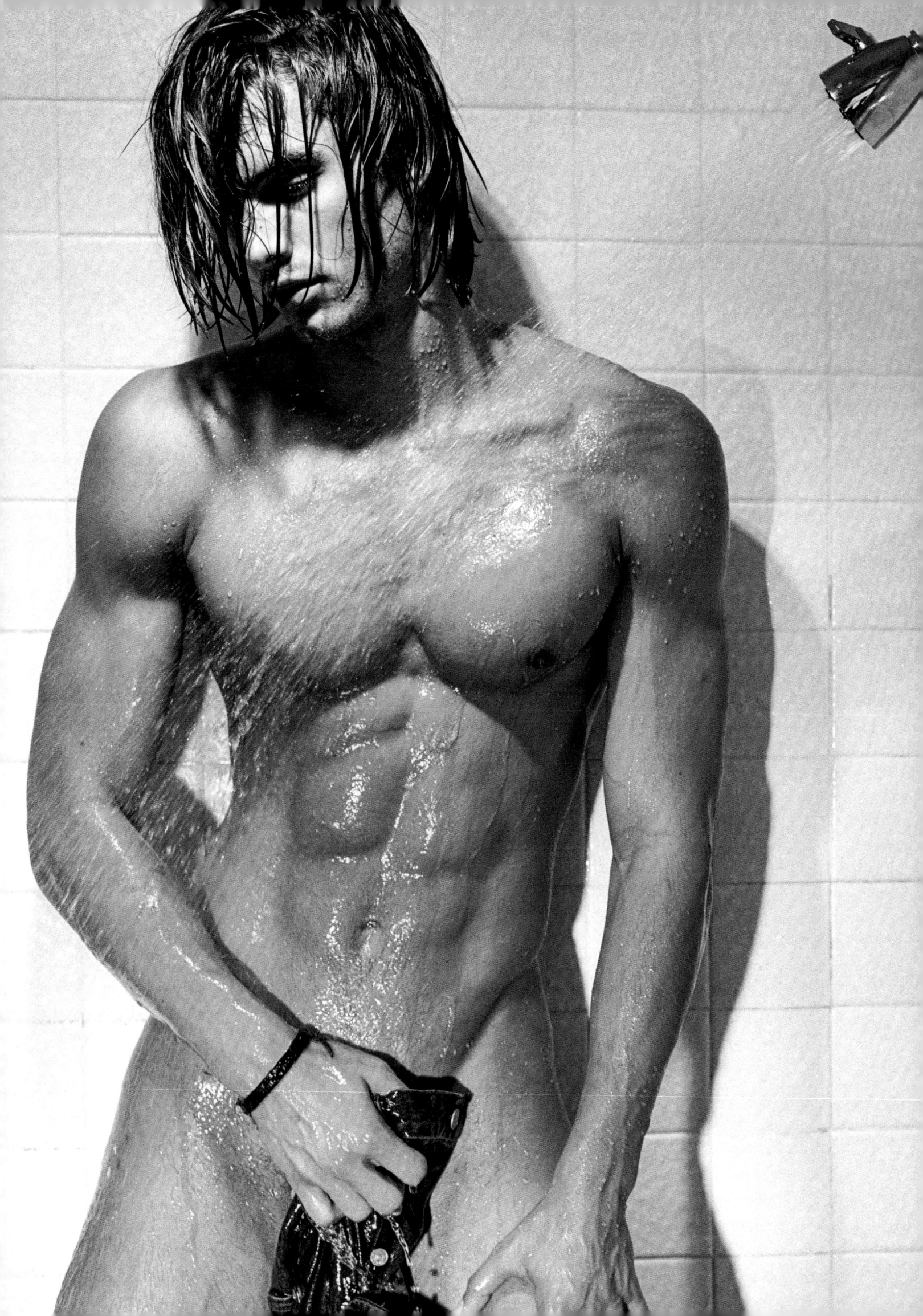

"FIVE DAYS WORKING WITH
FRANÇOIS, TOGETHER,
TO GATHER IDEAS AND
WORK, TRUST, AND JOY,
COMPLICITY AND SUPPORT,
MEMORIES AND FRIENDS.
IS IT CALLED WORK? IT WAS
SUCH A PLEASURE . . .
I AM STILL WONDERING."
– SARAH MOON

"SARAH IS A POET, A
SCULPTOR, A PAINTER. I HAVE
ALWAYS BEEN FASCINATED
BY HER WORK FOR SO MANY
YEARS. I LOVE HER VISION OF
BEAUTY, HER SENSIBILITY, AND
EXTREME PERFECTIONISM AND
REFINEMENT. WATCHING HER
TAKING PICTURES WAS A GREAT
LESSON OF LIFE. I DISCOVERED
ALSO THE SWEETEST HUMAN
BEING, FULL OF HUMOR AND
CHARM. COLLABORATING
TOGETHER WAS A BIG DREAM
FOR ME FOR SUCH A LONG
TIME, SO I GUESS DREAMS DO
COME TRUE SOMETIMES."
– FRANÇOIS NARS

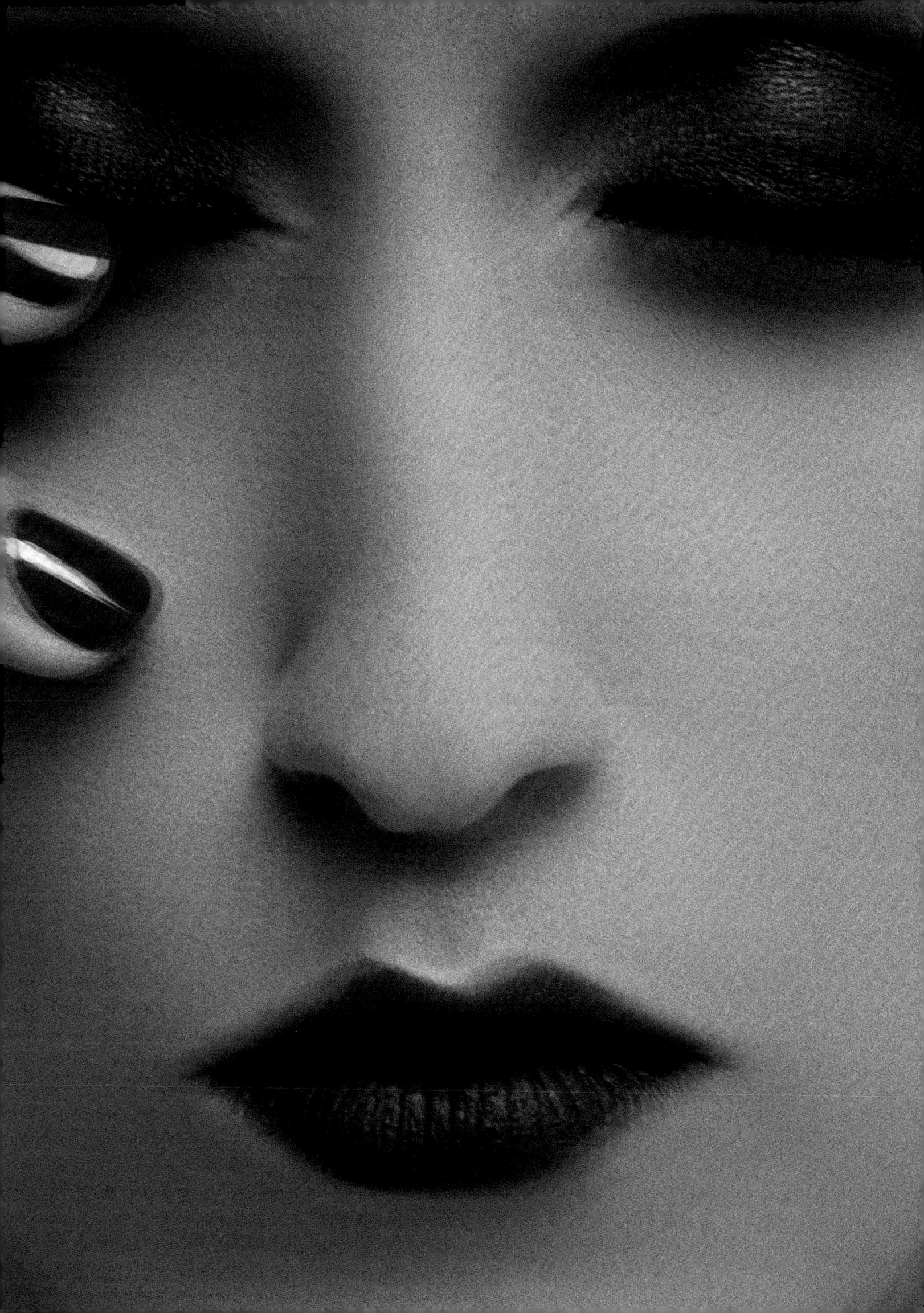

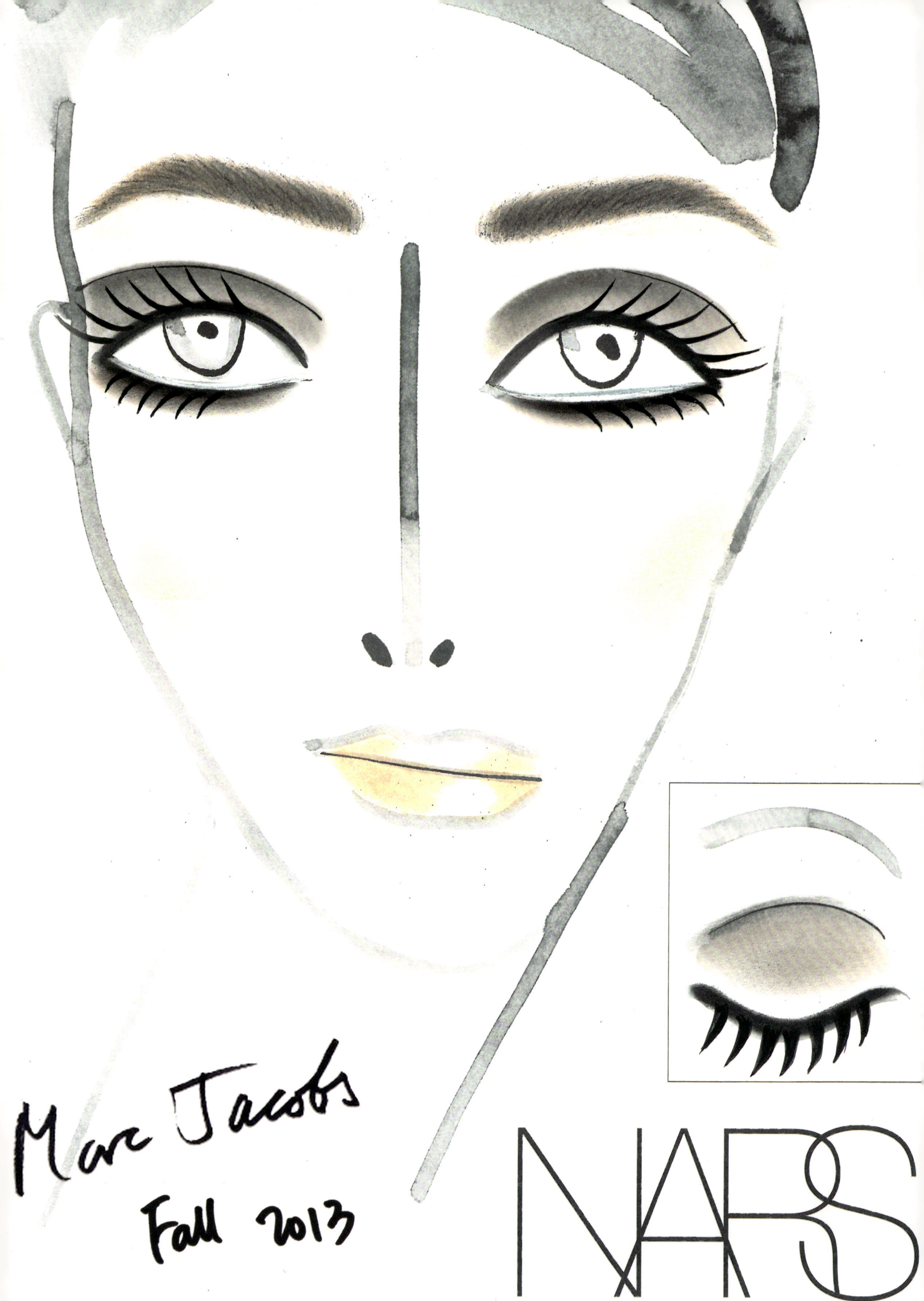

Marc Jacobs
Fall 2013

NARS

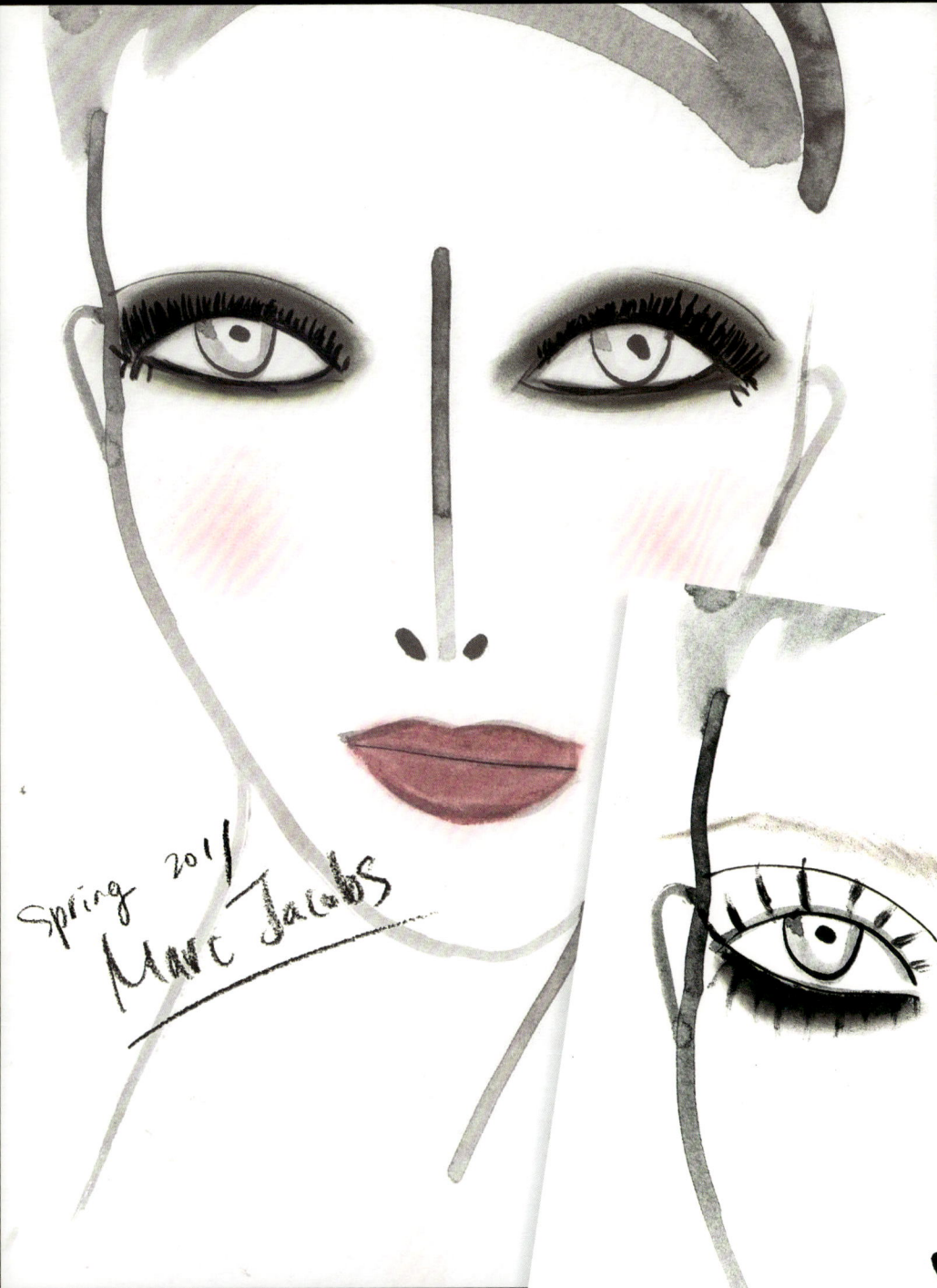

Spring 2011
Marc Jacobs

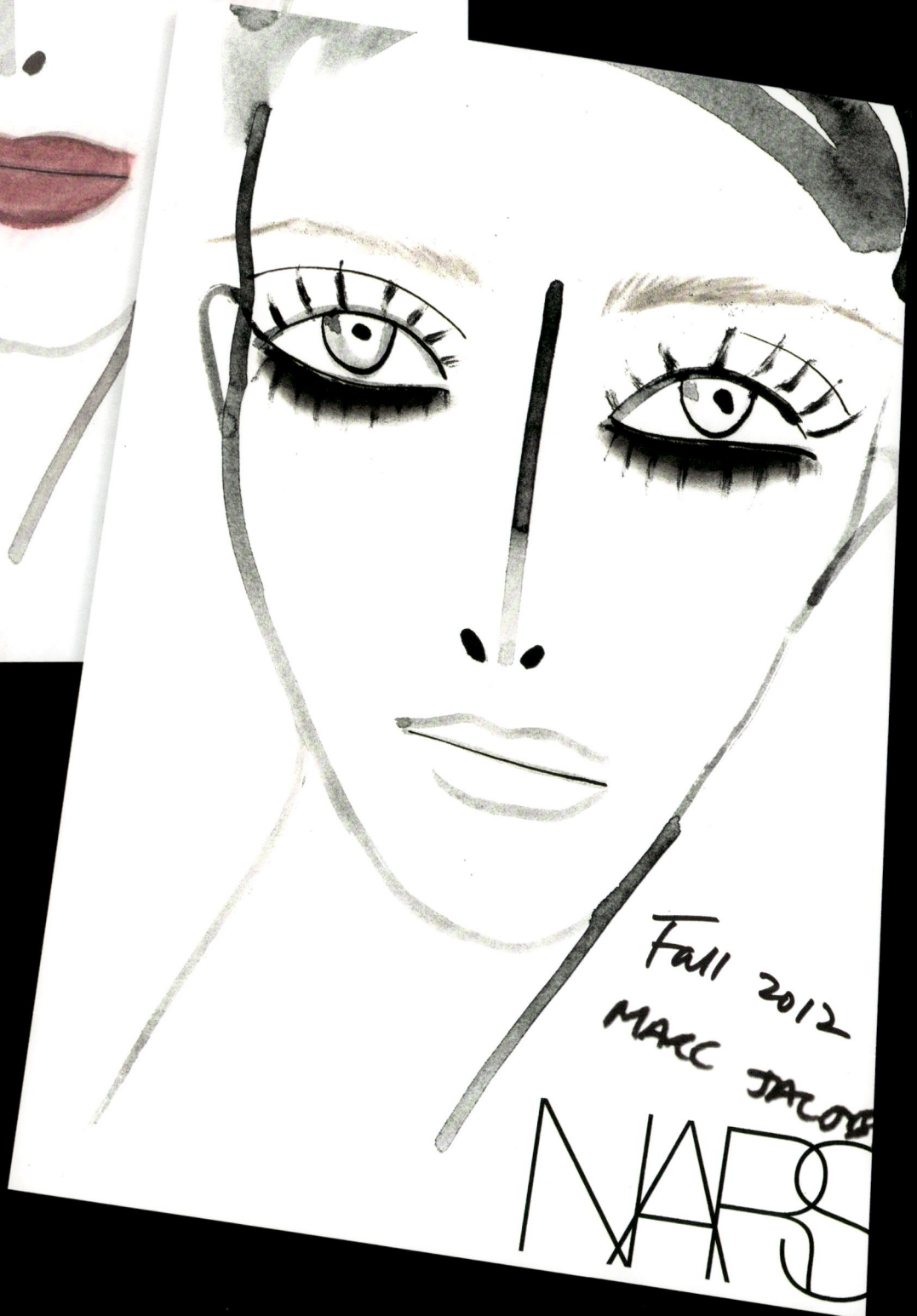

Fall 2012
MARC JACOBS

NARS

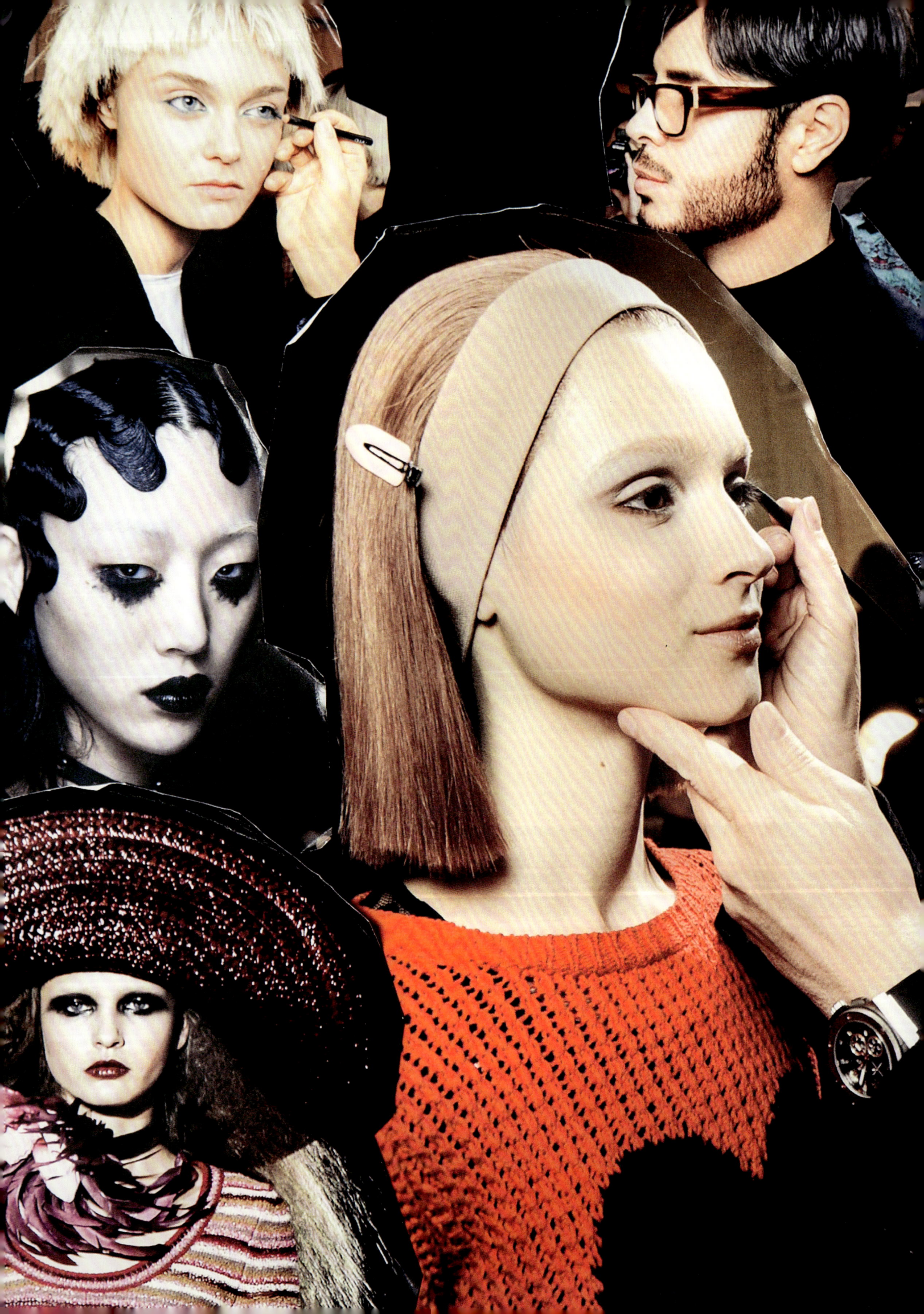

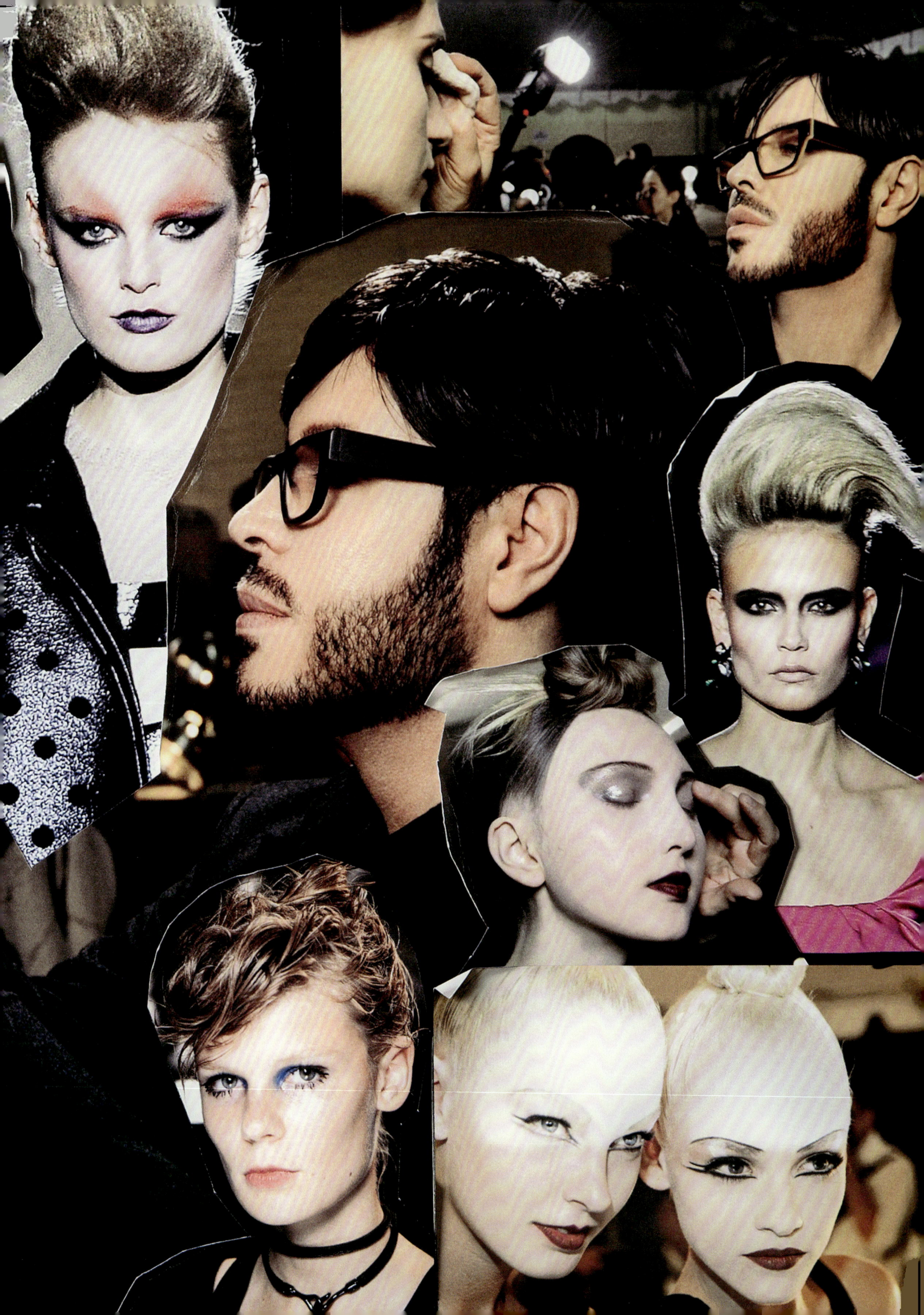

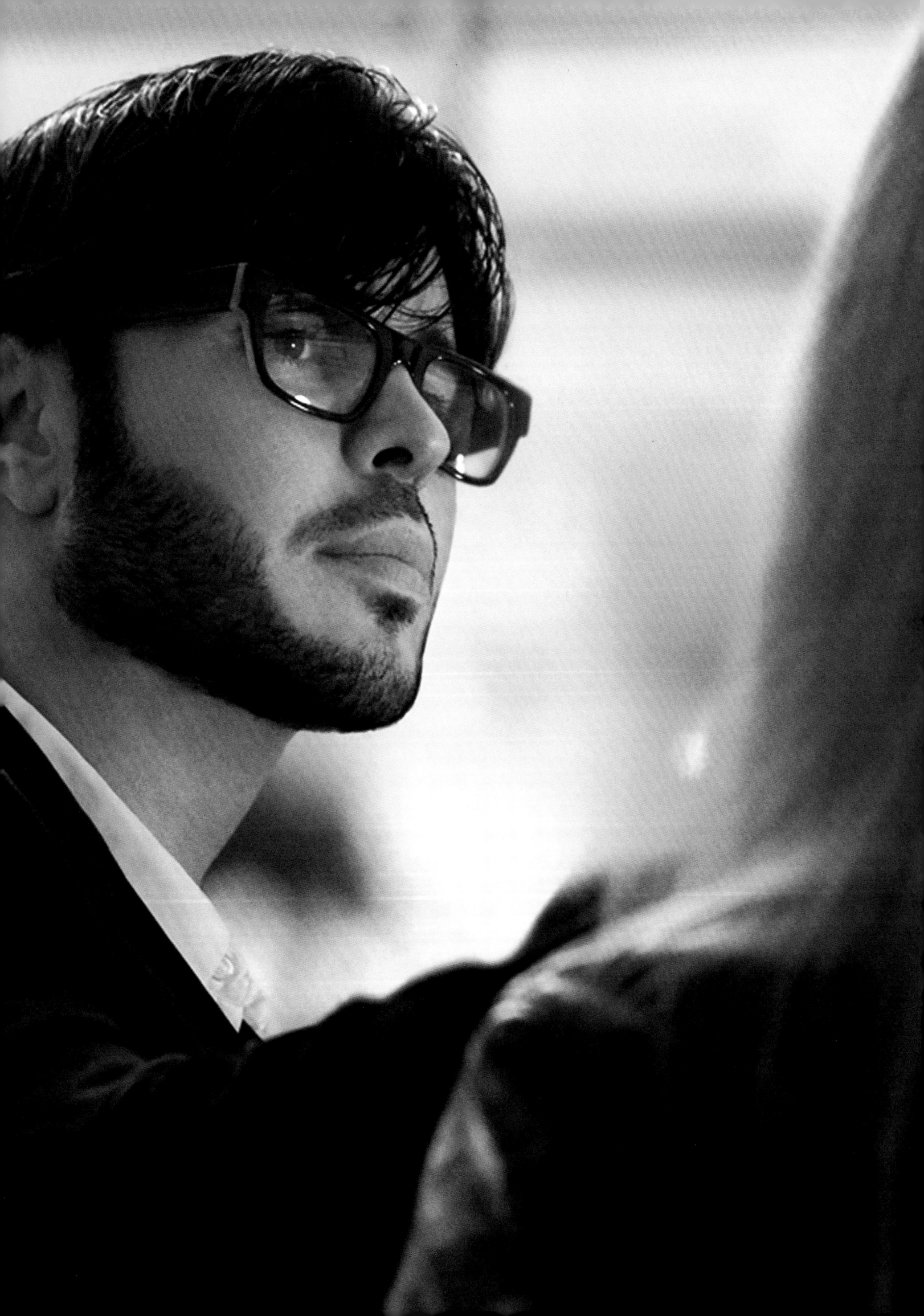

"I HAVE BEEN SO
LUCKY IN MY LIFE TO
BE ABLE TO PUT A
SMILE ON SO MANY
WOMEN'S FACES BY
JUST APPLYING SOME
MAKEUP ON THEM.
IT'S AMAZING TO
SEE WHAT A LITTLE
MAKEUP CAN DO."
– FRANÇOIS NARS

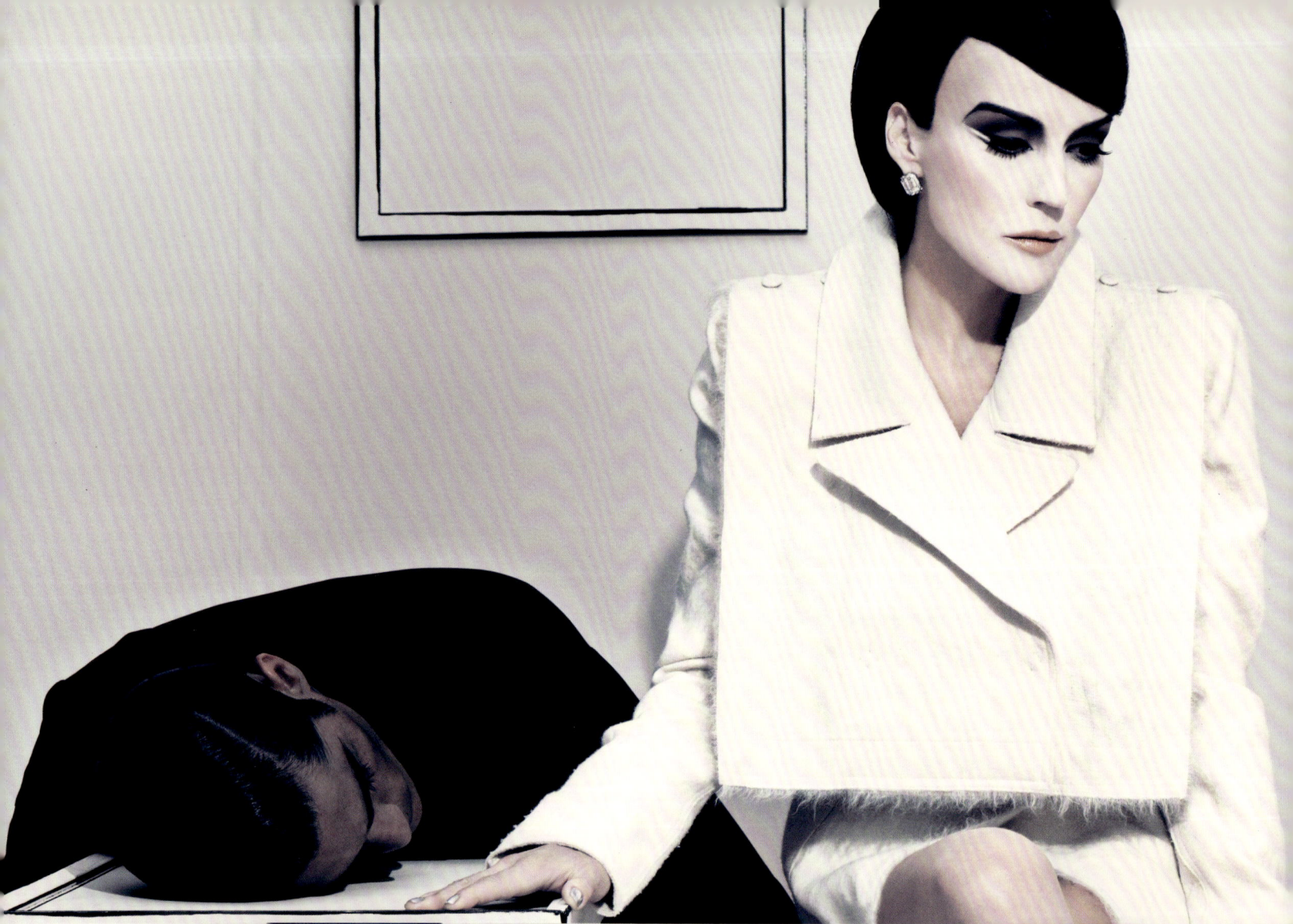

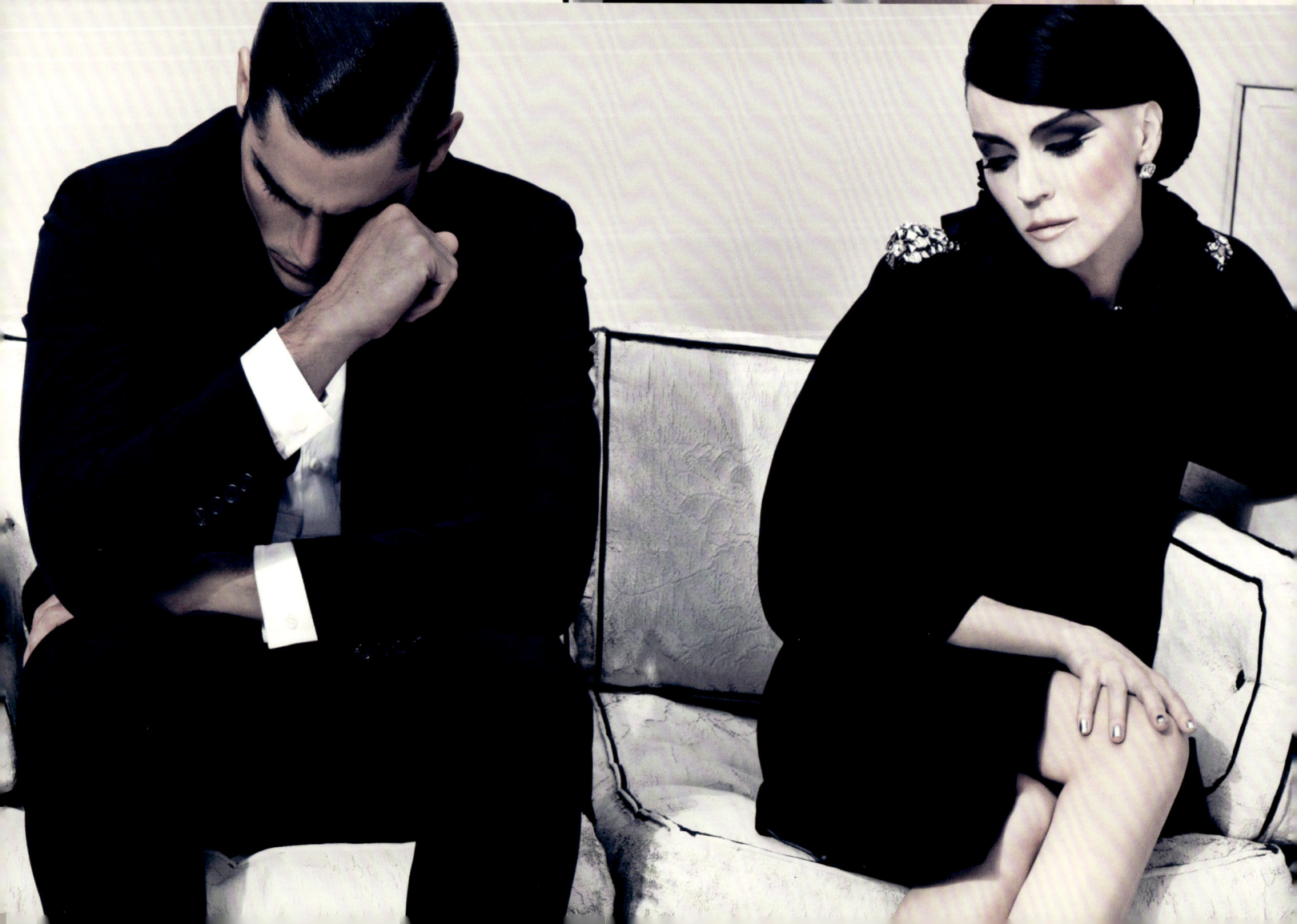

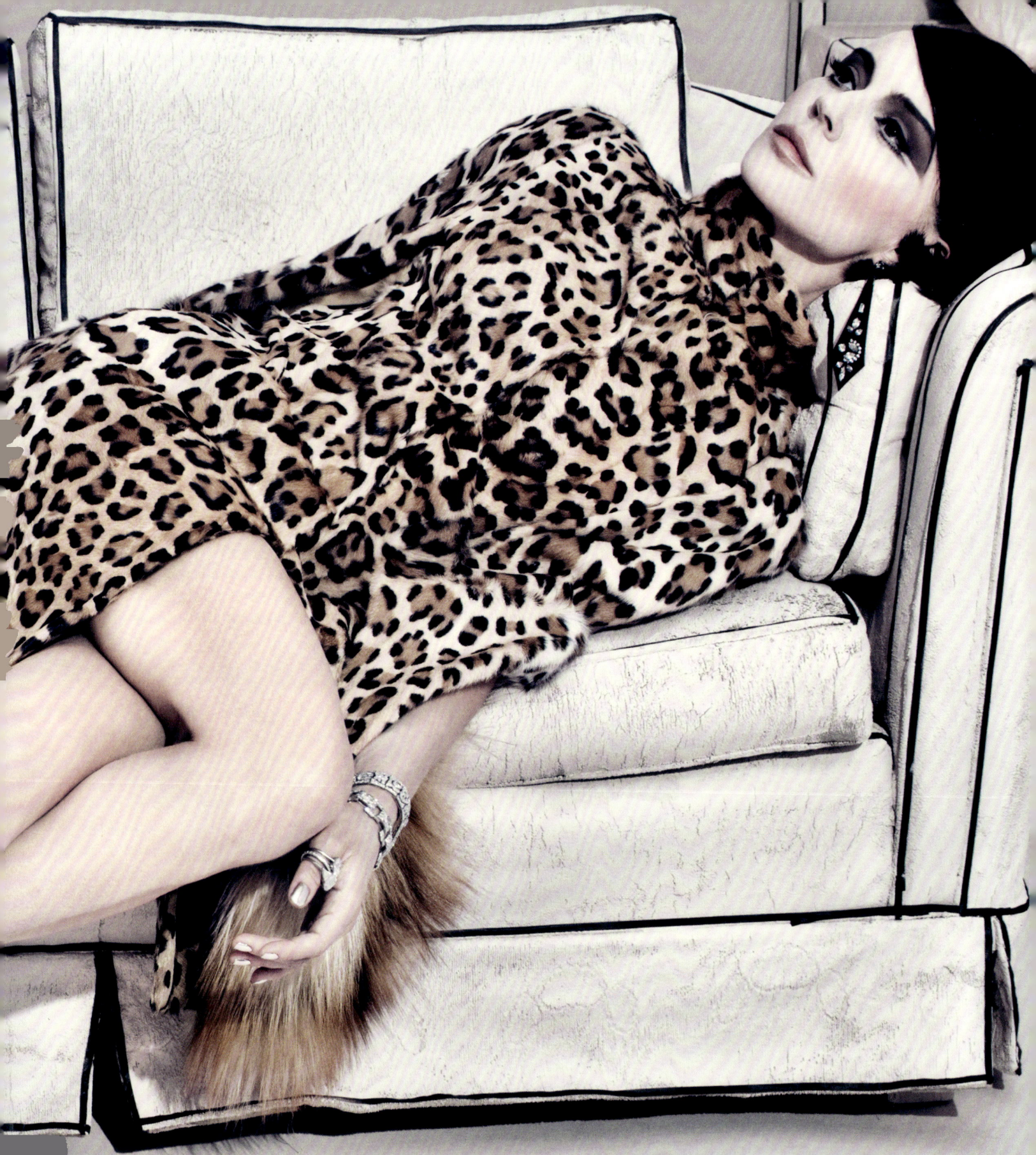

® VOGUE ITALIA

G I U.
2 0 1 5
N. 7 7 8
€ 5,00

中国特刊
THE CHINA ISSUE

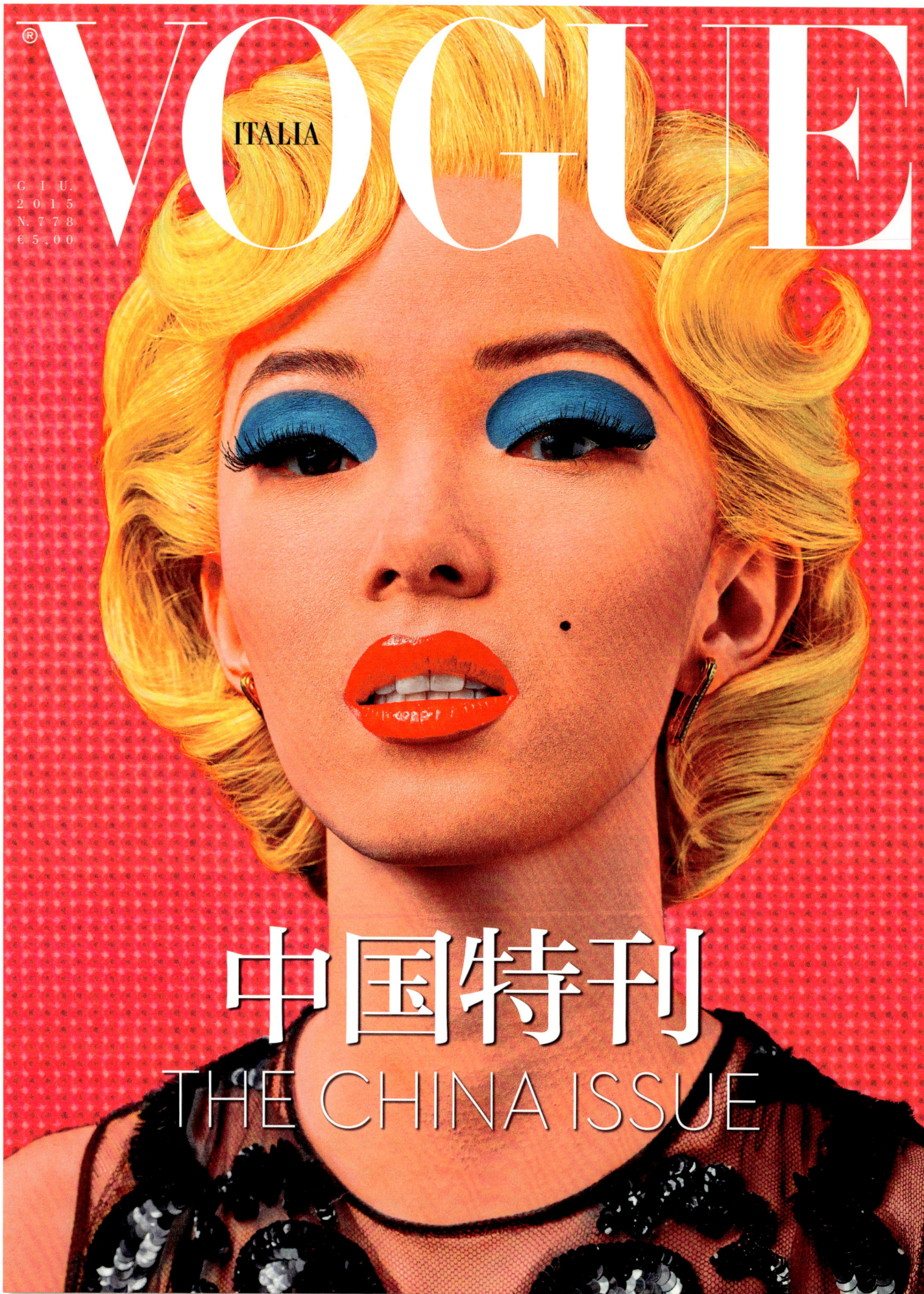

"WORKING WITH FRANÇOIS NARS RECENTLY FOR THE COVER OF *VOGUE* ITALIA, I WAS REMINDED ONCE MORE OF HOW HE TRANSCENDS BEING MERELY A MAKEUP PERSON. HE IS TRULY A MAGICIAN AND AN ARTIST, BENDING COLORS AND TEXTURES TO CREATE A HYPER-REALITY, A VIVID REPRESENTATION OF LIFE."
– STEVEN KLEIN

"I LOVE SO MUCH STEVEN KLEIN'S WORK. HE IS A TOTAL GENIUS AND A FANTASTIC ARTIST WITH AN INCREDIBLE VISION. A TRUE ARTIST. I LOVE HIS WORLD."
– FRANÇOIS NARS

UNCOND
LOVE

"I ATTENDED THE
CARITA SCHOOL
IN PARIS AFTER I
GRADUATED FROM
HIGH SCHOOL.
THE CARITA SISTERS
HAD BUILT UP A
FABULOUS EMPIRE
AND IT FELT VERY
GLAMOROUS TO
LEARN MAKEUP IN
THEIR SCHOOL."
– FRANÇOIS NARS

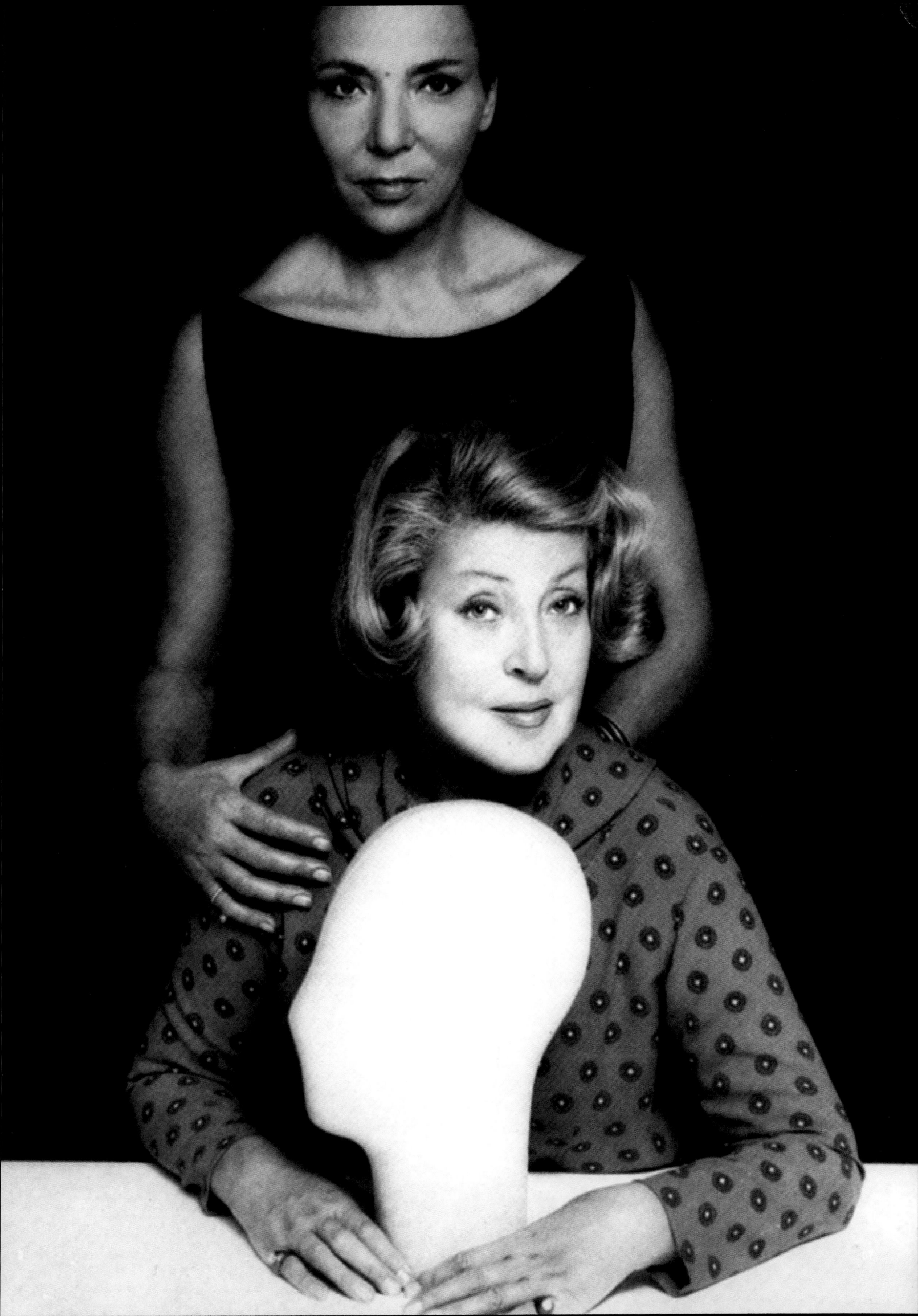

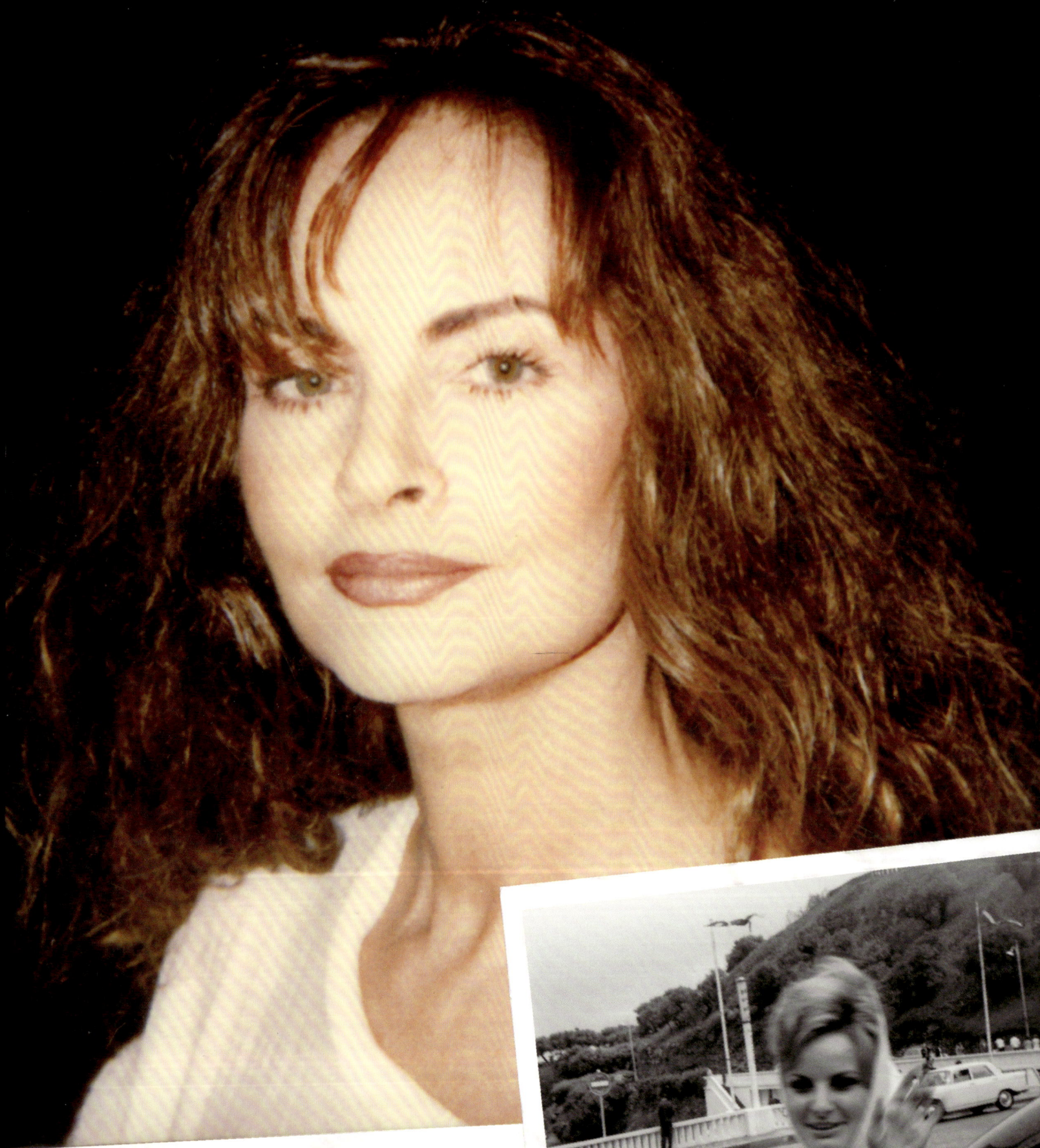

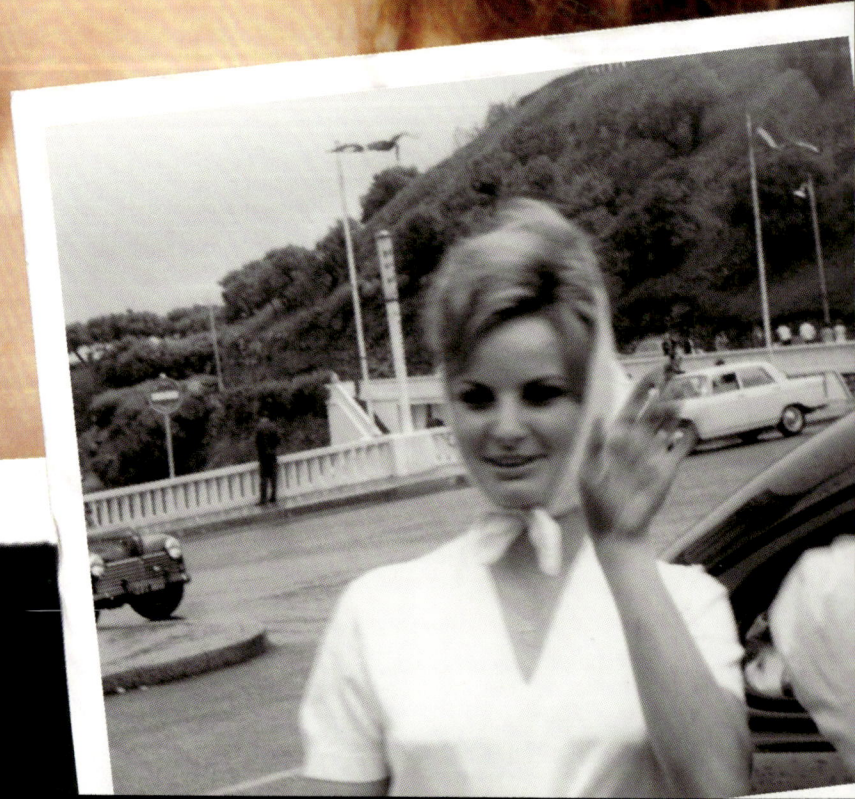

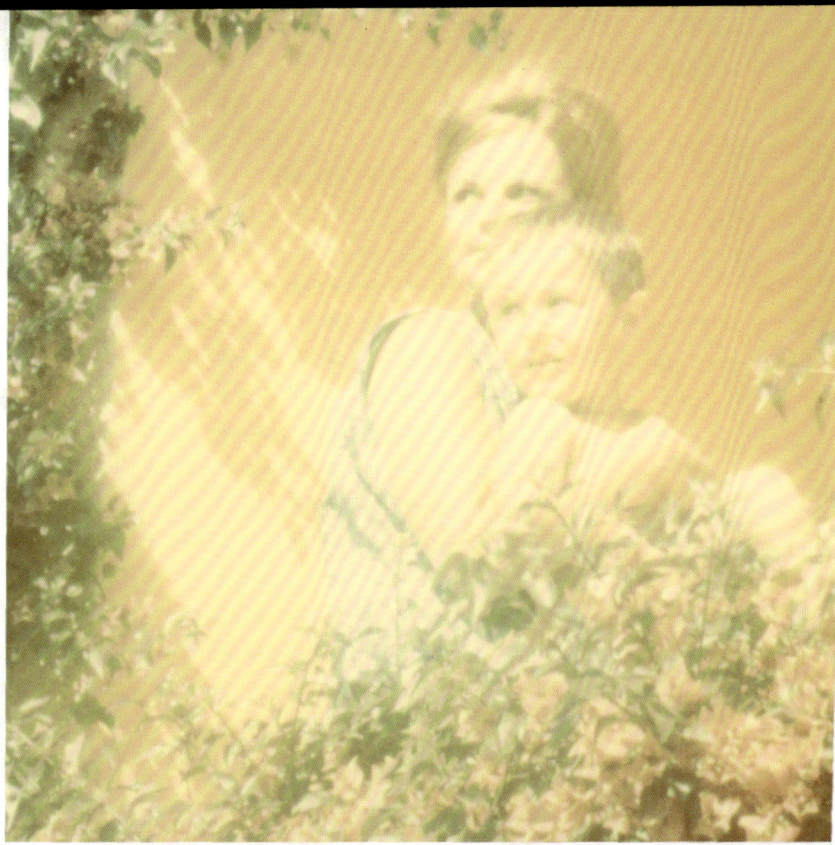

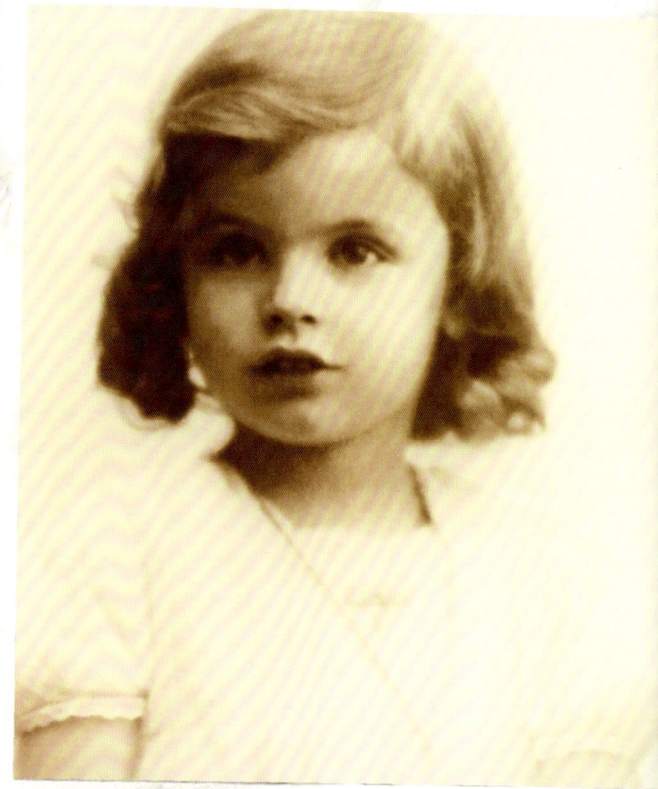

"MY BEAUTY ICONS ARE MY MOTHER, MY GRANDMOTHERS, GARBO, AND DIETRICH."
– FRANÇOIS NARS

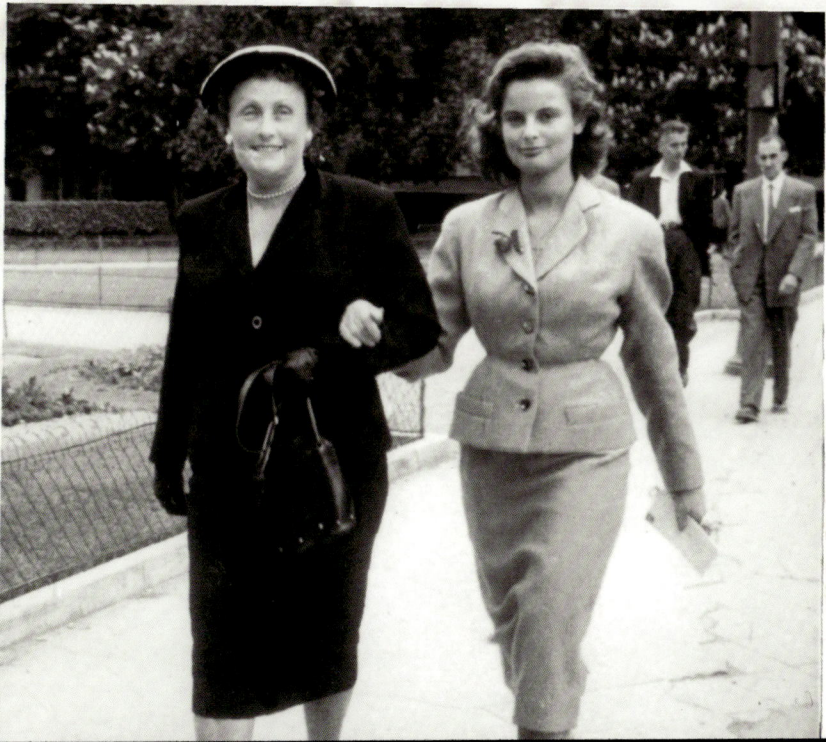

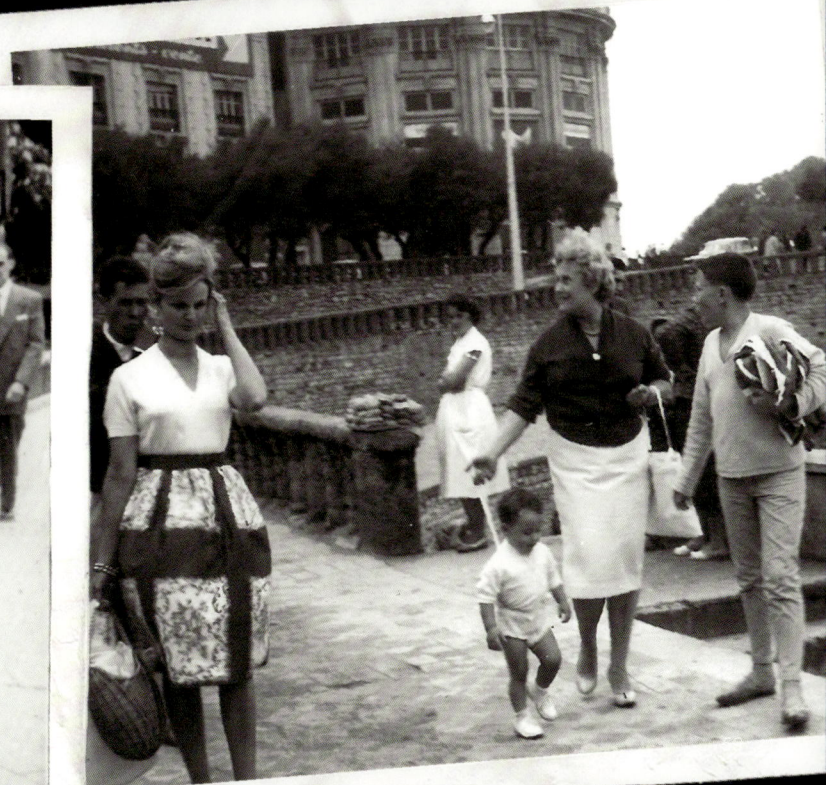

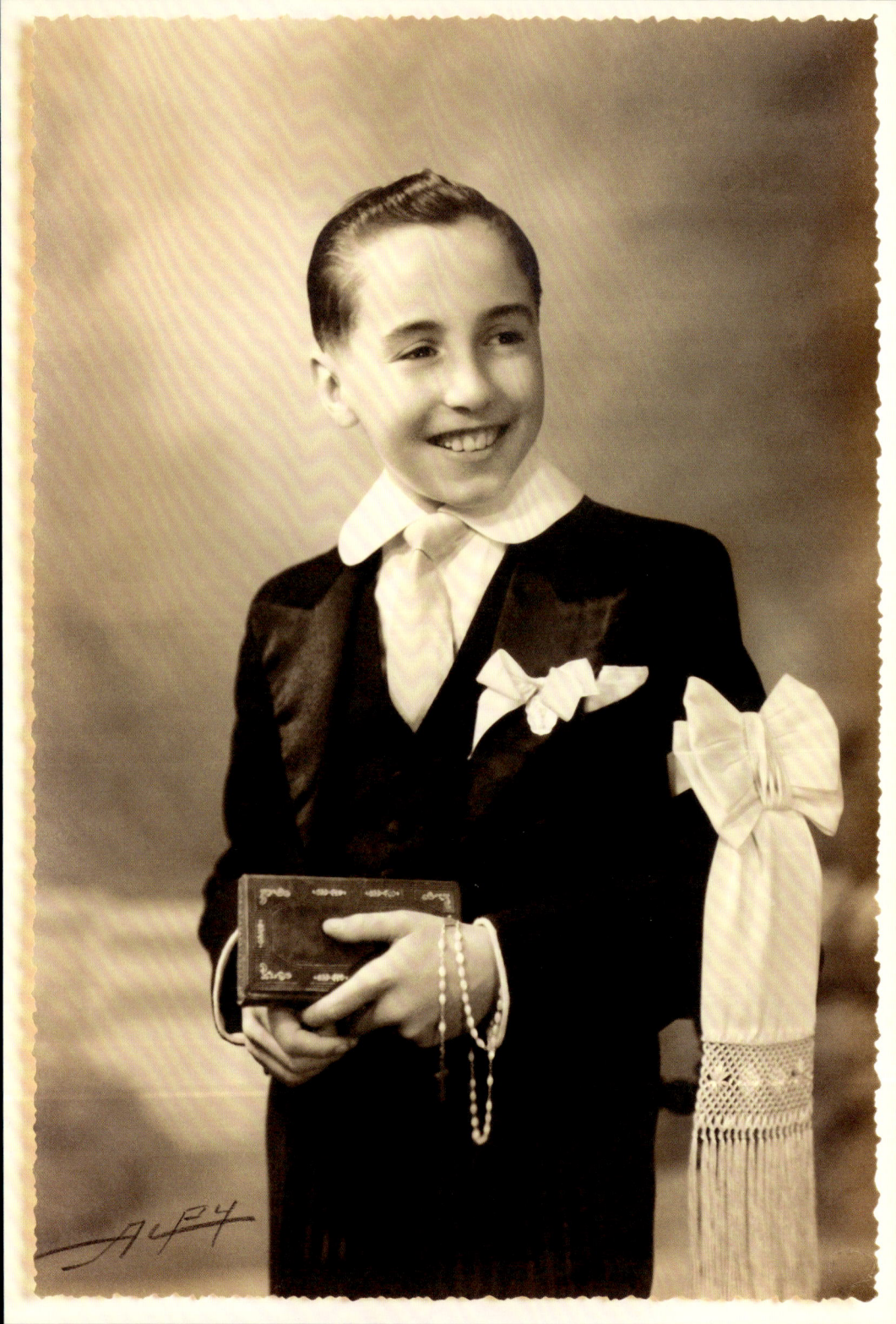

"MY PARENTS AT THEIR FIRST
COMMUNION LOOKING LIKE
TWO ANGELS."
– FRANÇOIS NARS

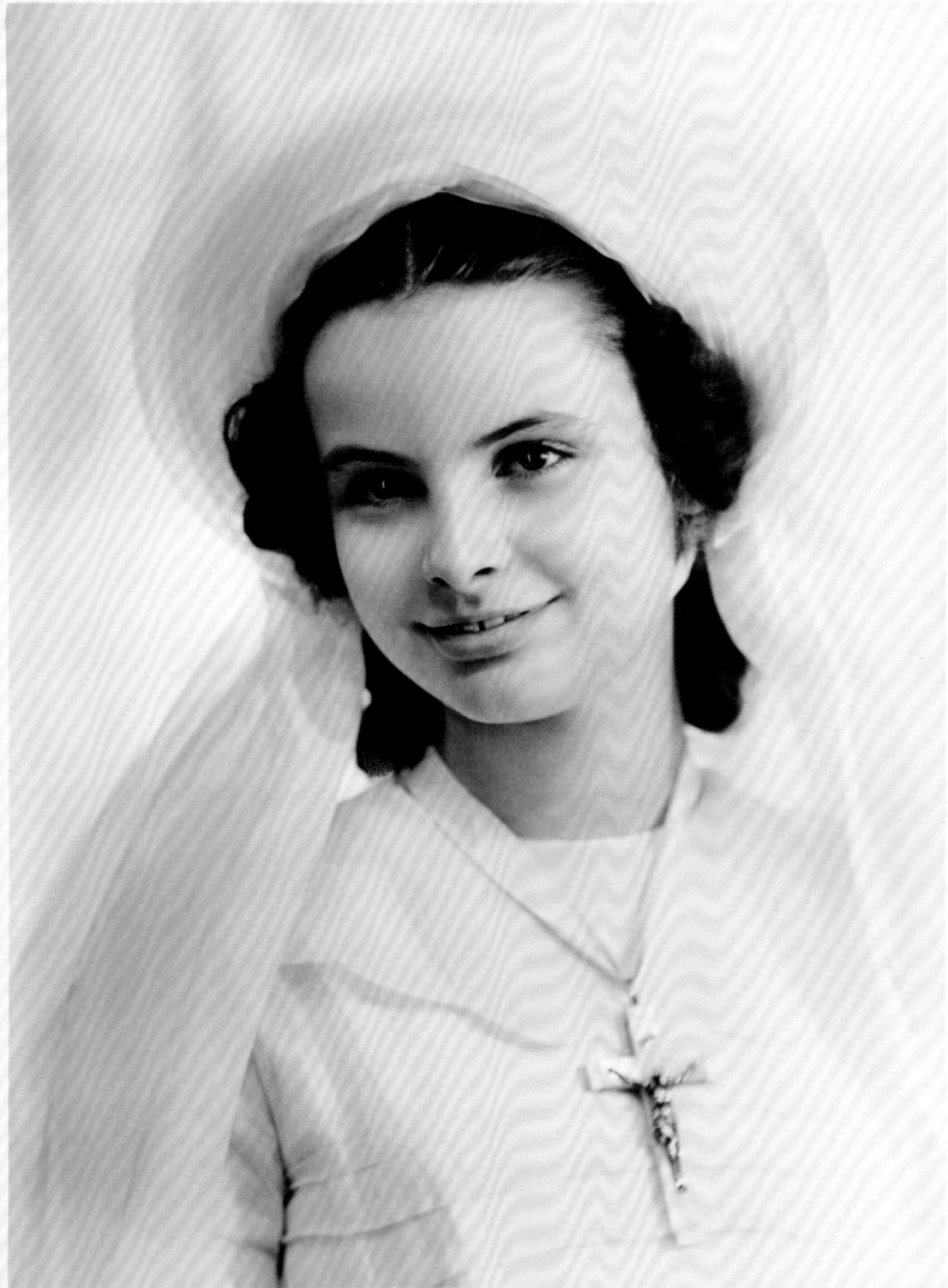

RIGASSI   PARIS

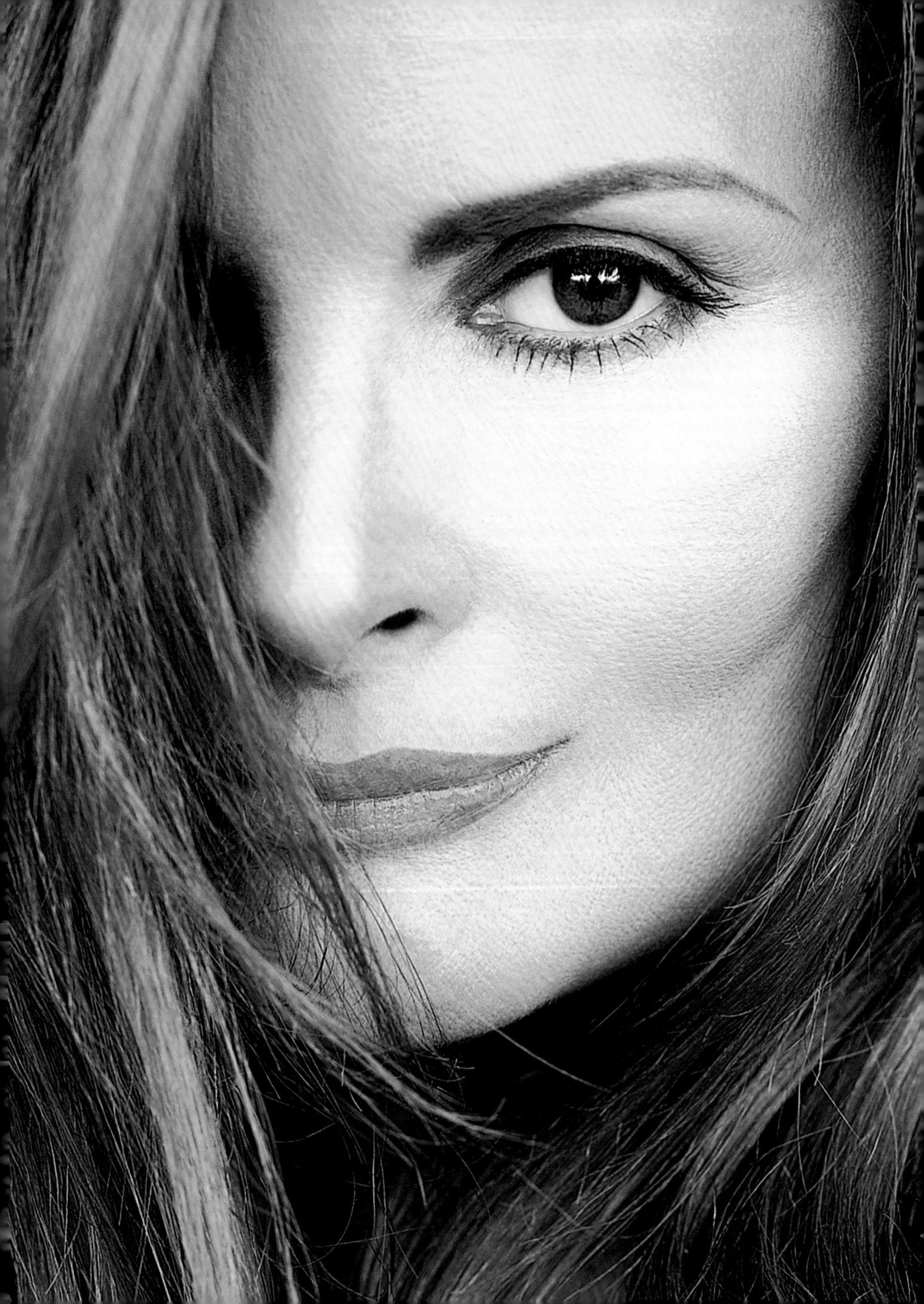

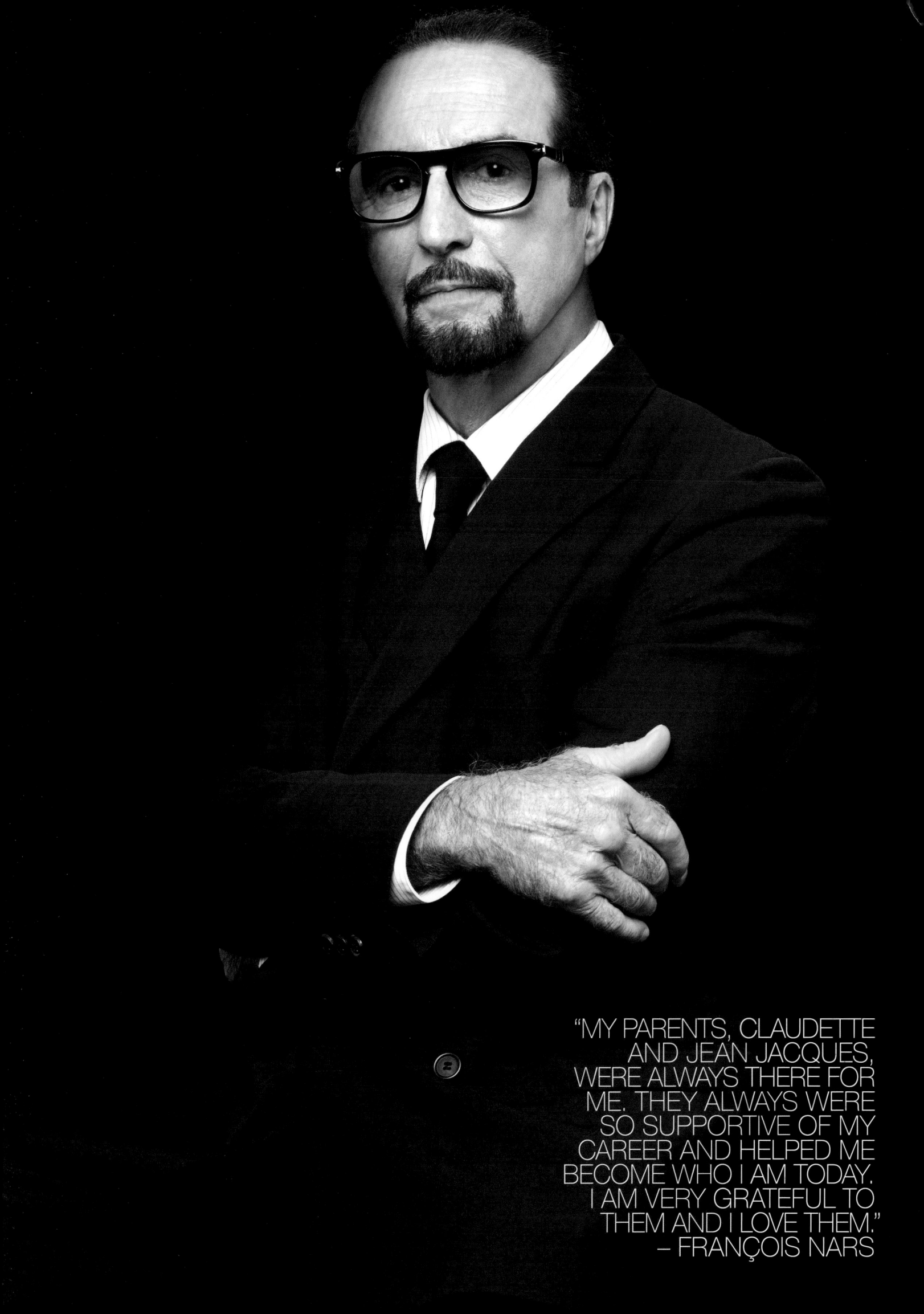

"MY PARENTS, CLAUDETTE AND JEAN JACQUES, WERE ALWAYS THERE FOR ME. THEY ALWAYS WERE SO SUPPORTIVE OF MY CAREER AND HELPED ME BECOME WHO I AM TODAY. I AM VERY GRATEFUL TO THEM AND I LOVE THEM."
– FRANÇOIS NARS

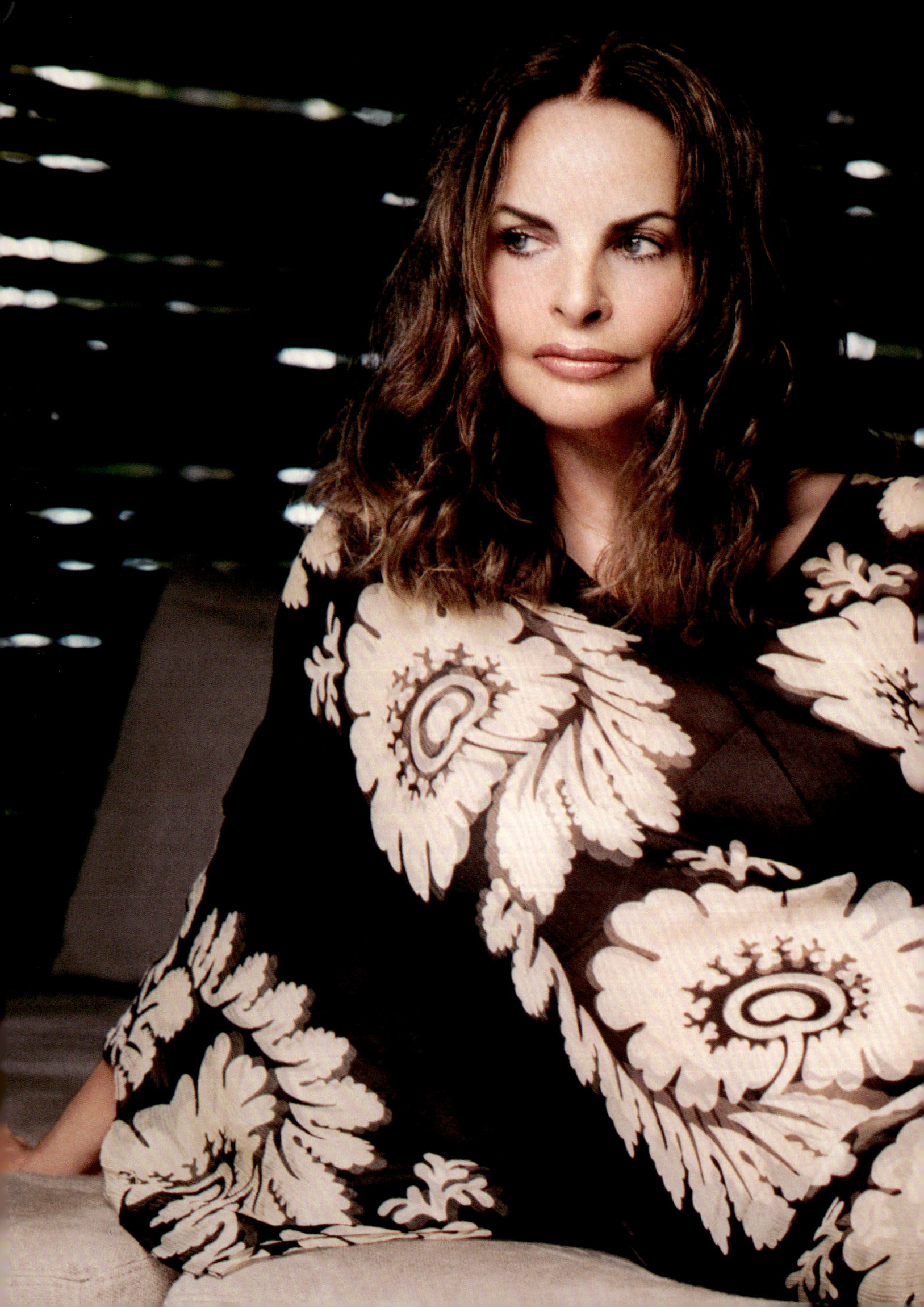

"MY MOTHER IN BORA BORA, ON MOTU TANÉ,
LOOKING LIKE A TROPICAL PRINCESS."
– FRANÇOIS NARS

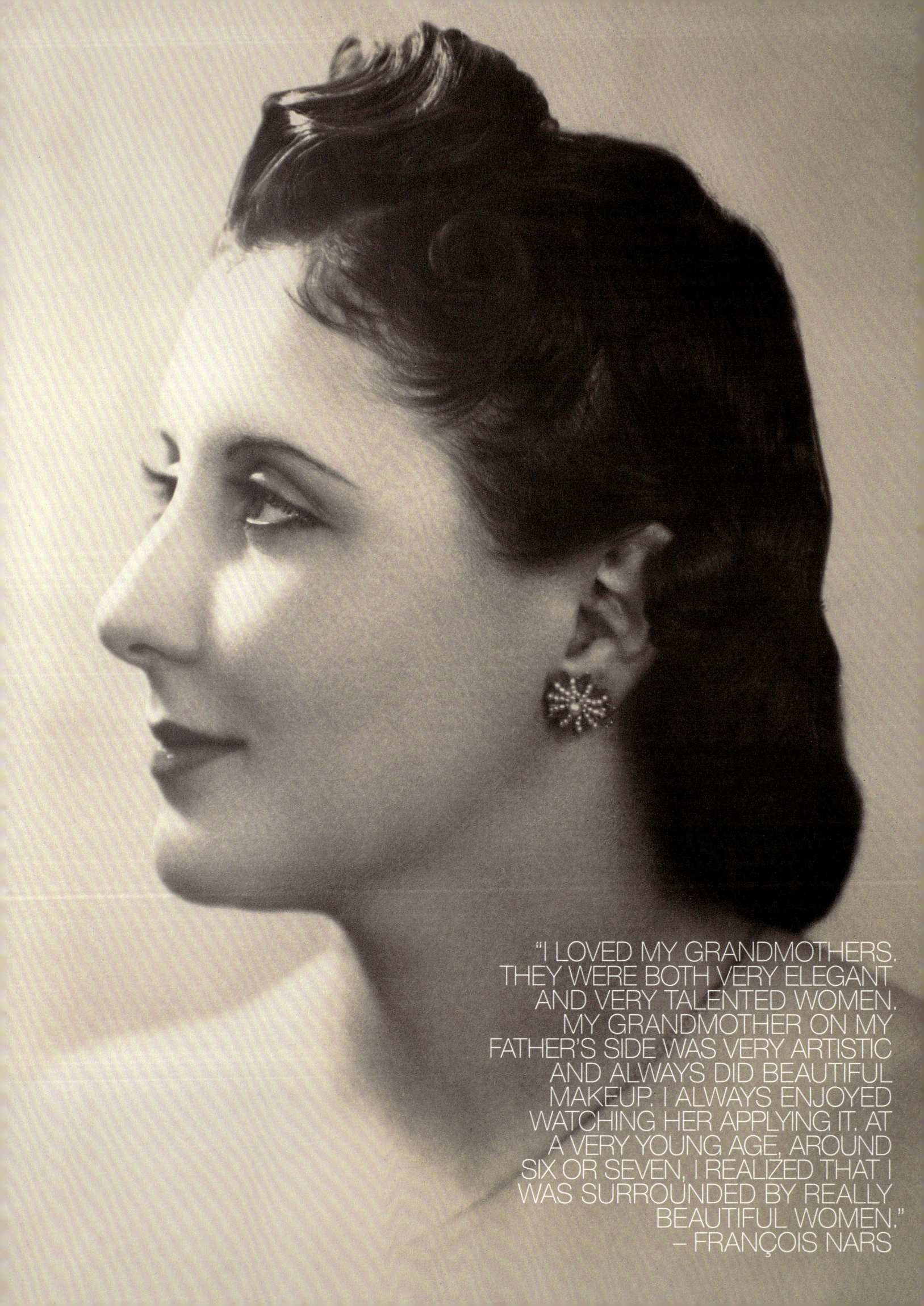

"I LOVED MY GRANDMOTHERS.
THEY WERE BOTH VERY ELEGANT
AND VERY TALENTED WOMEN.
MY GRANDMOTHER ON MY
FATHER'S SIDE WAS VERY ARTISTIC
AND ALWAYS DID BEAUTIFUL
MAKEUP. I ALWAYS ENJOYED
WATCHING HER APPLYING IT. AT
A VERY YOUNG AGE, AROUND
SIX OR SEVEN, I REALIZED THAT I
WAS SURROUNDED BY REALLY
BEAUTIFUL WOMEN."
– FRANÇOIS NARS

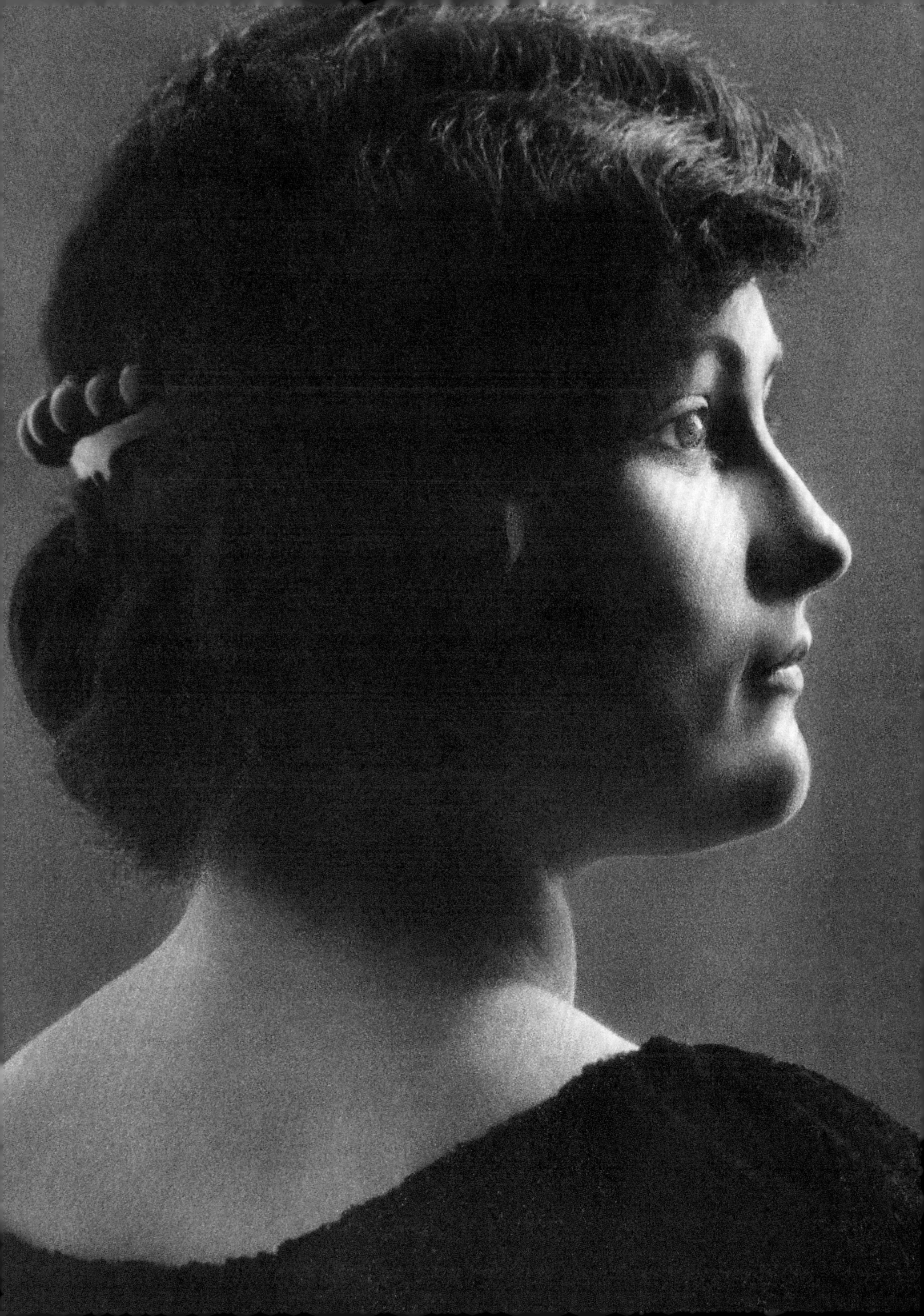

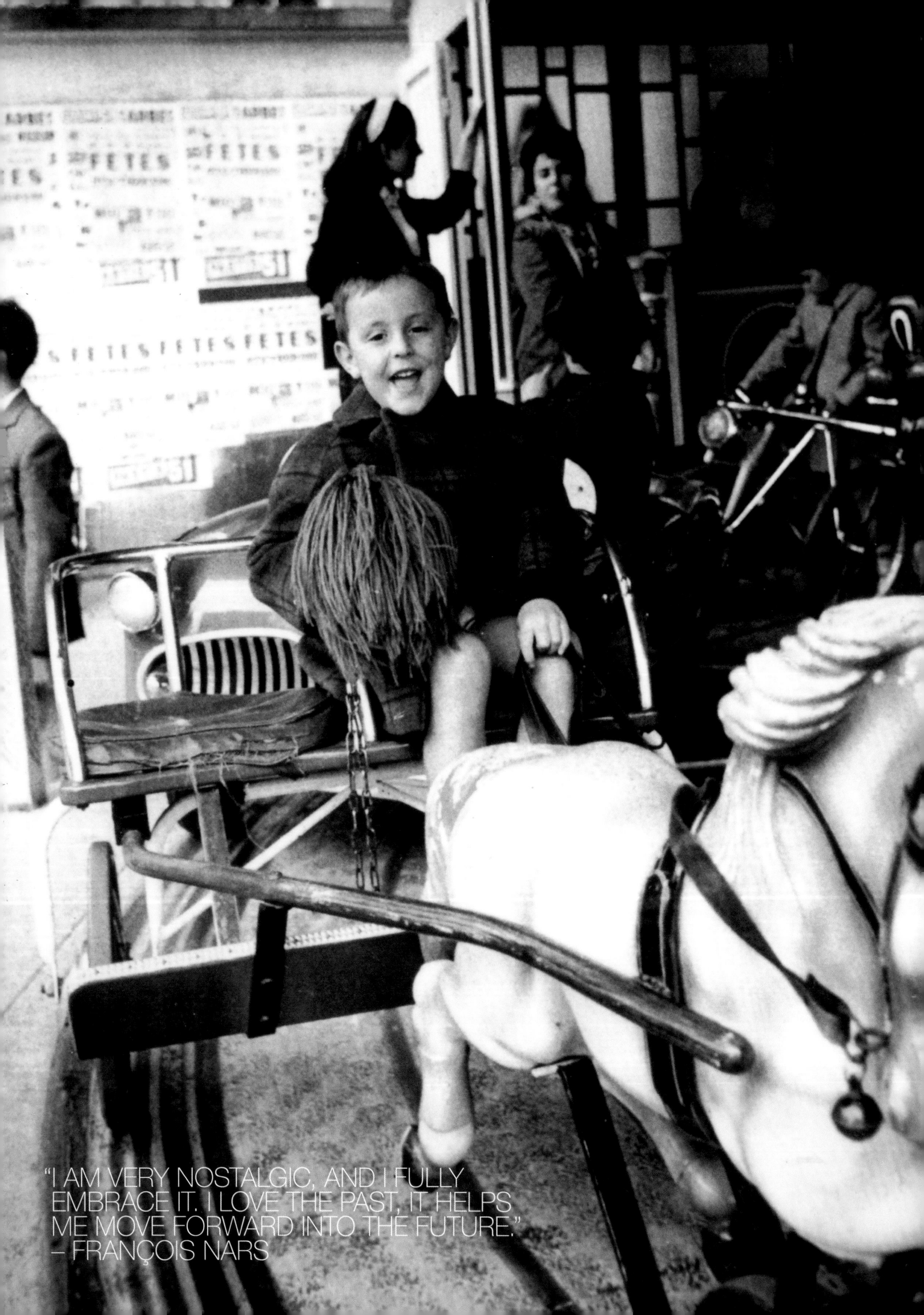

"I AM VERY NOSTALGIC, AND I FULLY EMBRACE IT. I LOVE THE PAST, IT HELPS ME MOVE FORWARD INTO THE FUTURE."
– FRANÇOIS NARS

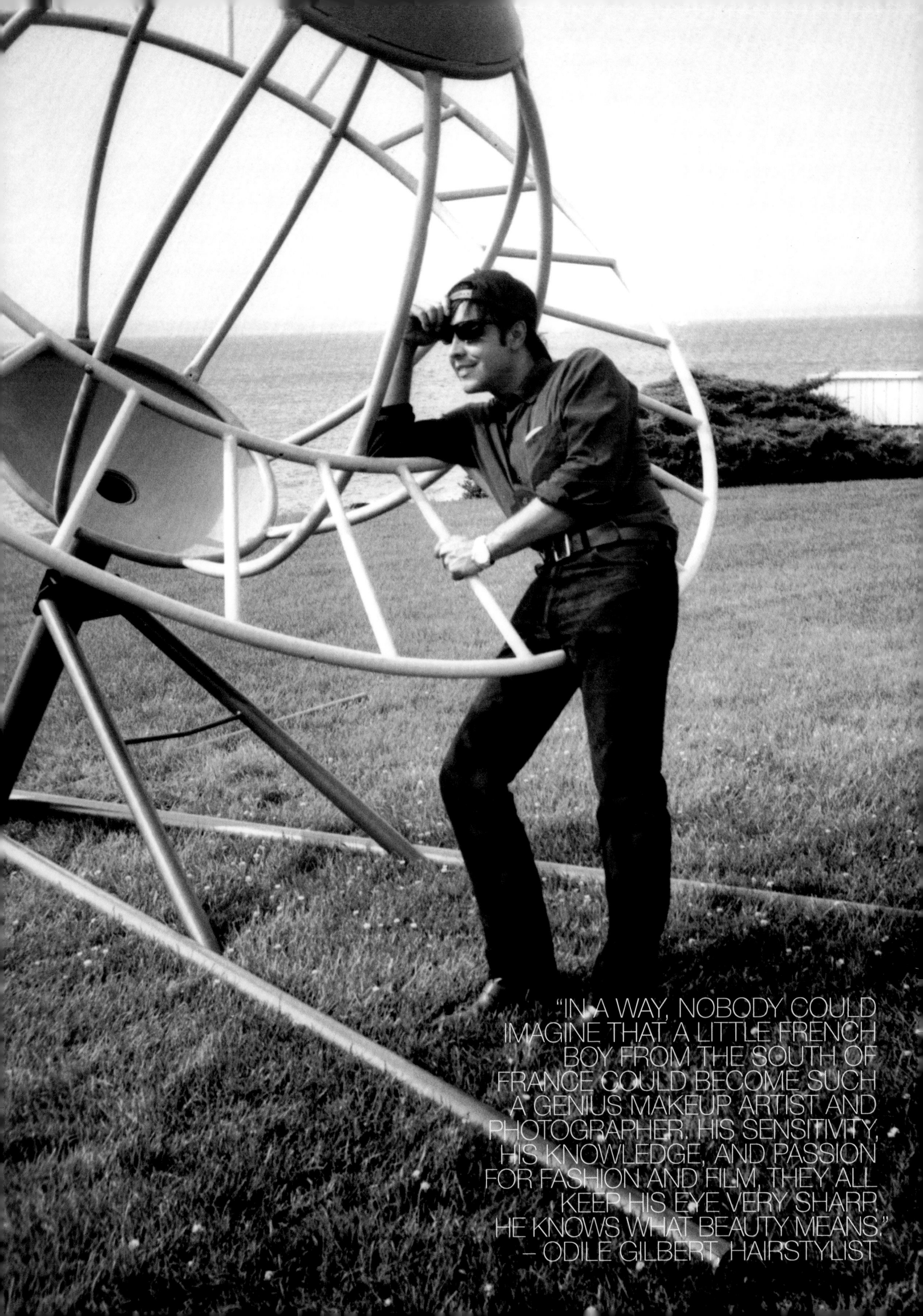

"IN A WAY, NOBODY COULD IMAGINE THAT A LITTLE FRENCH BOY FROM THE SOUTH OF FRANCE COULD BECOME SUCH A GENIUS MAKEUP ARTIST AND PHOTOGRAPHER. HIS SENSITIVITY, HIS KNOWLEDGE, AND PASSION FOR FASHION AND FILM, THEY ALL KEEP HIS EYE VERY SHARP. HE KNOWS WHAT BEAUTY MEANS."
– ODILE GILBERT, HAIRSTYLIST

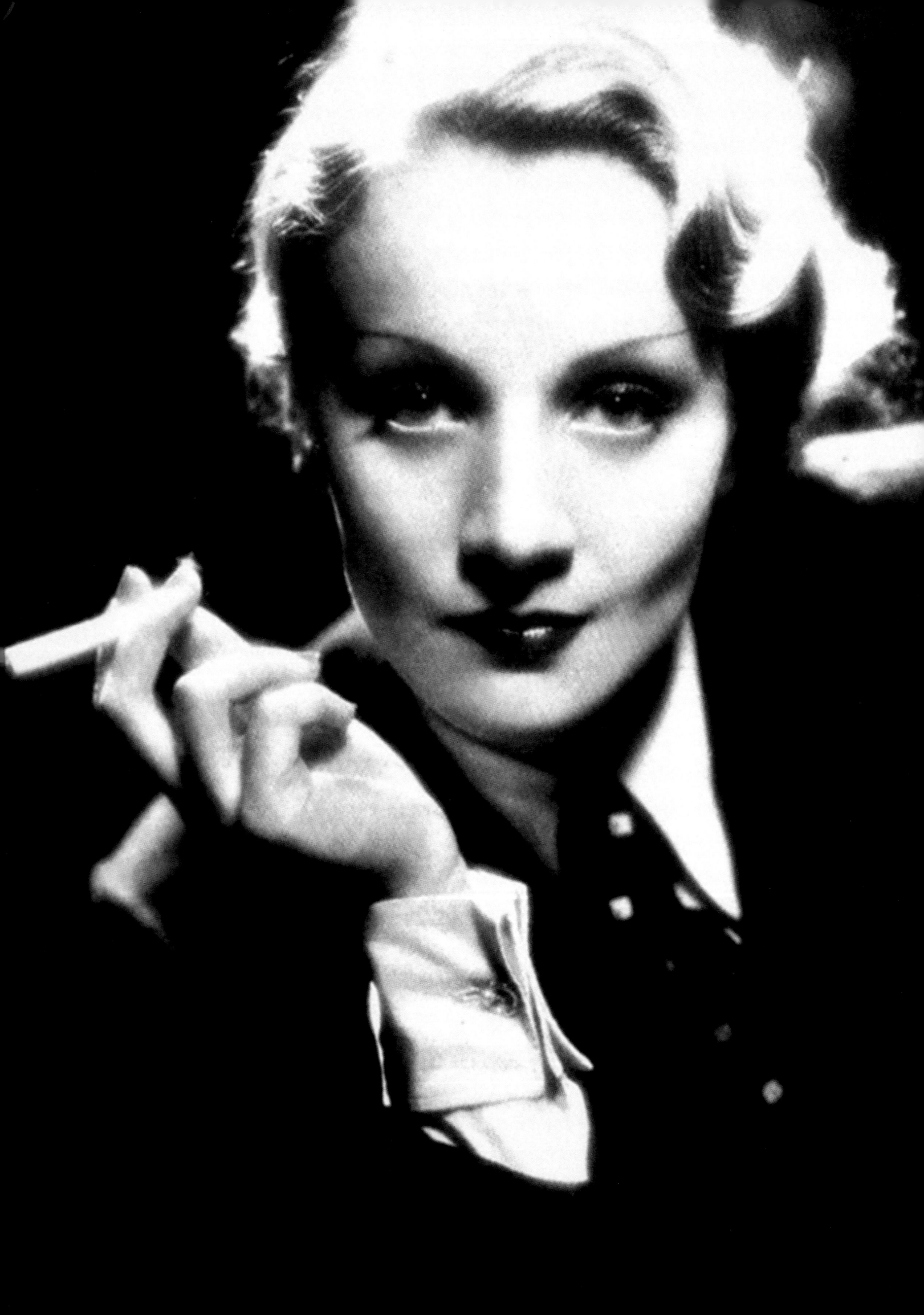

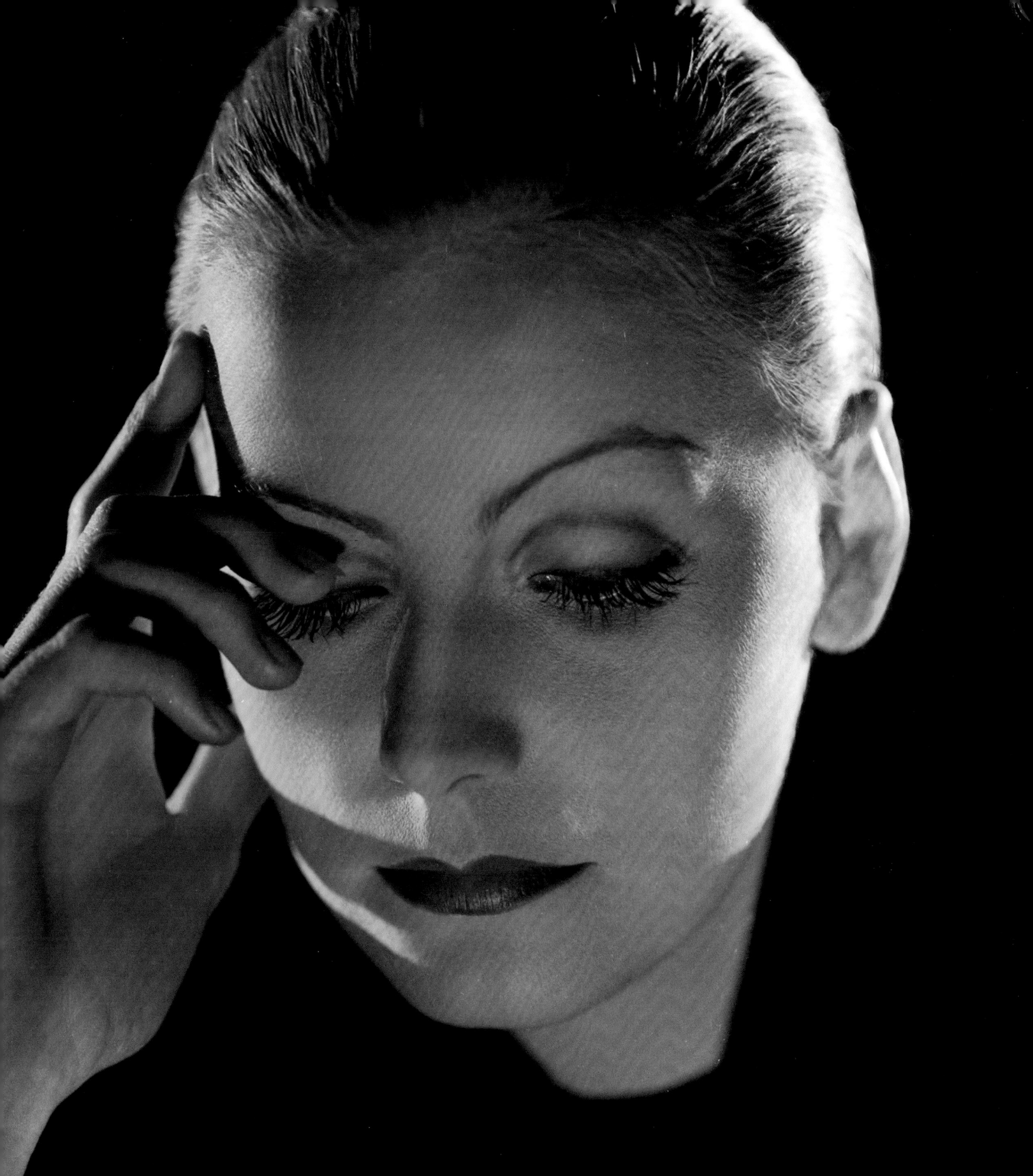

"GARBO AND DIETRICH WERE INCREDIBLY INSPIRING. I REMEMBER STAYING UP VERY LATE AT NIGHT WHEN I WAS A KID WATCHING THOSE FABULOUS SILENT MOVIES. I WAS ALREADY LEARNING ABOUT MAKEUP, LIGHT, AND STYLE."
– FRANÇOIS NARS

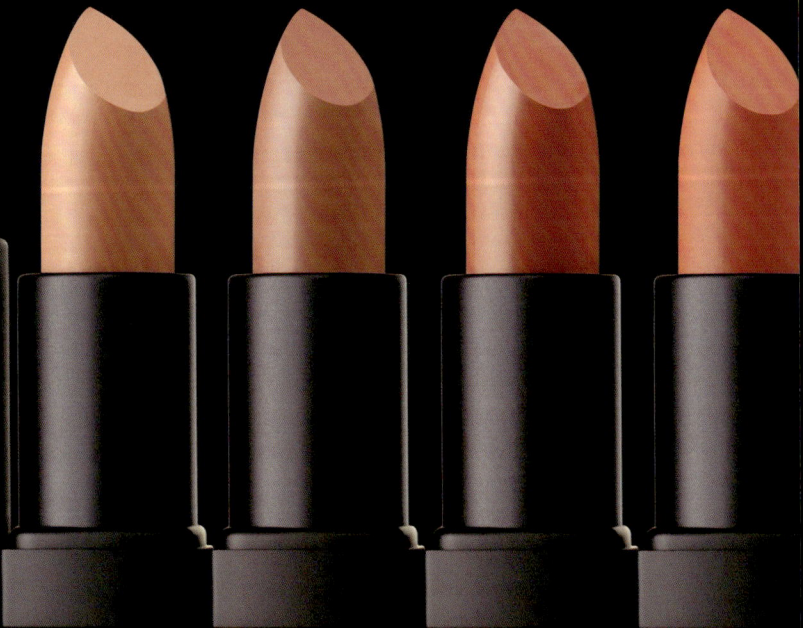

HONOLULU HONEY

BLONDE VENUS

MOROCCO

CASABLANCA

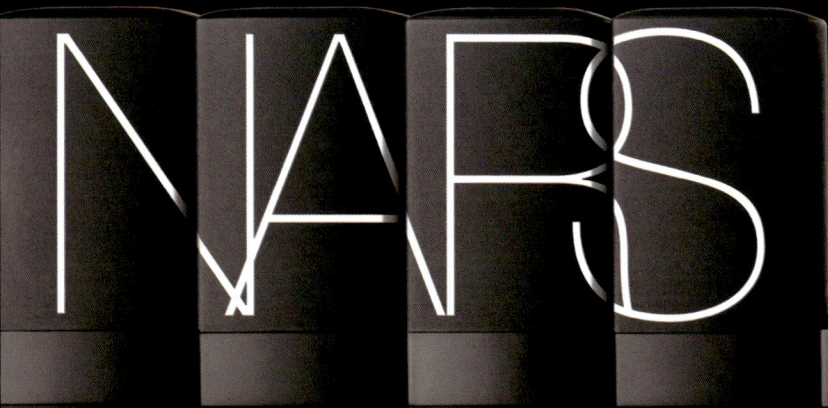

RED LIZARD

SHANGHAI EXPRESS

TRANS SIBERIAN

SCARLET EMPRESS

FUNNY FACE

HEAT WAVE

JUNGLE RED

TRANSEUROPE EXPRESS

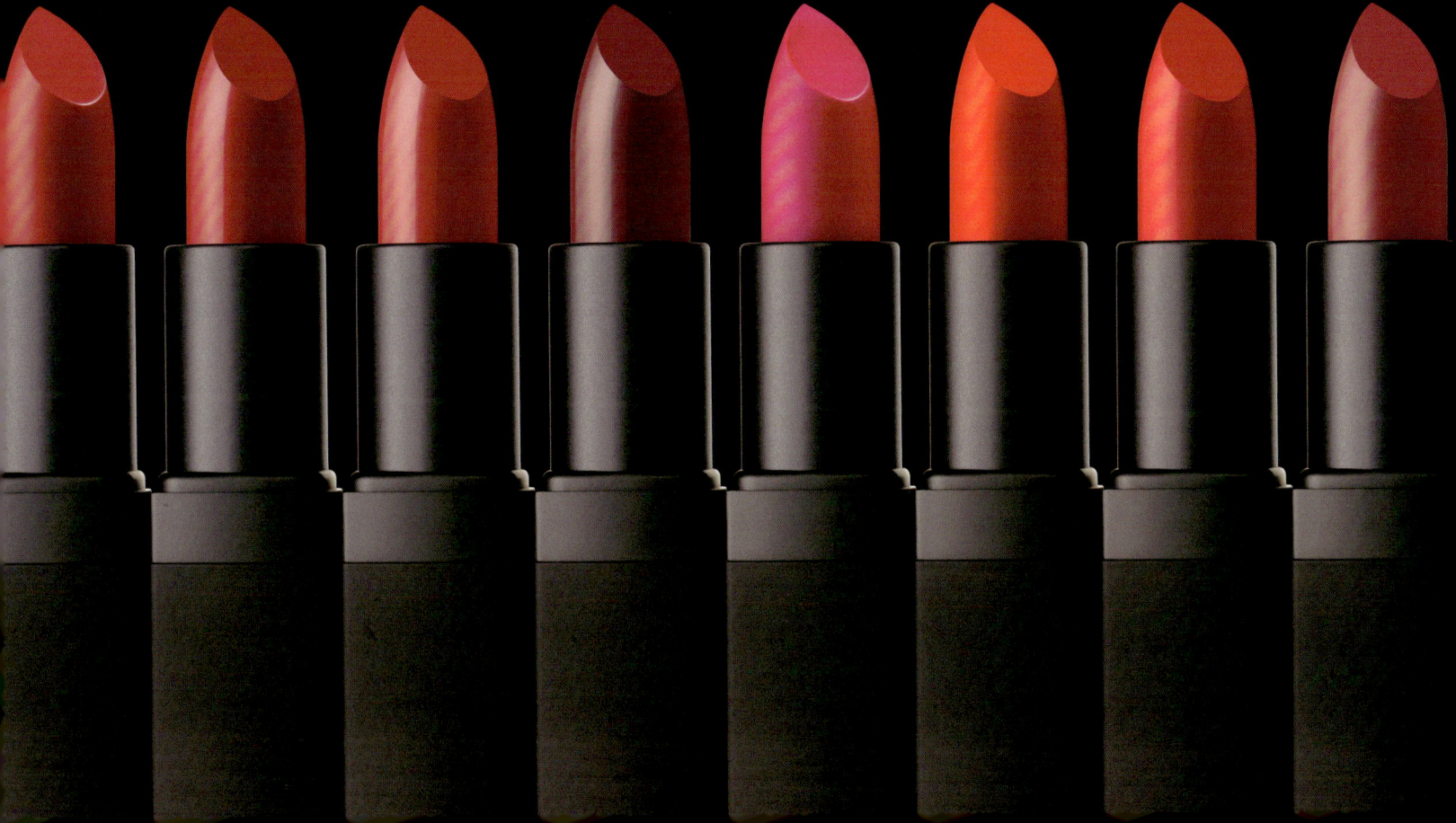

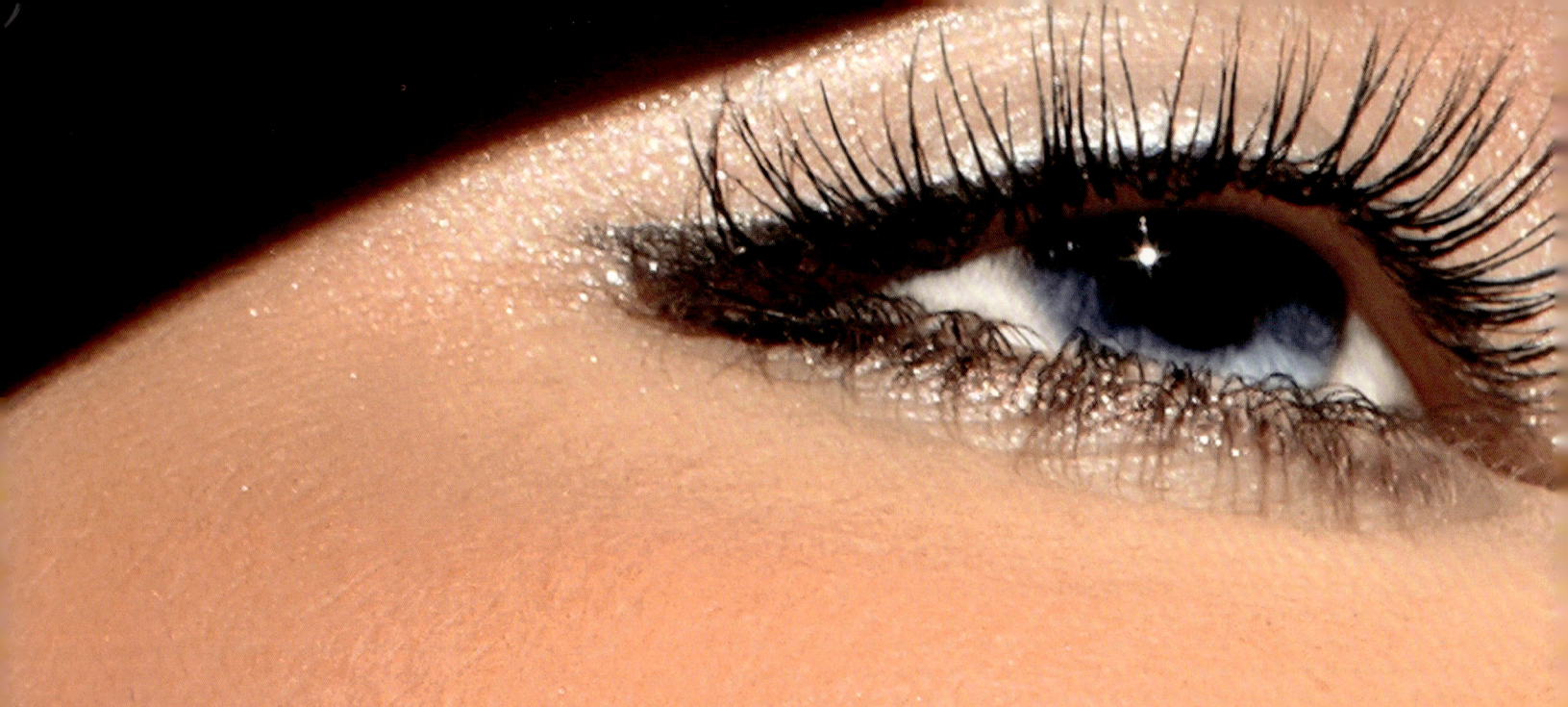

CHIHUAHUA GIZA PAPUA TONGA NIAGARA PAGO VOLGA BANGKOK TONKIN TERRE DE FEU TASHKENT VESUVIO MADE
CARTHAGE MASCATE MONTEGO BAY VALPARAISO MOSCOW AMSTERDAM PELOPONNESE LA PAZ PAIMPOL BUENOS AIR
BILBAO VENICE TANGIER NAPOLI LUXOR PAIMPOL CHANTACO CORINTHE BELIZE SARDINIA CORSICA MALTA BAHAMA PIGAL
POSITANO CARAIBE PORTE VECCHIO REVOLT TOLEDE CASABLANCA TRAIN BLEU TRANS SIBERIAN TRANSEUROPE EXPRES
HAPPY DAYS HARLOW TRIPLE X SUNSET STRIP HUSTLER SWEET DREAMS BABE SCANDAL BILITIS FOUL PLAY STEL
BLOODWORK FRISKY SUMMER DIRTY SHAME PILLOW TALK GOTHIKA SANDPIPER METIS ROSE BIRMAN STOLEN KISSE
MOON FLEET TEMPEST BAD EDUCATION GREEK HOLIDAY SUPERVIXEN MISBEHAVE FEMALE TROUBLE ALL NIGHT LON
SWEET REVENGE OPHELIA EASY LOVER COUP DE COEUR STRAWBERRY FIELDS BOUGAINVILLE ALBATROSS ANGELIKA OAS
SUPER ORGASM LUSTER NANA WONDER ODALISQUE PIREE COMO PLACE VENDOME SPRING BREAK GOLD DIGGER COEU
SUCRE BORN THIS WAY TRIBAL RED PENNY ARCADE INTERNATIONAL VELVET TIBER VIVA CANDY SAYS HOLLYWOODLAW
PARIS FOLLIES PENNY ARCADE INTERNATIONAL VELVET VIVA CANDY SAYS MORE HOLLY WOODLAWN BABY DOLL SWE
CHARITY BUTTERFIELD CABIRIA BEWITCHED GALACTICA HOT WIRED VAGABOND HELLFIRE MEDEA DIABLO AFRICA
QUEEN ROSEBUD AMAZON FANTASIA HUSH MARNIE JILTED LOVE CREOLE NEW LOVER HOPI BAROQUE CLUB MIX CYTHE
SEX MACHINE SIERRA CRUELLA RED SQUARE DAMNED TORTOLA MARINA HONOLULU HONEY BETTINA CAFE CON LEC
TOUNDRA POP LIFE NEVER SAY NEVER 413 BLKR MYSTERIOUS RED AFGHAN RED MASAI FIRST BITE CHRISTINA ROU
D ENFER TAMANGO PROMISCUOUS LARA SUCCESS ROUGE BASQUE PETIT MONSTRE BLONDE VENUS MOROCCO RE
LIZARD HEAT WAVE JUNGLE RED CONGO RED FIRE DOWN BELOW MONGOLIAN RED TANGANYKA GIPSY VIVA LAS VEGA
ANGELIQUE RAIN HOT VOODOO BARBARELLA GALAXY GIRL BIANCA MITZI TOBAGO CATFIGHT VIRIDIANA JOYOUS R
FLAME FLAIR DAMAGE KLUTE KISS NOUBA RUSSIAN DOLL SPANISH RED HINDU CRUISING TUTTI FRUTTI SEXUAL HEALI
MANHUNT MINDGAME BEAUTIFUL LIAR SENORITA CANAILLE SHRINAGAR OUTSIDER FALBALA FAST RIDE LOVE DEVOTIC
LITTLE DARLING TZIGANE MAYFLOWER VENDANGES TABOO AUTUMN LEAVES CHIHUAHUA GIZA PAPUA TONGA NIAGARA PAG
VOLGA BANGKOK TONKIN TERRE DE FEU TASHKENT VESUVIO MADERE CARTHAGE MASCATE MONTEGO BAY VALPARAI
MOSCOW AMSTERDAM PELOPONNESE LA PAZ PAIMPOL BUENOS AIRES BILBAO VENICE TANGIER NAPOLI LUXOR PAIMPO
CHANTACO CORINTHE BELIZE SARDINIA CORSICA MALTA BAHAMA PIGALLE POSITANO CARAIBE PORTE VECCHIO REVO
TOLEDE CASABLANCA TRAIN BLEU TRANS SIBERIAN TRANSEUROPE EXPRESS HAPPY DAYS HARLOW TRIPLE X SUNSET STR
HUSTLER SWEET DREAMS BABE SCANDAL BILITIS FOUL PLAY STELLA BLOODWORK FRISKY SUMMER DIRTY SHAME PILL
TALK GOTHIKA SANDPIPER METIS ROSE BIRMAN STOLEN KISSES MOON FLEET TEMPEST BAD EDUCATION GREEK HOLIDA
SUPERVIXEN MISBEHAVE FEMALE TROUBLE ALL NIGHT LONG SWEET REVENGE OPHELIA EASY LOVER COUP DE COEU
STRAWBERRY FIELDS BOUGAINVILLE ALBATROSS ANGELIKA OASIS SUPER ORGSM LUSTER NANA WONDER ODALISQU
PIREE COMO PLACE VENDOME SPRING BREAK GOLD DIGGER COEUR SUCRE BORN THIS WAY TRIBAL RED PENNY ARCAD
INTERNATIONAL VELVET TIBER VIVA CANDY SAYS HOLLYWOODLAWN PARIS FOLLIES PENNY ARCADE INTL VELVET VI
CANDY SAYS MORE HOLLY WOODLAWN BABY DOLL SWEET CHARITY BUTTERFIELD CABIRIA BEWITCHED GALACTICA HC
WIRED VAGABOND HELLFIRE MEDEA DIABLO AFRICAN QUEEN ROSEBUD AMAZON FANTASIA HUSH MARNIE JILTED LO
CREOLE NEW LOVER HOPI BAROQUE CLUB MIX CYTHERE SEX MACHINE SIERRA CRUELLA RED SQUARE DAMNED TORTO
MARINA HONOLULU HONEY BETTINA CAFE CON LECHE TOUNDRA POP LIFE NEVER SAY NEVER 413 BLKR MYSTERIOUS RE
AFGHAN RED MASAI FIRST BITE CHRISTINA ROUGE D ENFER TAMANGO PROMISCUOUS LARA SUCCESS ROUGE BASQU
PETIT MONSTRE BLONDE VENUS MOROCCO RED LIZARD HEAT WAVE JUNGLE RED CONGO RED FIRE DOWN BELO
MONGOLIAN RED TANGANYKA GIPSY VIVA LAS VEGAS ANGELIQUE RAIN HOT VOODOO BARBARELLA GALAXY GIRL BIANC
MITZI TOBAGO CATFIGHT VIRIDIANA JOYOUS RED FLAME FLAIR DAMAGE KLUTE KISS NOUBA RUSSIAN DOLL SPANISH R
HINDU CRUISING TUTTI FRUTTI SEXUAL HEALING MANHUNT MINDGAME BEAUTIFUL LIAR SENORITA CANAILLE SHRINAG
OUTSIDER FALBALA FAST RIDE LOVE DEVOTION LITTLE DARLING TZIGANE MAYFLOWER VENDANGES TABOO AUTUMN LEA

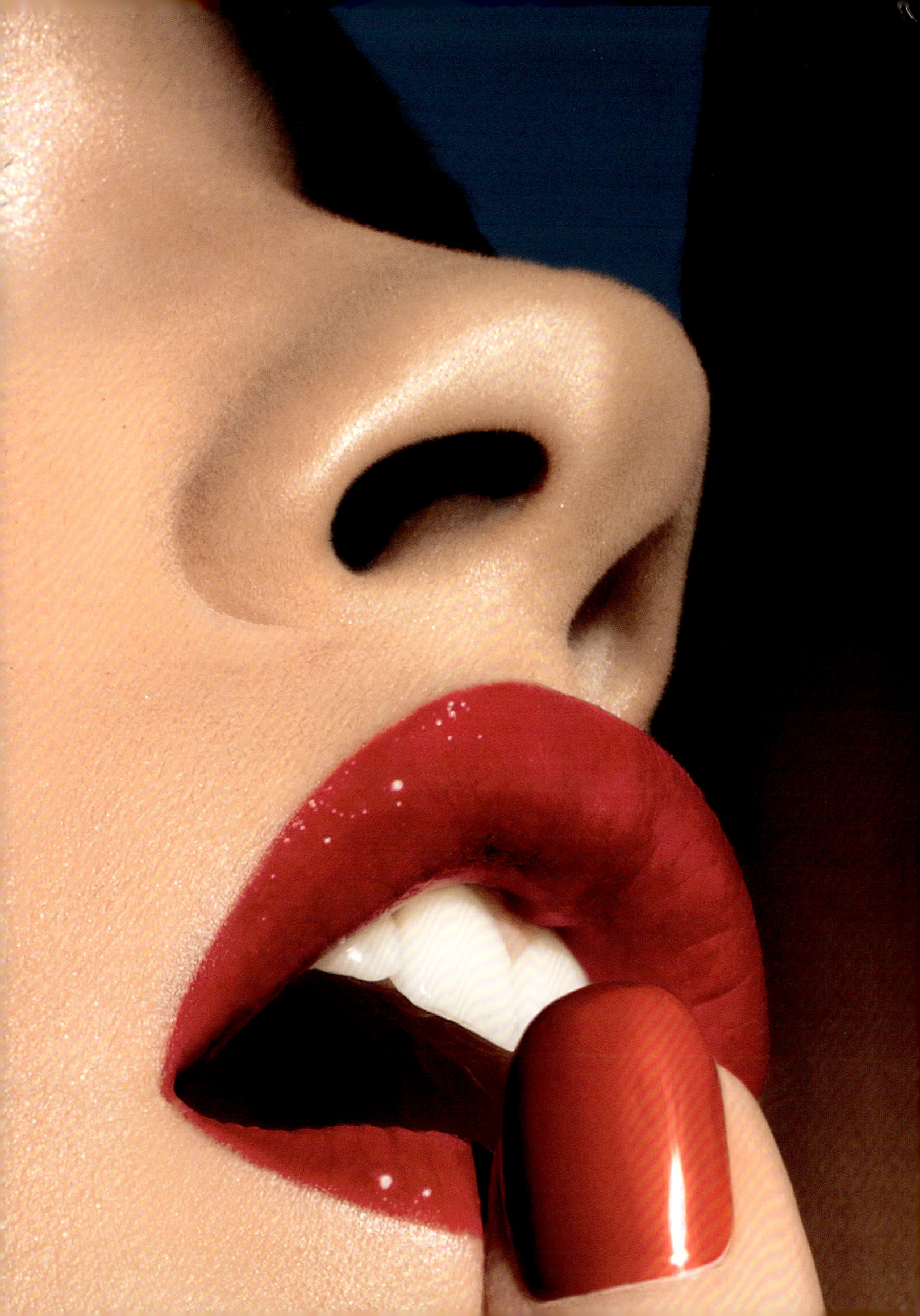

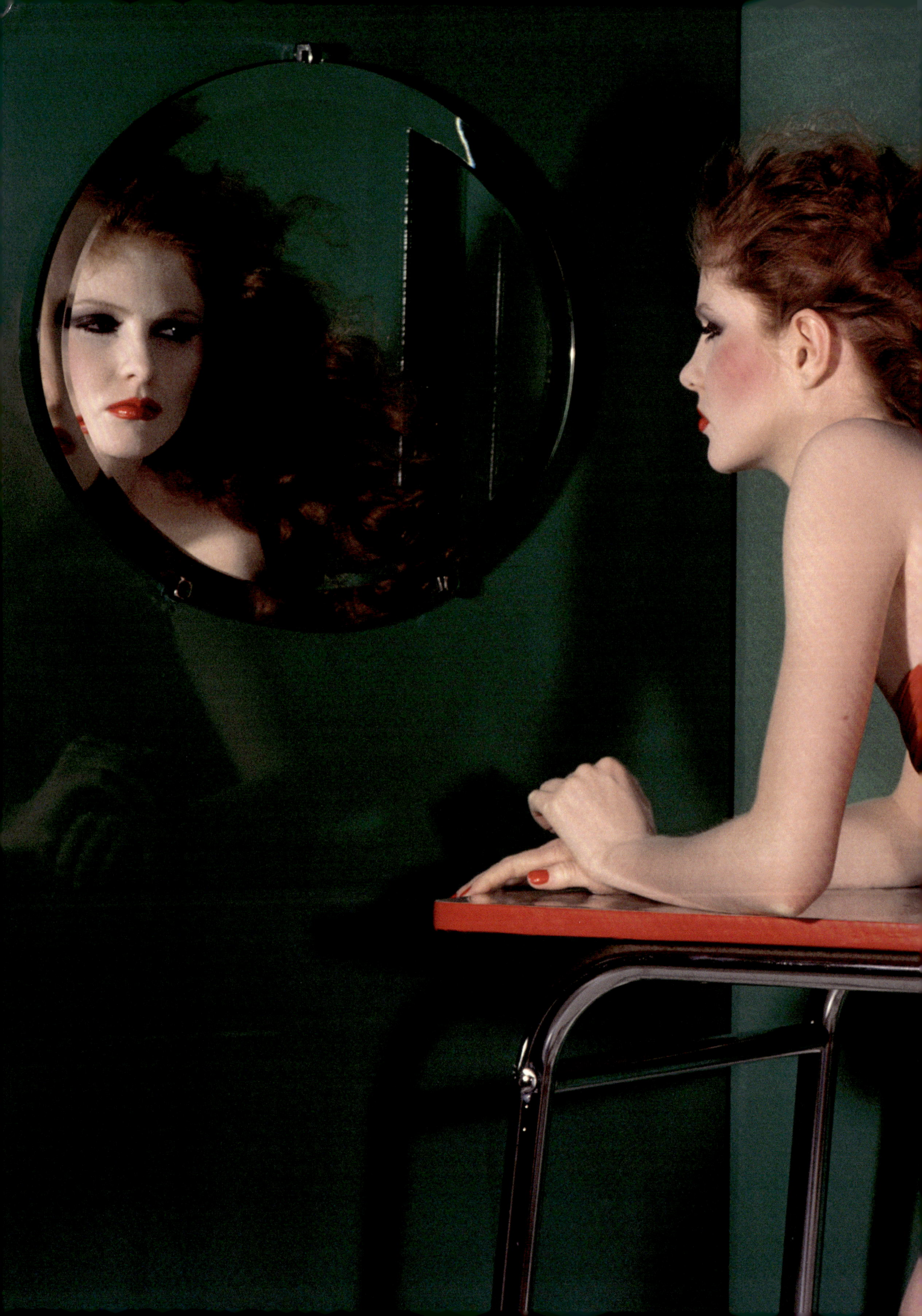

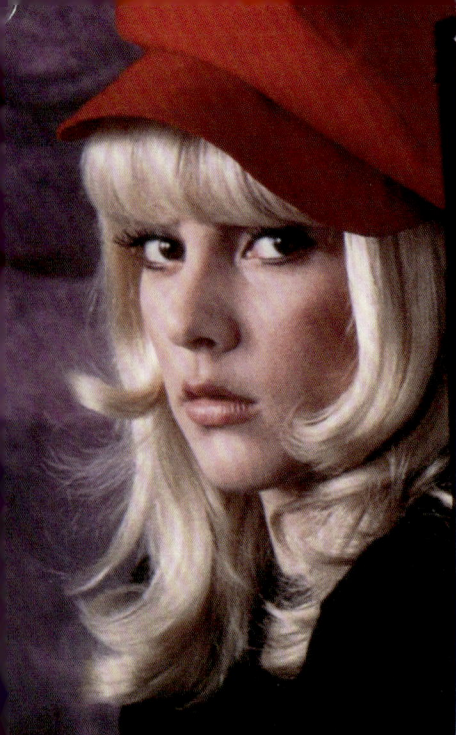

BURT LANCASTER | SILVANA MANGANO | HELMUT BERGER

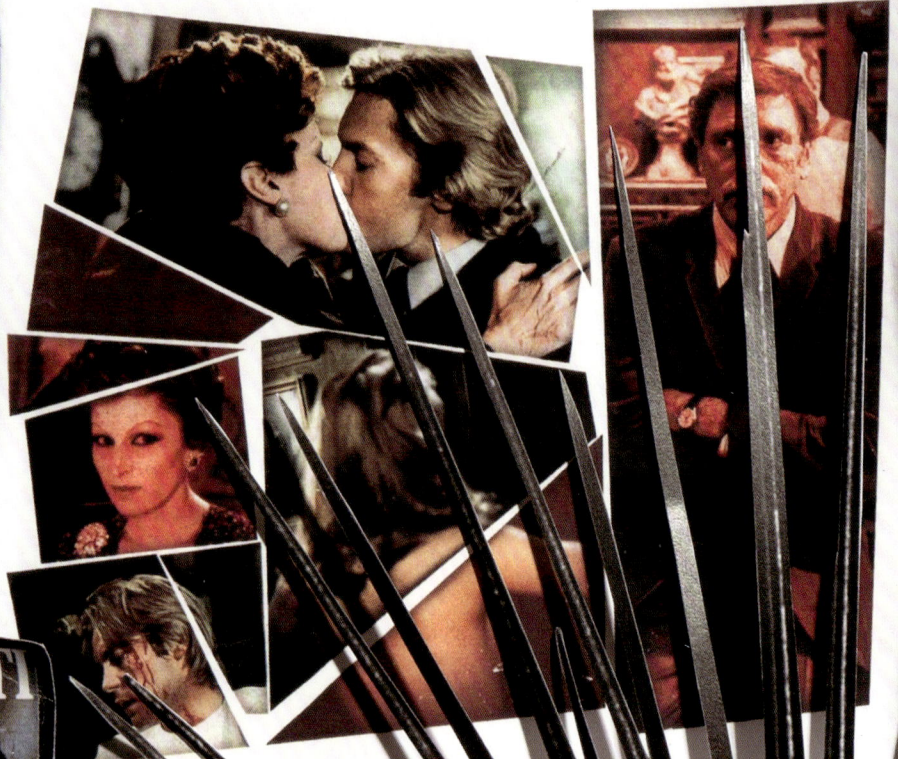

LUDWIG VISCONTI

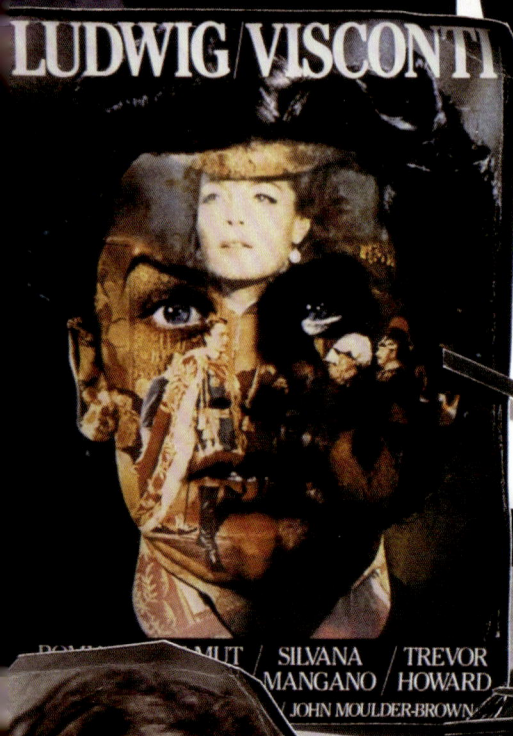

VIOLENCE ET PASSION

UN FILM DE LUDWIG VISCONTI

...MUT / SILVANA MANGANO / TREVOR HOWARD
JOHN MOULDER-BROWN

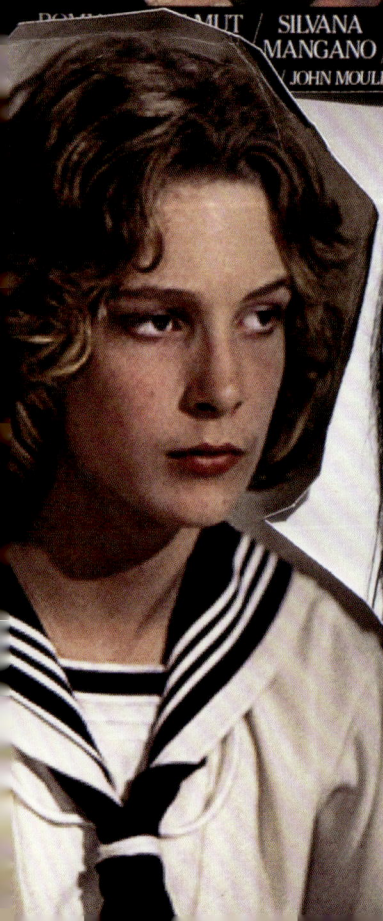

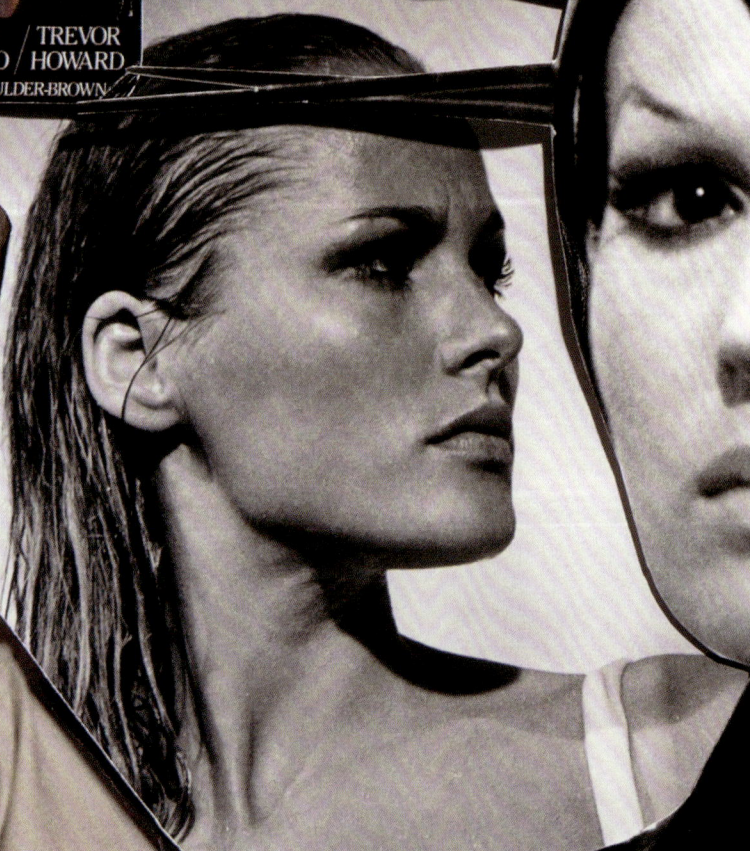

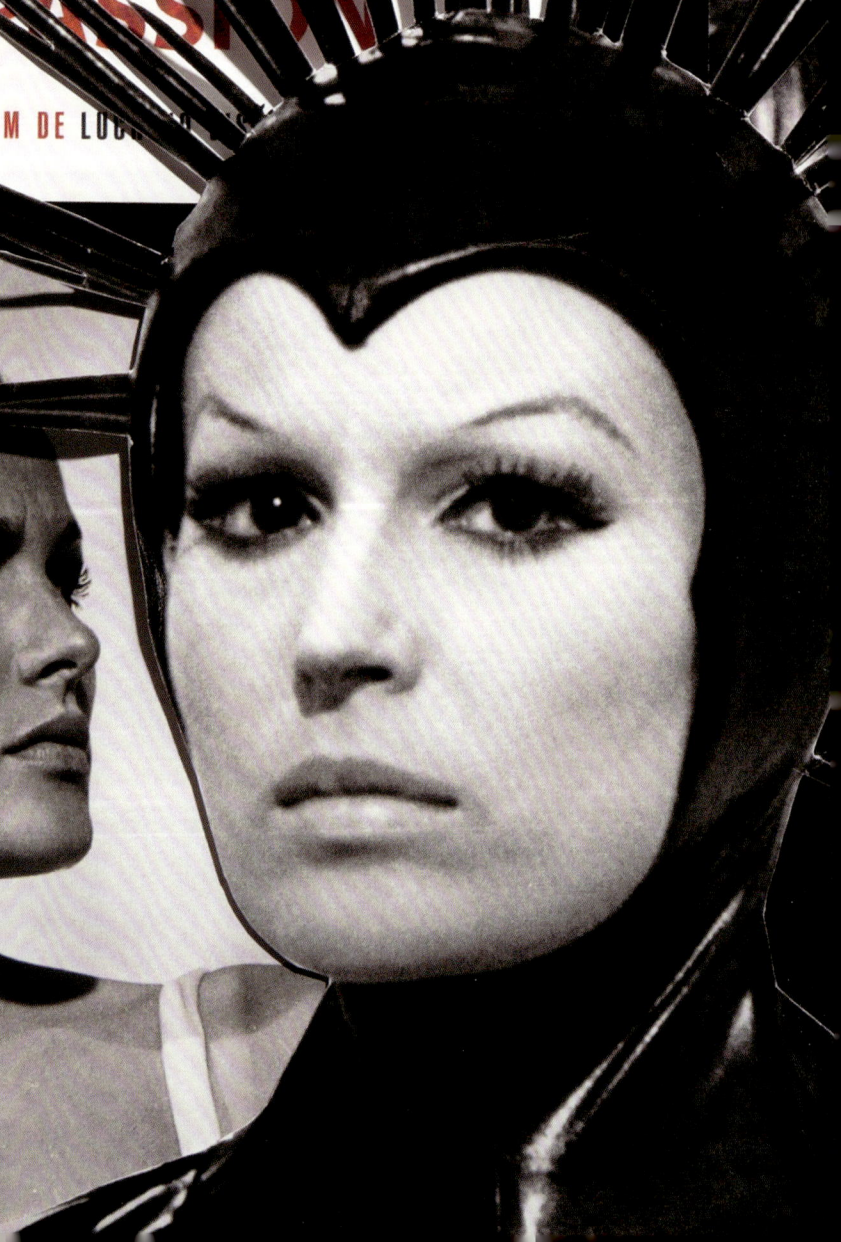

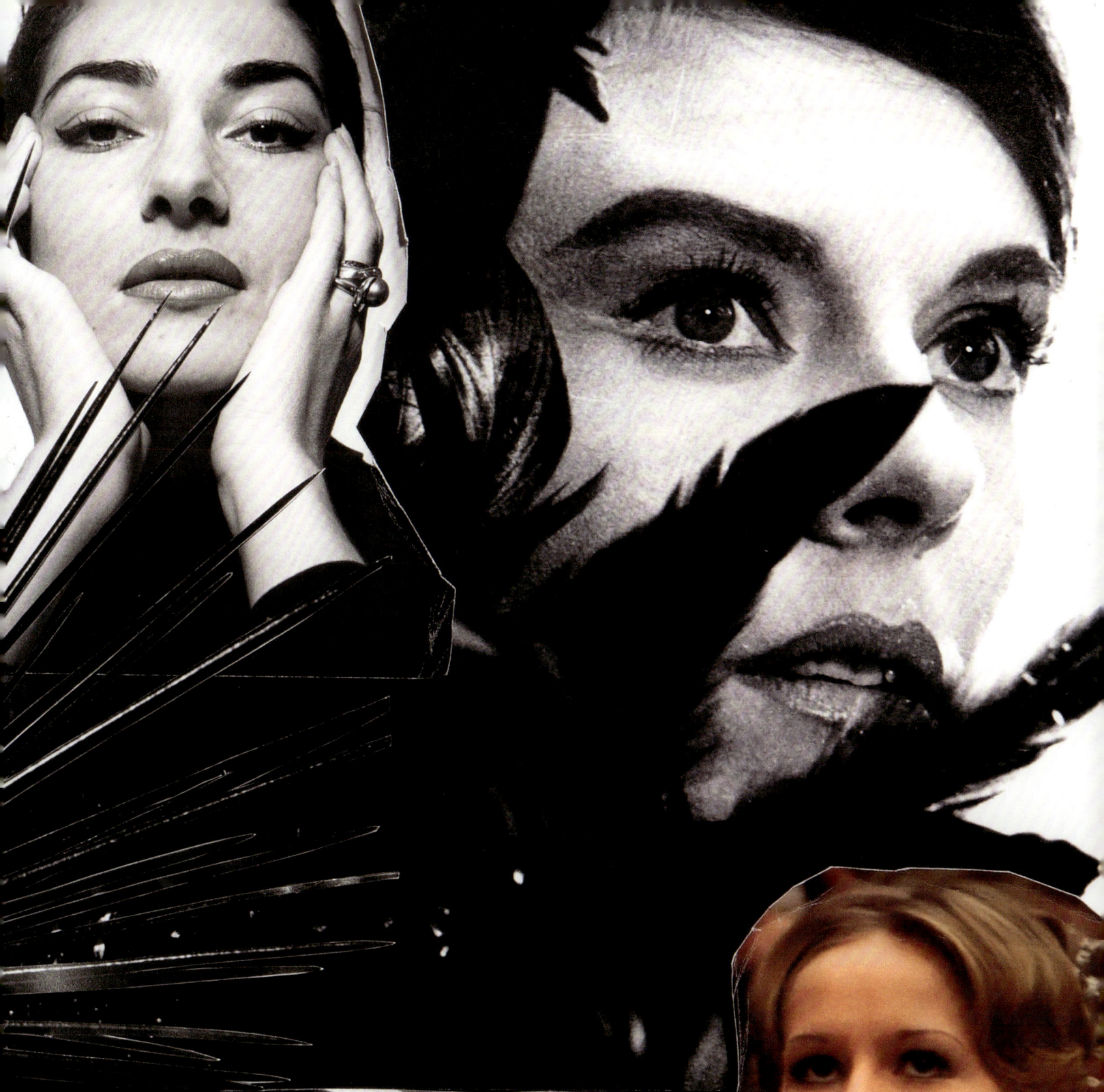

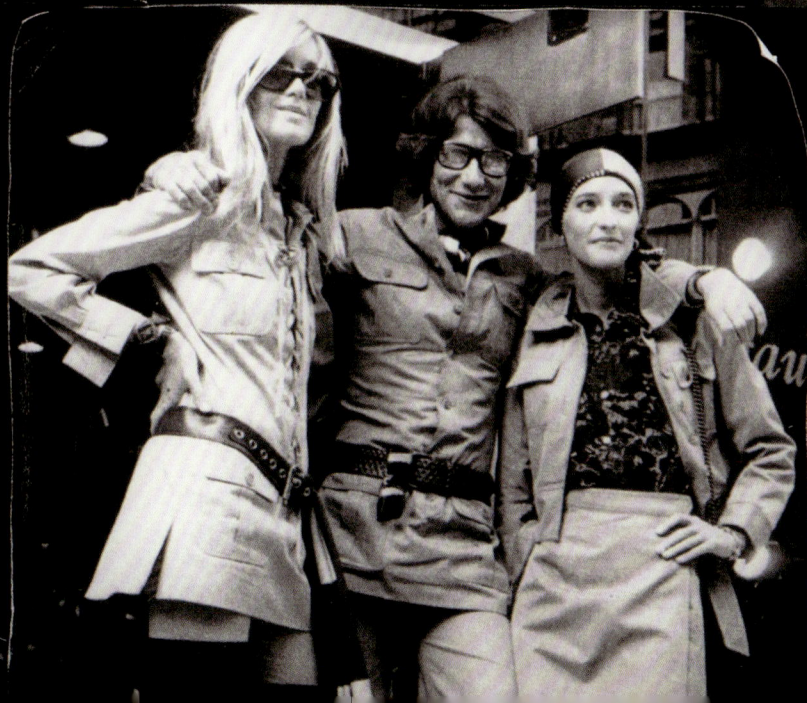

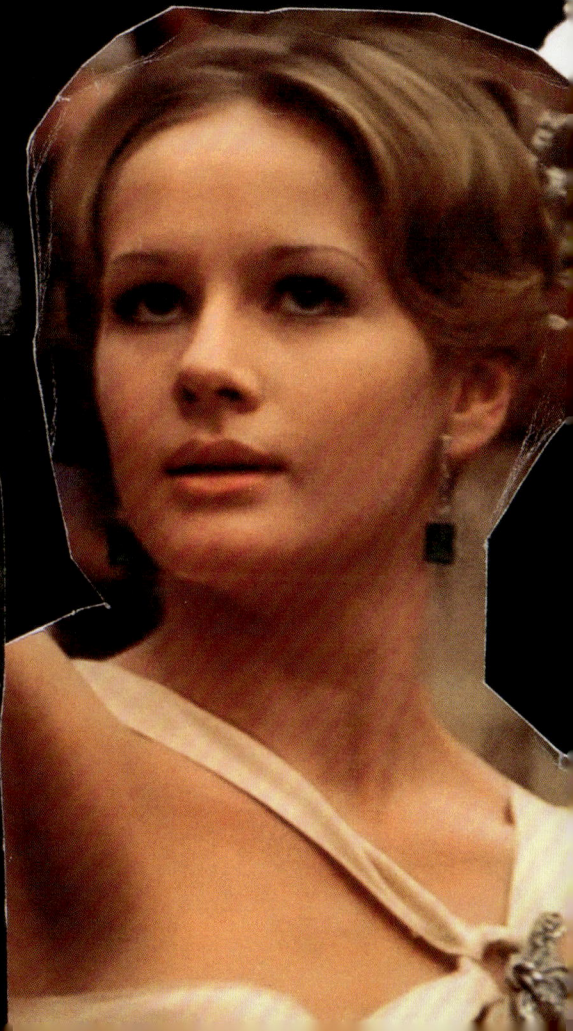

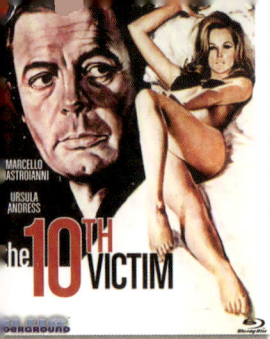

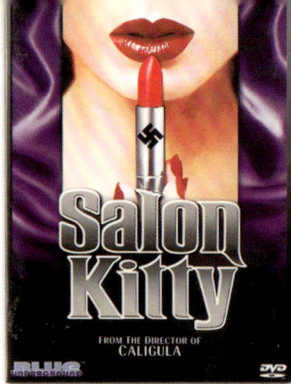

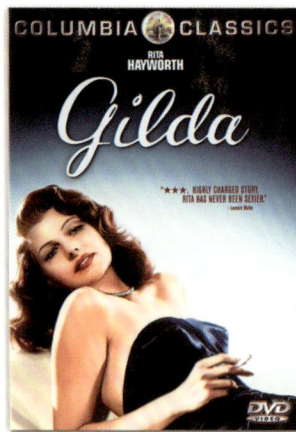

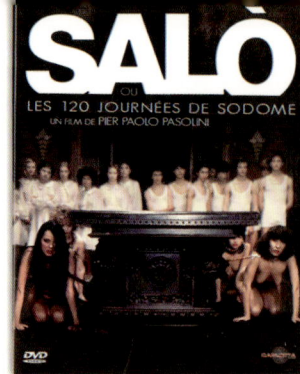

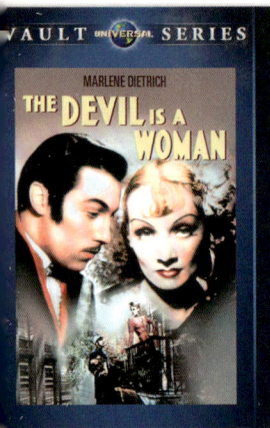

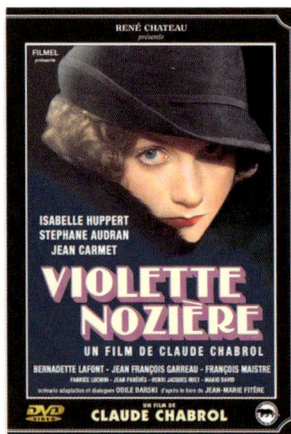

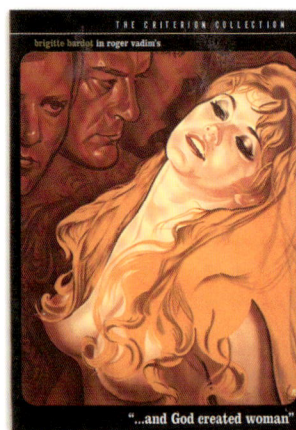

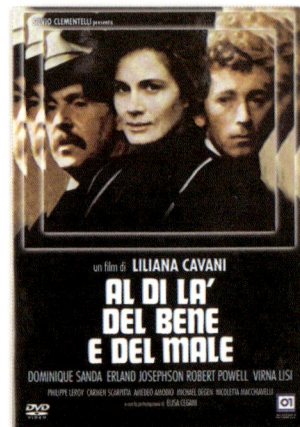

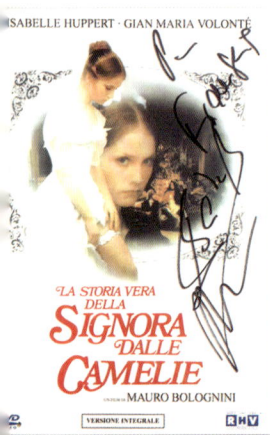

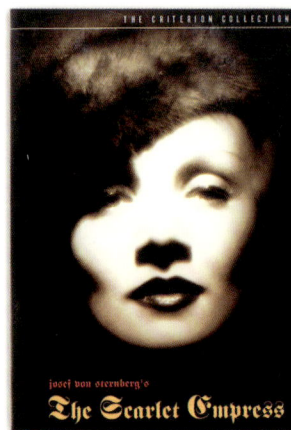

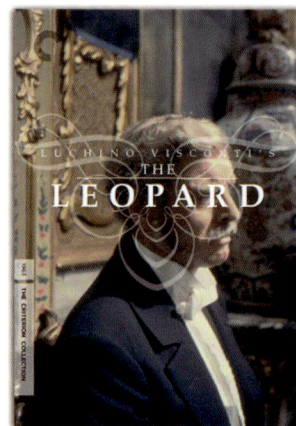

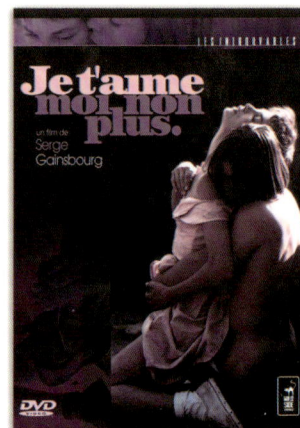

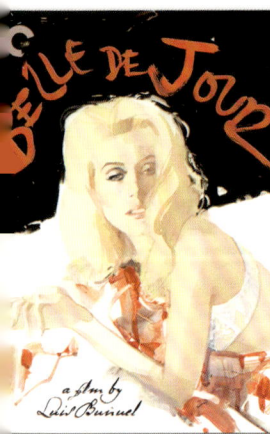

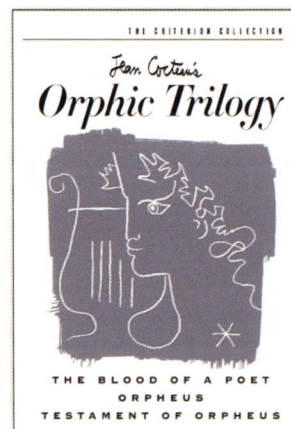

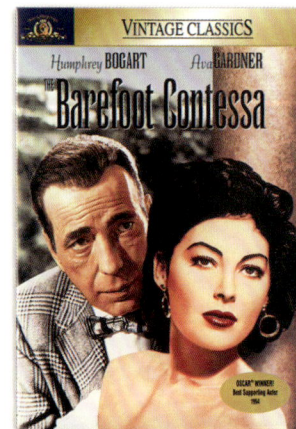

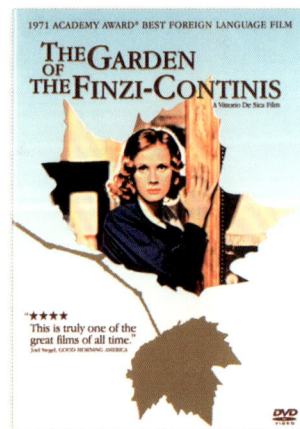

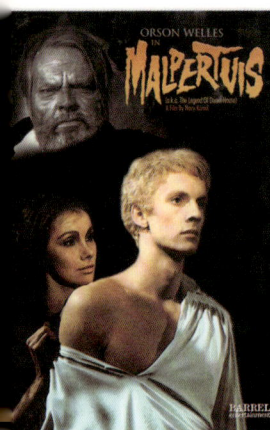

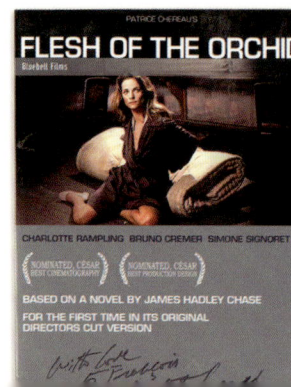

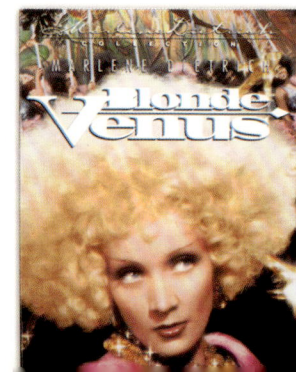

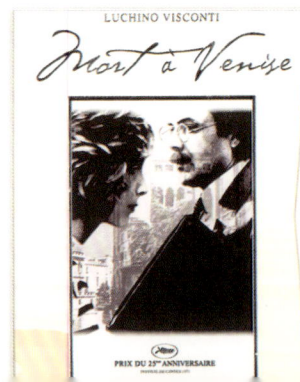

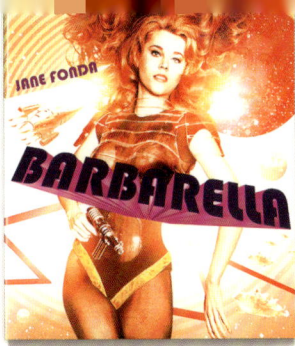

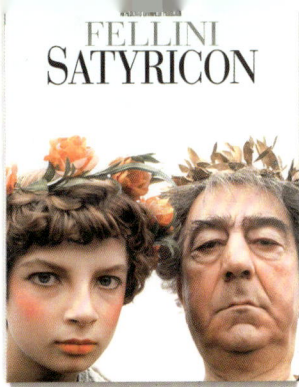

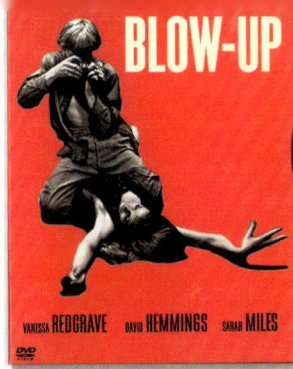

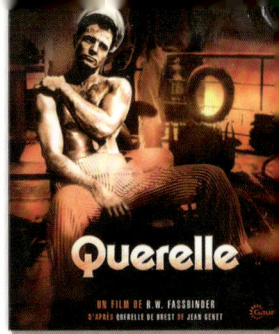

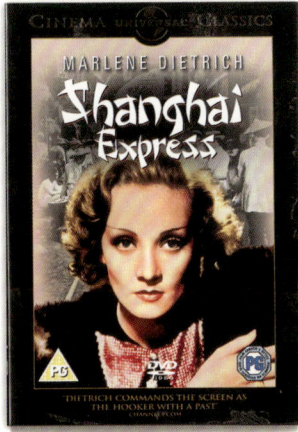

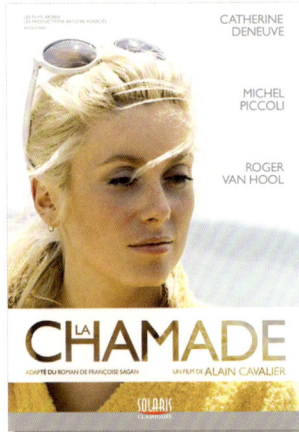

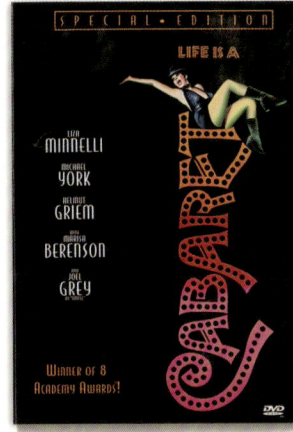

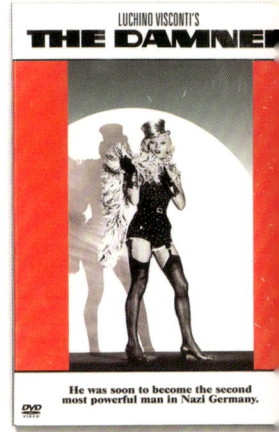

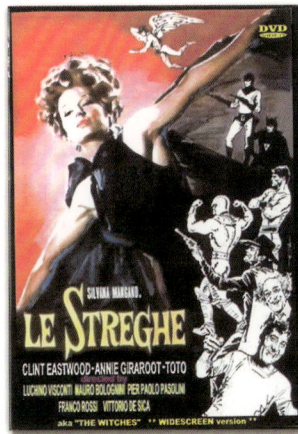

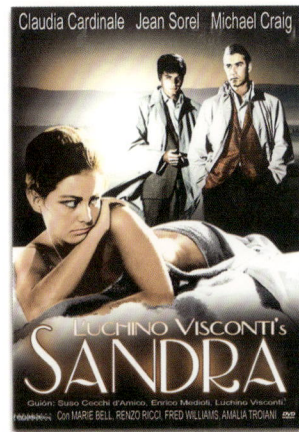

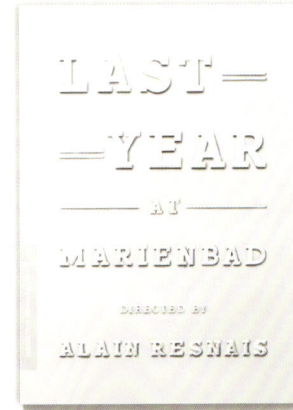

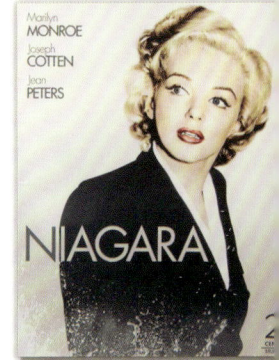

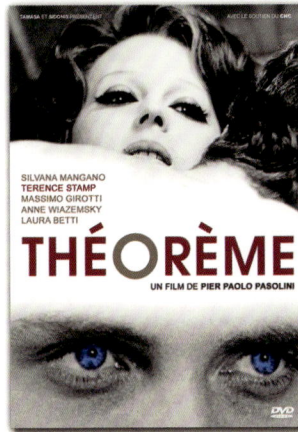

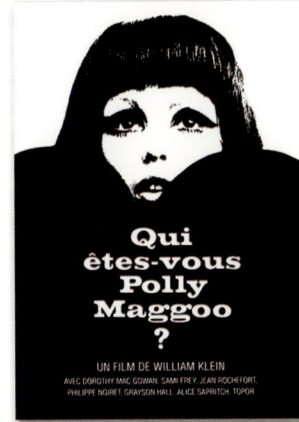

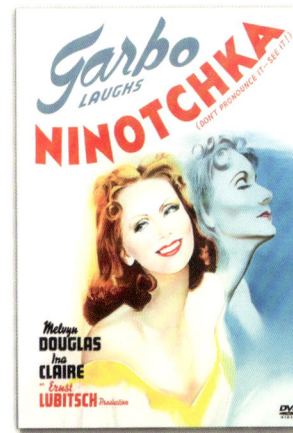

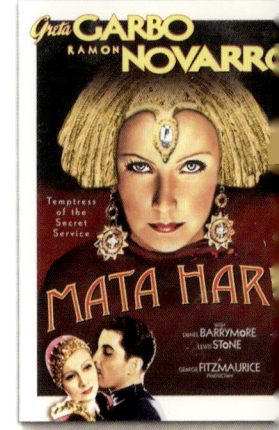

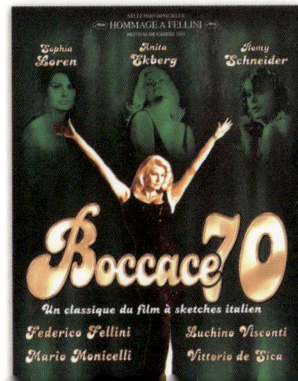

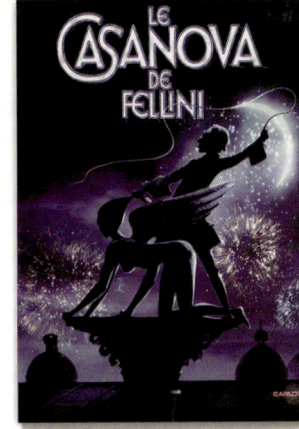

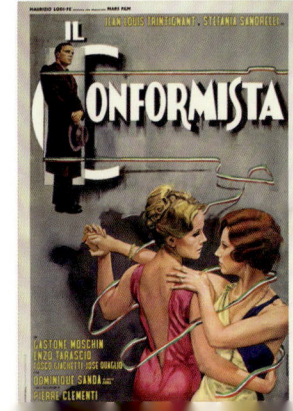

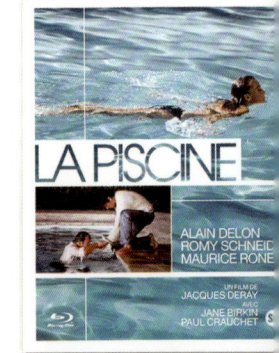

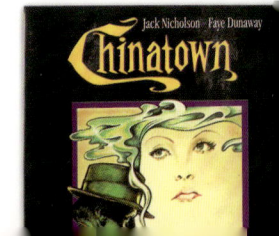

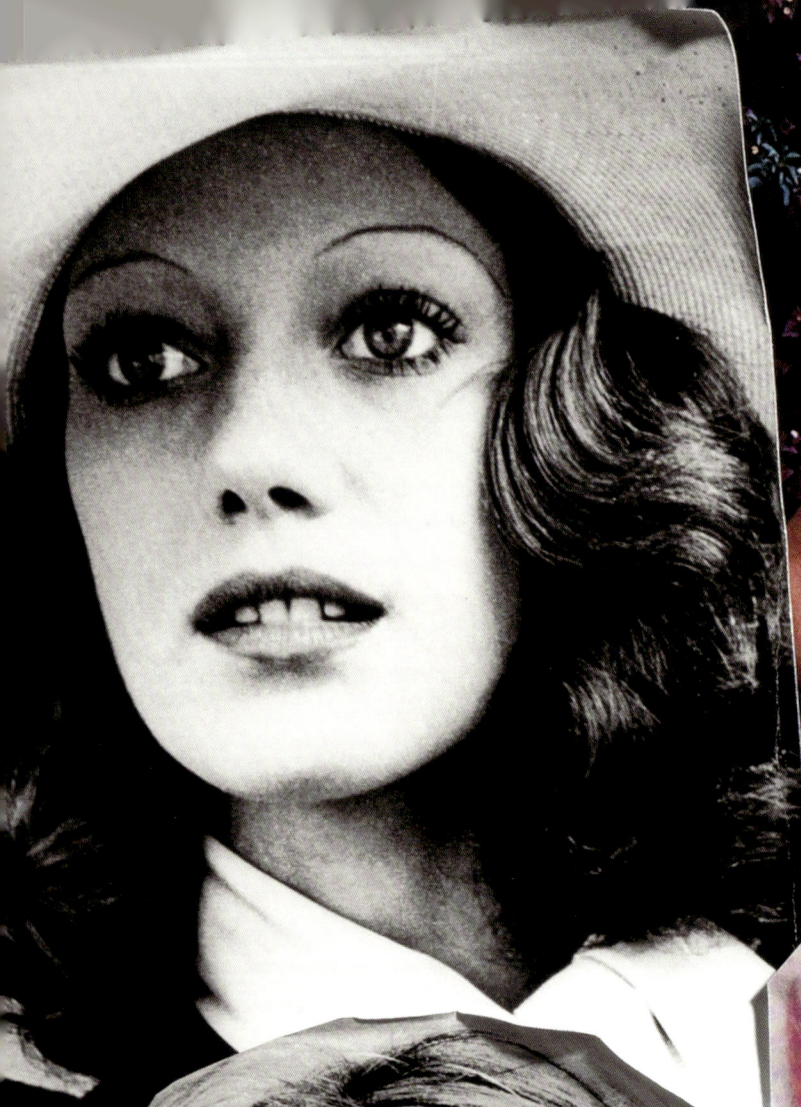

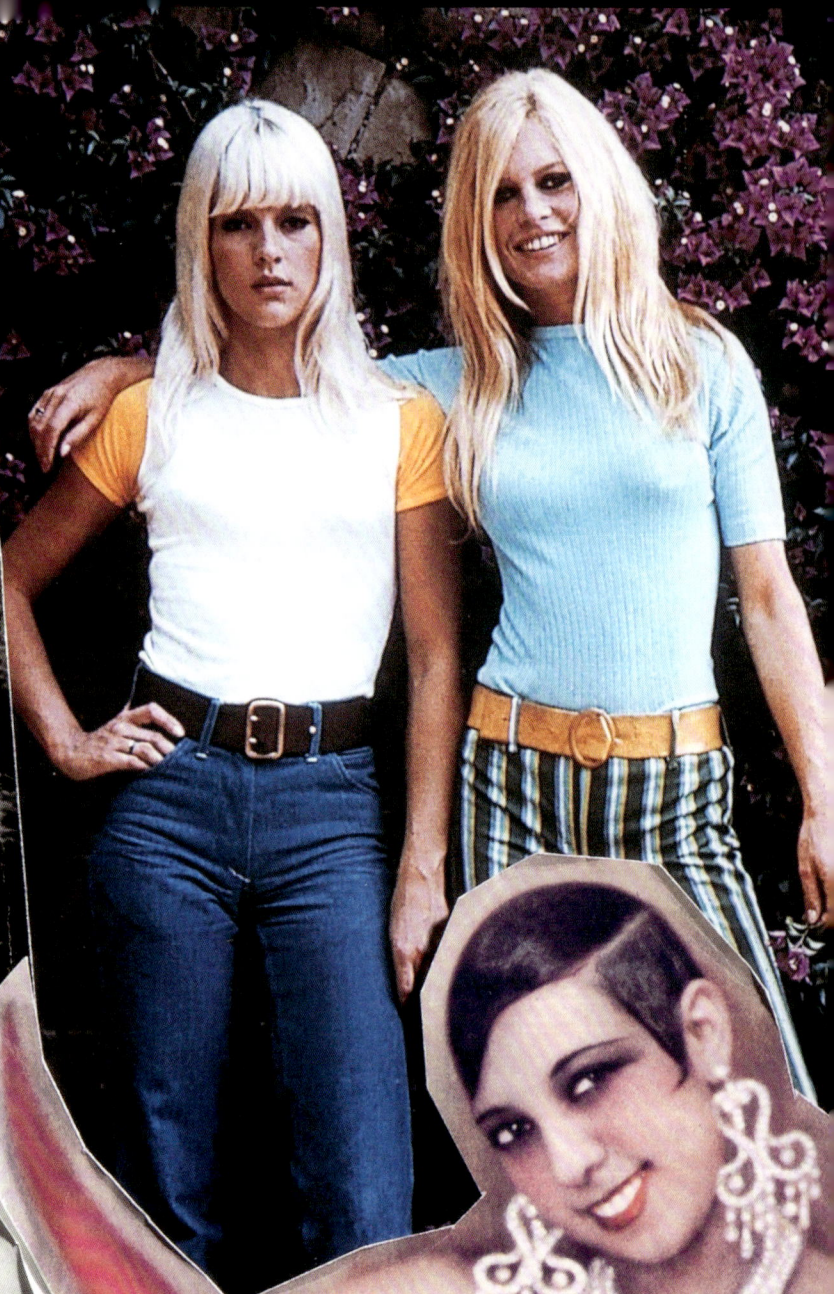

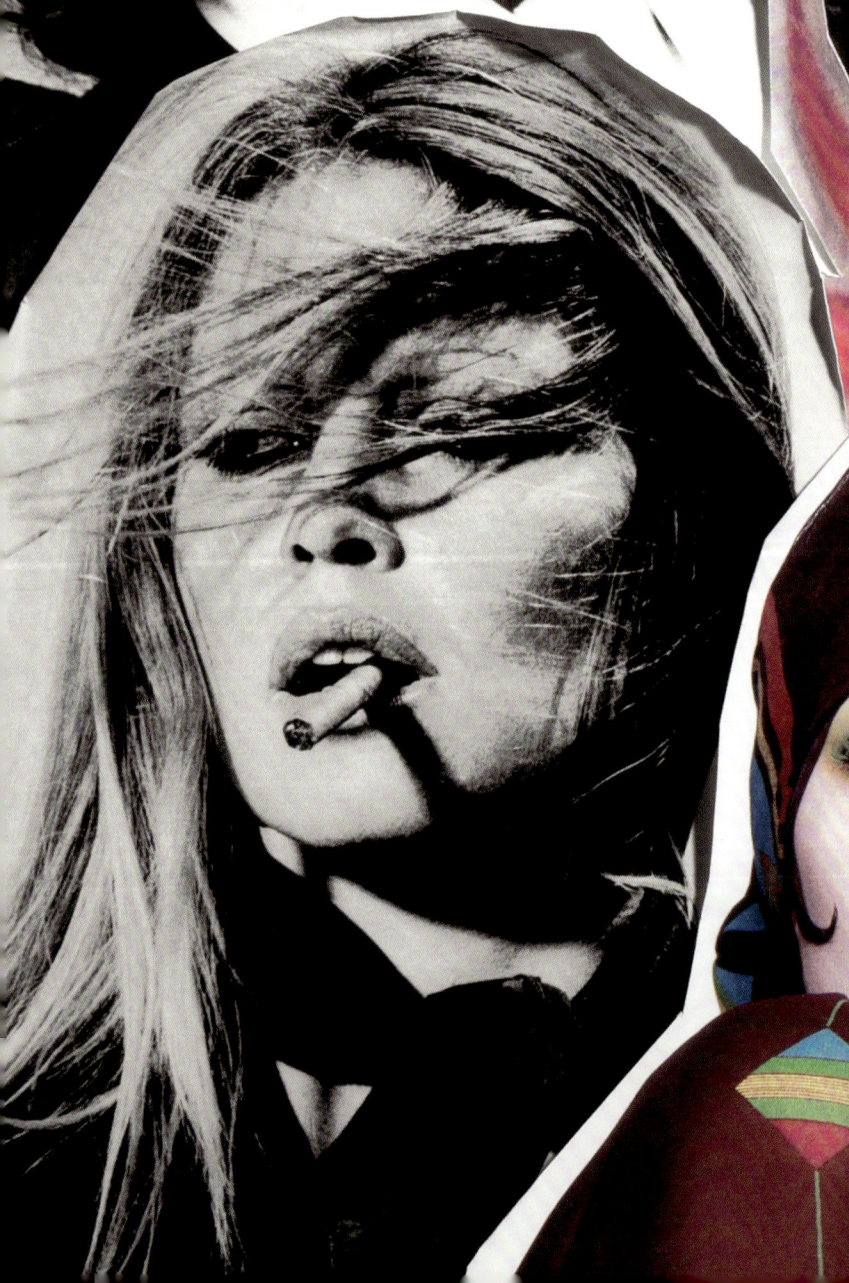

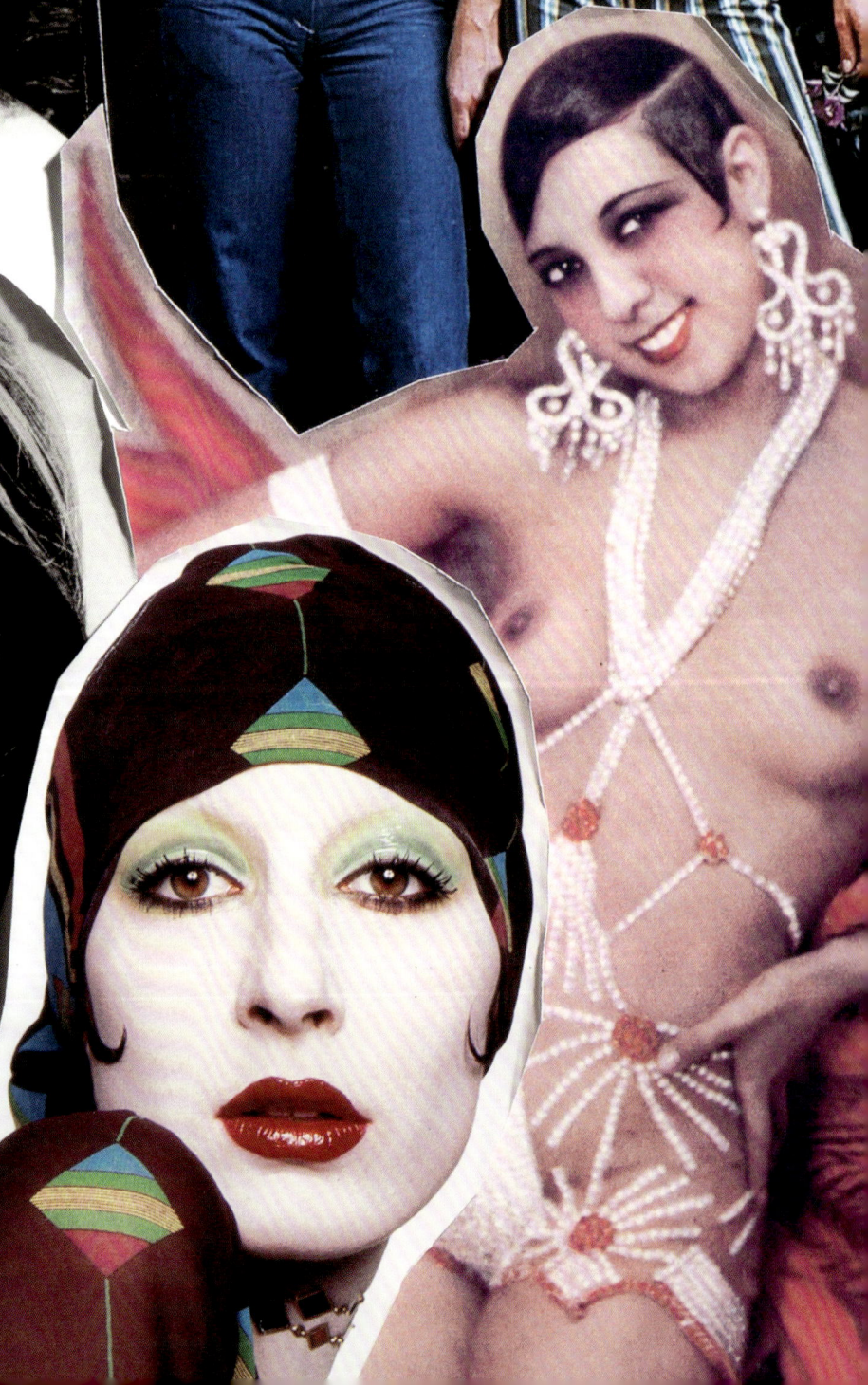

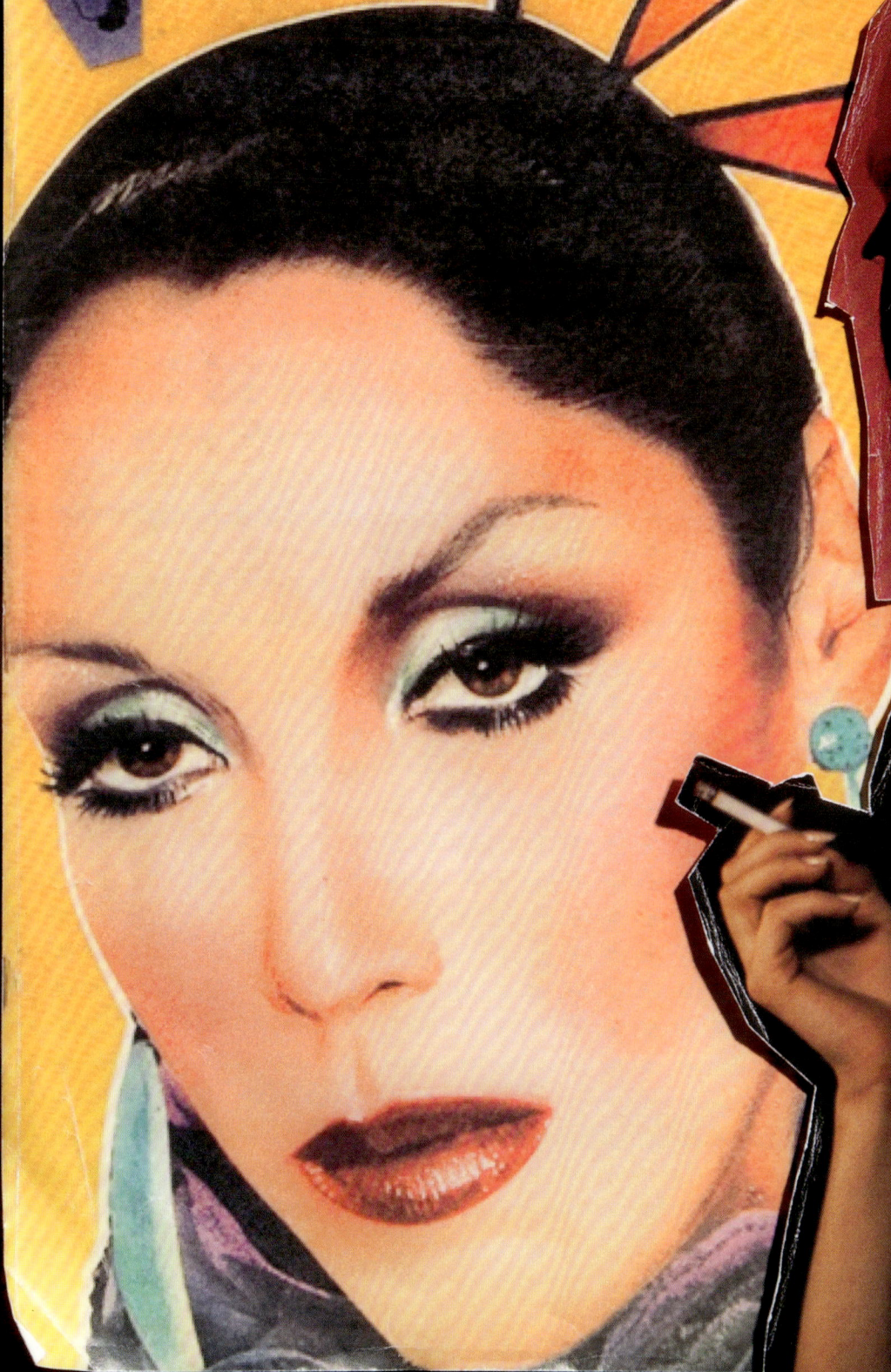

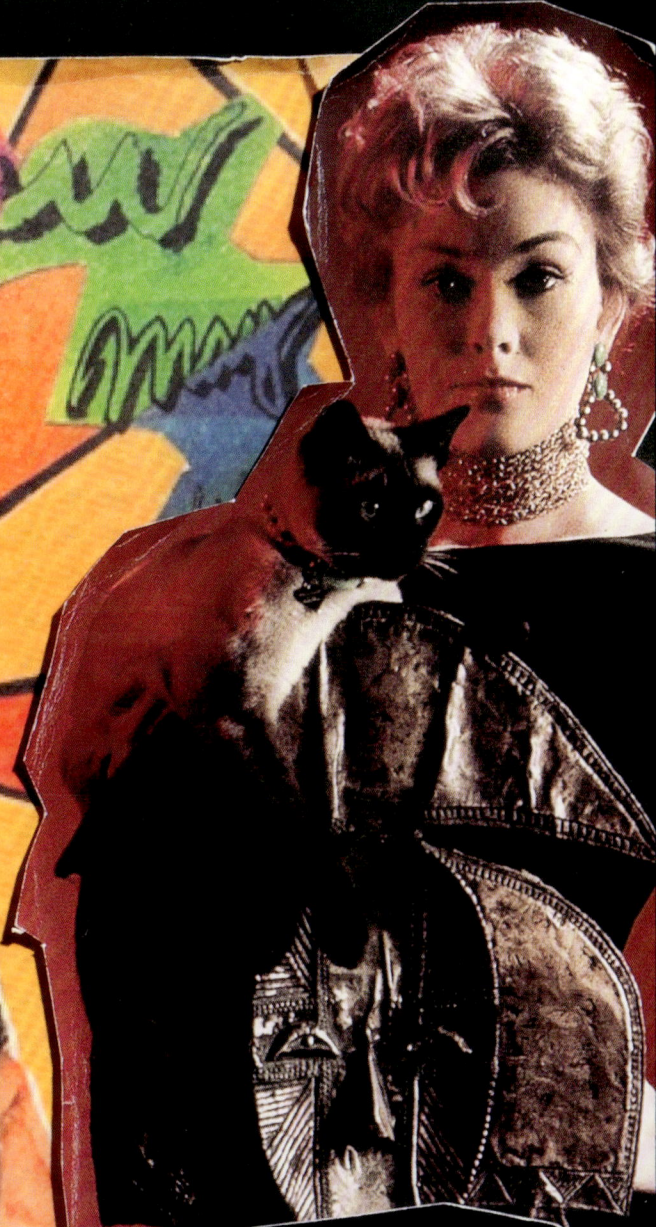

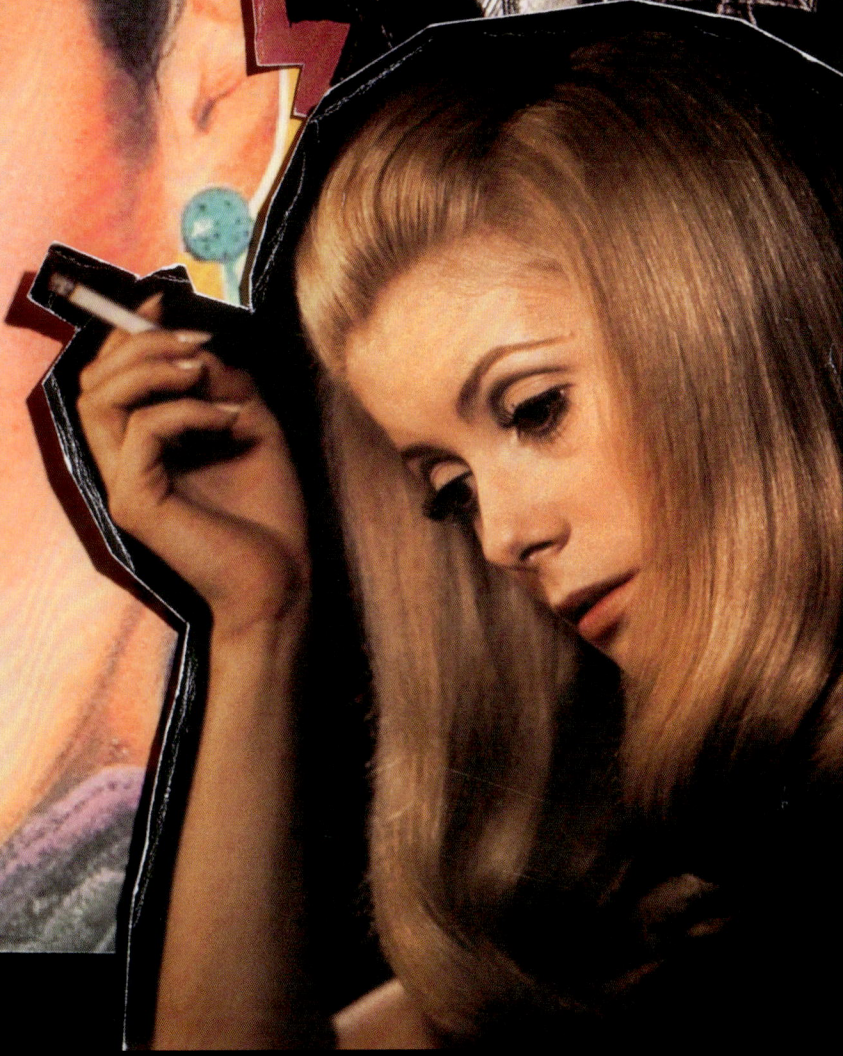

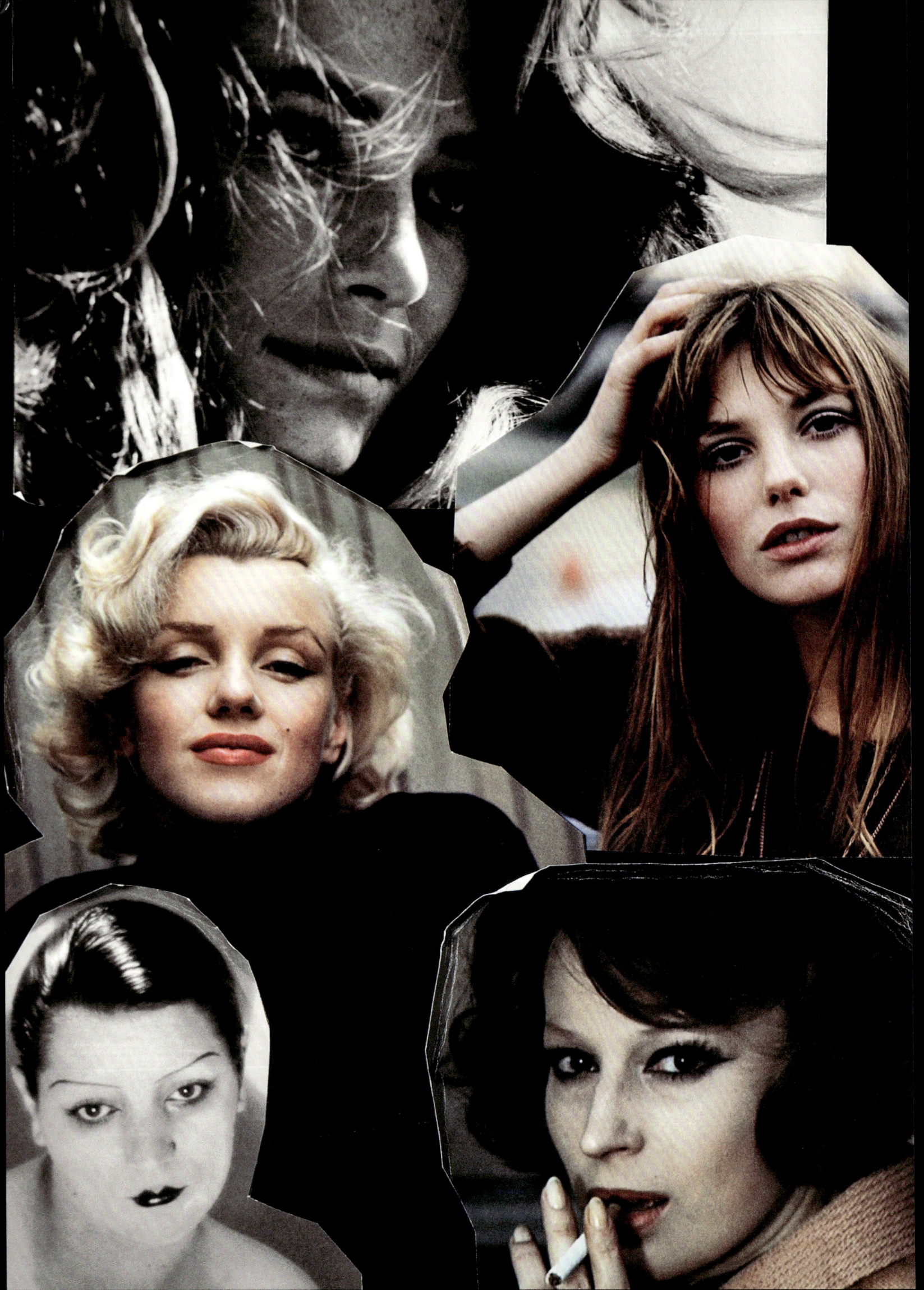

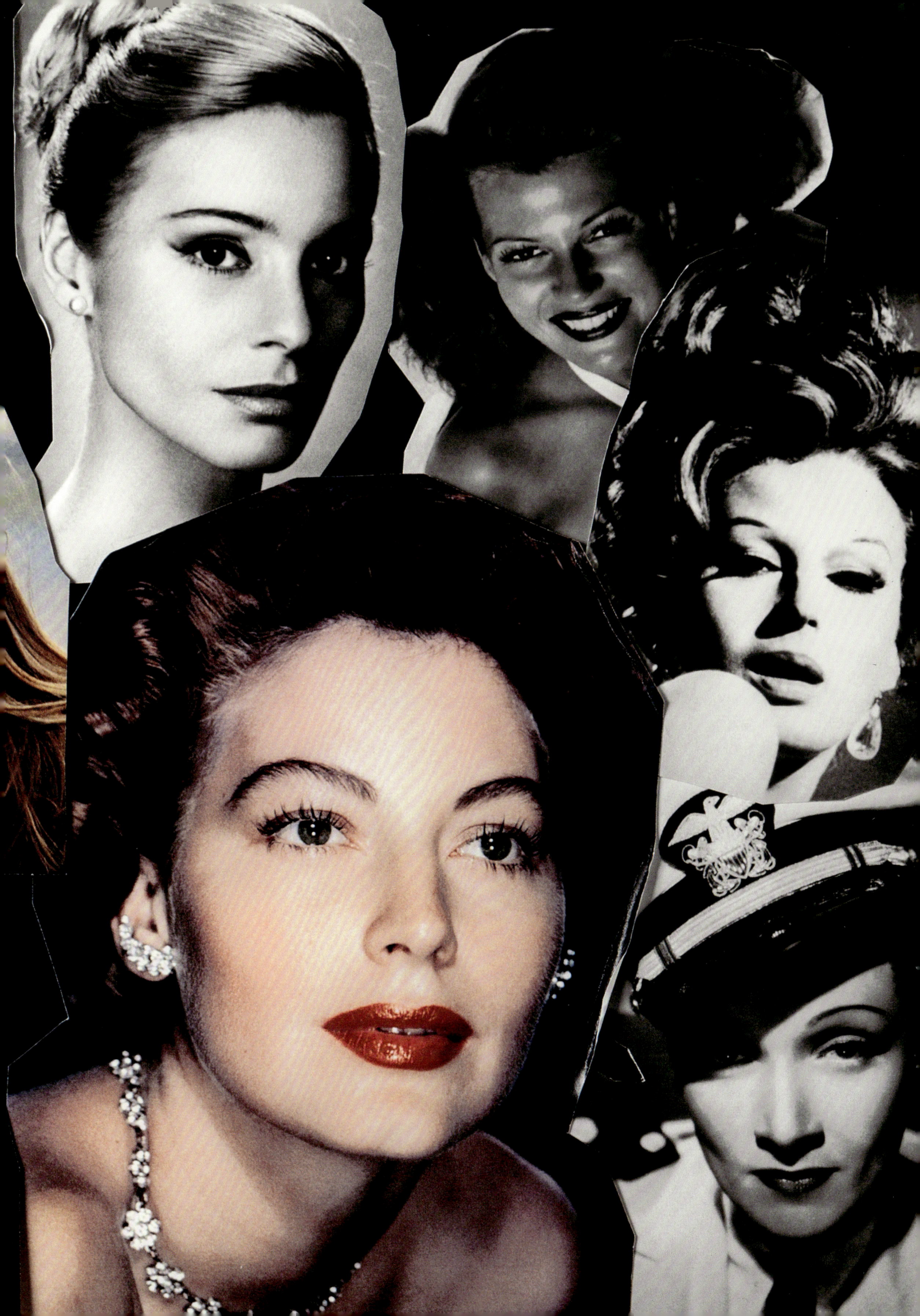

"FRANÇOIS IS THE MOST
TALENTED AND MOST FUN!
HIS MAKEUP DOESN'T
SIMPLY MAKE US MORE
BEAUTIFUL BUT IT IS FULL
OF REFERENCES TO ART,
HISTORY, ICONS OF PAST,
AND FUTURE FANTASIES.
HIS PRODUCTS REFLECT HIS
PLAYFULNESS, ELEGANCE,
AND SOPHISTICATION. IN
MY BAG I ALWAYS CARRY
A NARS PRODUCT LIKE HIS
MARVELOUS LIPSTICK."
— ISABELLA ROSSELLINI

"ISABELLA IS A GREAT
FRIEND, I LOVE HER SO
MUCH. SHE HAS THE
GREATEST, WITTIEST
SENSE OF HUMOR. WE
ALWAYS LAUGH SO
MUCH TOGETHER. SHE IS
ALSO ONE OF THE MOST
BEAUTIFUL WOMEN I
EVER WORKED WITH,
SHE IS JUST WONDERFUL."
— FRANÇOIS NARS

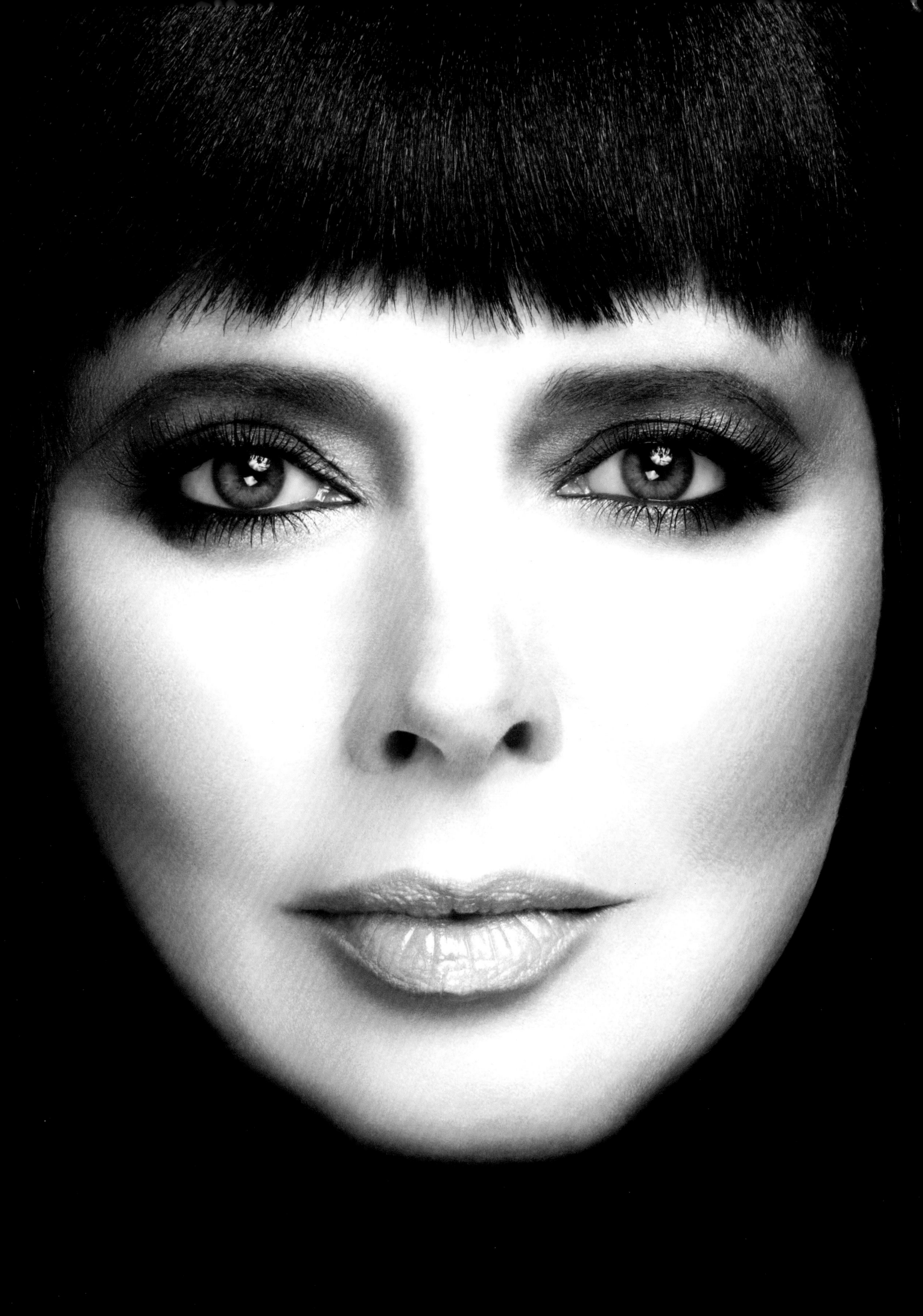

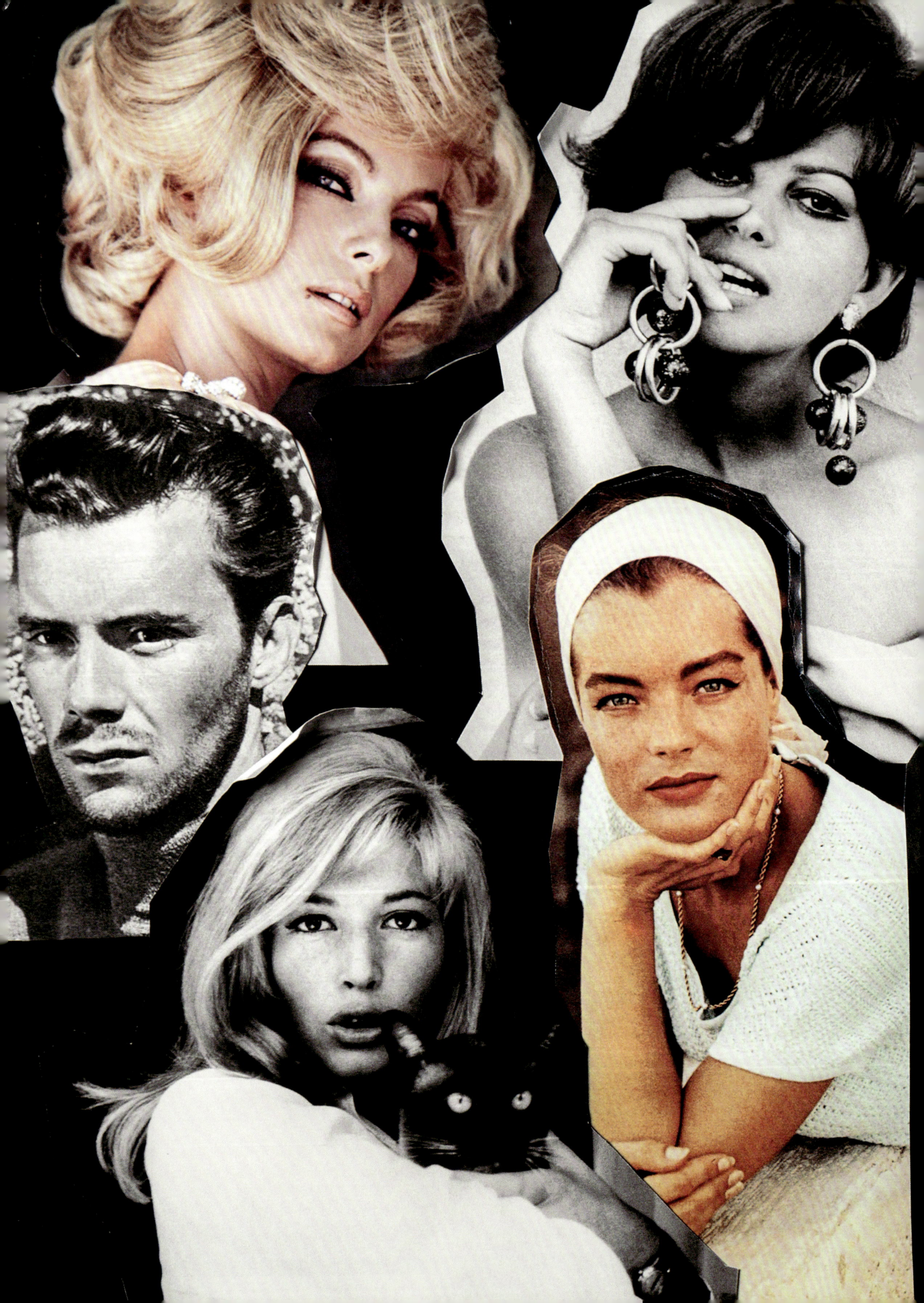

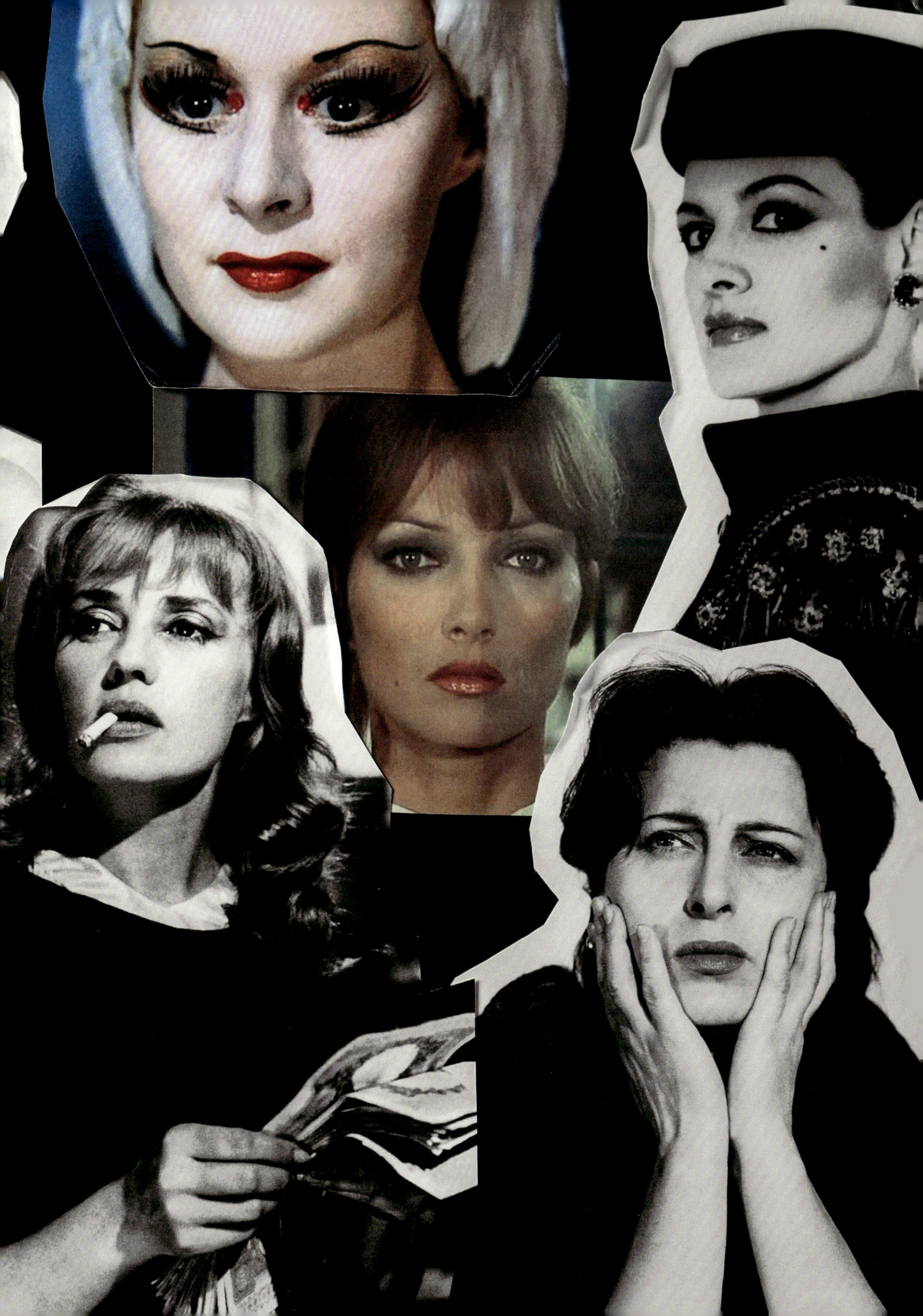

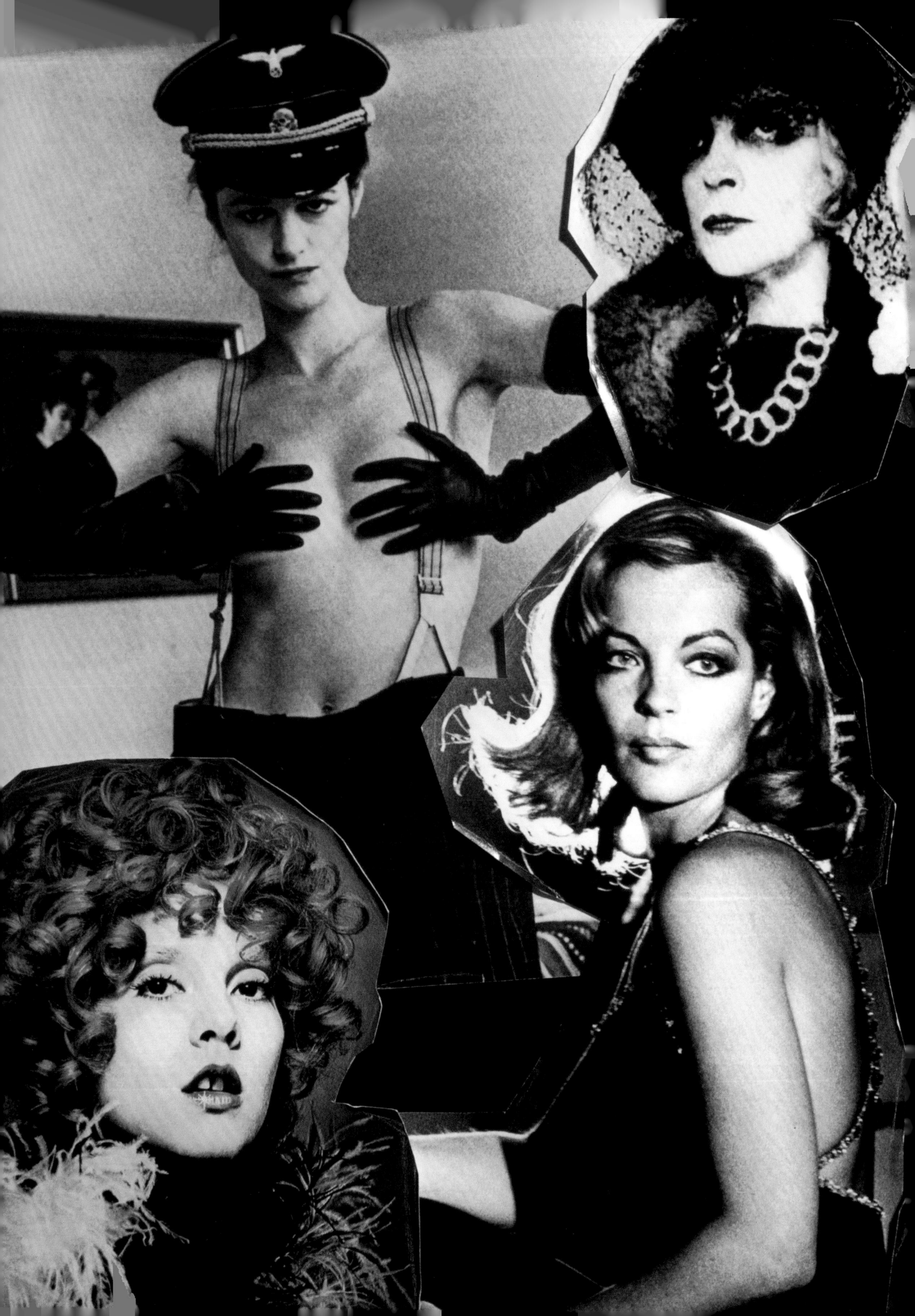

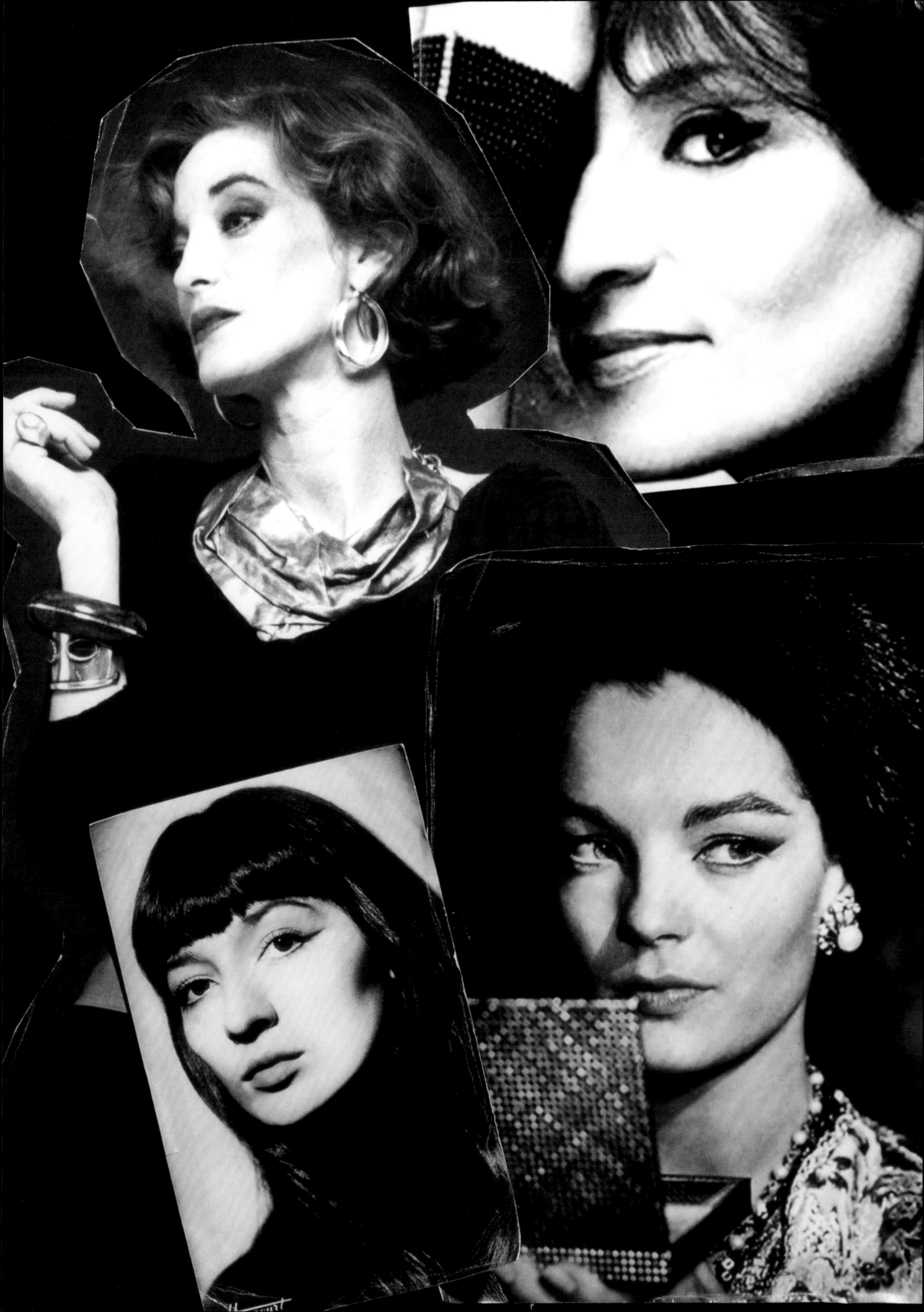

"I WAS PROBABLY TWELVE YEARS OLD WHEN I FIRST 'FELL IN LOVE' WITH HELMUT BERGER, AFTER HAVING SEEN HIM IN *THE DAMNED* AND *LUDWIG* BY LUCHINO VISCONTI. I, LIKE MILLIONS OF PEOPLE, FELL UNDER THE CHARM AND CHARISMA OF HELMUT. LATER ON, WE MET WHEN I WAS SHOOTING MY BOOK *X-RAY* AND I MUST SAY I WAS NOT DISAPPOINTED. HELMUT IS EXTREMELY SMART, FUNNY, WITTY, WITH A GREAT SENSE OF HUMOUR. HE IS REALLY ONE OF A KIND."
— FRANÇOIS NARS

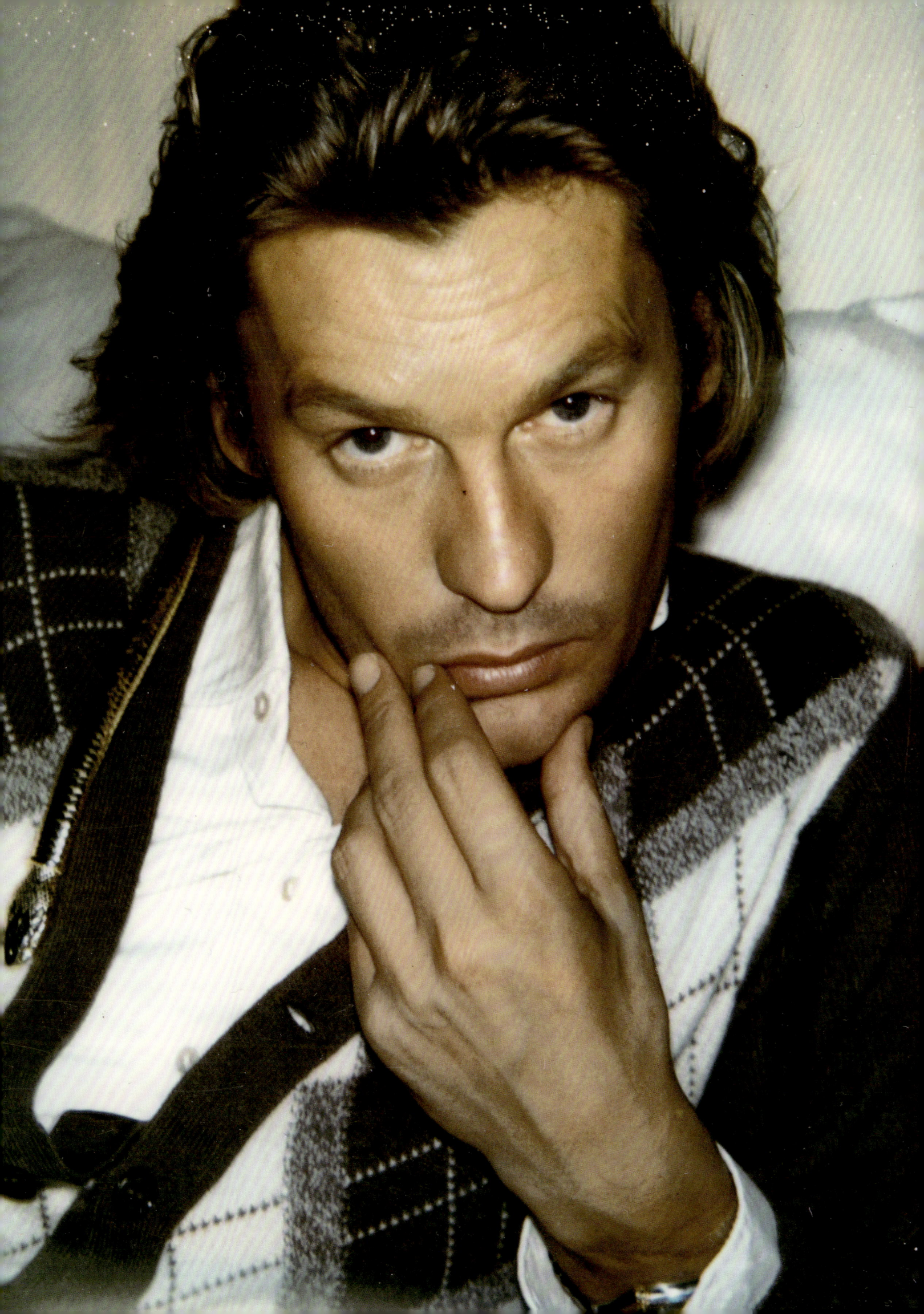

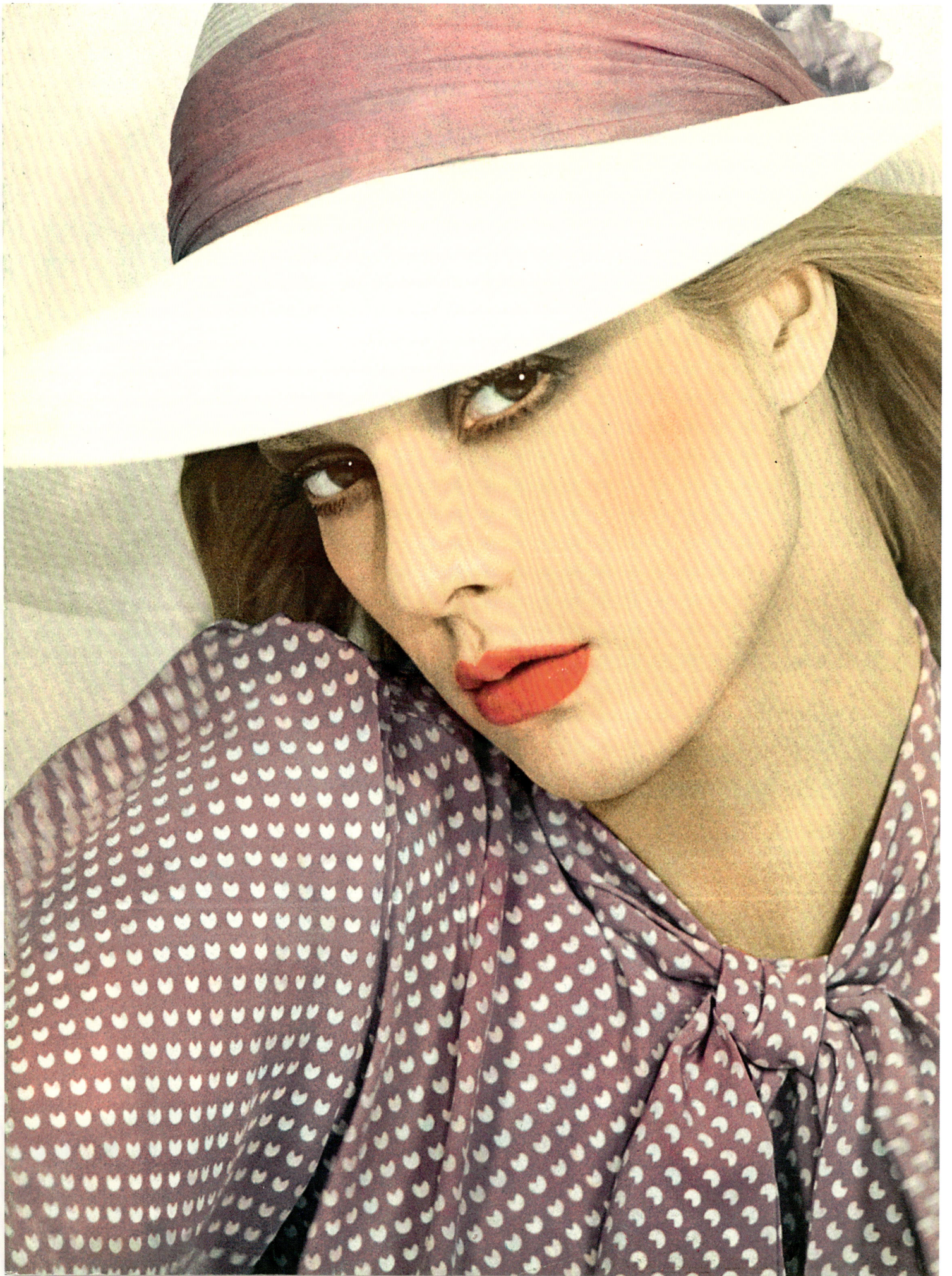

"THE FIRST TIME I MET YOU FRANÇOIS, I RECOGNIZED THAT YOU WERE AN EXCEPTIONAL PERSON. YOU HAD CHARM, TALENT, AND CREATIVITY LIKE VERY FEW PEOPLE I'VE KNOWN THROUGHOUT MY CAREER. AS AN ARTIST YOU ARE A MAGICIAN AND YOU HAVE ALWAYS BEEN MAGIC FOR ME. I CHERISH OUR FRIENDSHIP. MY LOVE ALWAYS."
– SYLVIE VARTAN

"SYLVIE HAS ALWAYS BEEN IN MY HEART, AS LONG AS I CAN REMEMBER. SHE IS FOR ME A SYMBOL OF FEMININITY, CHARM, TALENT, AND INTELLIGENCE. SHE IS SENSITIVE, FULL OF STRENGTH, BEAUTIFUL, AND HER MUSIC IS A POTION FOR LOVE AND HAPPINESS. SYLVIE, *TU ES DIVINE*."
– FRANÇOIS NARS

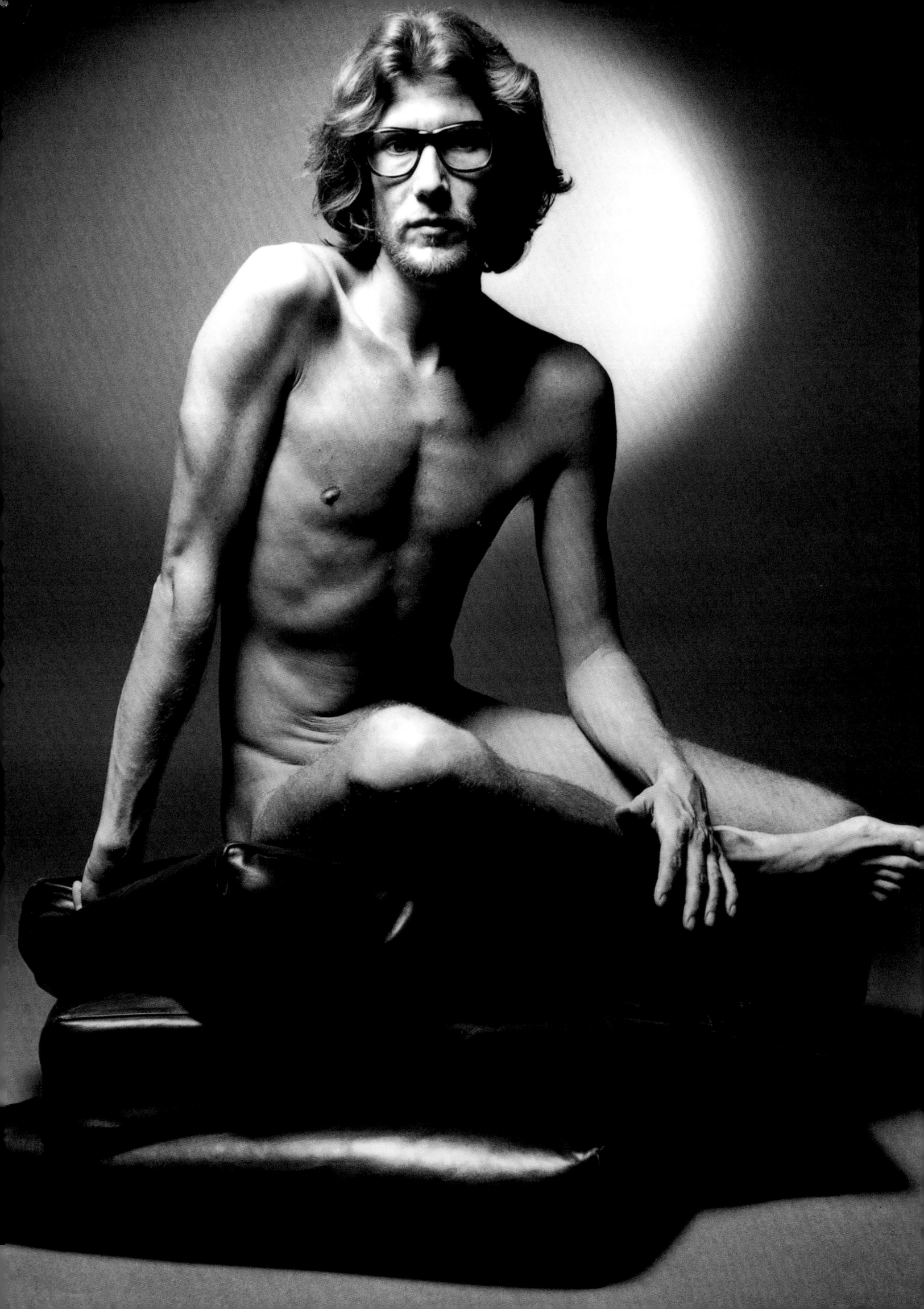

"YVES SAINT LAURENT, THE ONLY ONE! HE LOVED WOMEN SO MUCH AND LOVED MAKING THEM BEAUTIFUL. WHAT A GREAT PHILOSOPHY! A PHILOSOPHY A LOT OF DESIGNERS TEND TO FORGET TODAY." — FRANÇOIS NARS

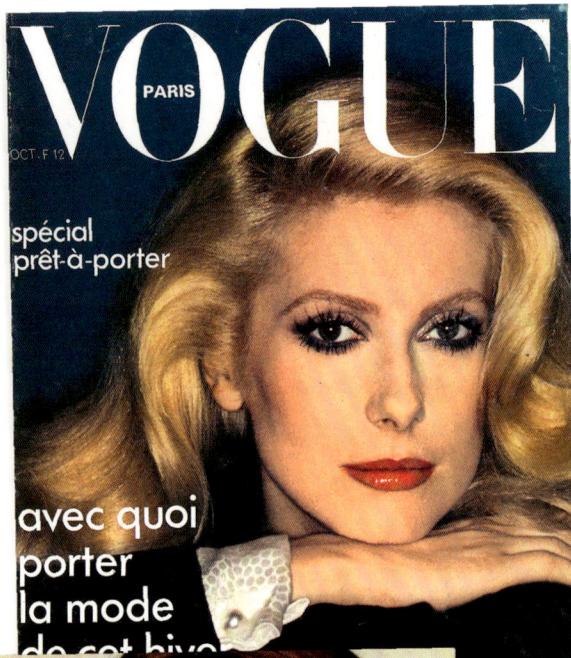

VOGUE PARIS
OCT - F 12
spécial
prêt-à-porter
avec quoi
porter
la mode
de cet hiver

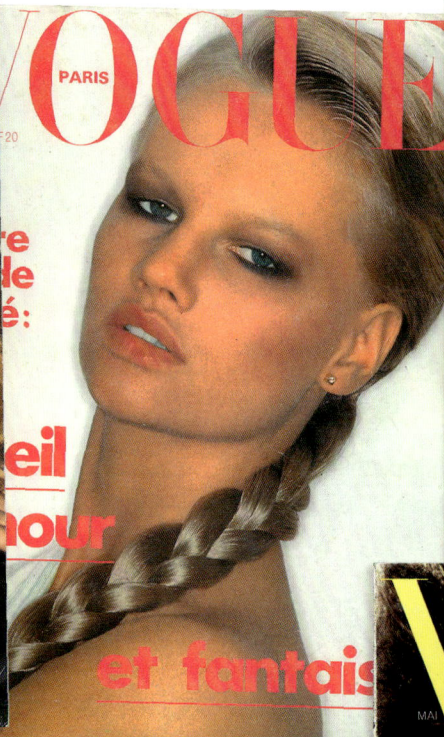

VOGUE PARIS
F 20
...eil
...our
et fantais...

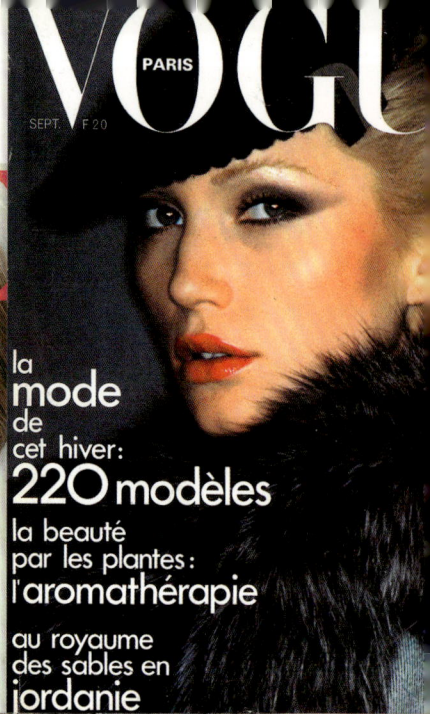

VOGUE PARIS
SEPT. F 20
la mode
de
cet hiver:
220 modèles
la beauté
par les plantes:
l'aromathérapie
au royaume
des sables en
jordanie

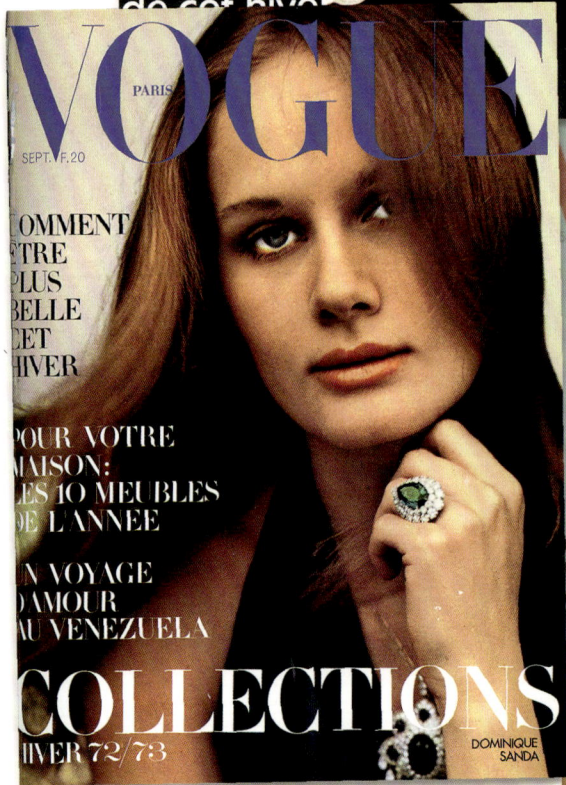

VOGUE PARIS
SEPT. F 20
COMMENT
ÊTRE
PLUS
BELLE
CET
HIVER
POUR VOTRE
MAISON:
LES 10 MEUBLES
DE L'ANNÉE
UN VOYAGE
D'AMOUR
AU VENEZUELA
COLLECTIONS
HIVER 72/73
DOMINIQUE SANDA

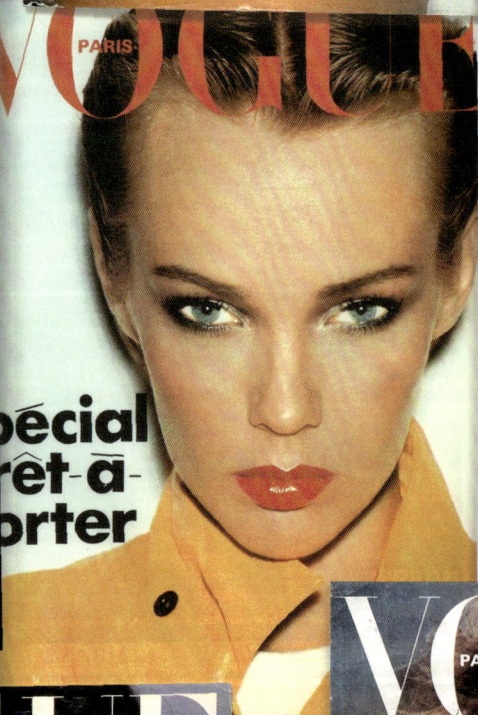

VOGUE PARIS
spécial
prêt-à-
porter

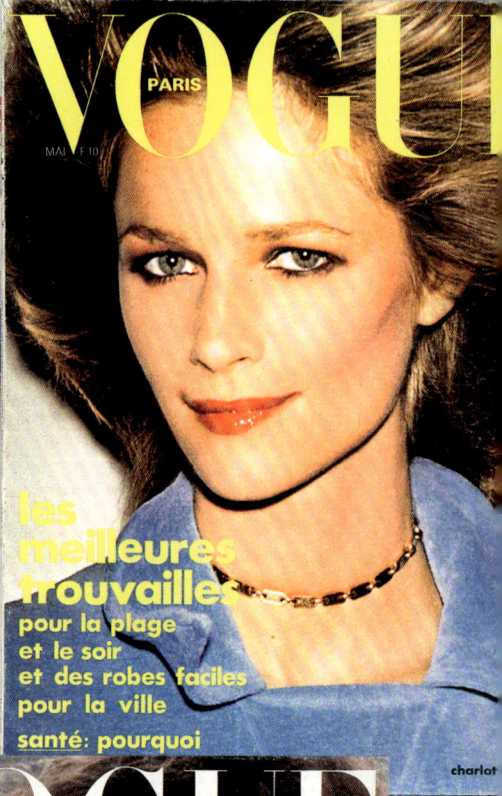

VOGUE PARIS
MAI F 10
les
meilleures
trouvailles
pour la plage
et le soir
et des robes faciles
pour la ville
santé: pourquoi
charlot...

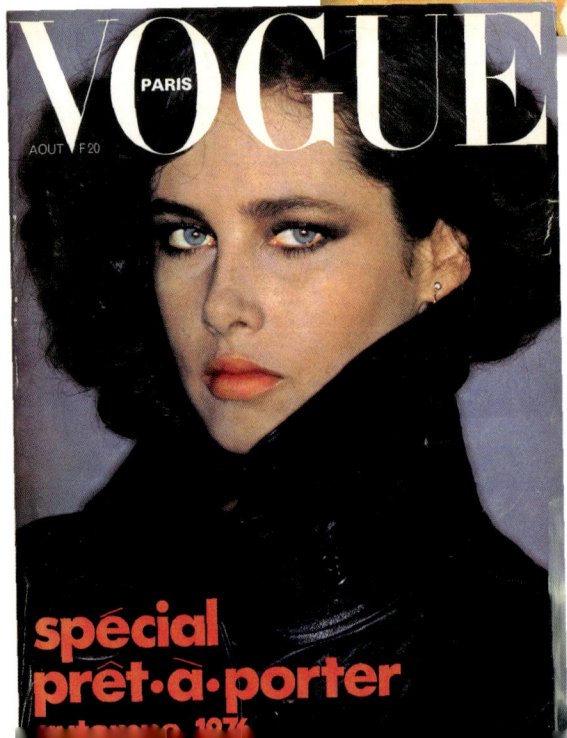

VOGUE PARIS
AOUT F 20
spécial
prêt-à-porter
...ternes 1974

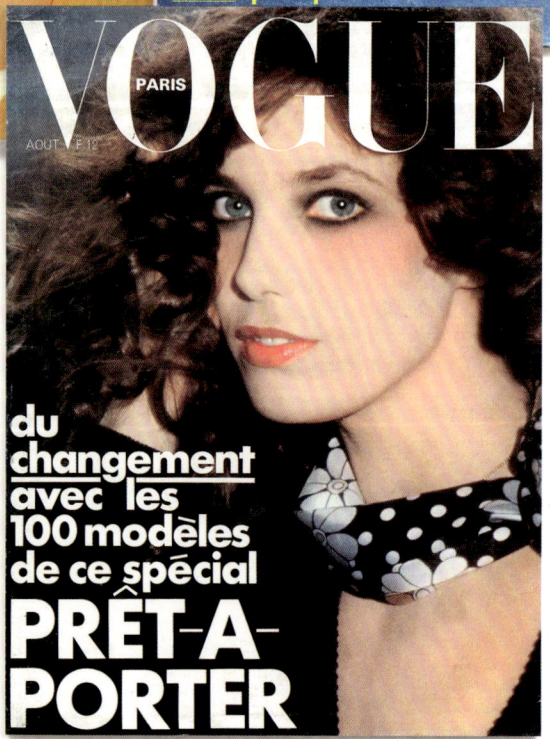

VOGUE PARIS
AOUT F 12
du
changement
avec les
100 modèles
de ce spécial
PRÊT-A-
PORTER

VOGUE PARIS

VOGUE PARIS

JUNGLE LOOK

55 MODÈLES «NATURE» POUR TOUT L'ÉTÉ

VOGUE PARIS

PAR MARLENE DIETRICH

VOGUE PARIS

special prêt-à-porter

135 modeles

VOGUE PARIS

la mode de printemps: 250 modèles

du soleil très près en tunisie

VOGUE PARIS

SPÉCIAL PRÊT-À-PORTER

PRINTEMPS/ÉTÉ 1977

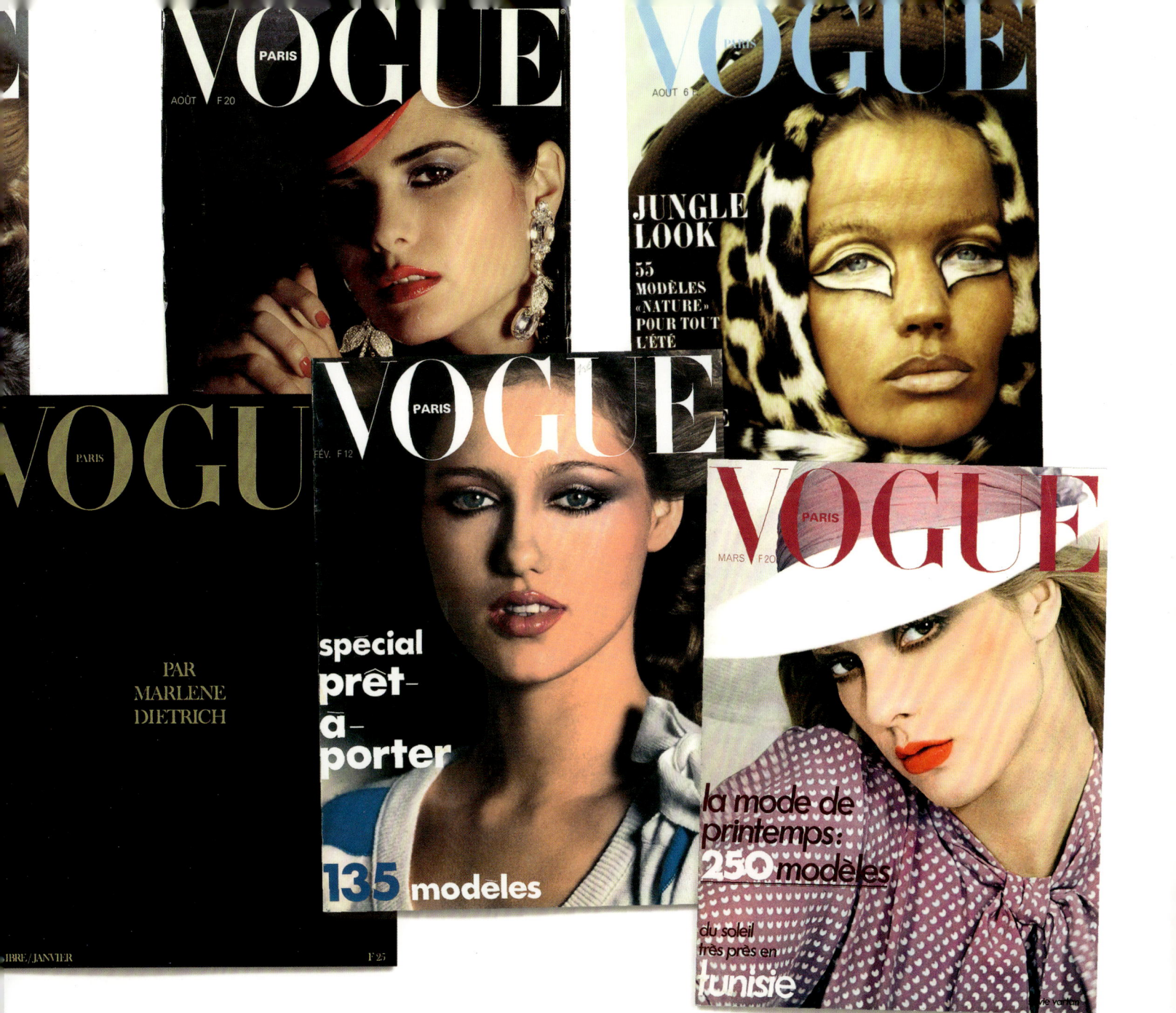

"AS A LITTLE BOY I WAS POURING OVER FASHION MAGAZINES: EVERY MONTH MY MOTHER WOULD BUY FRENCH *VOGUE* AND I WOULD COMB THROUGH IT FOR HOURS LOOKING AT PHOTOS AND MAKEUP LOOKS. FRENCH *VOGUE* FROM THE 70s REALLY INSPIRED ME, AS IT EPITOMIZED THE WORLD OF SOPHISTICATION, GLAMOUR, AND BEAUTY. I COULD NOT WAIT TO GROW UP AND MOVE TO PARIS." – FRANÇOIS NARS

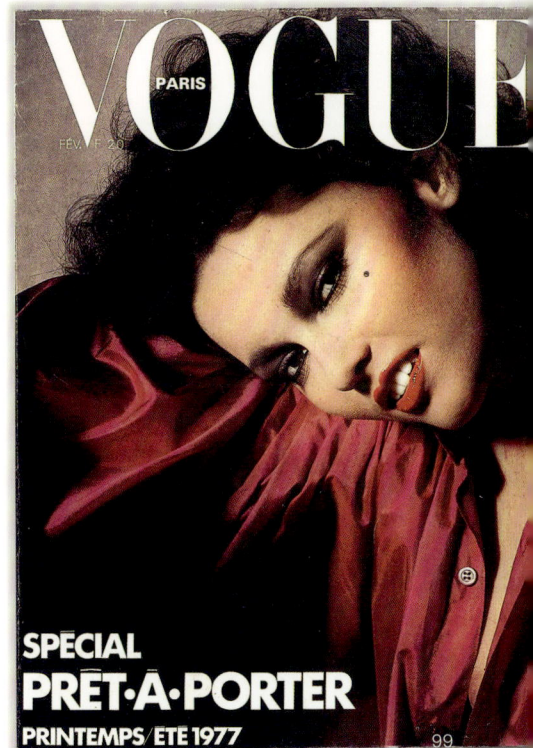

99

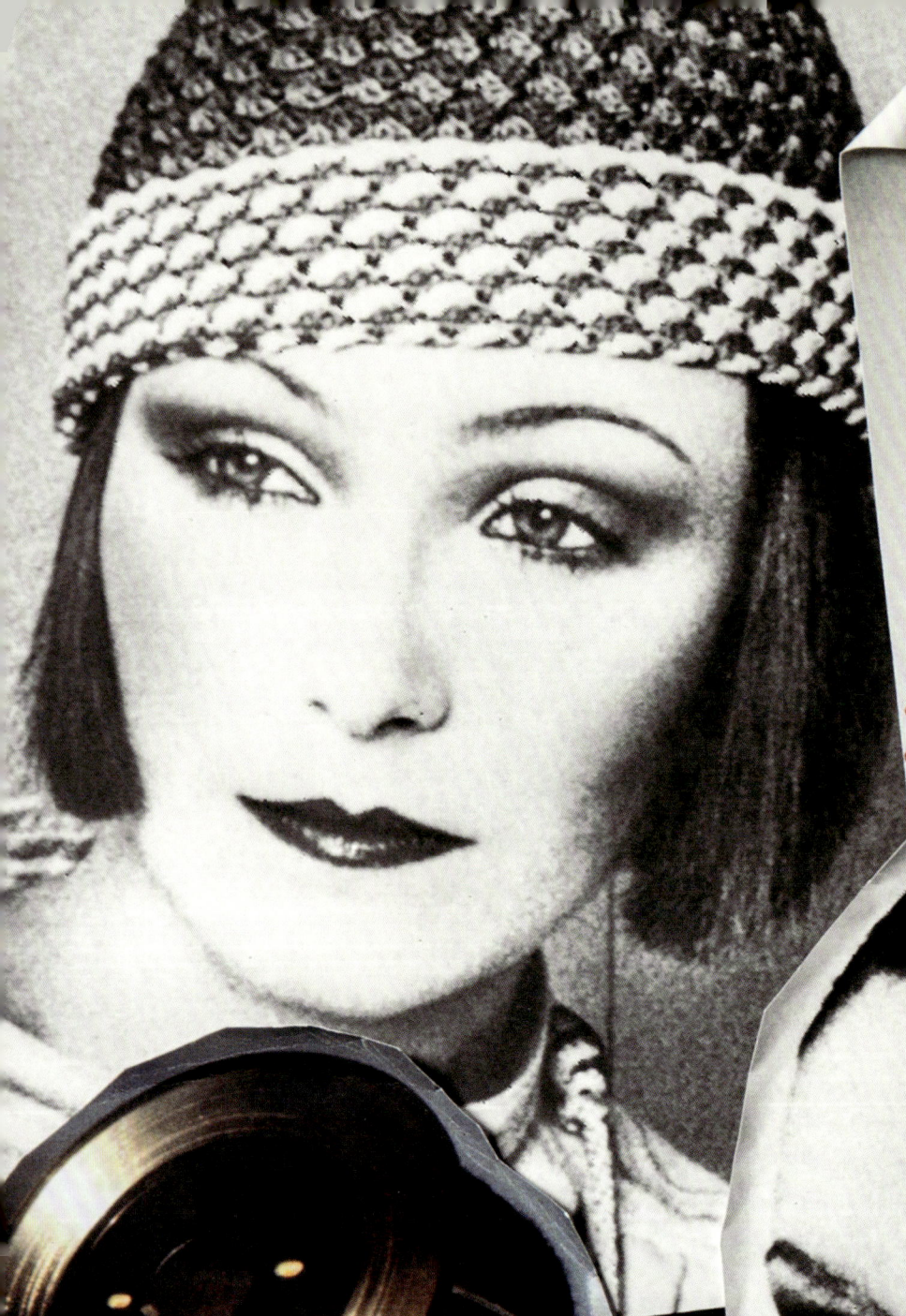

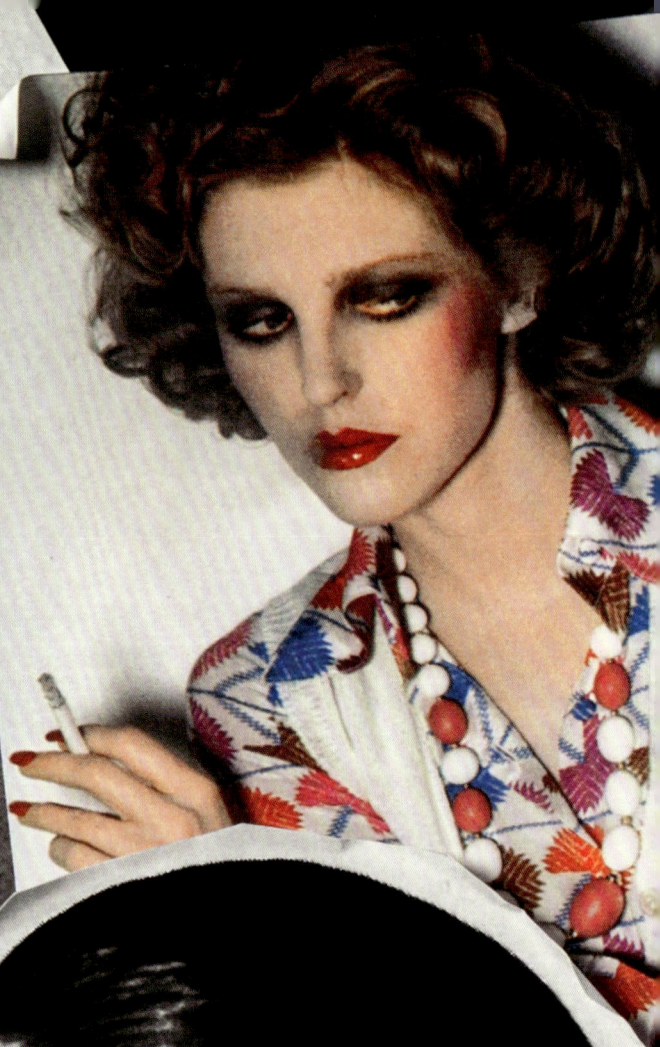

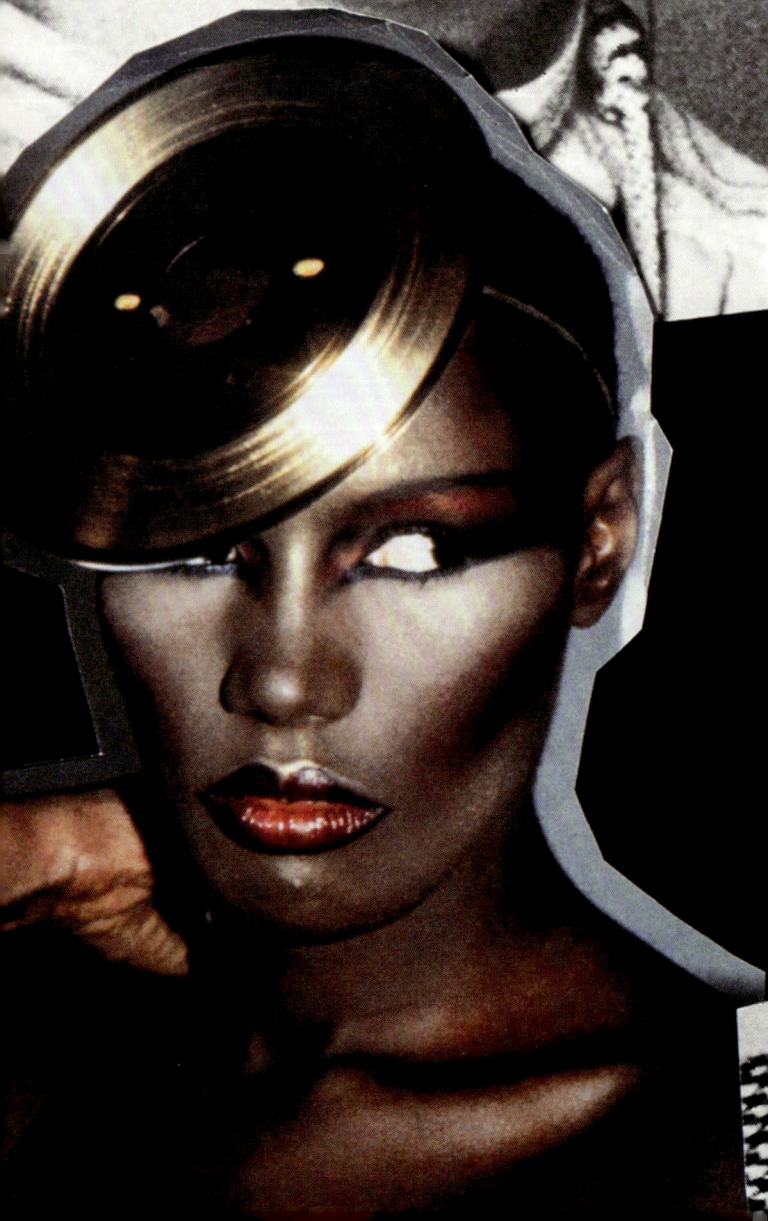

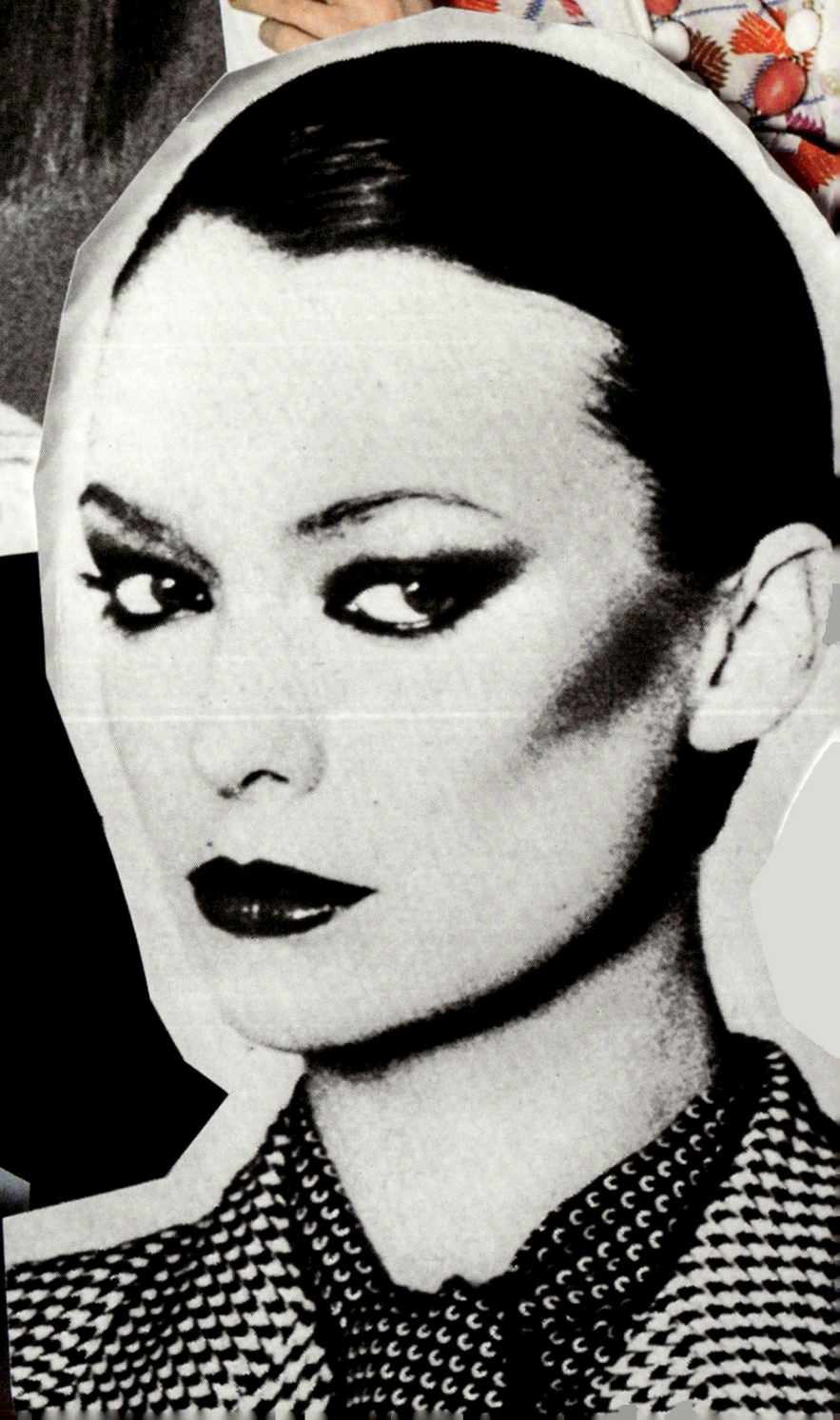

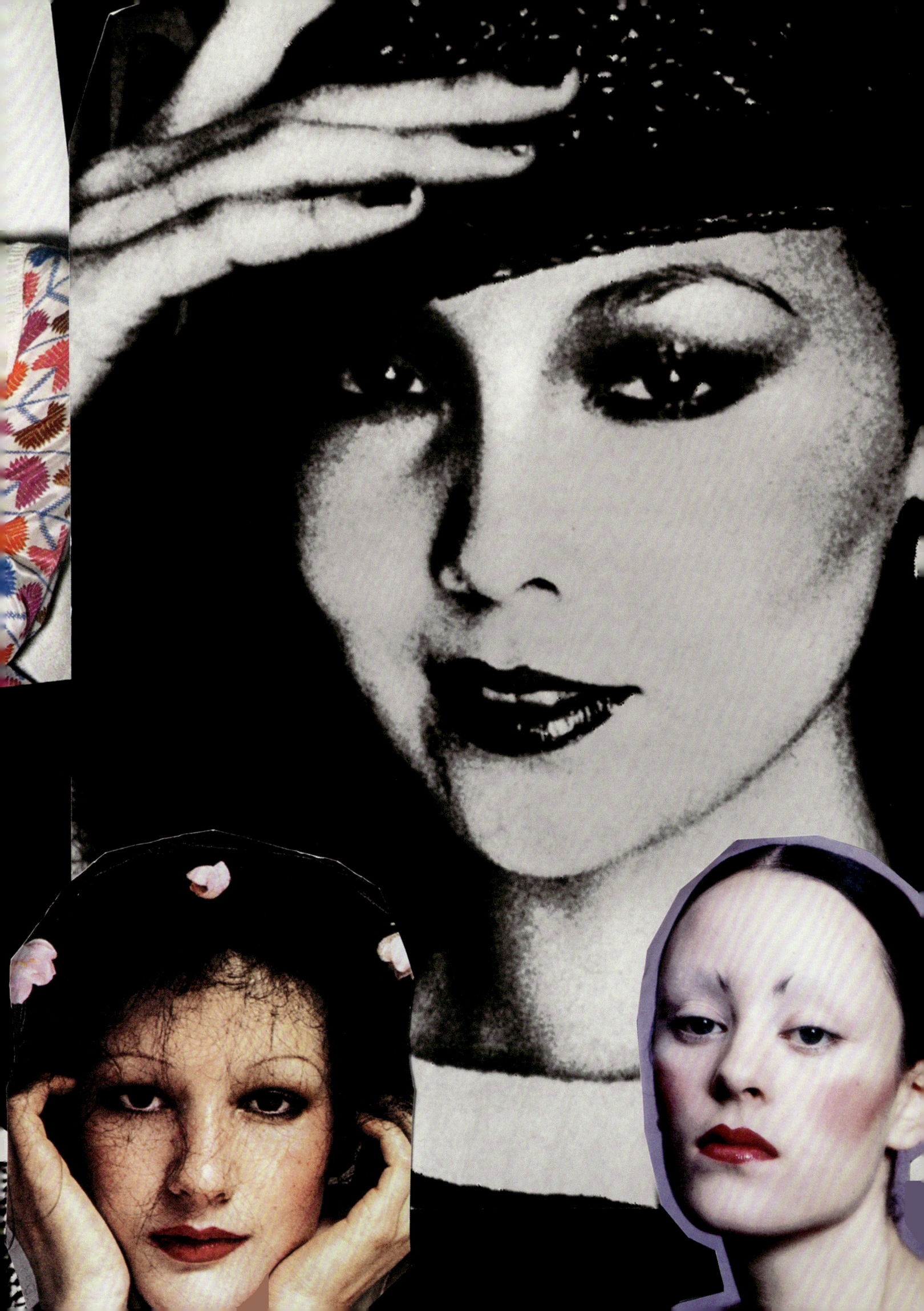

"A BIG THANK YOU
TO ALL THE GREAT
MAKEUP ARTISTS AND
HAIRDRESSERS I WORK
WITH AND LOVE; THEY
UNFORTUNATELY DO
NOT ALWAYS GET THE
CREDIT THEY DESERVE
FOR THE SUCCESS OF
A BEAUTIFUL IMAGE."
– FRANÇOIS NARS

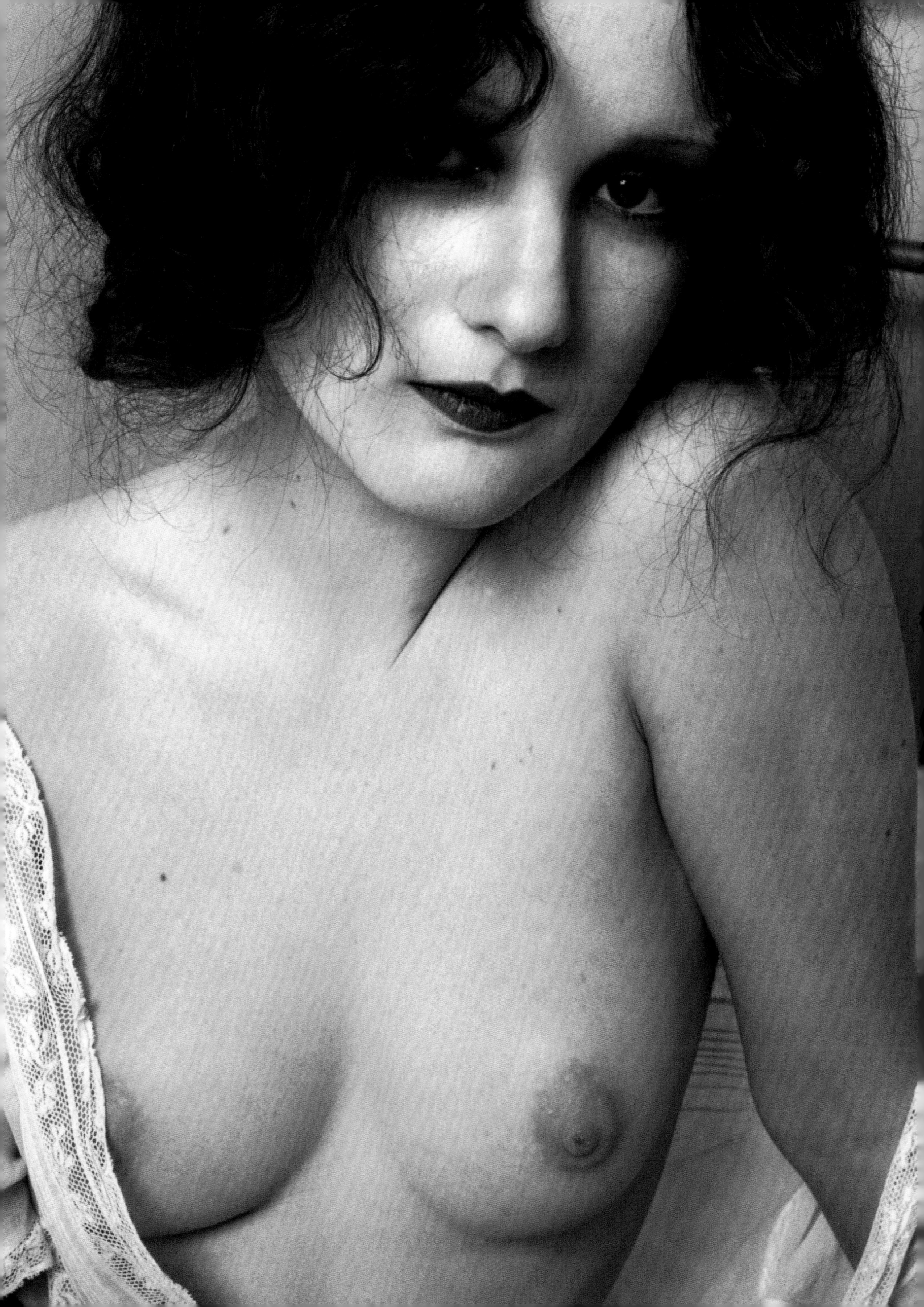

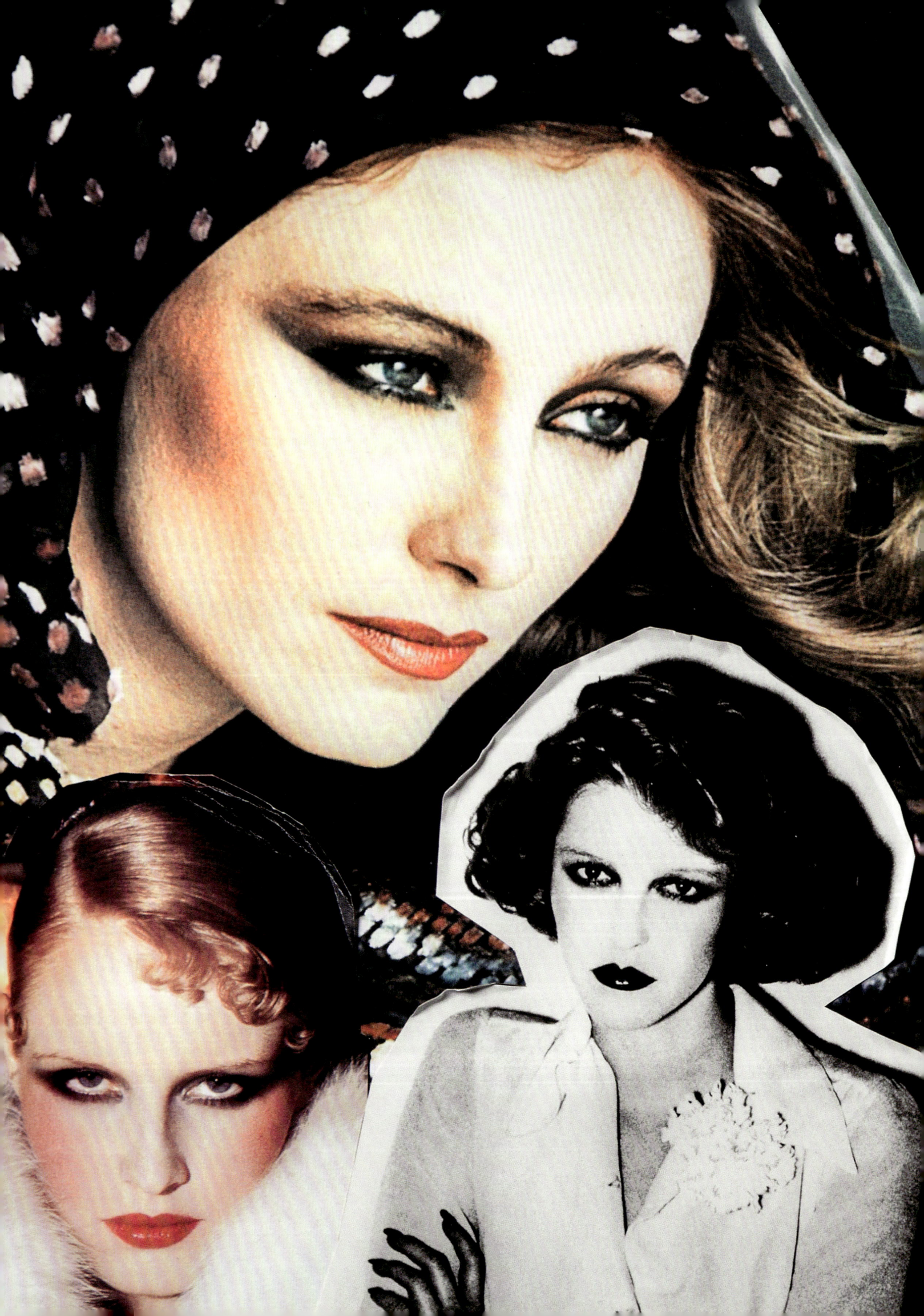

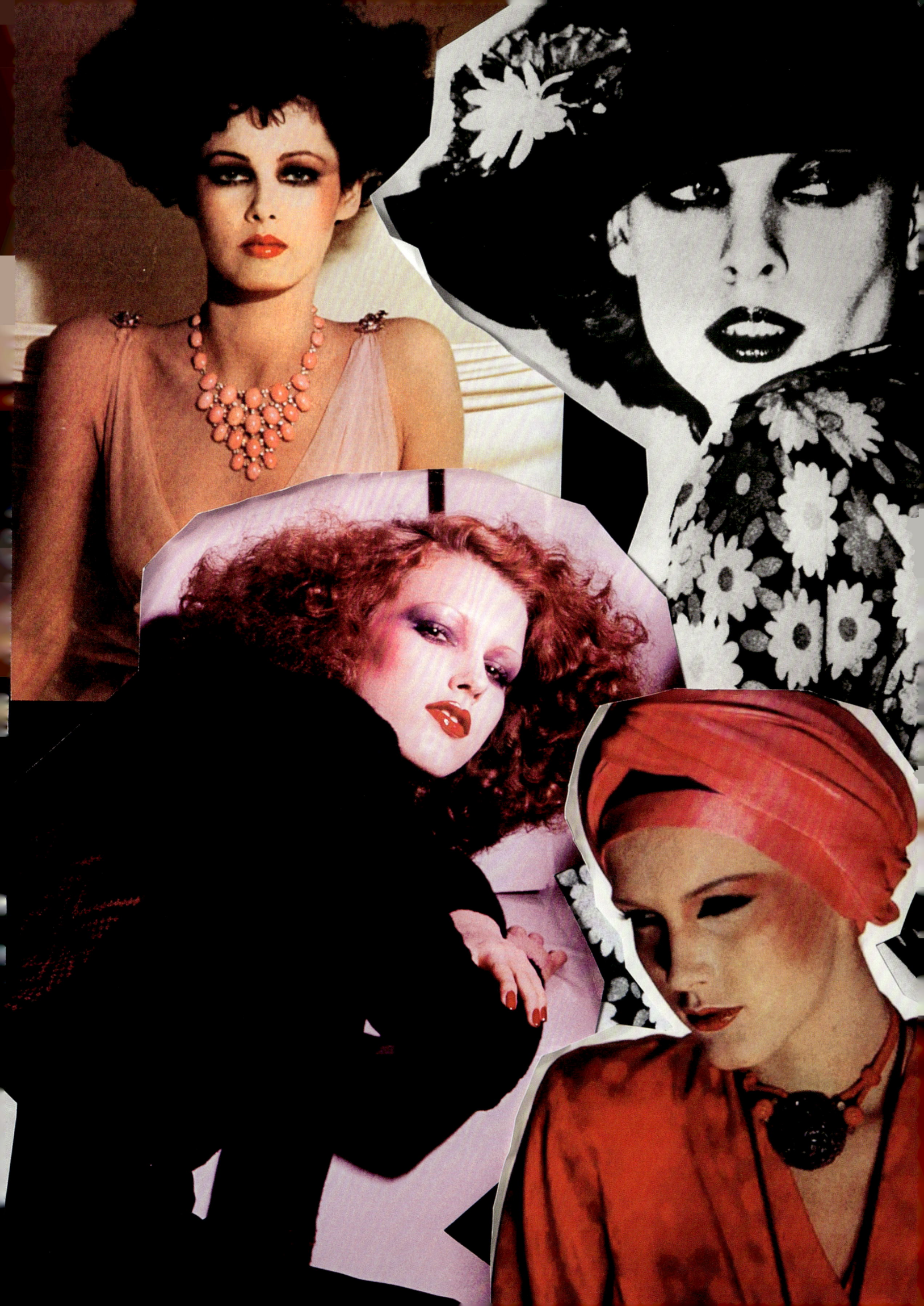

"I LOVED SO MUCH THE MODELS FROM THE 70s, THEY WERE AMAZING: VIBEKE KNUDSEN, DAYLE HADDON, CARRIE NYGREN, NICOLE MEYER, KAREN HOWARD, MARIE HELVIN, SUSAN MONCUR, LOUISE DESPOINTES, GUNILLA LINDBLAD, EVA MALMSTROM, PAT CLEVELAND, MARCIE HUNT, APOLONIA VON RAVENSTEIN, CAROLE SINGLETON, KATHY QUIRK, ANNA ANDERSON, ISABELLE WEINGARTEN, DONNA JORDAN, JANE FORTH, GRACE JONES, JEANETTE CHRISTIANSEN, ANJELICA HUSTON, INGMARI LAMY, VERUSCHKA, SOFIA KIUKKONEN, MARISA BERENSON, WILLY VAN ROY, JERRY HALL, ARJA TOYRYLA, TRACY WEED, AND MANY OTHERS. ALSO, ALL THE WONDERFUL MAKEUP ARTISTS: SERGE LUTENS, HEIDI MORAWETZ, JOSE LUIS, OLIVIER ECHAUDEMAISON, JACQUES CLEMENTE, AND NAIK. THEY MADE ME DREAM AND INSPIRED ME TO BECOME A MAKEUP ARTIST AND A PHOTOGRAPHER. I WANT TO THANK THEM TODAY." — FRANÇOIS NARS

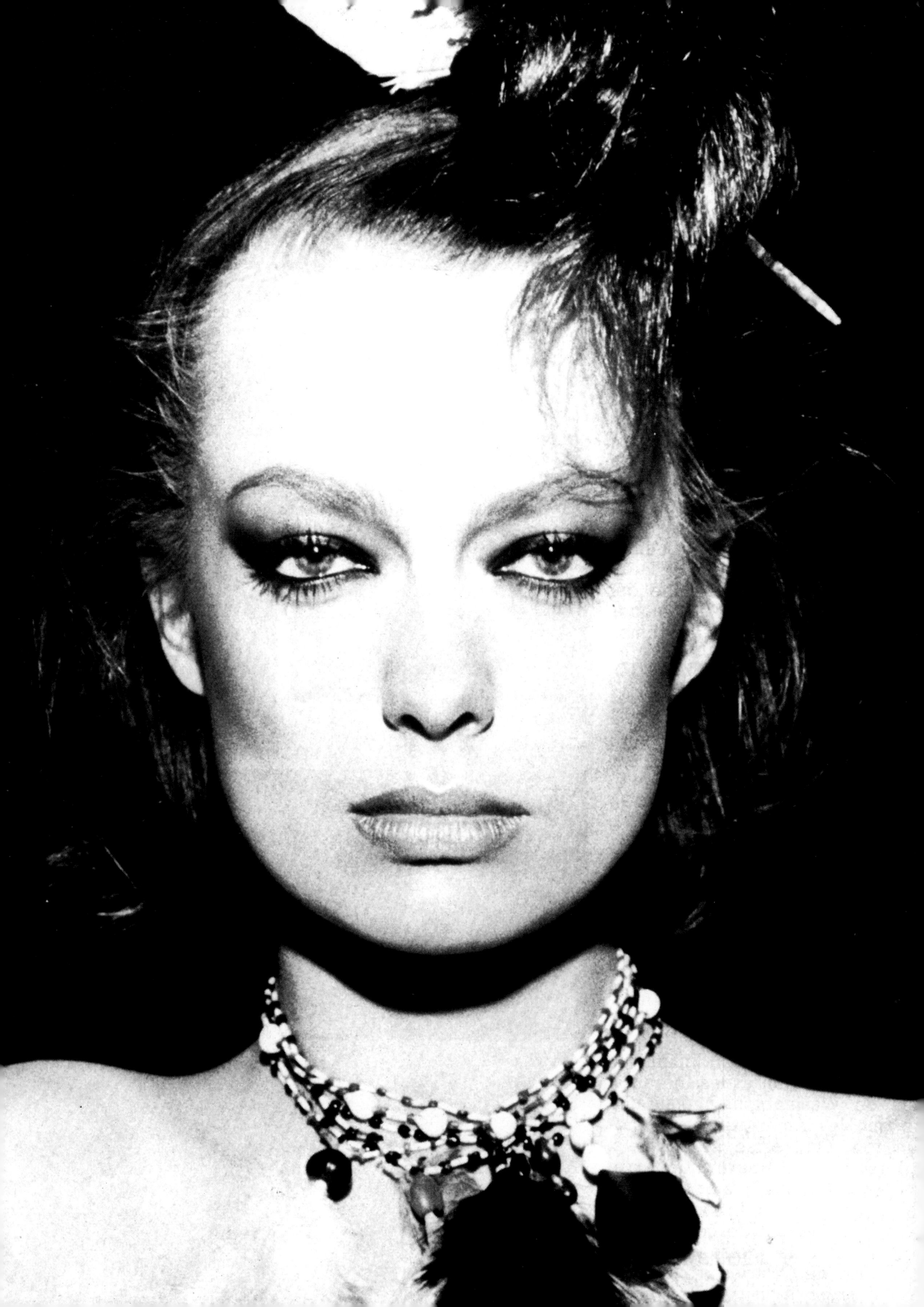

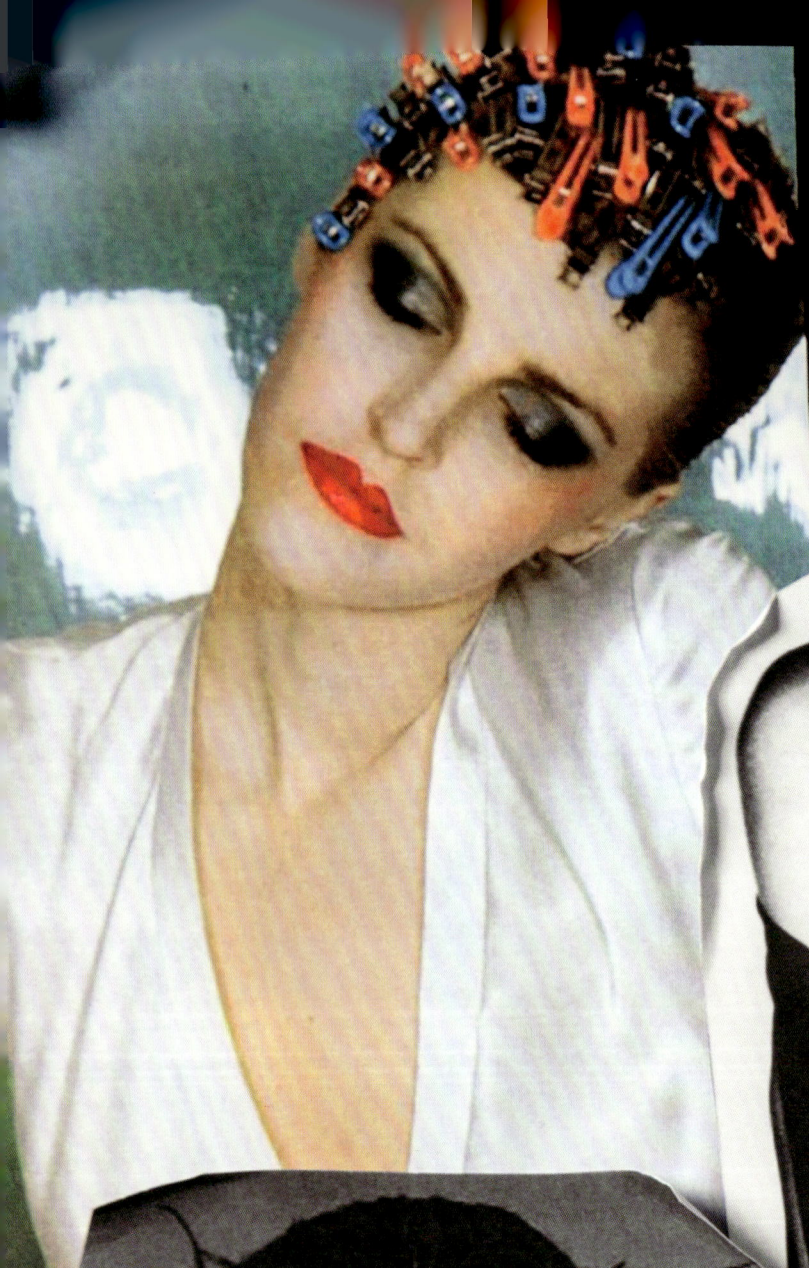

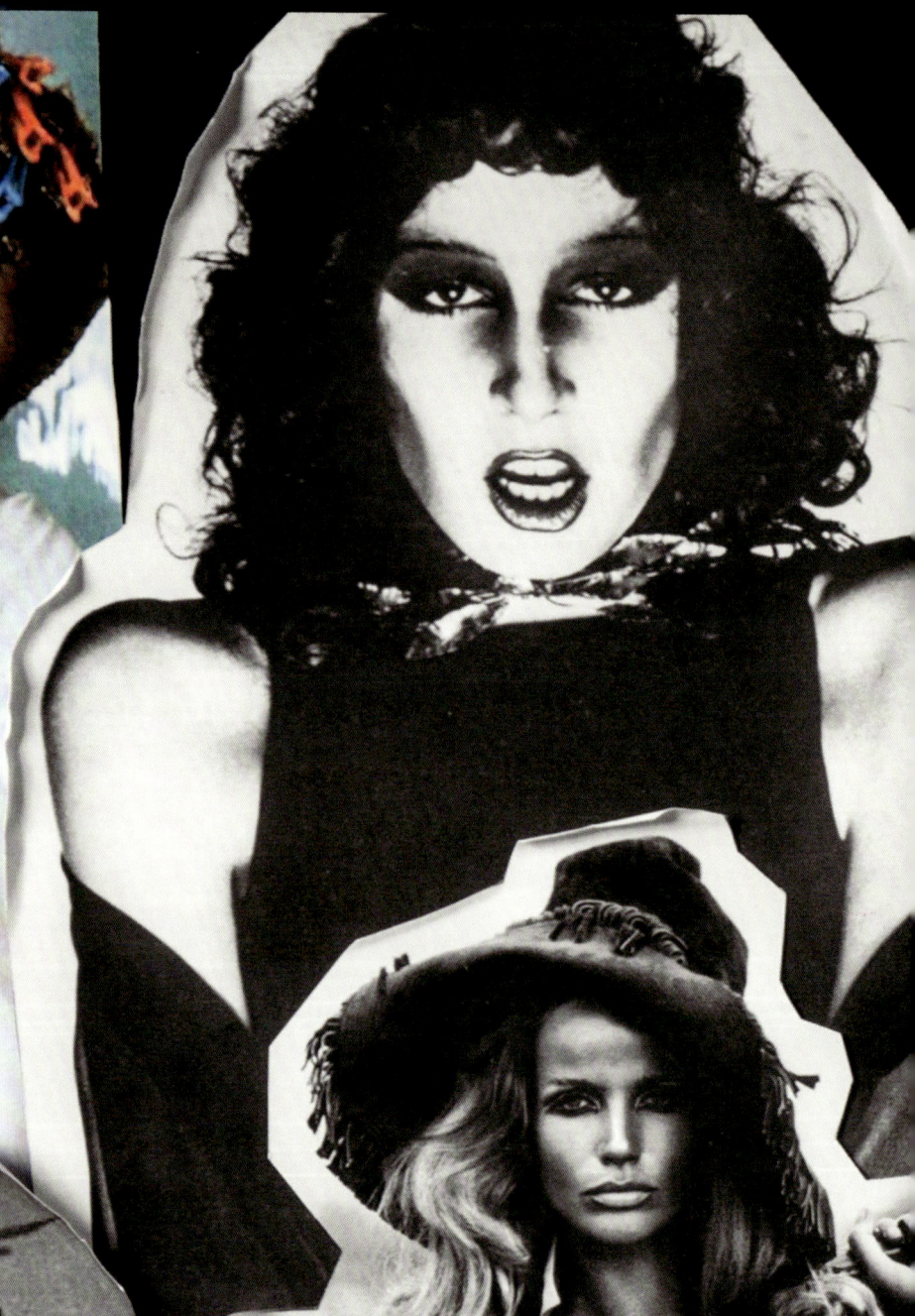

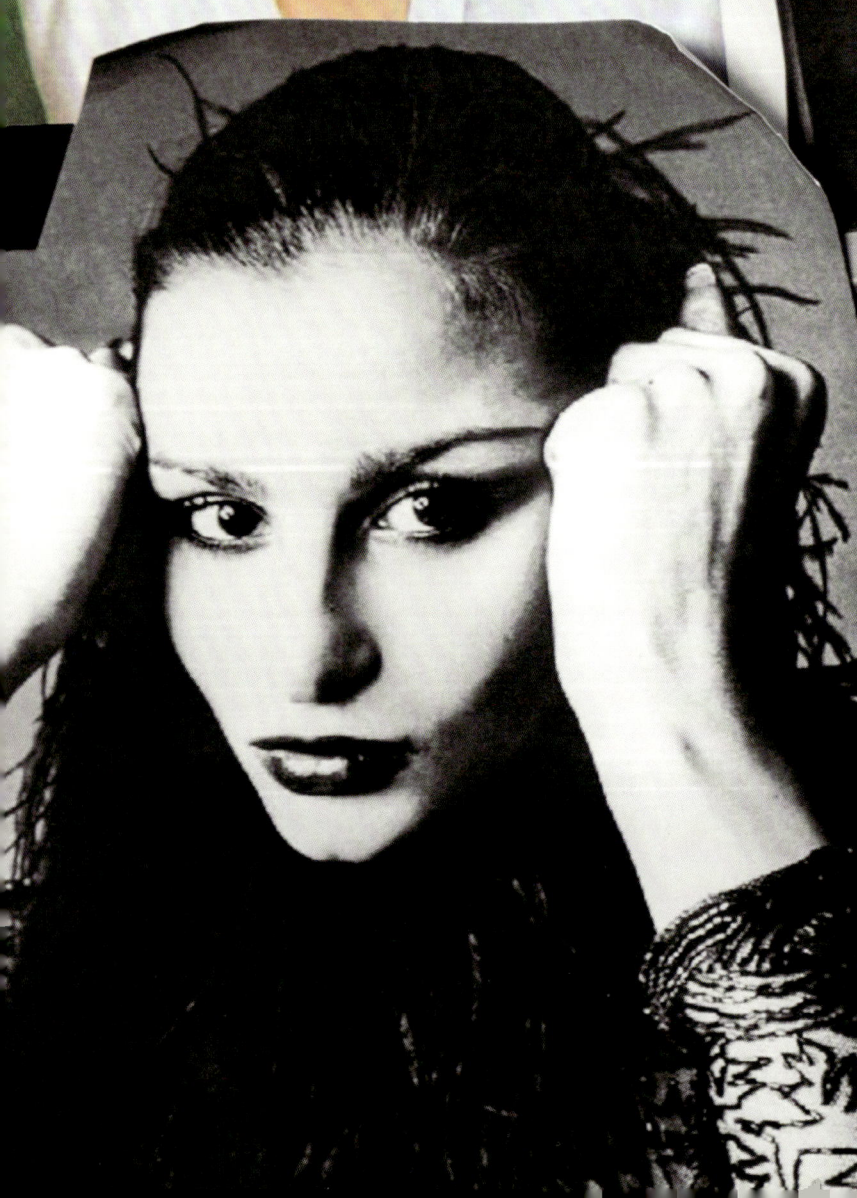

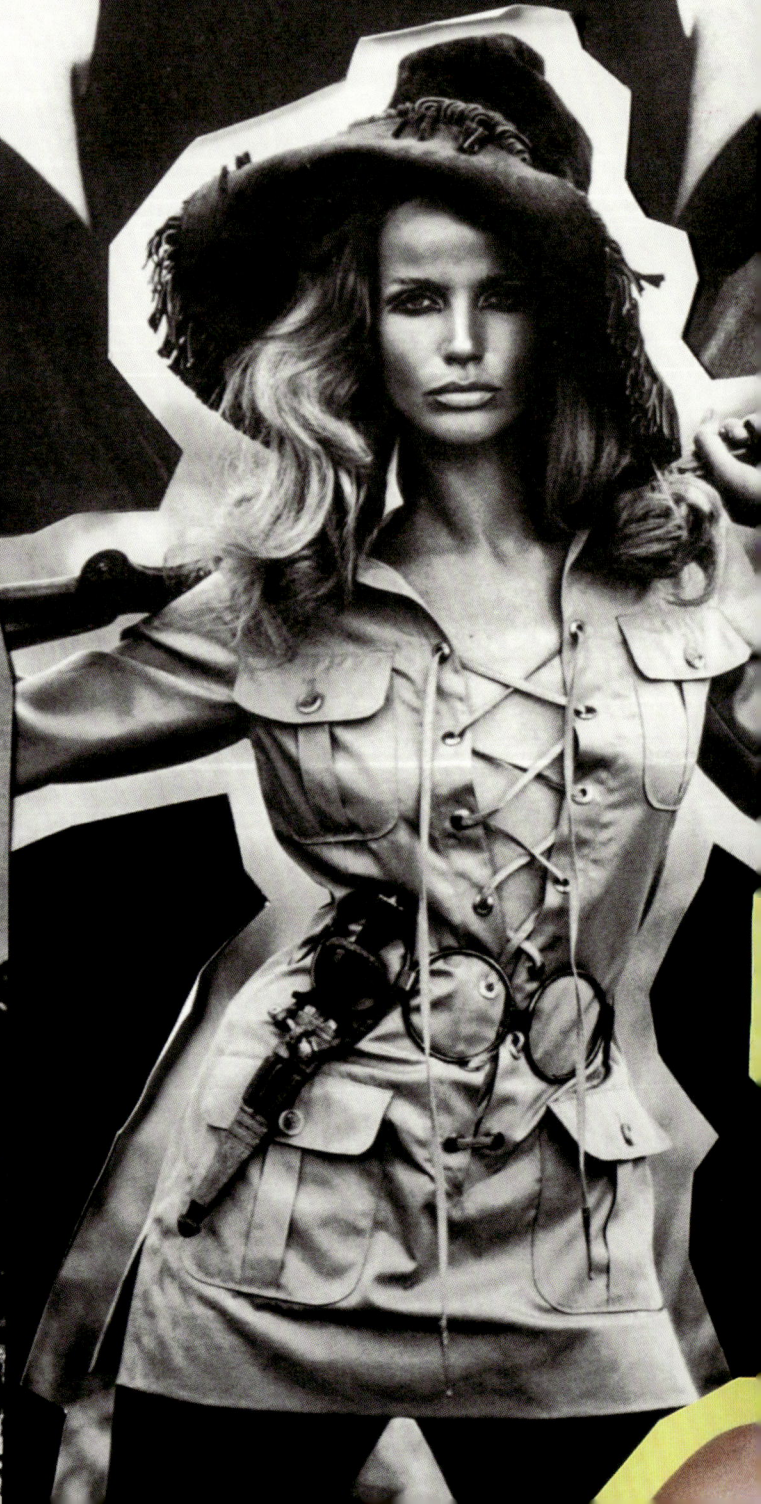

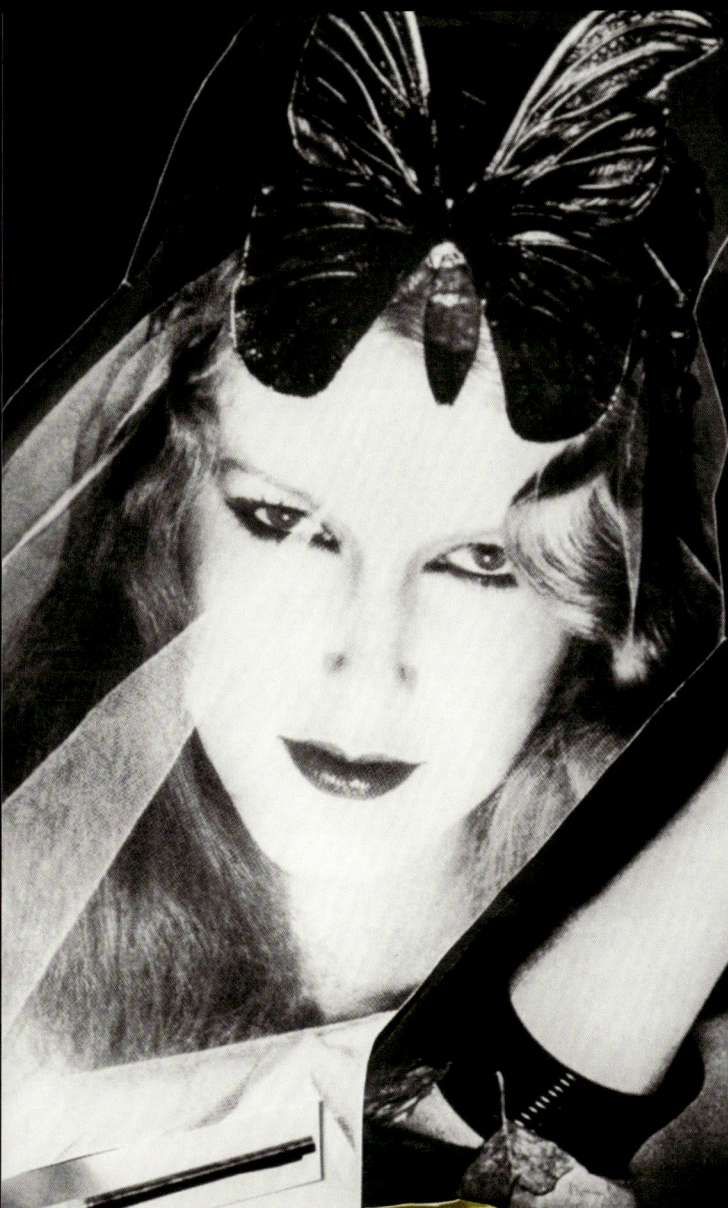

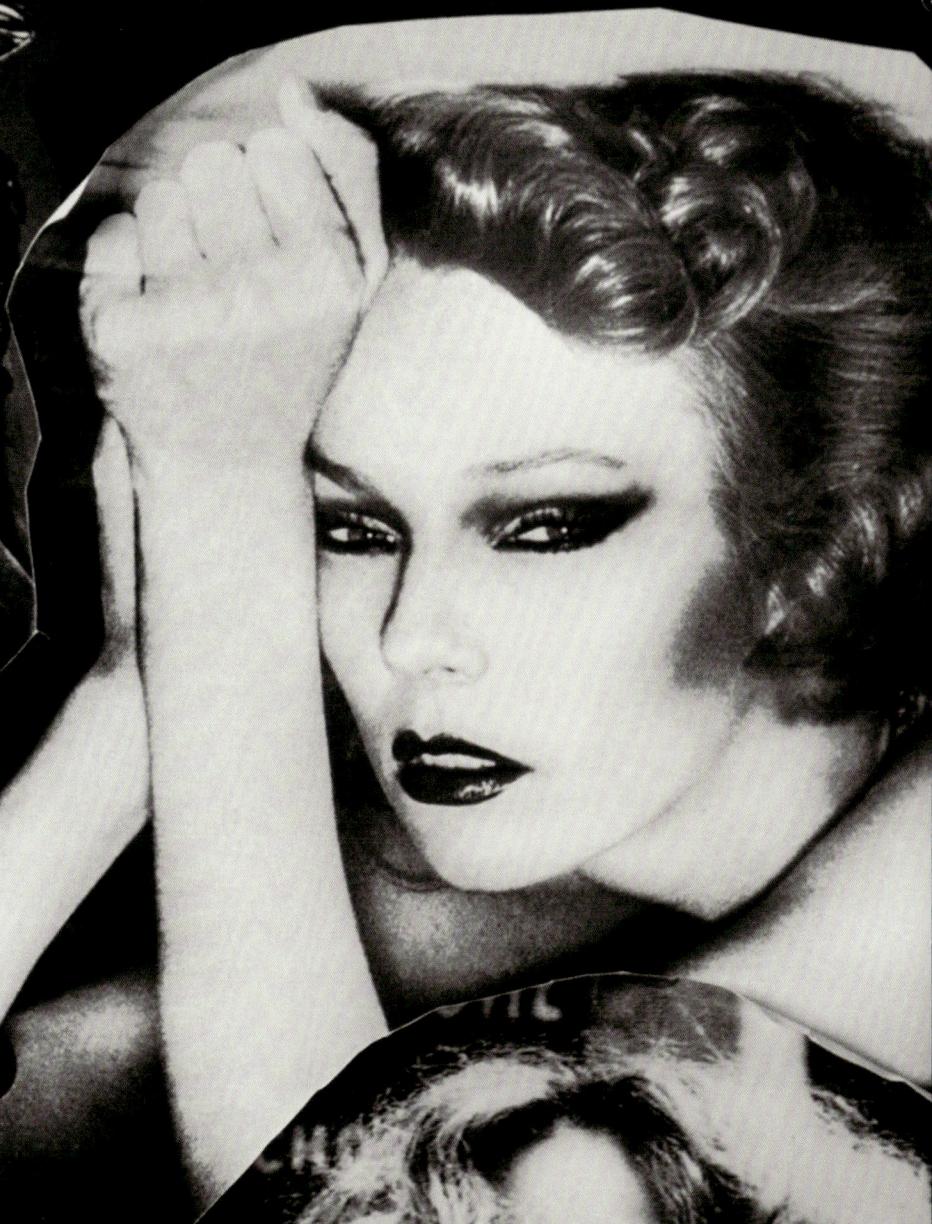

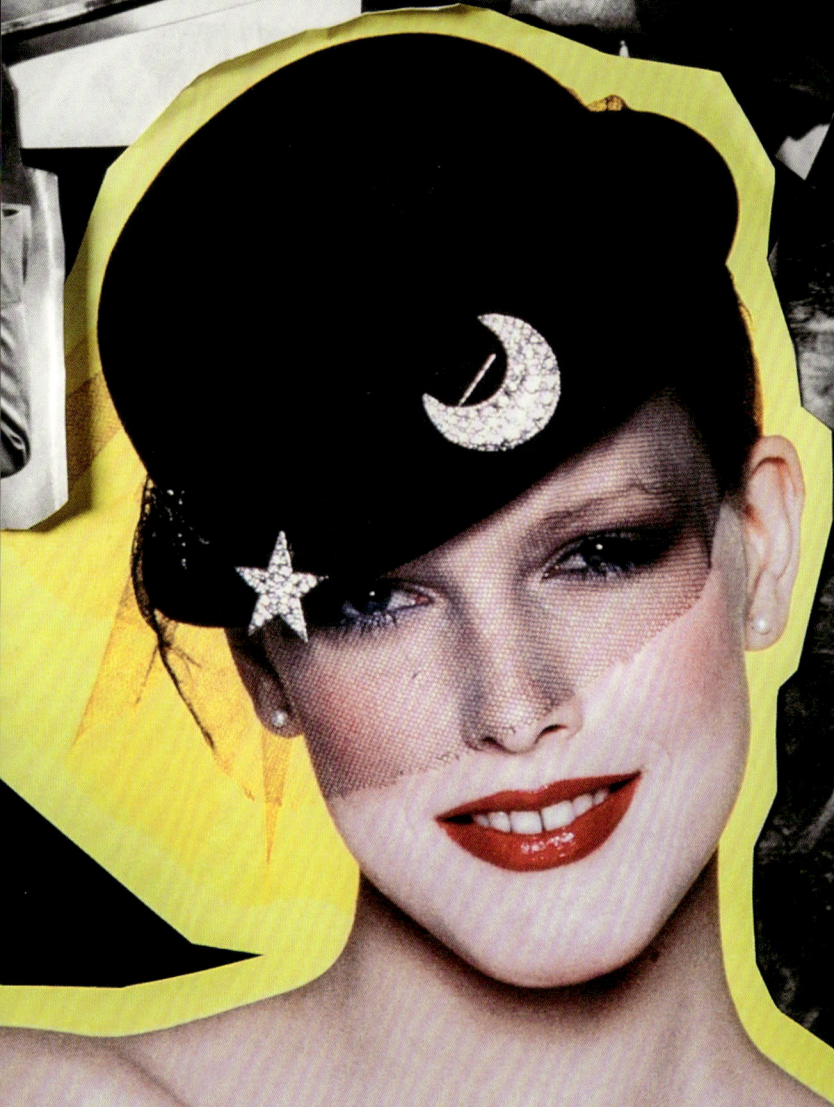

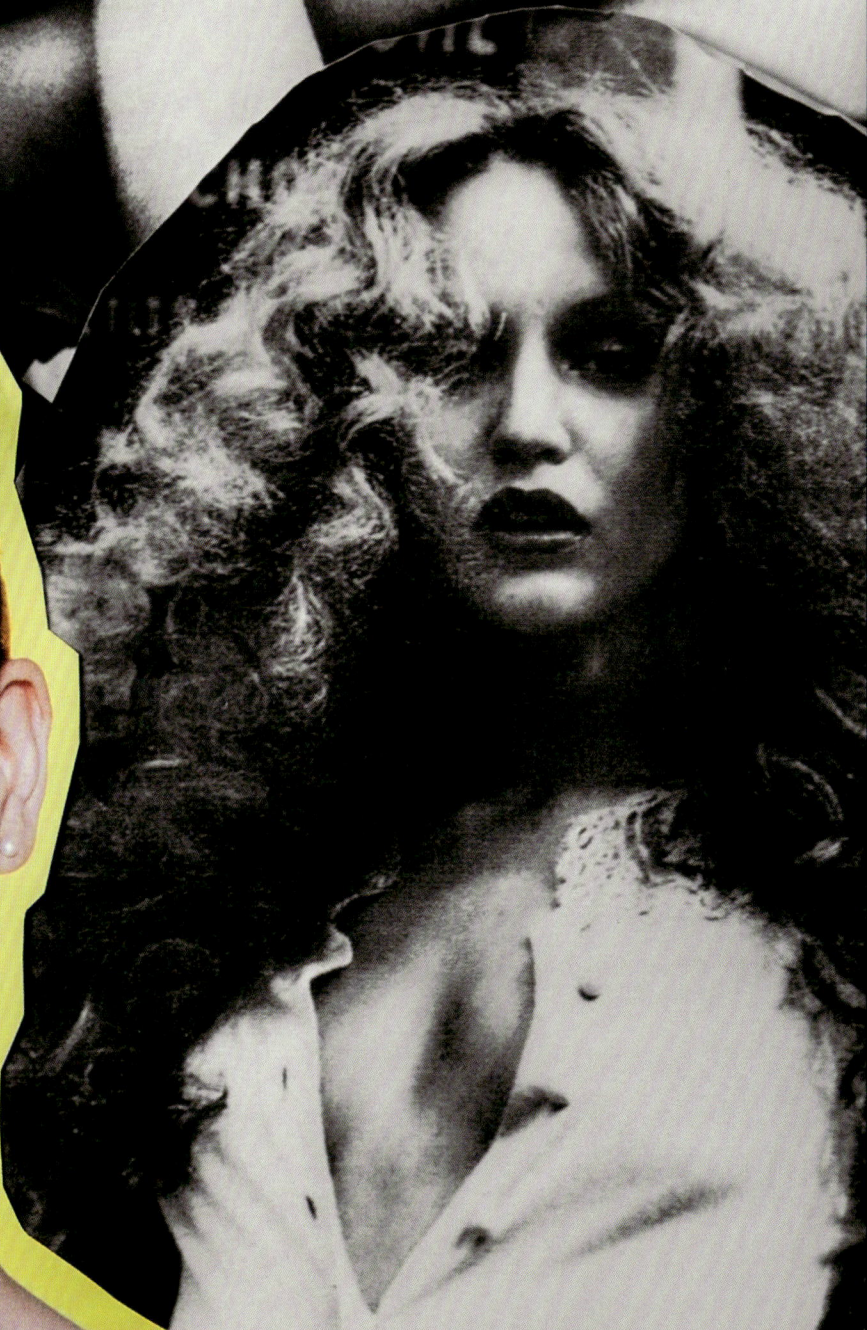

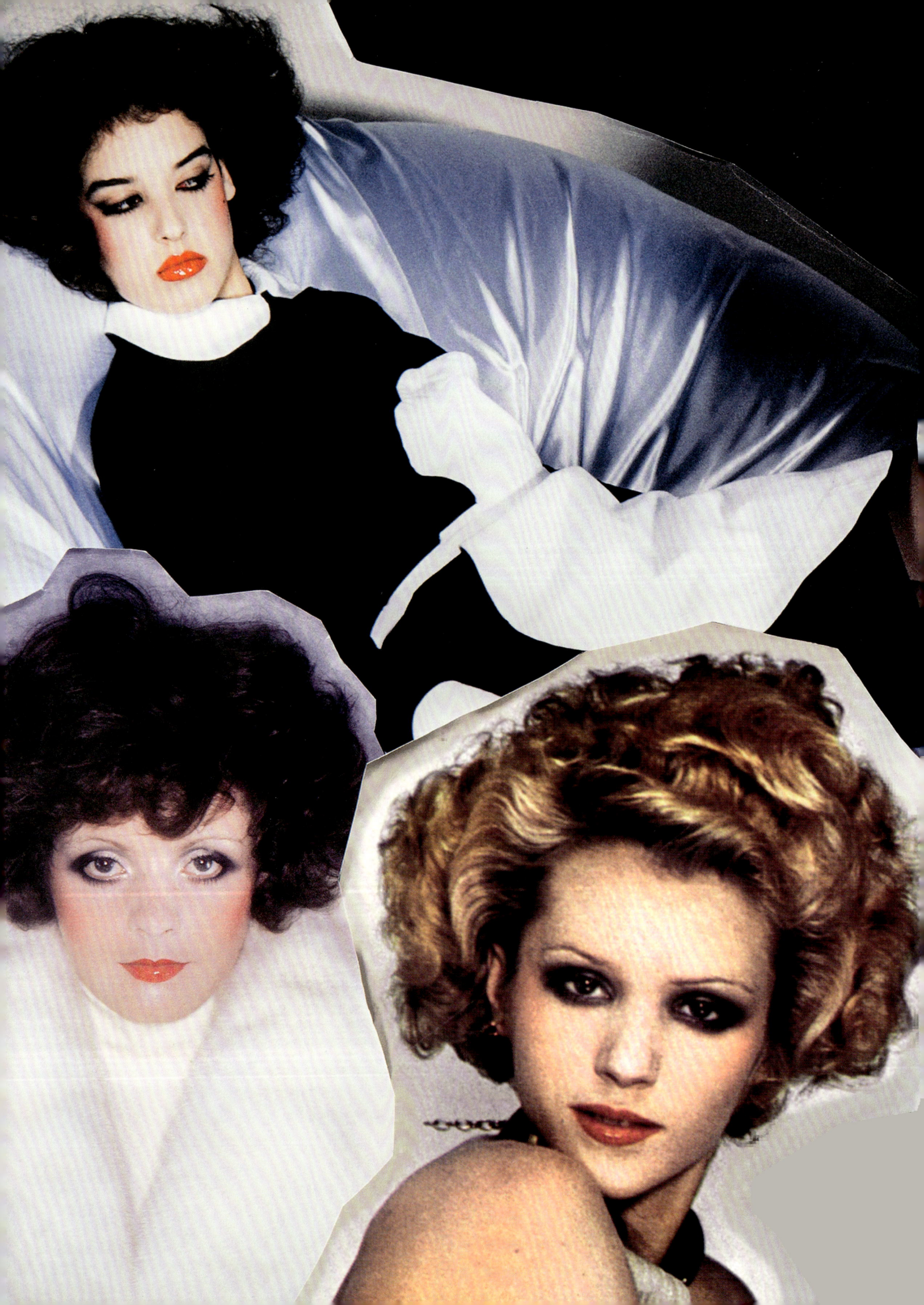

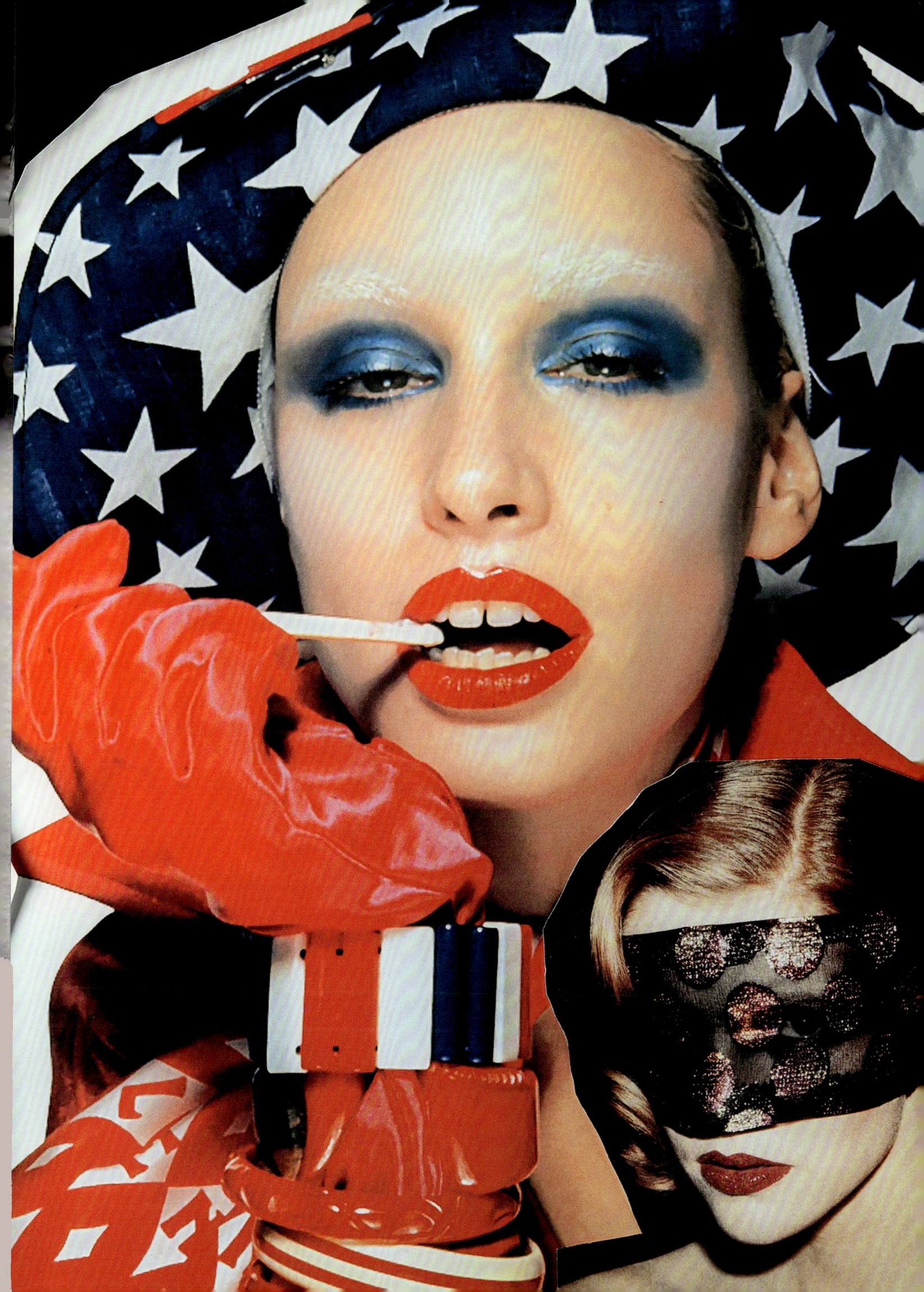

"WHEN I WAS THIRTEEN OR FOURTEEN YEARS OLD, I HAD A PICTURE OF DAYLE ON MY CLASSBOOK AND USED TO STARE AND DREAM AT IT WHEN I WAS BORED IN MATH CLASS. DAYLE'S EYES TOOK ME TO A MAGICAL WORLD THAT MADE SCHOOL MORE BEARABLE. TODAY, DAYLE STILL MAKES ME DREAM BUT IN ANOTHER WAY. HER REMARKABLE WORK FOR UNICEF ON BEHALF OF WOMEN AND HER ACTIONS IN THE FIELD GIVE HOPE TO ALL THOSE YOUNG BEAUTIFUL GIRLS IN AFRICA. SHE IS JUST INCREDIBLE! IT'S HER SWEETNESS THAT TOUCHES ME TODAY MORE THAN ANYTHING ELSE, EVEN THOUGH HER AMAZING EYES STILL MAKE ME DREAM."
— FRANÇOIS NARS

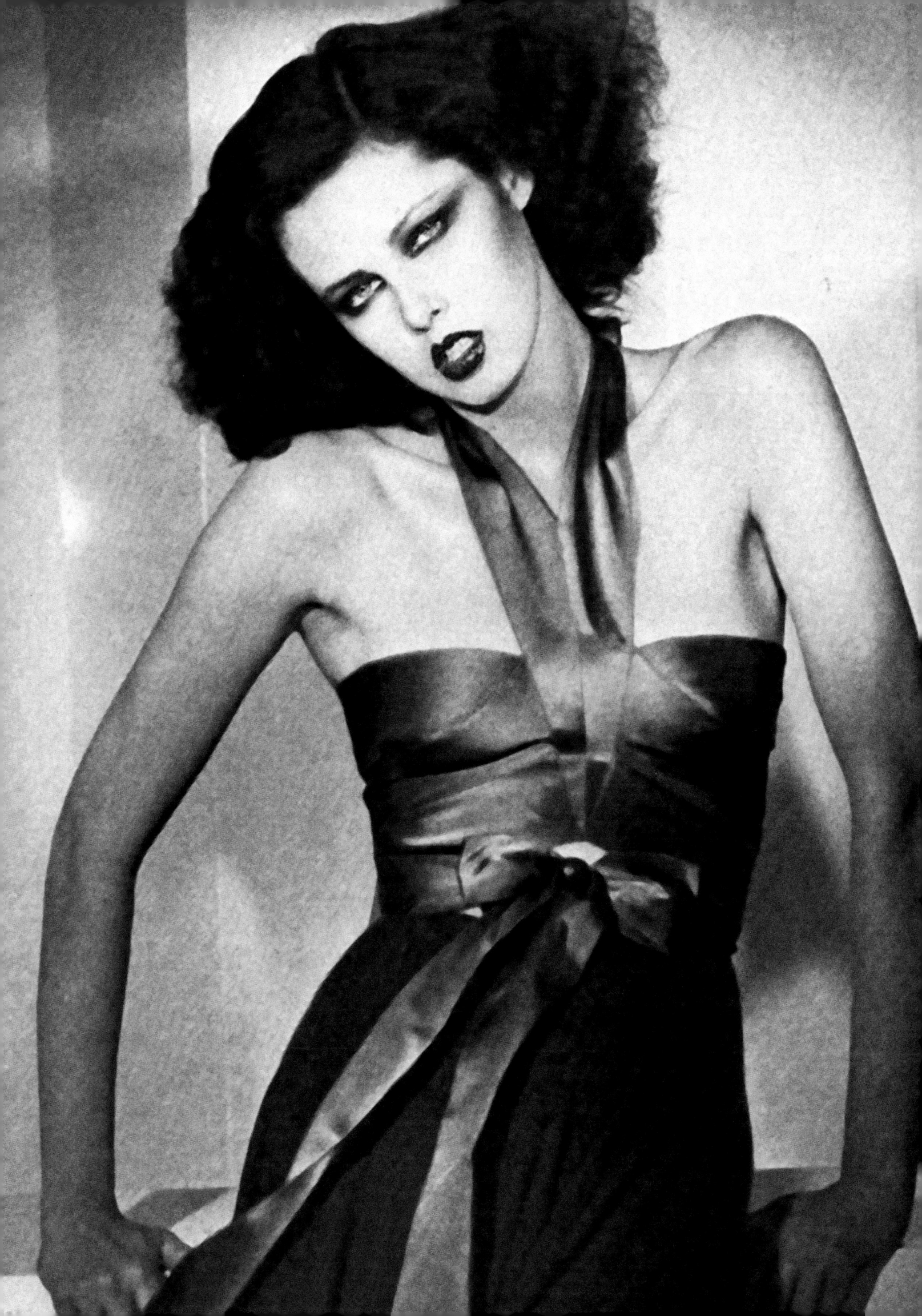

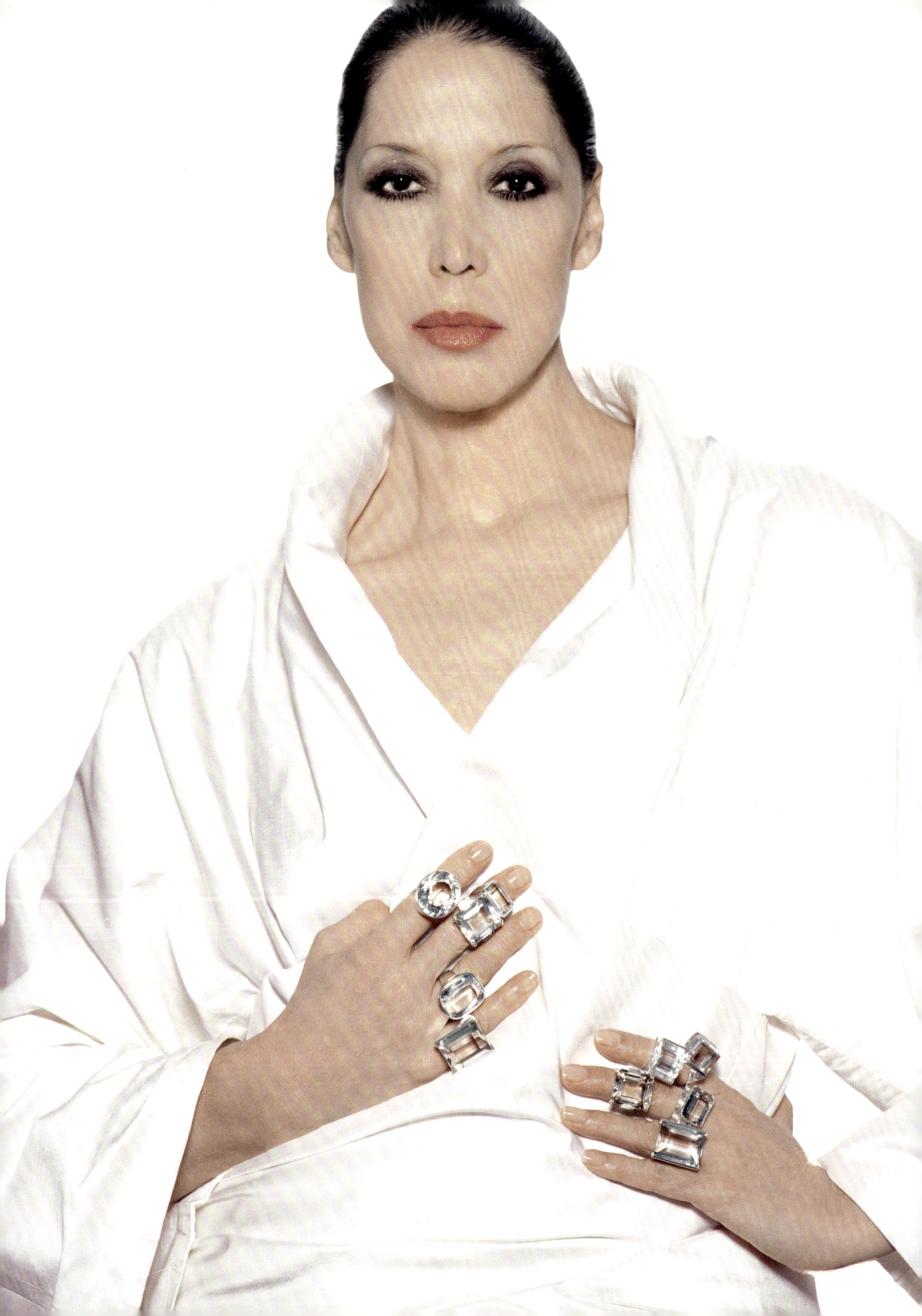

"HE IS A KALEIDOSCOPIC
TALENT: A COLOR MASTER,
A CINEMA CONNOISSEUR, A
BRILLIANT PHOTOGRAPHER.
HE MAKES WOMEN'S DREAMS
COME TRUE, AND ABOVE ALL
HE HAS A GREAT SENSE OF
HUMOR. HE IS MY BEST FRIEND."
– MARINA SCHIANO

"THE FIRST TIME I SAW MARINA WAS IN THE
MID-70s IN A DIVINE LITTLE RESTAURANT
IN PARIS CALLED 'LOUS LANDES.' SHE
WAS HAVING DINNER WITH PIERRE BERGÉ
AND WAS WEARING A FABULOUS PILOT
JACKET BY YVES WITH A SILK SCARF TIED
AROUND HER NECK. I WAS STRICKEN BY
HER ENERGY, CONFIDENCE, ELEGANCE,
AND STRENGTH. MANY YEARS LATER,
WE WORKED TOGETHER WHEN MARINA
WAS AN EDITOR AT VANITY FAIR. RIGHT
AWAY WE STARTED LAUGHING TOGETHER
AND HAVEN'T STOPPED SINCE. MARINA IS
SO MUCH FUN. NOBODY ELSE LIKE HER
KNOWS HOW TO CHEER ME UP WHEN
I FEEL DEPRESSED. I LOVE HER!"
– FRANÇOIS NARS

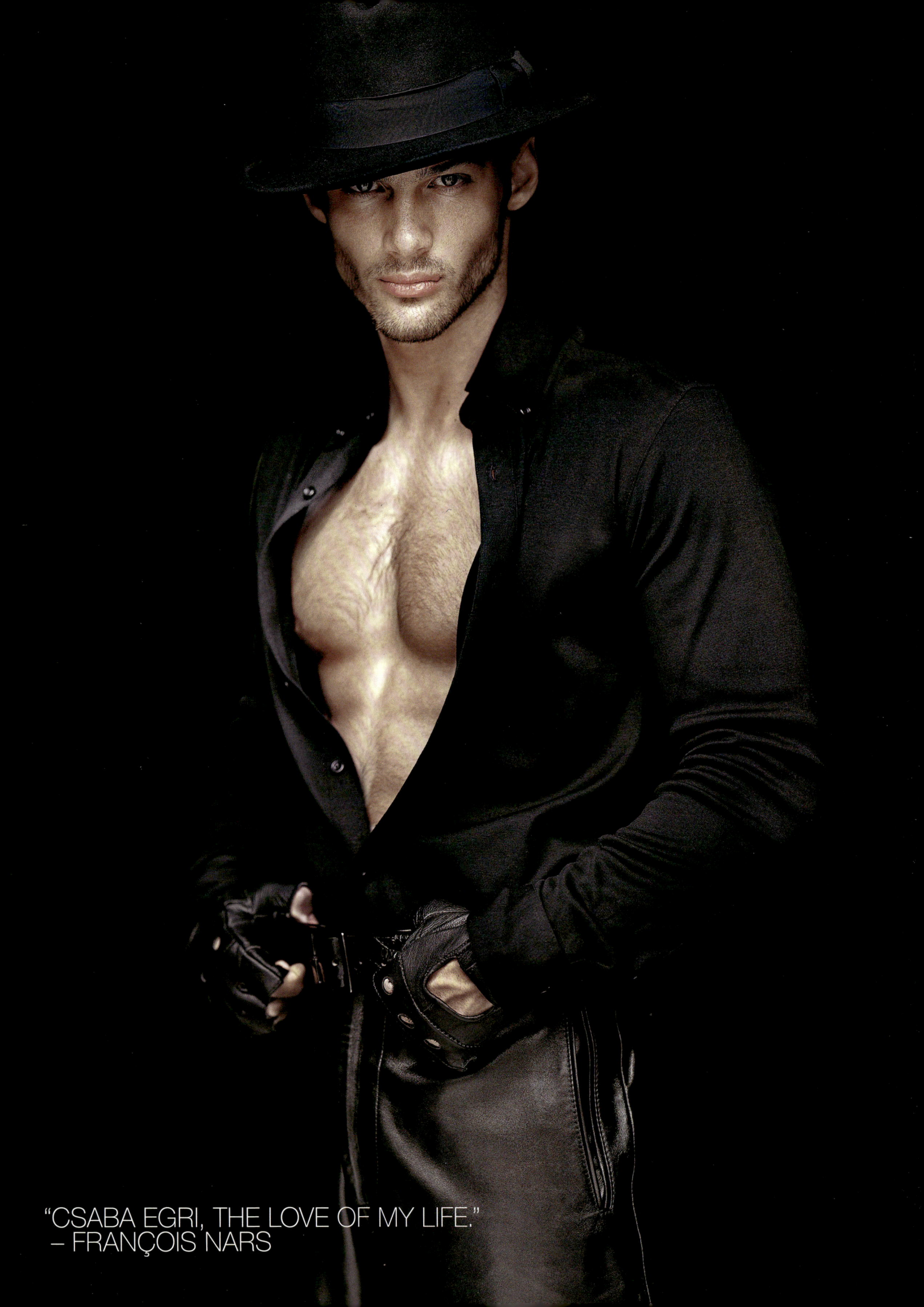

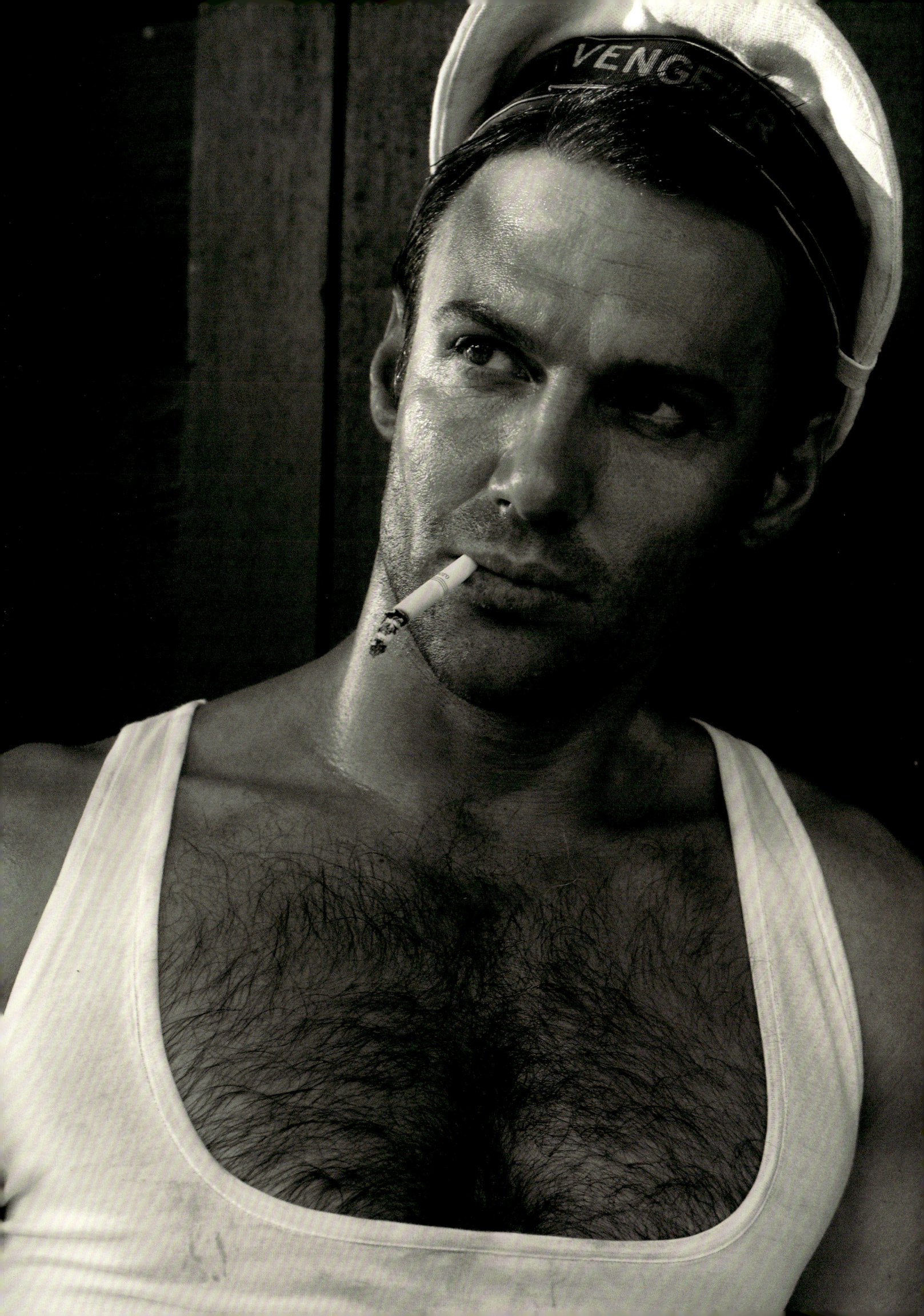

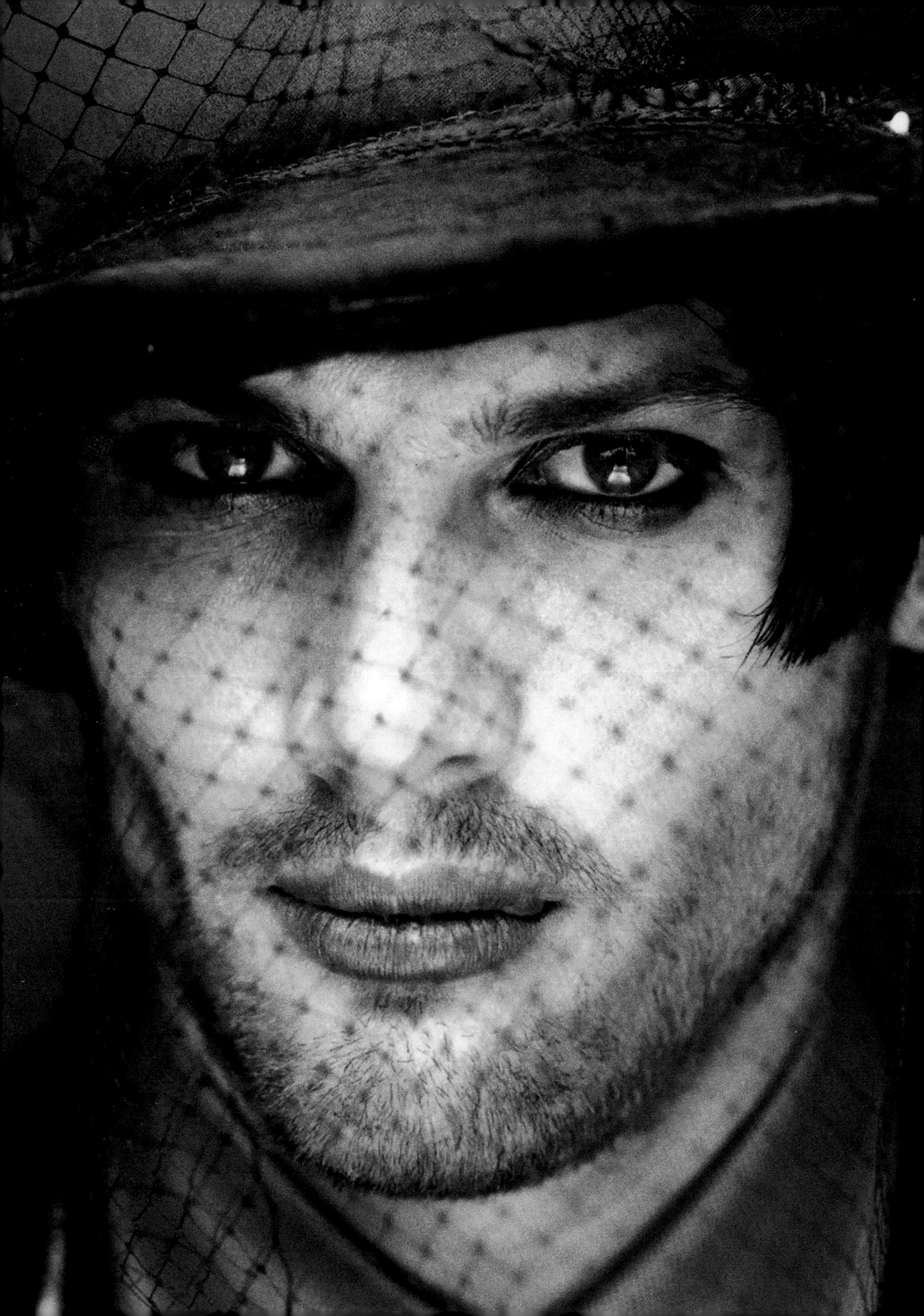

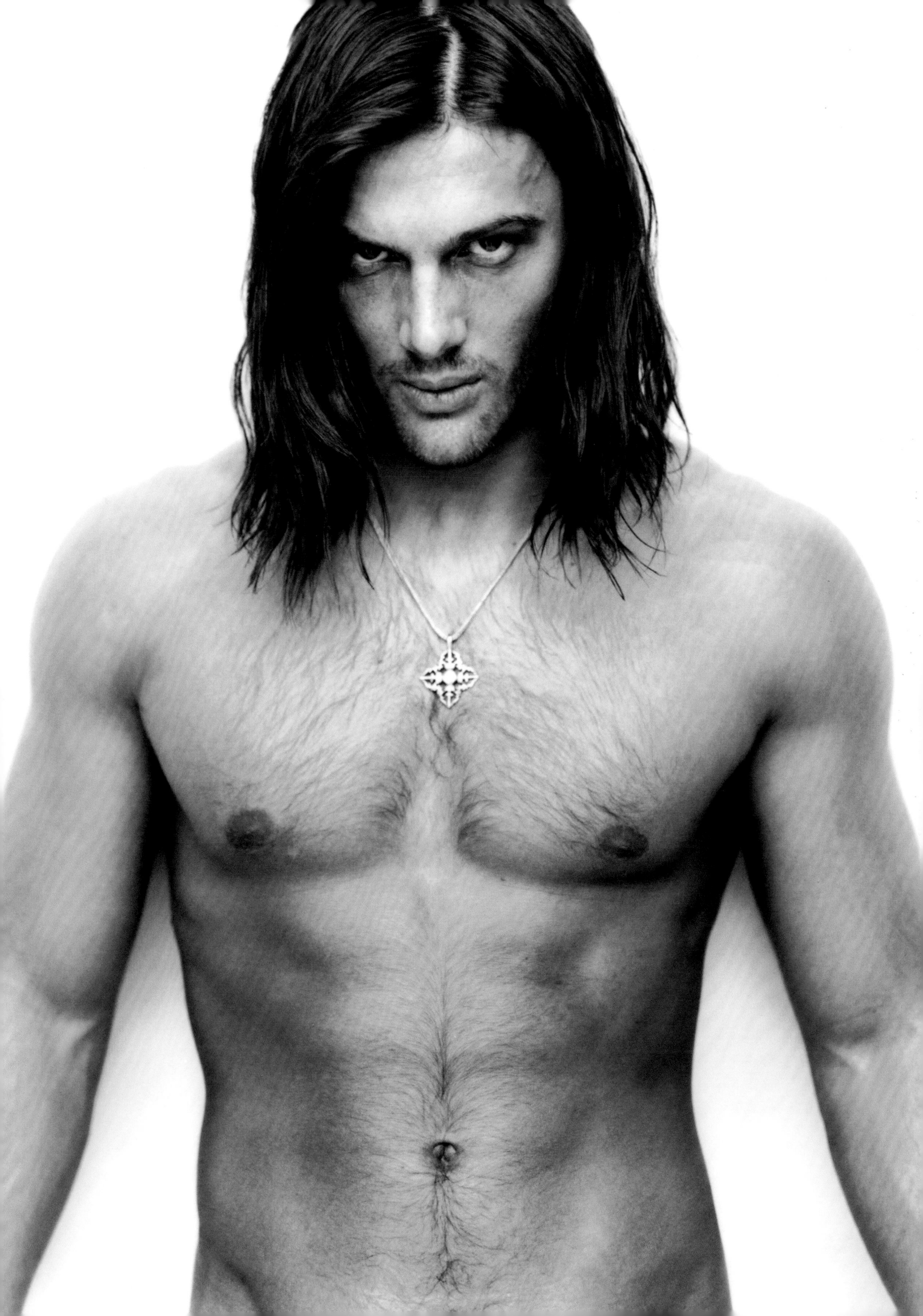

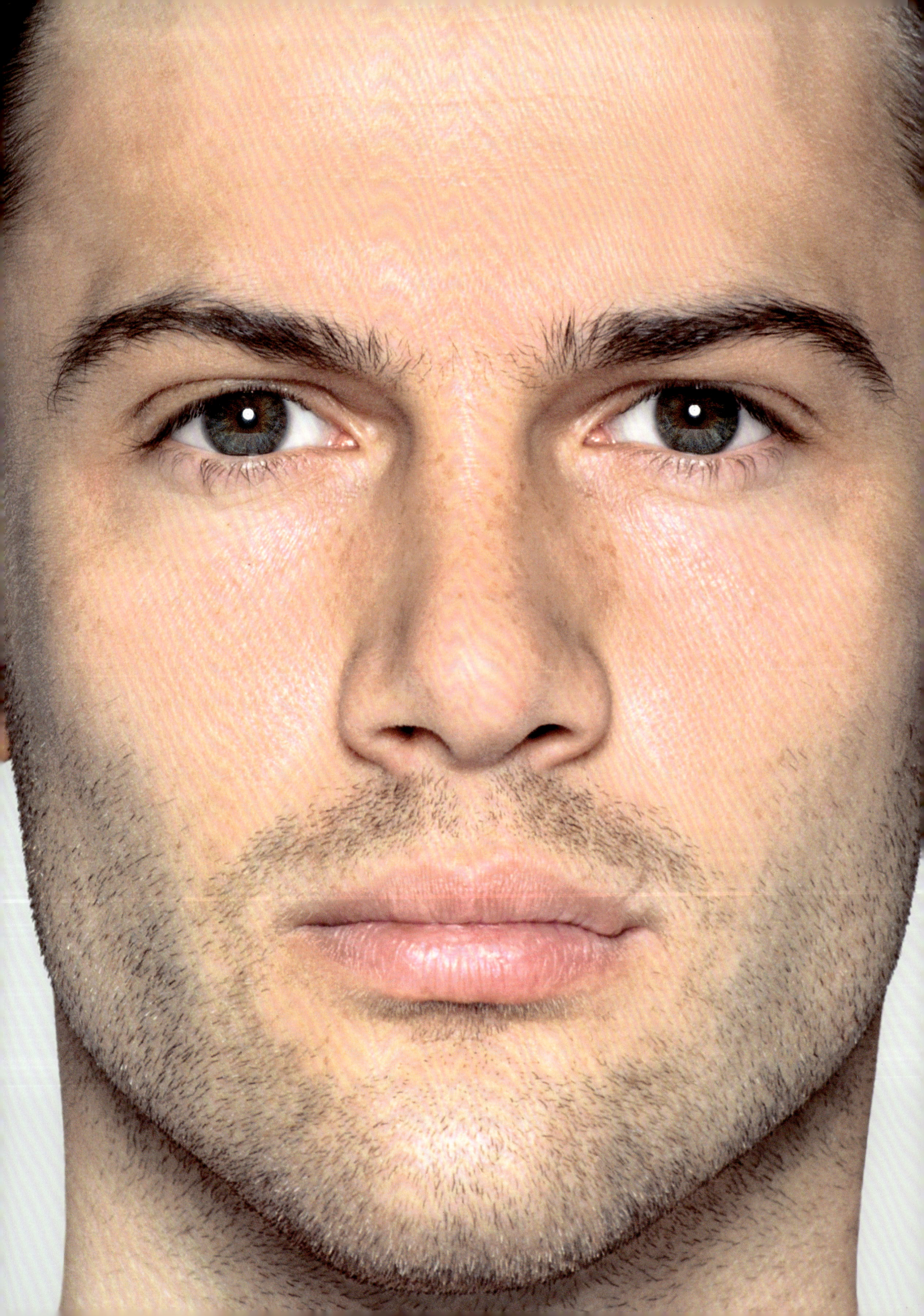

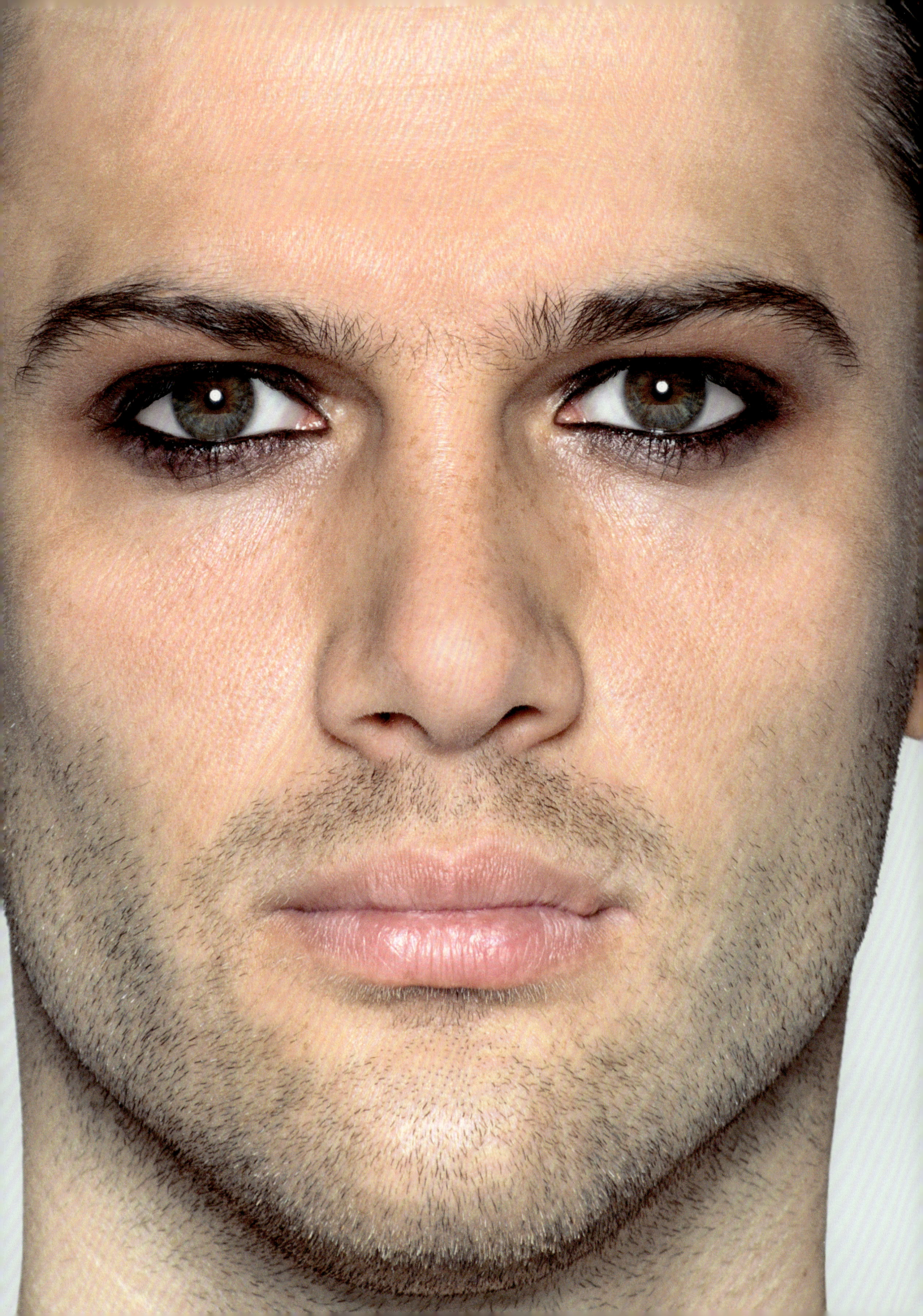

THE POP LIFE

AS EXTRAORDINARY DAYS TURNED TO NIGHTS, FRANÇOIS NARS AND HIS FELLOW AESTHETES DISCOVERED THAT EVERYTHING GOOD HAPPENS AFTER DARK. HIS PEERS ON SET QUICKLY BECAME HIS SOCIAL SET—LINDA, NAOMI, GARREN, ODILE, ORIBE, AND STEVEN, AMONG OTHERS. "WE WERE A FAMILY. MODELS, MAKEUP ARTISTS, AND HAIRSTYLISTS. WE PRACTICALLY LIVED TOGETHER WHEN WE DID SHOWS. WE HAD SO MUCH FUN, LAUGHED SO MUCH," SAYS FRANÇOIS.

THIS NEW WAVE OF IMAGINEERS FOUND THEMSELVES AT THE VERY CENTER OF THE CULTURE THEY HELPED CREATE—ALL LUMINARIES IN THEIR OWN RIGHT, RISING FURIOUSLY IN FASHION'S NEW MOMENT. NOTABLES TRANSFORMED INTO HOUSEHOLD NAMES NEARLY OVERNIGHT, WINKING THROUGH EXCESS AS THE PRESS WATCHED ON IN FASCINATION. THEIR UNSTOPPABLE AURA IN THE 80s AND 90s DEFINED THE HEIGHT OF NEW YORK'S DOWNTOWN GLAMOUR.

SUPERMODELS, DESIGNERS, PHOTOGRAPHERS, MAKEUP ARTISTS, AND HAIRSTYLISTS NOW JOINED THE HOLLYWOOD ELITE AS FRONT-PAGE PERSONALITIES IN FANTASY AND FOLLY. THIS WAS A TIME OF PLAY, EXPRESSION, AND NO RULES—A PHILOSOPHY FRANÇOIS HOLDS TRUE TODAY. "FASHION IS IN CONSTANT MOVEMENT, AND MAKEUP SHOULD BE THE SAME," HE SAYS.

IT CAUSED MORE THAN A SCENE. IT INSPIRED A FAST, NEW LIFESTYLE AND INTRODUCED A FASHIONABLE DAYDREAM: WHY WORK AND PLAY WHEN YOU CAN PLAY AT WORK?

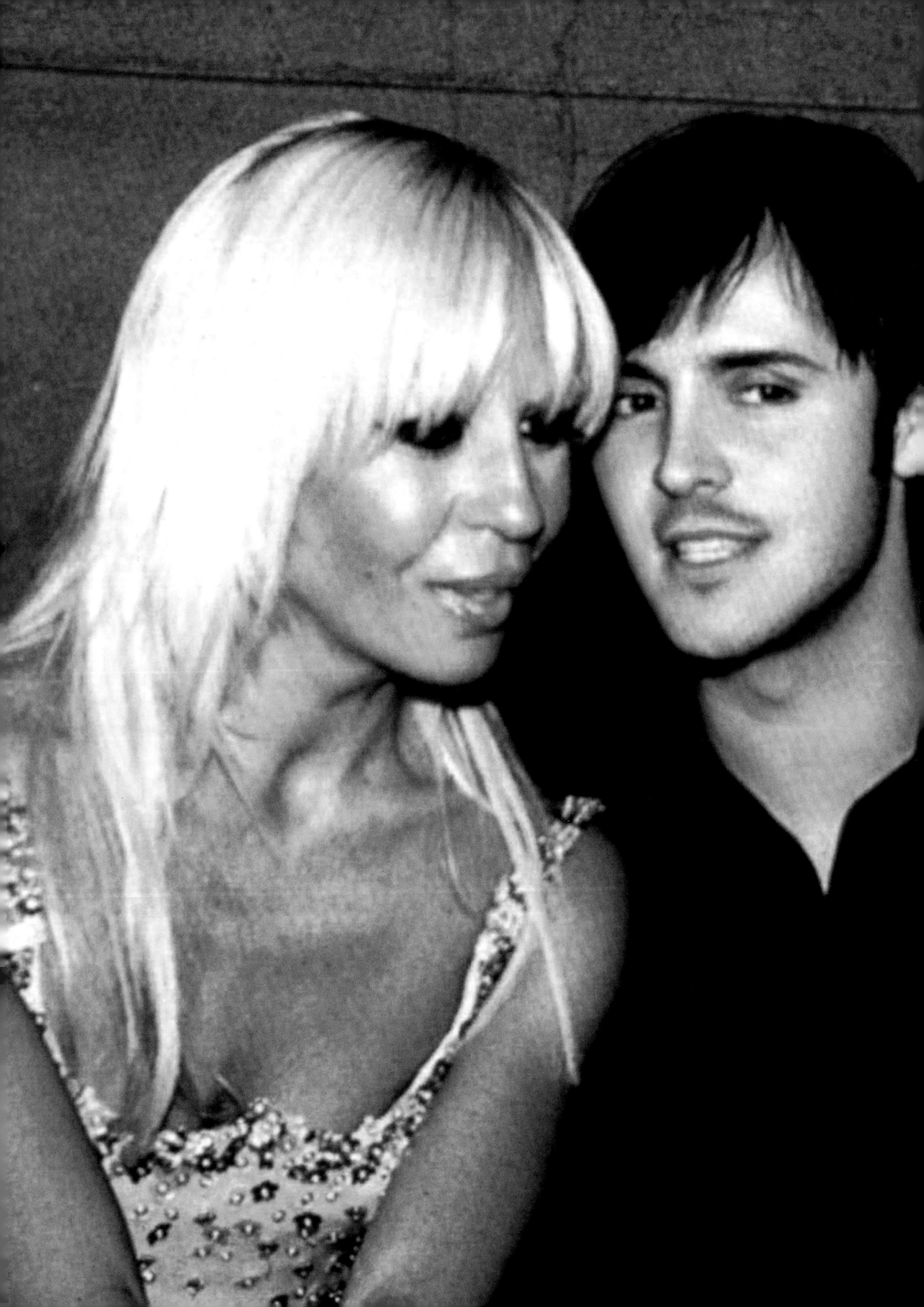

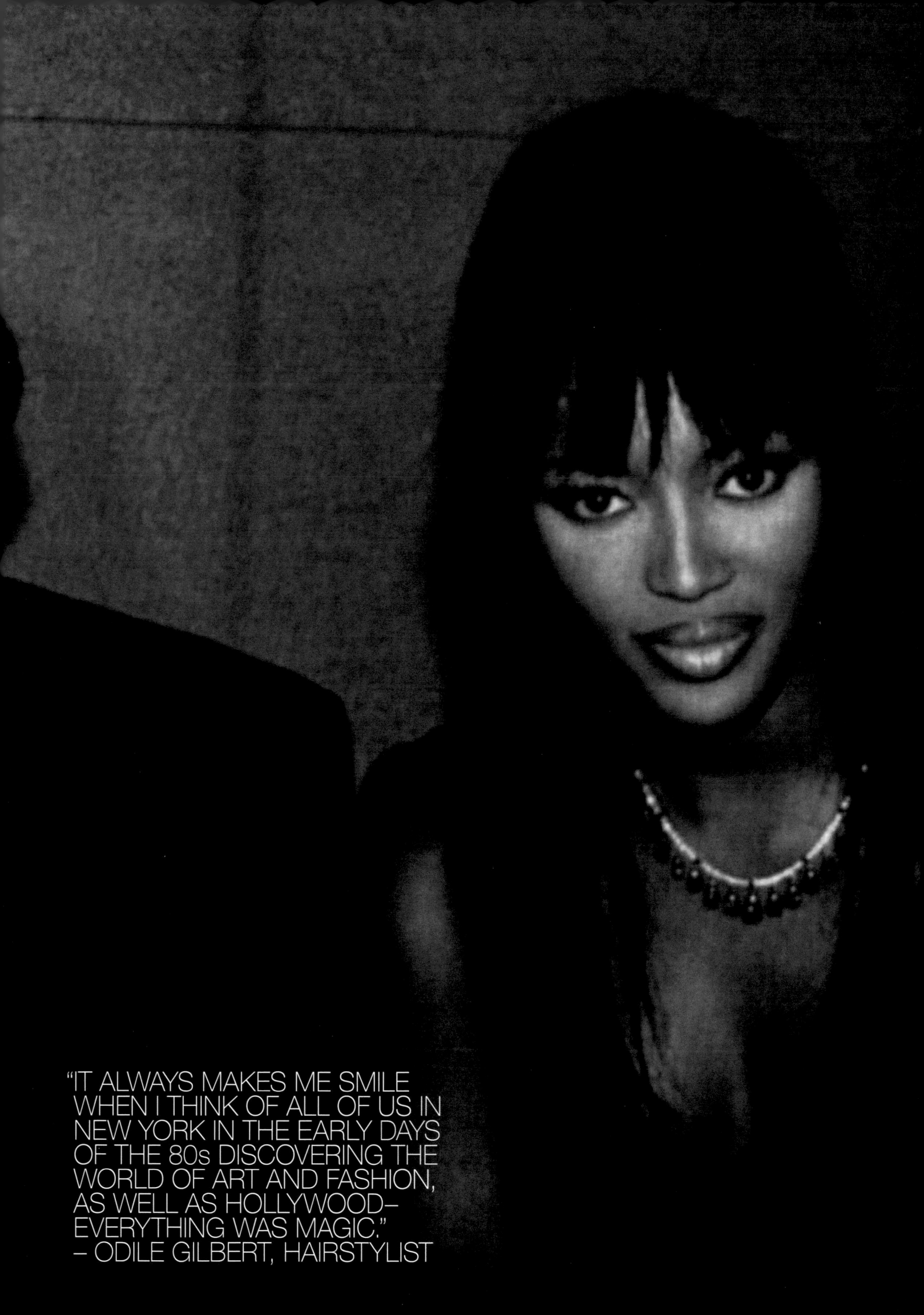

"IT ALWAYS MAKES ME SMILE
WHEN I THINK OF ALL OF US IN
NEW YORK IN THE EARLY DAYS
OF THE 80s DISCOVERING THE
WORLD OF ART AND FASHION,
AS WELL AS HOLLYWOOD–
EVERYTHING WAS MAGIC."
– ODILE GILBERT, HAIRSTYLIST

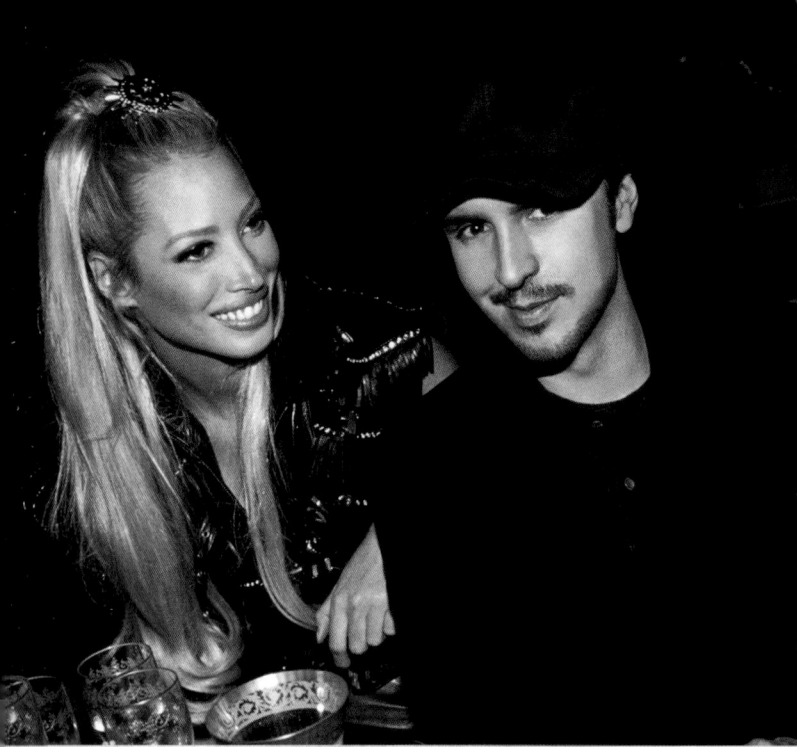

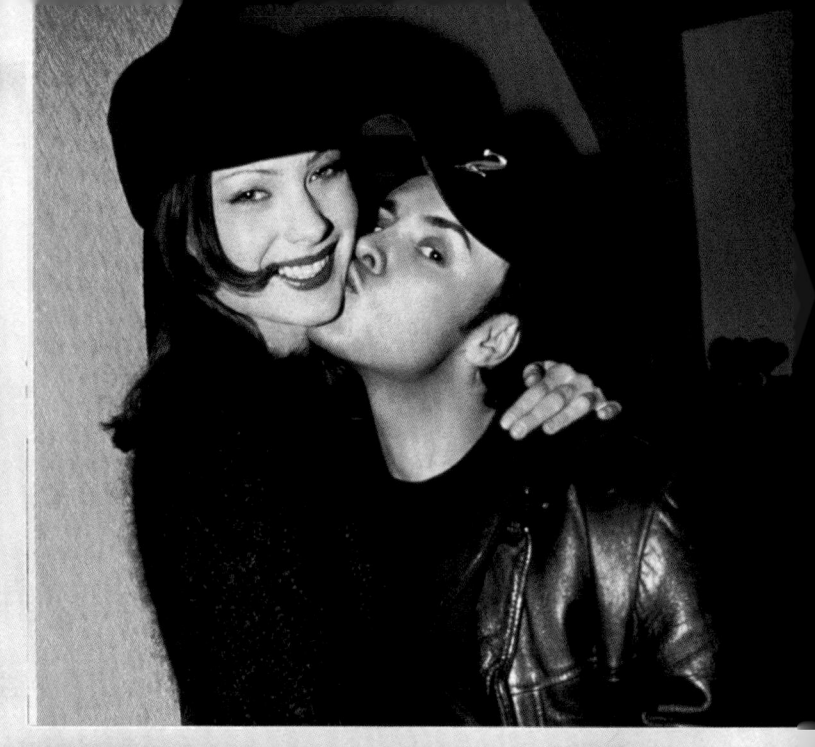

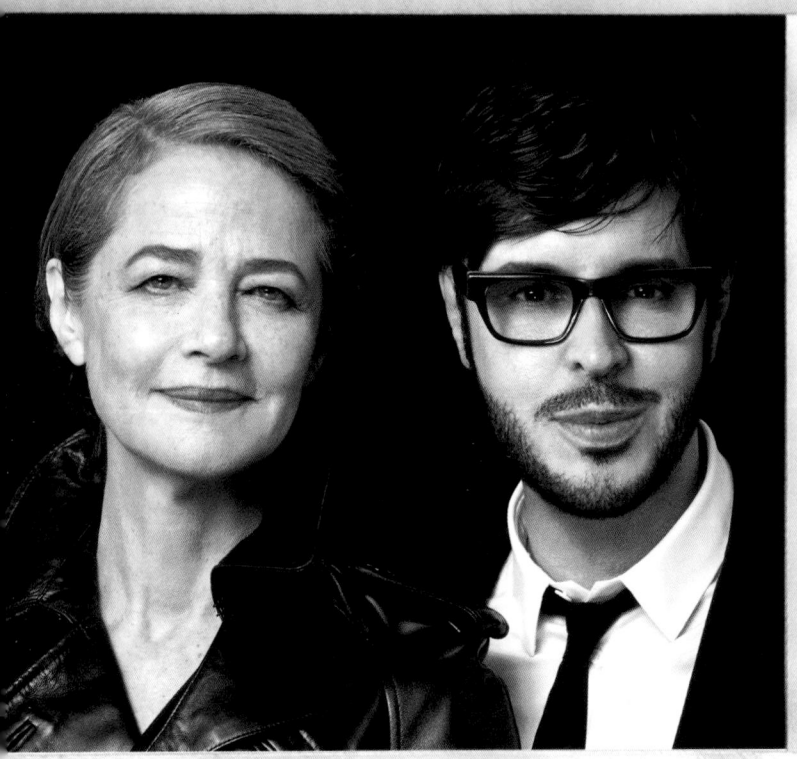

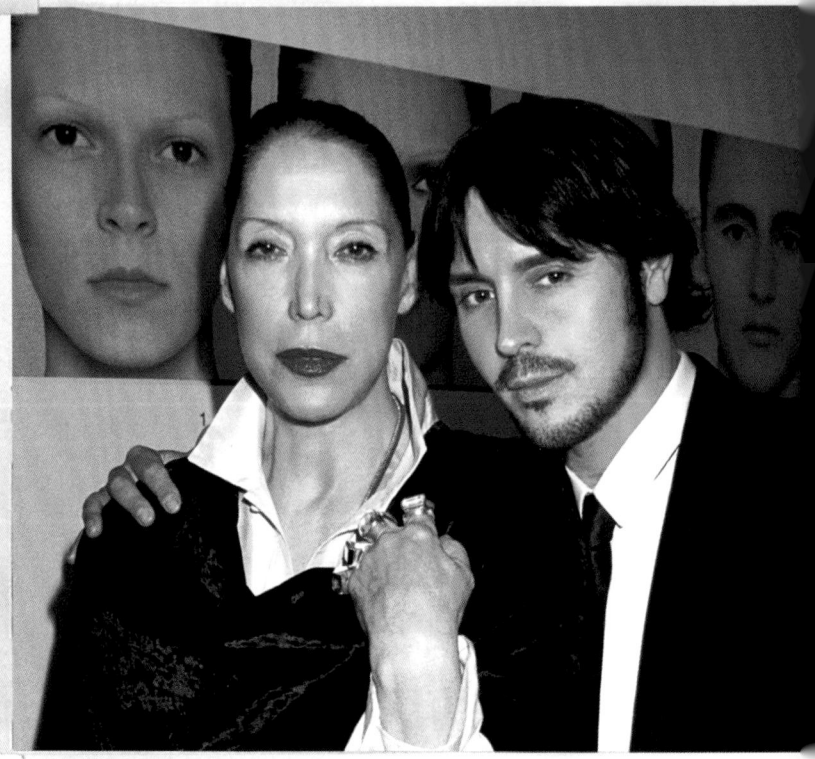

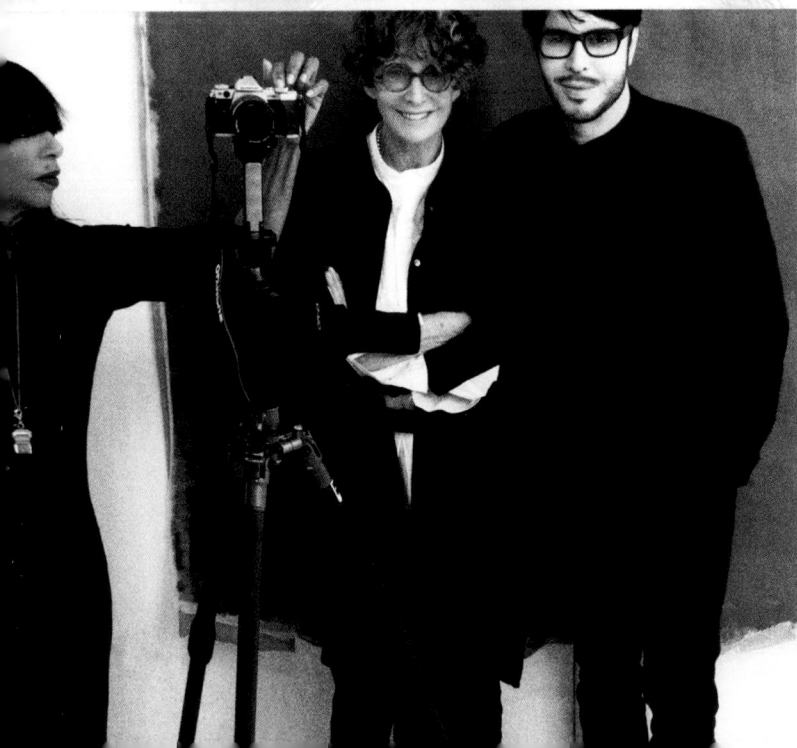

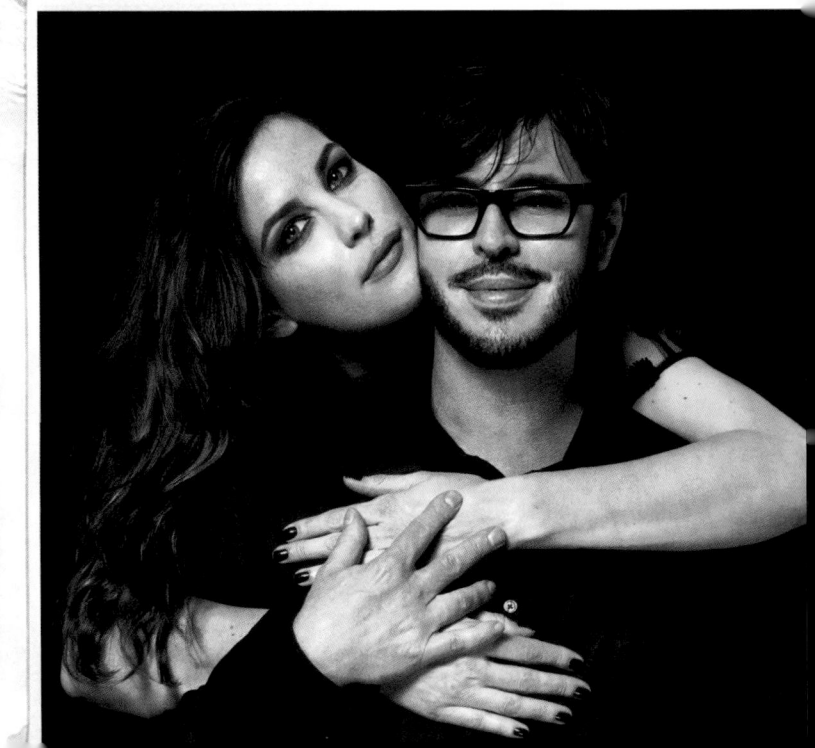

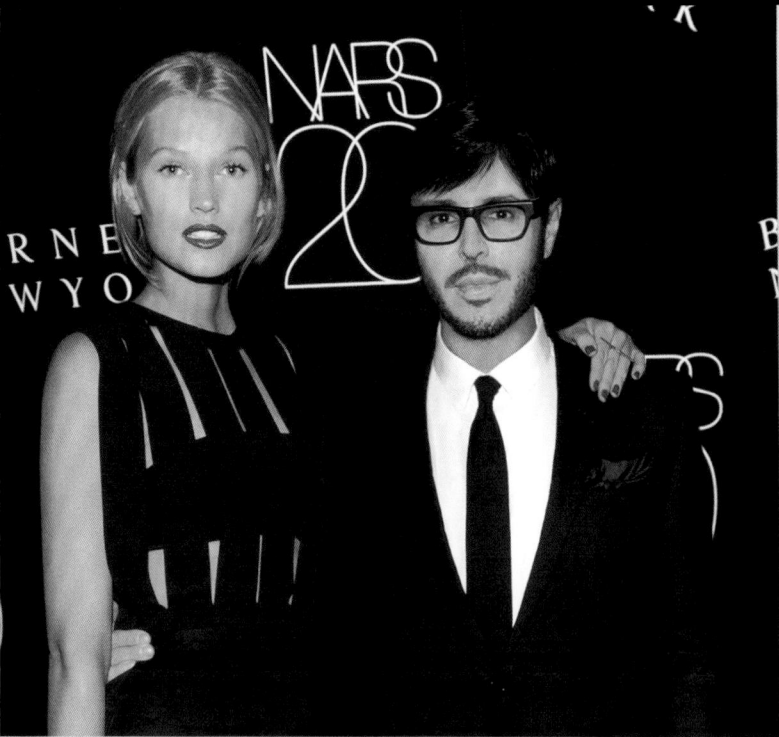

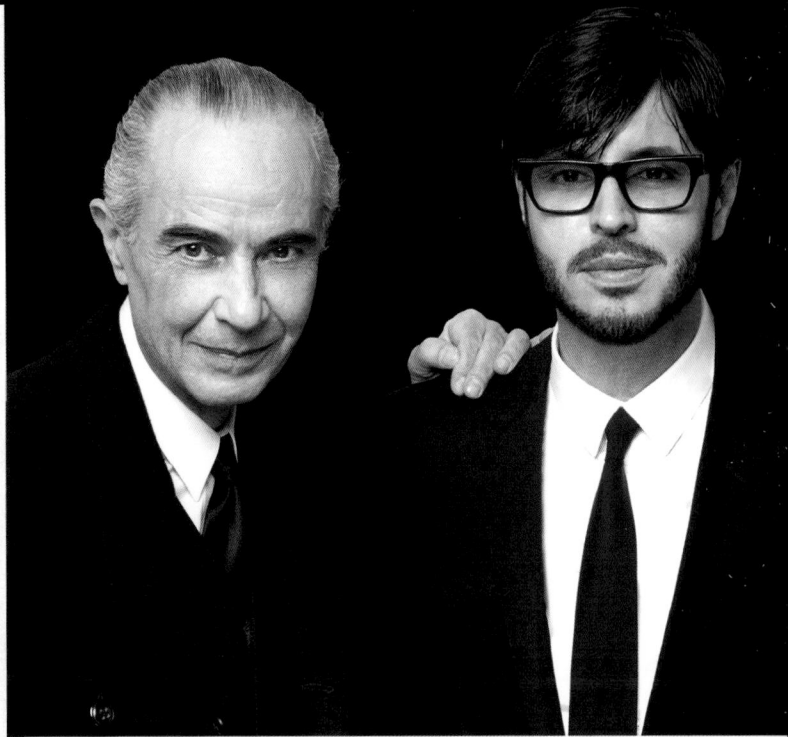

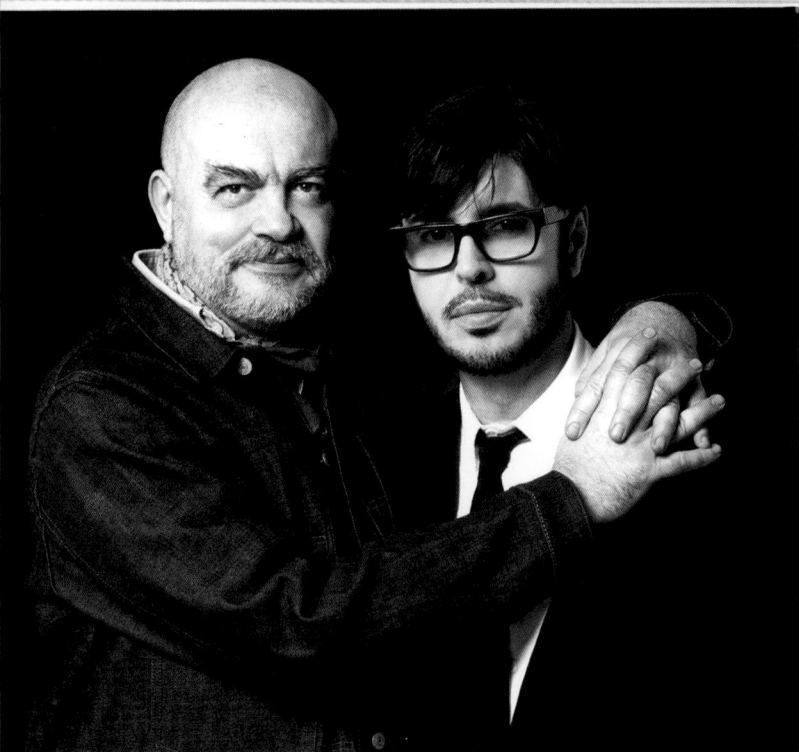

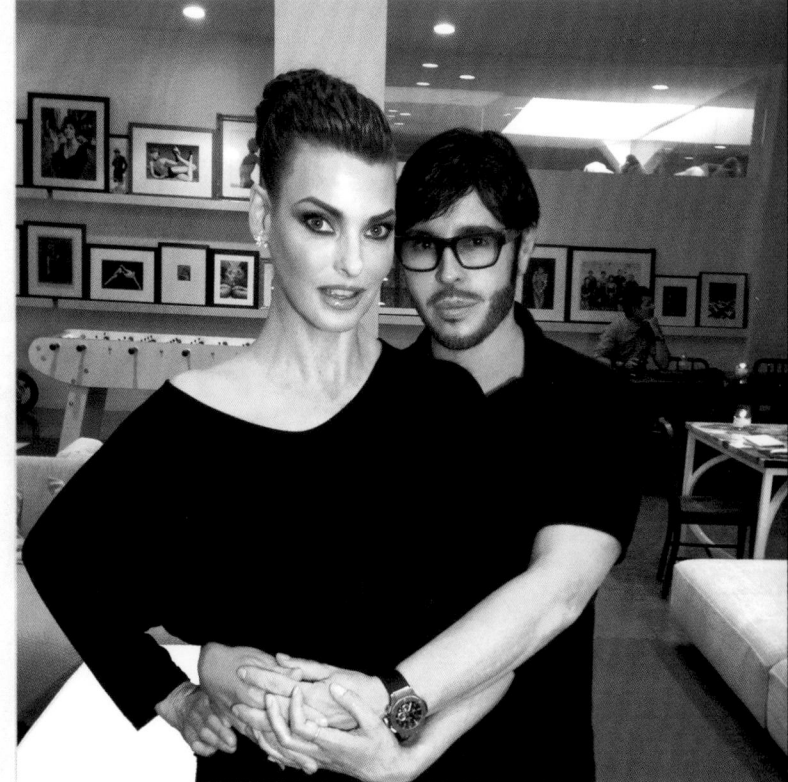

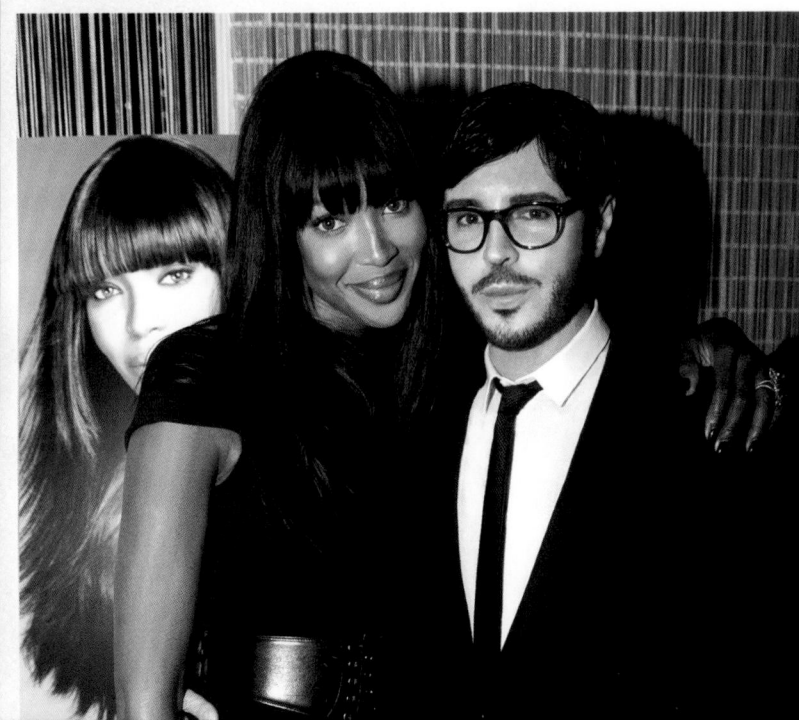

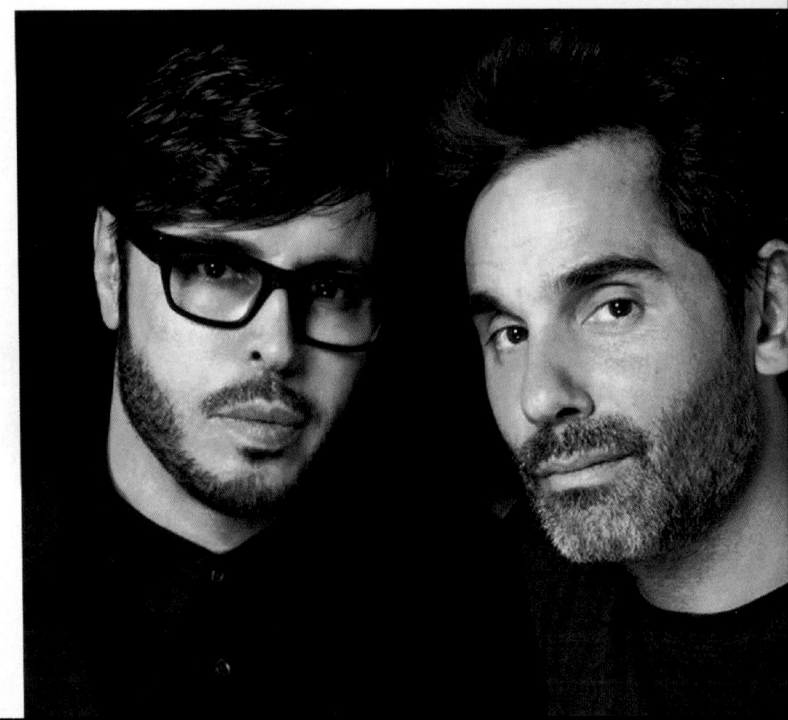

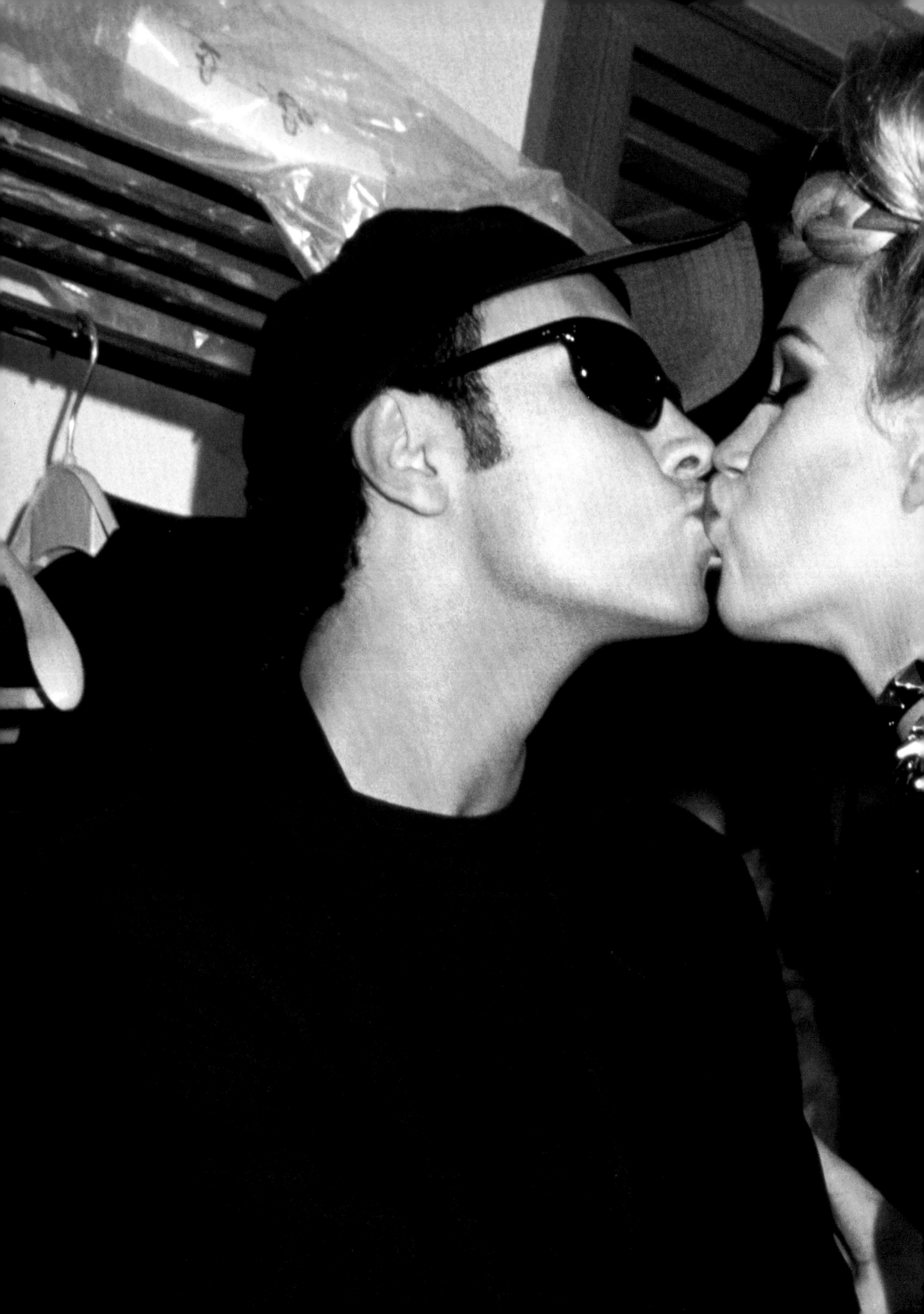

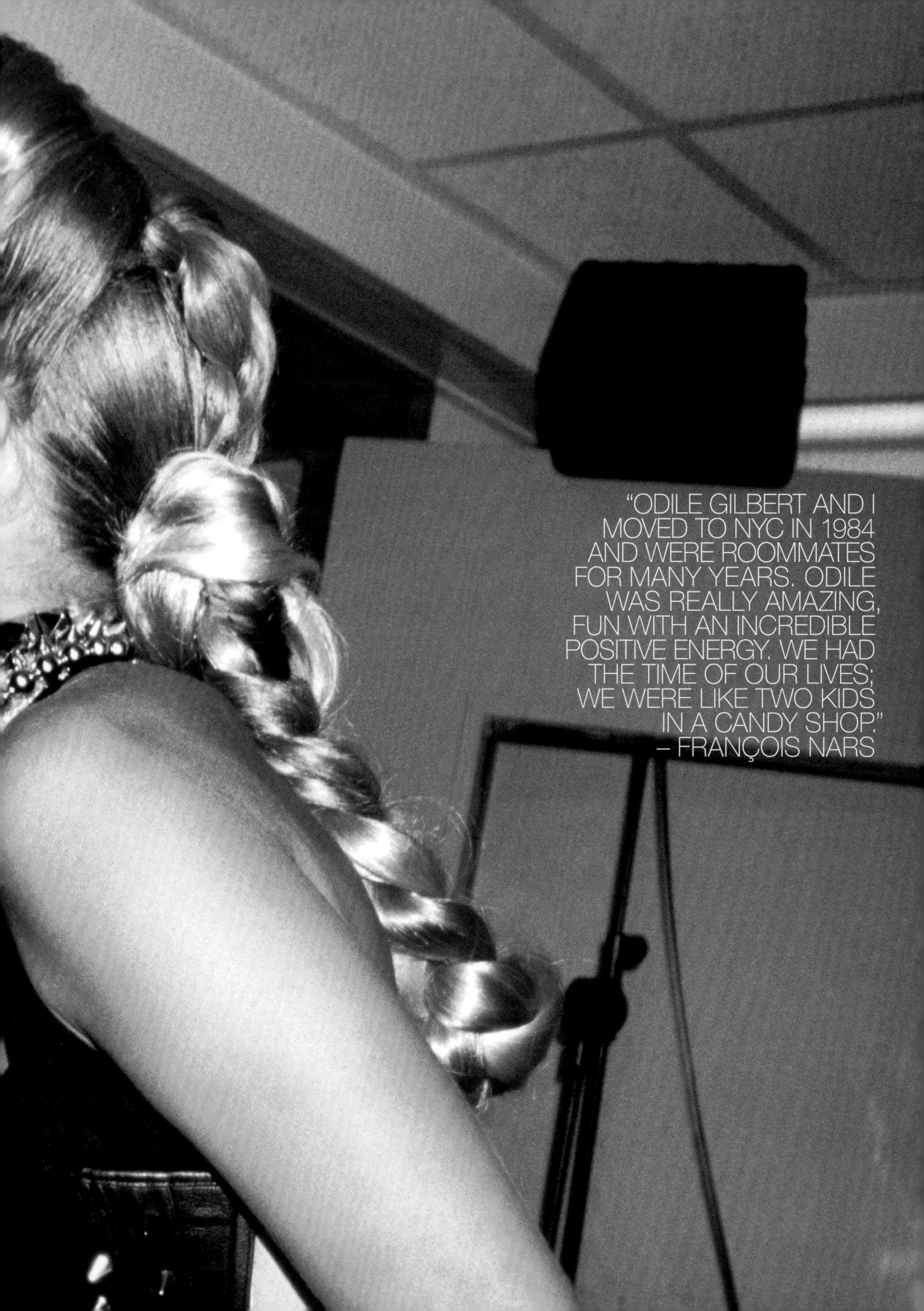

"ODILE GILBERT AND I MOVED TO NYC IN 1984 AND WERE ROOMMATES FOR MANY YEARS. ODILE WAS REALLY AMAZING, FUN WITH AN INCREDIBLE POSITIVE ENERGY. WE HAD THE TIME OF OUR LIVES; WE WERE LIKE TWO KIDS IN A CANDY SHOP."
— FRANÇOIS NARS

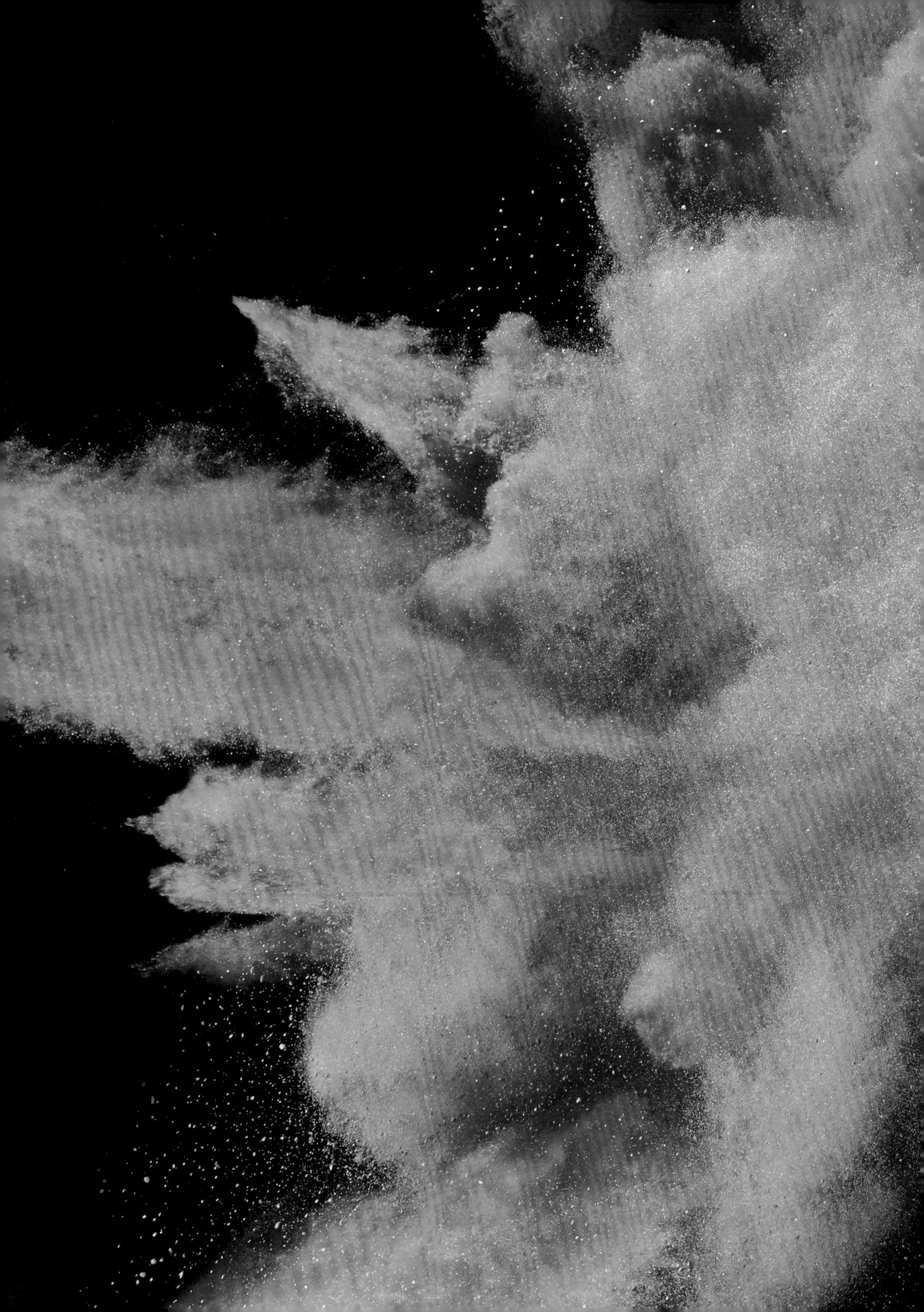

"LOOKING BACK, I THINK THE COMBINATION OF ITS AUDACIOUS NAME AND ITS UNIVERSALLY FLATTERING SHADE MADE IT SO POPULAR. EVEN GRANDMOTHERS LIKE ORGASM."
– FRANÇOIS NARS

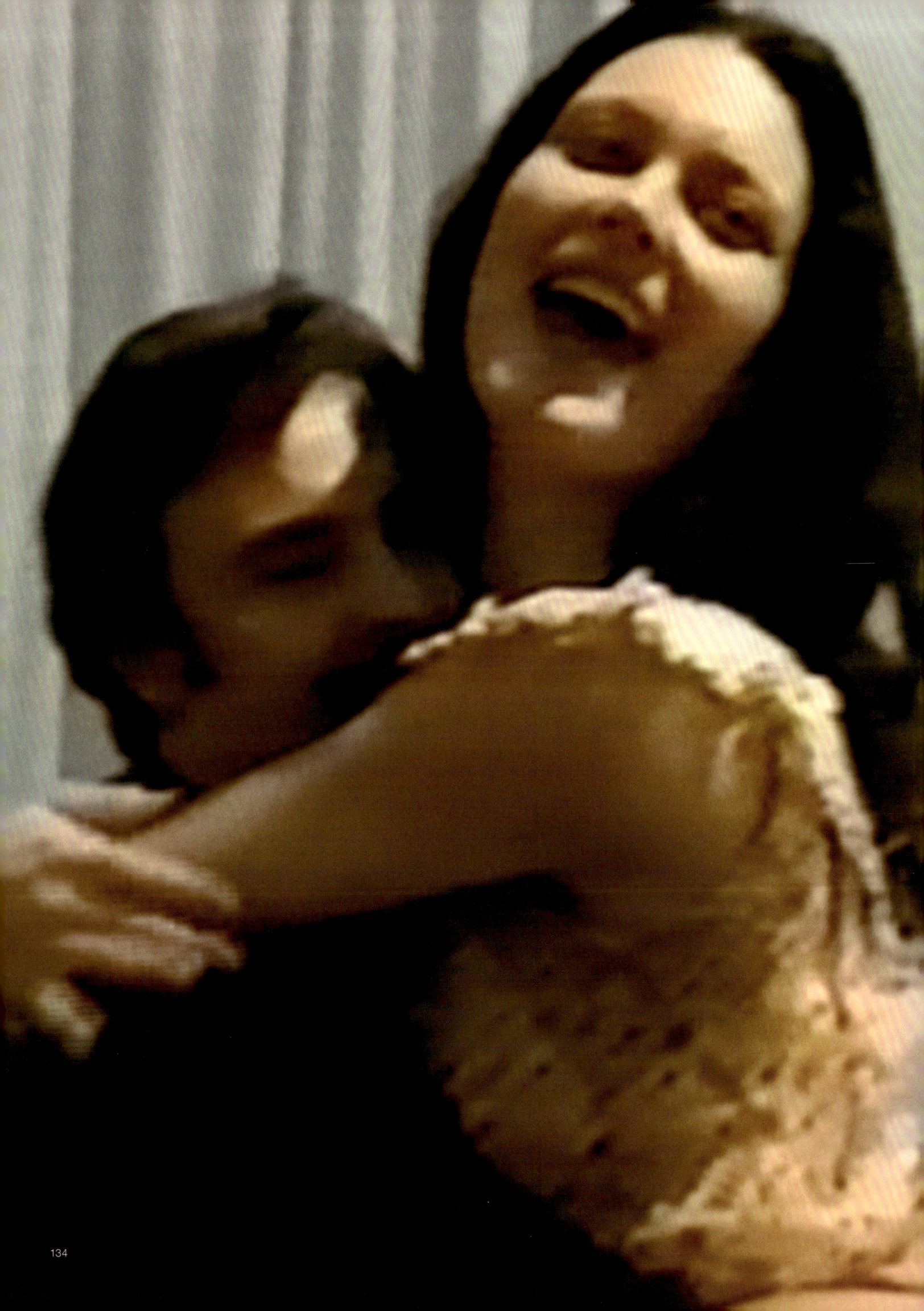

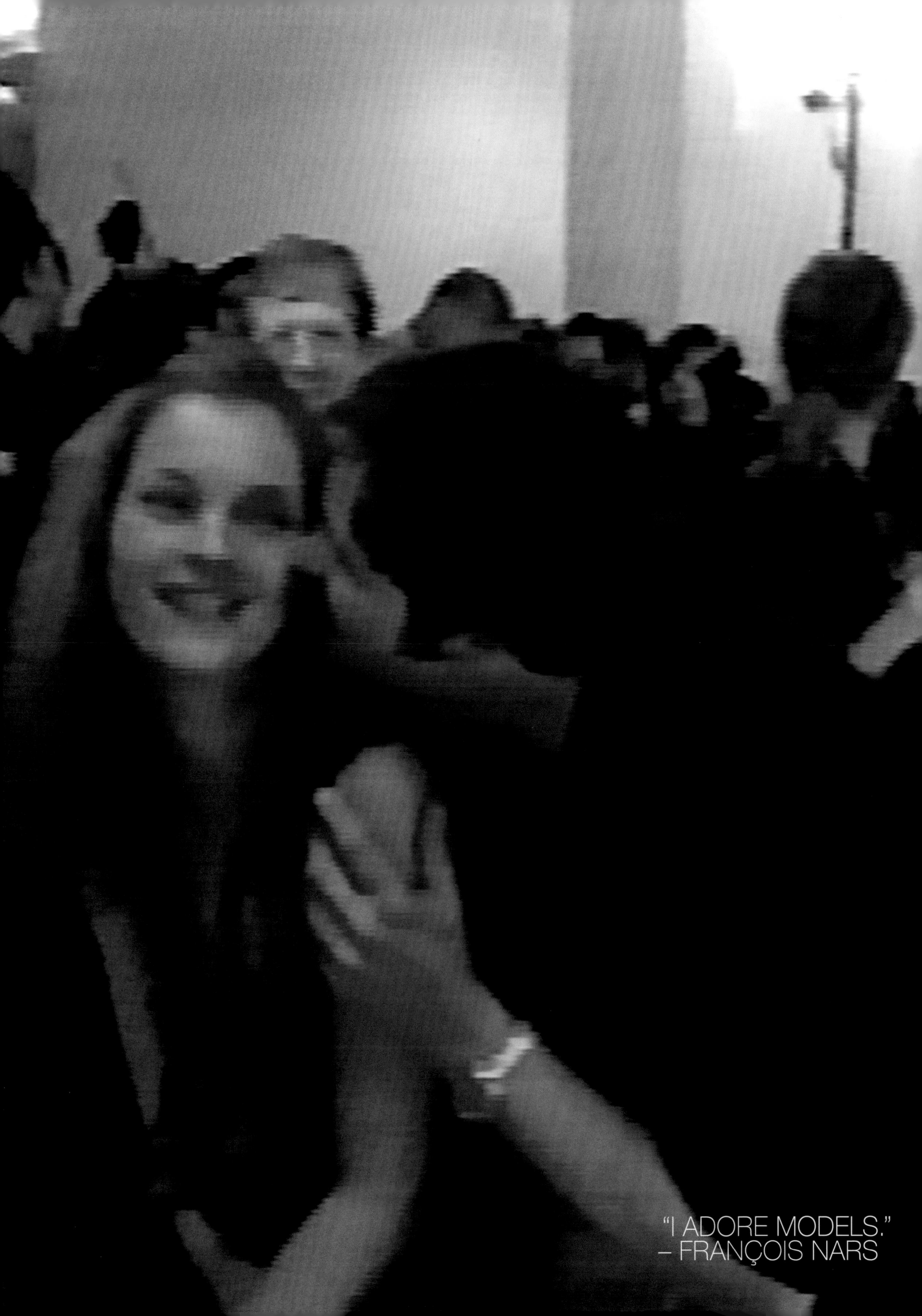

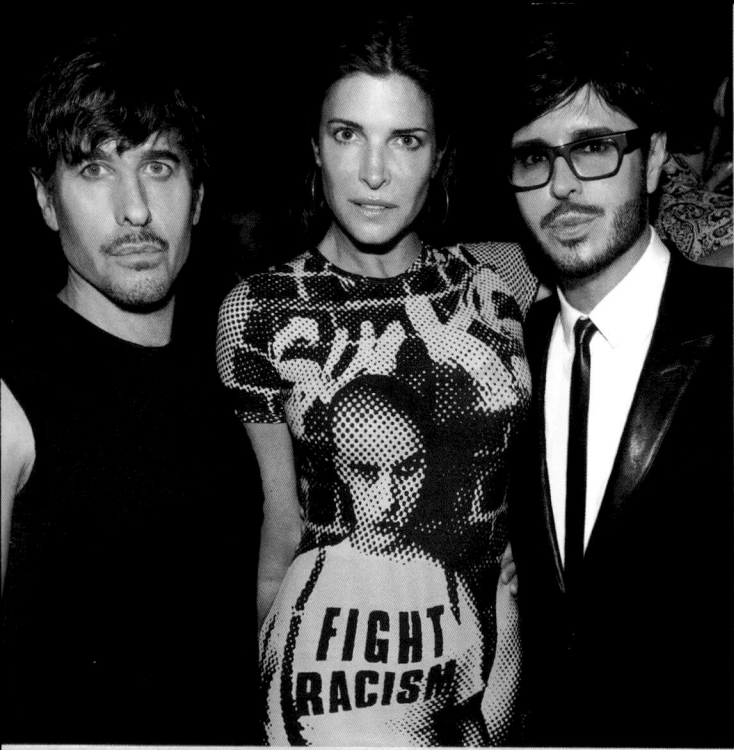

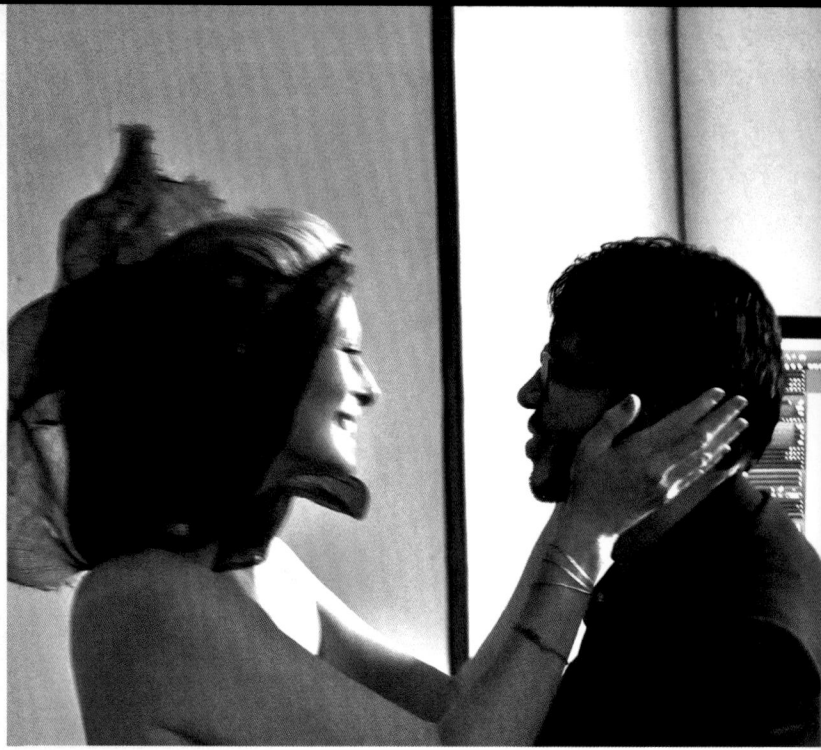

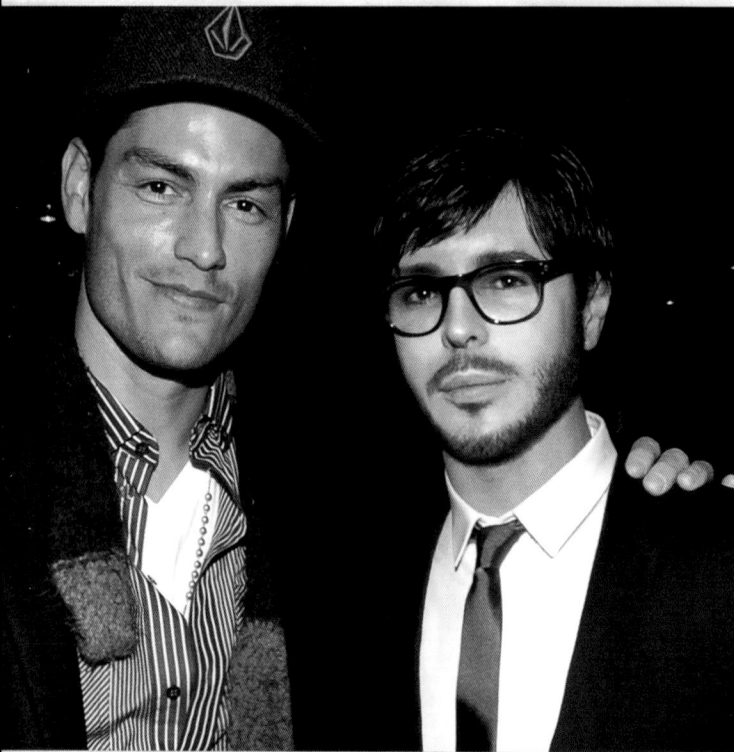

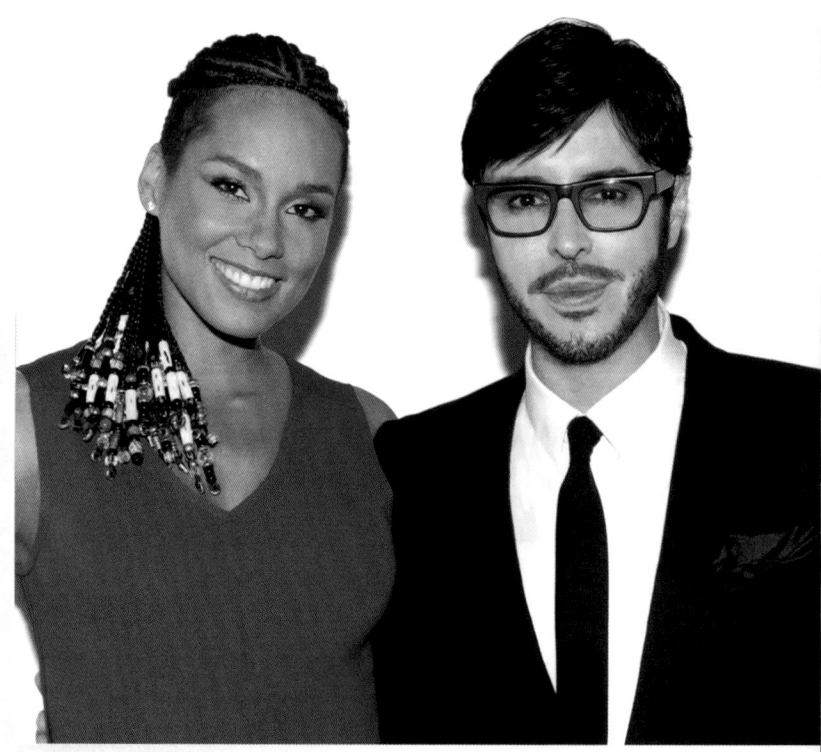

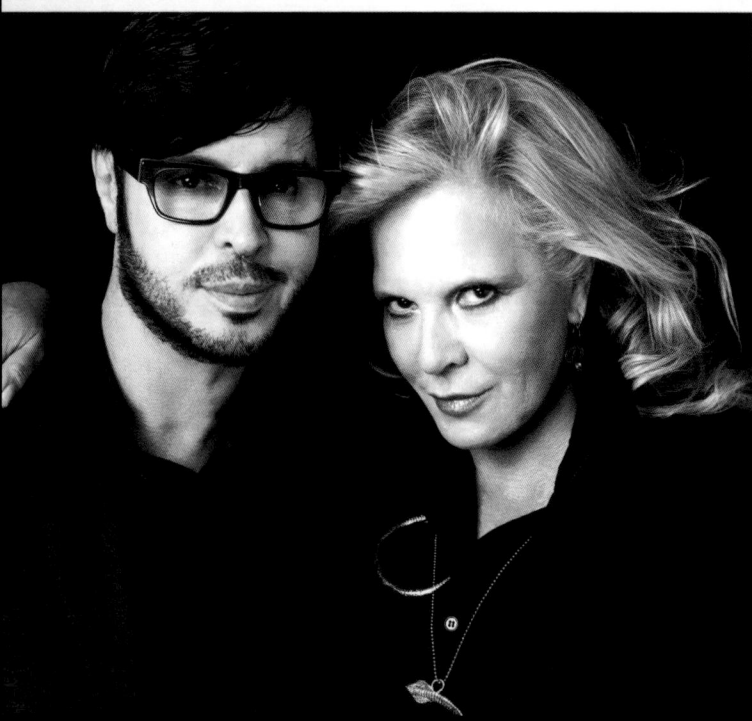

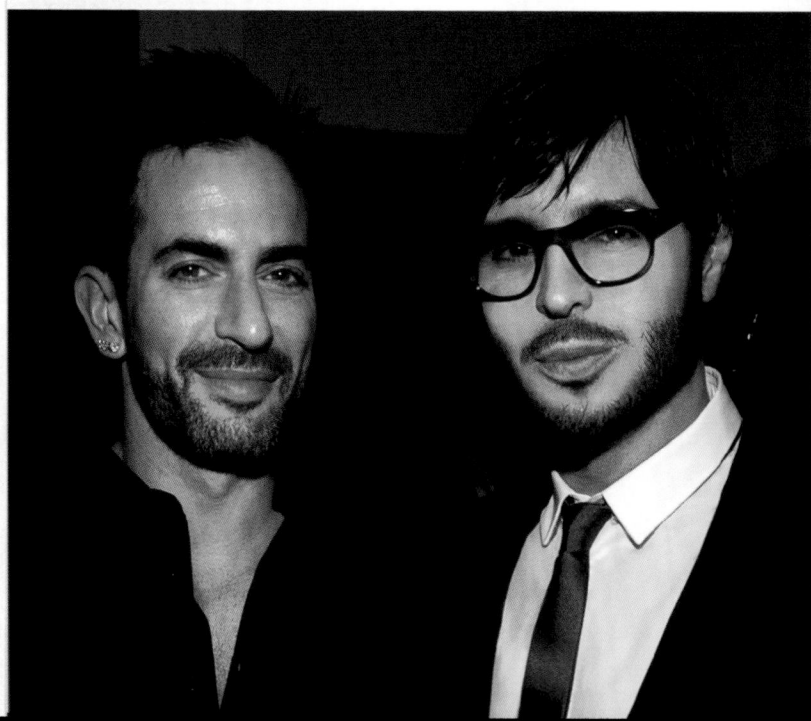

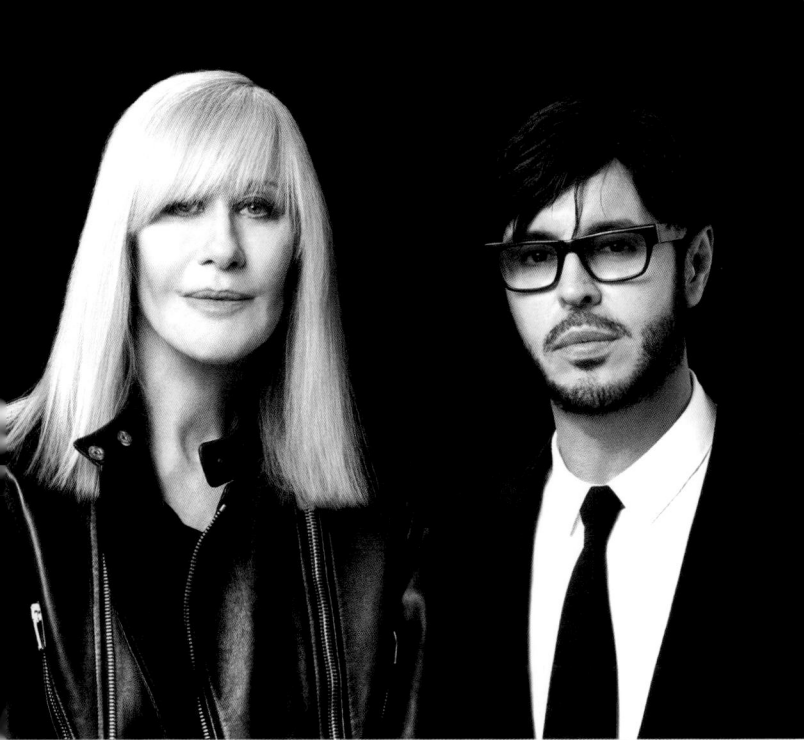

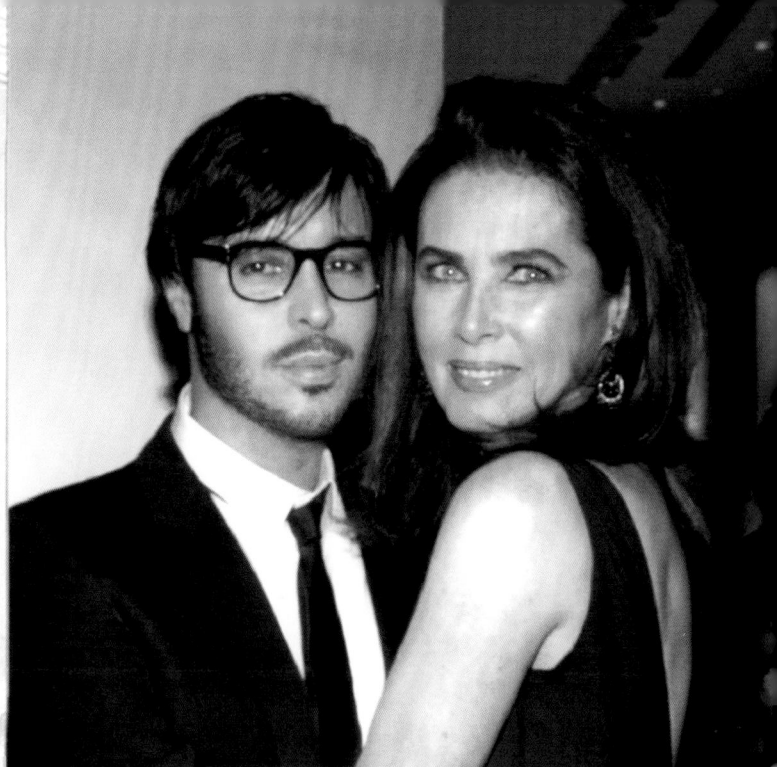

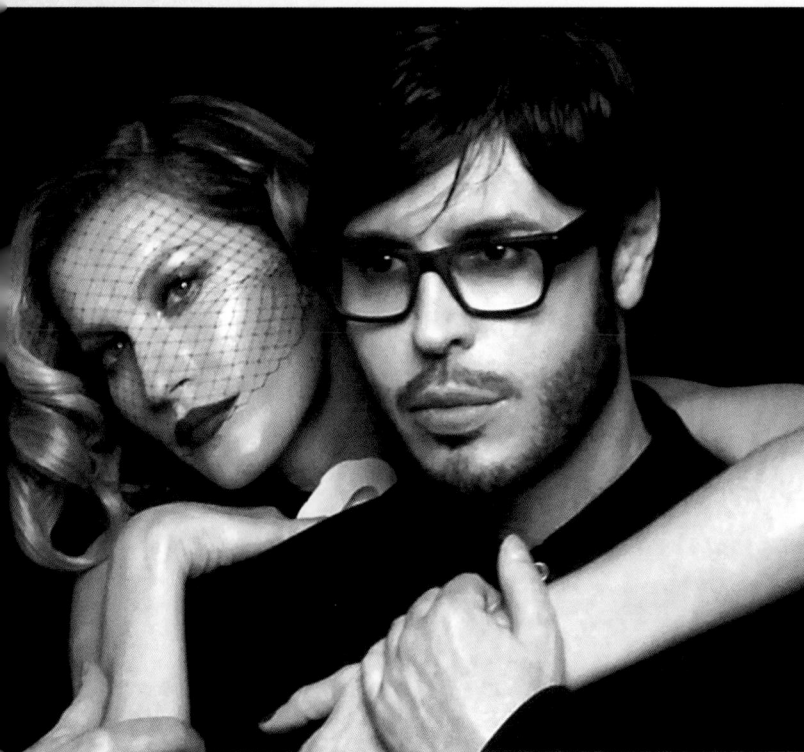

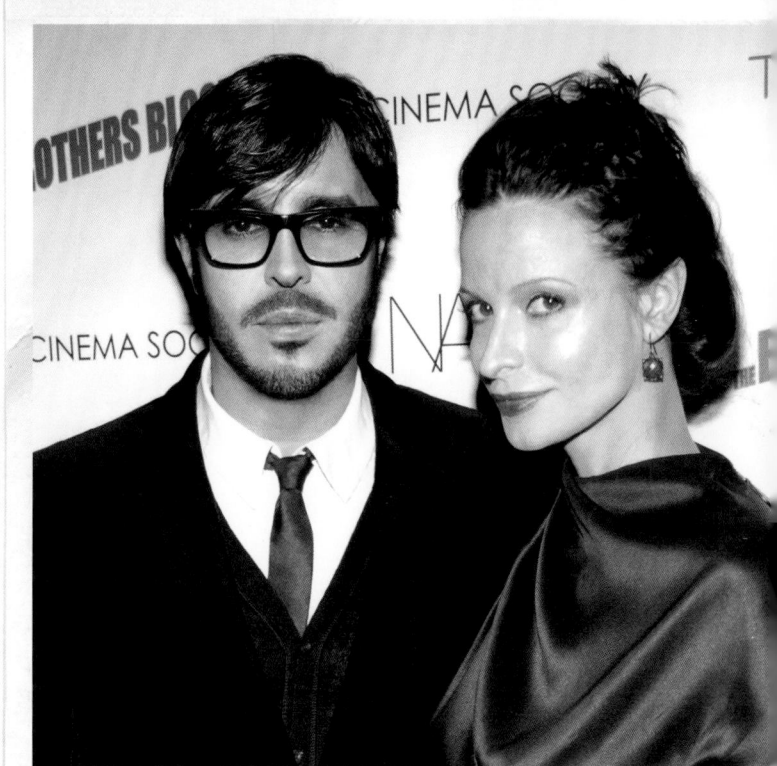

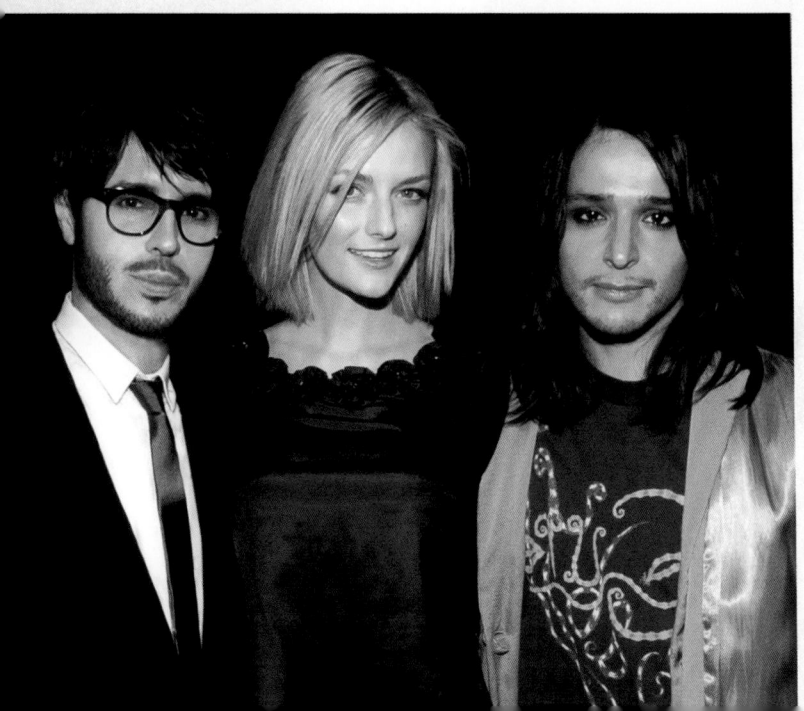

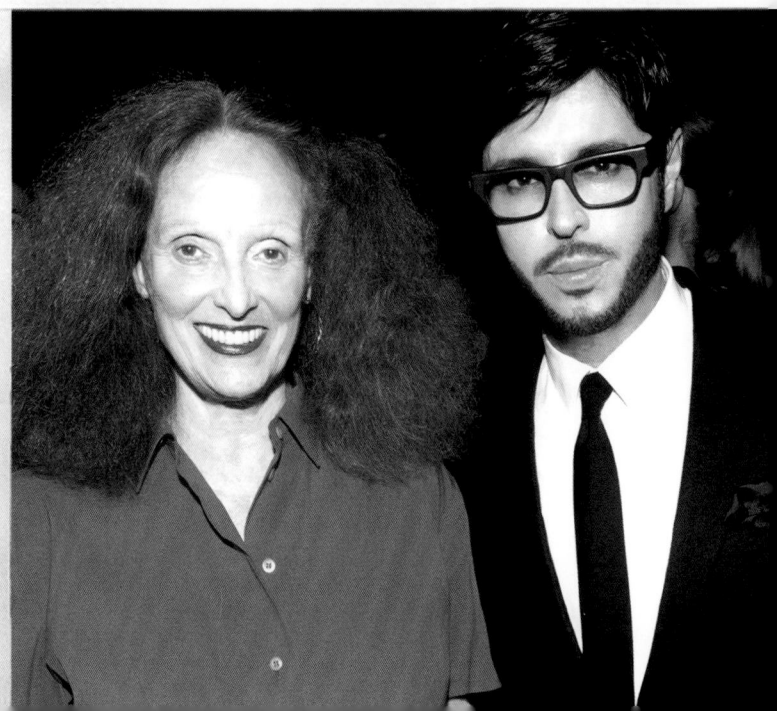

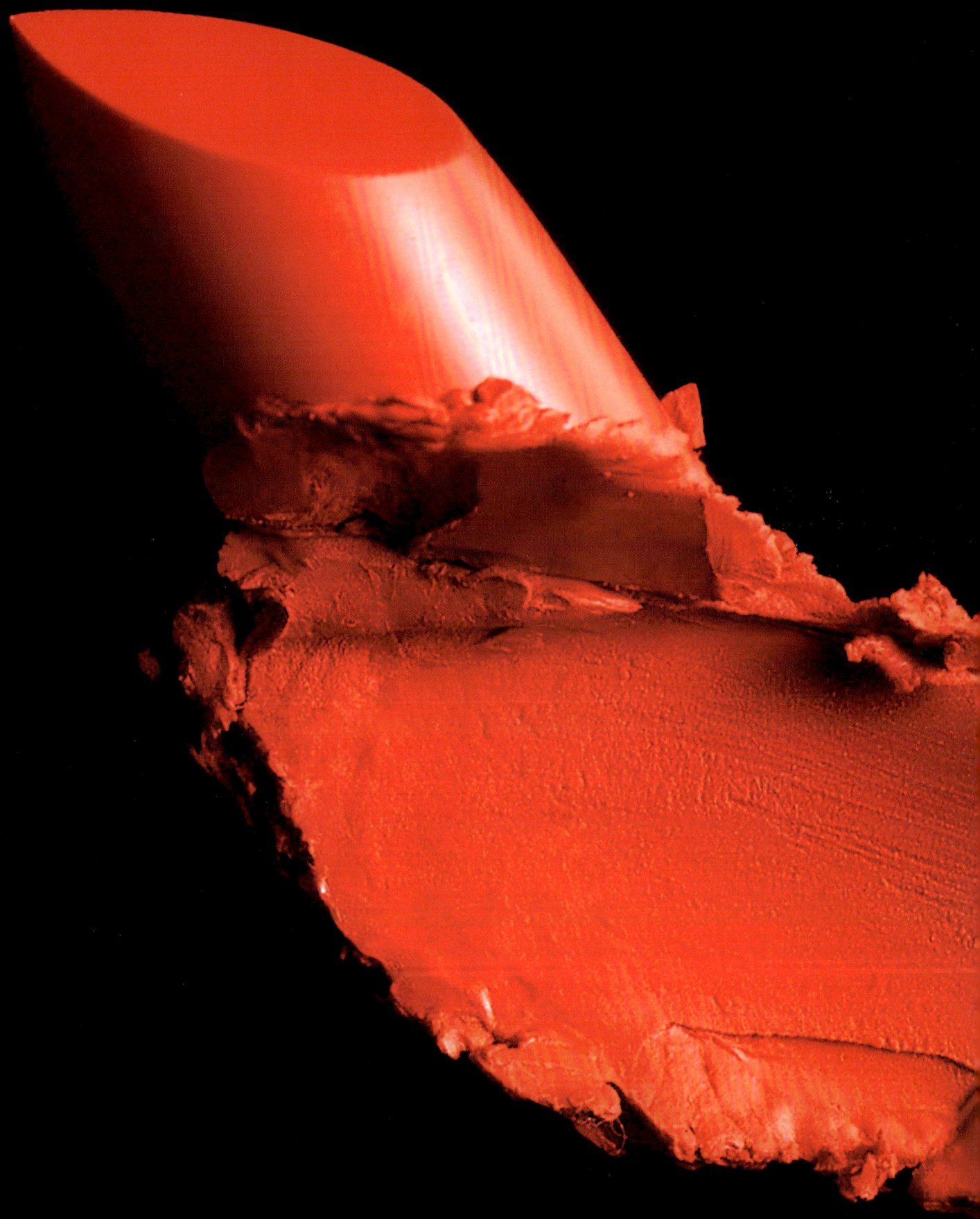

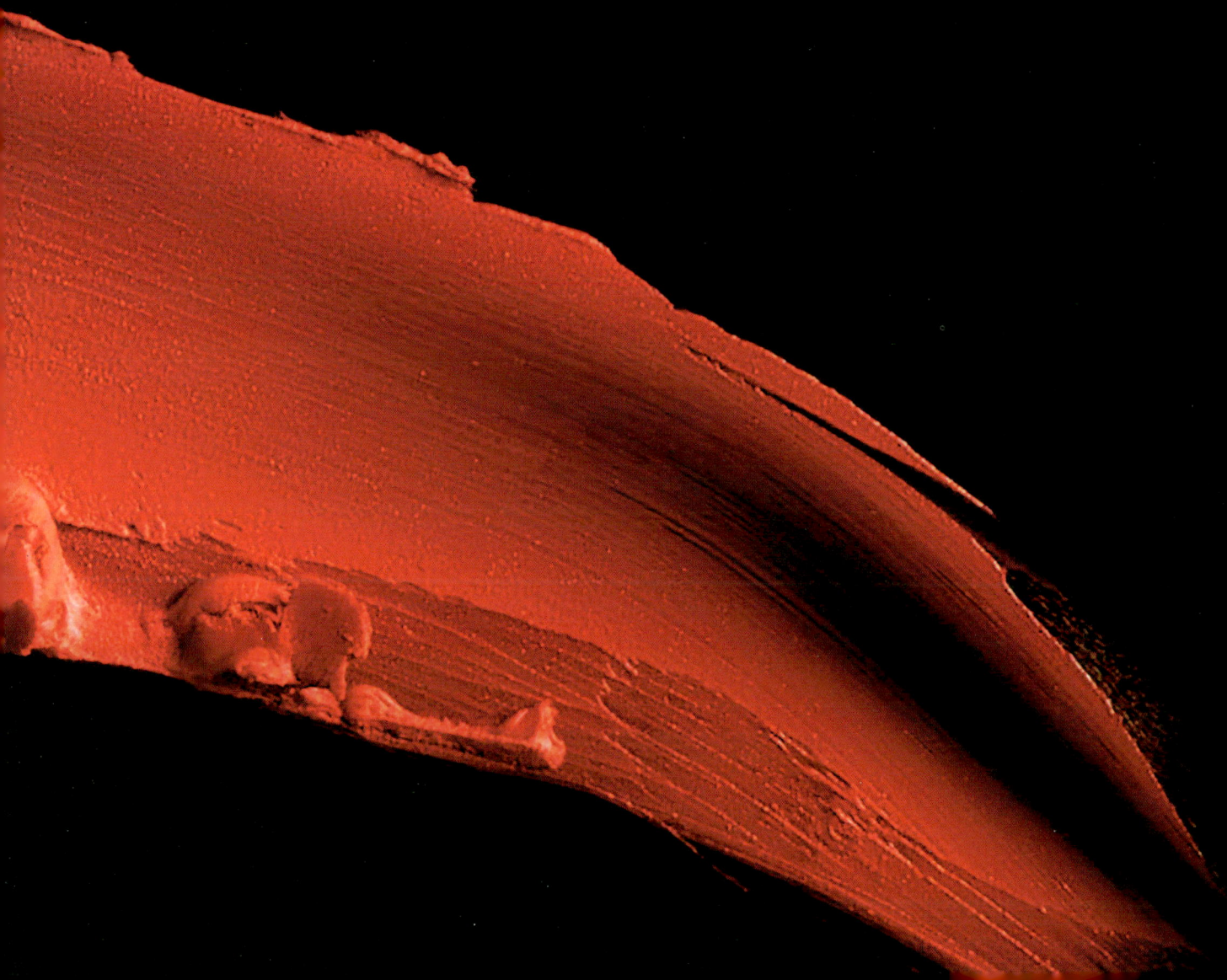

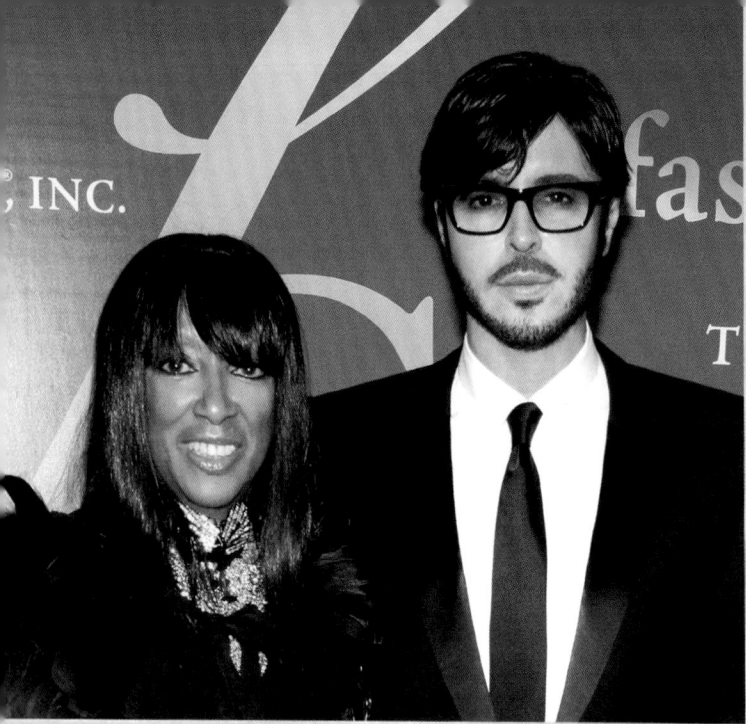

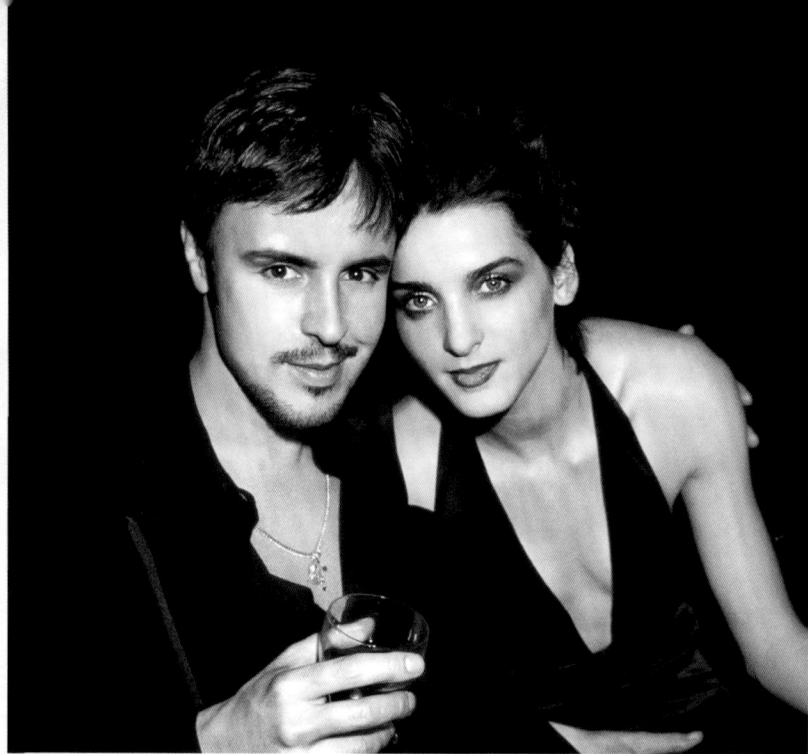

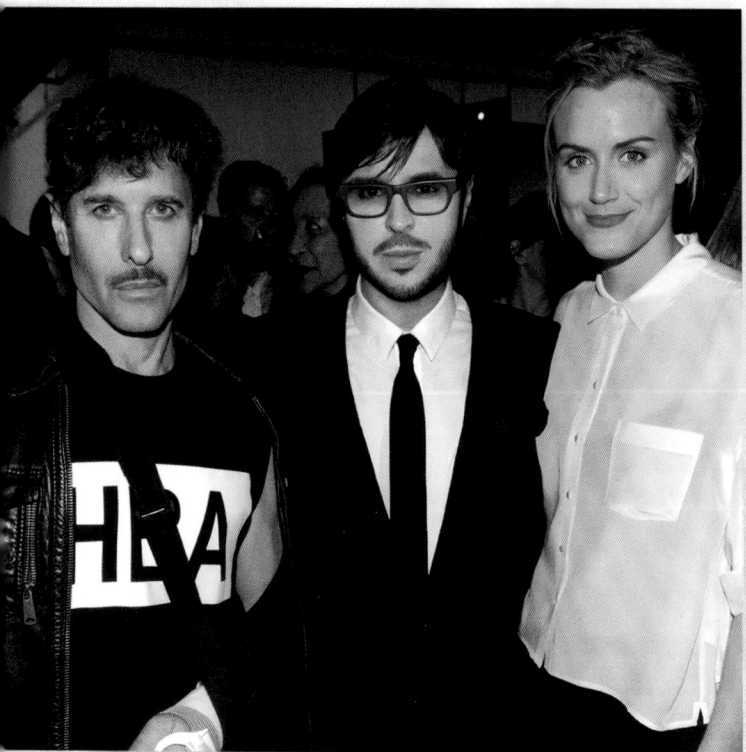

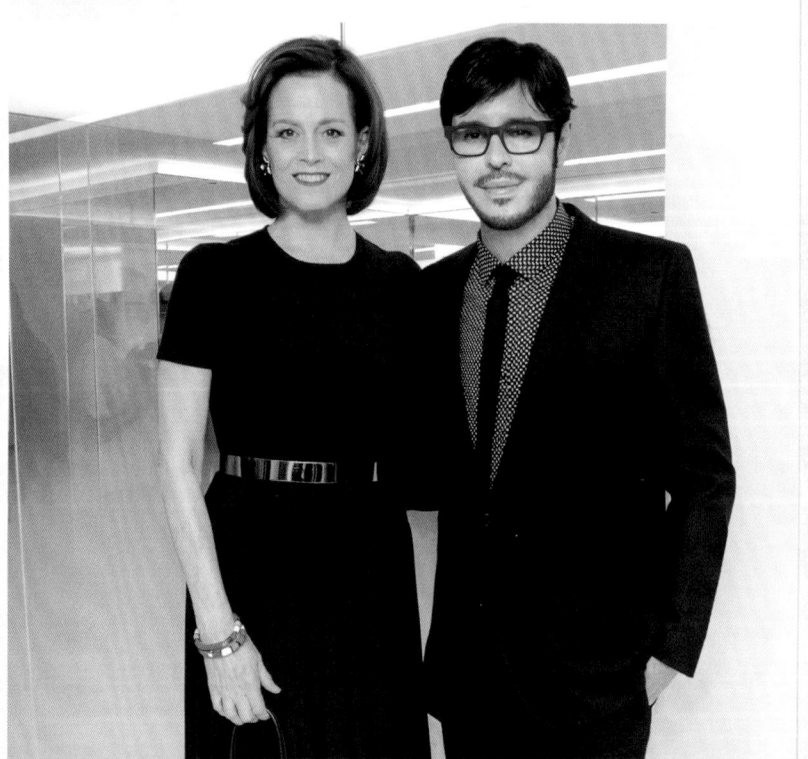

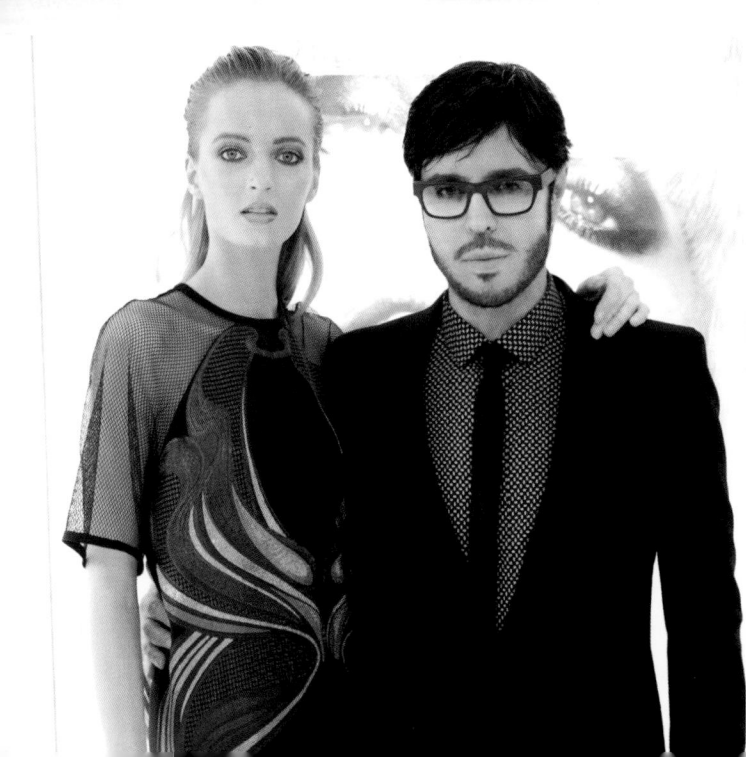

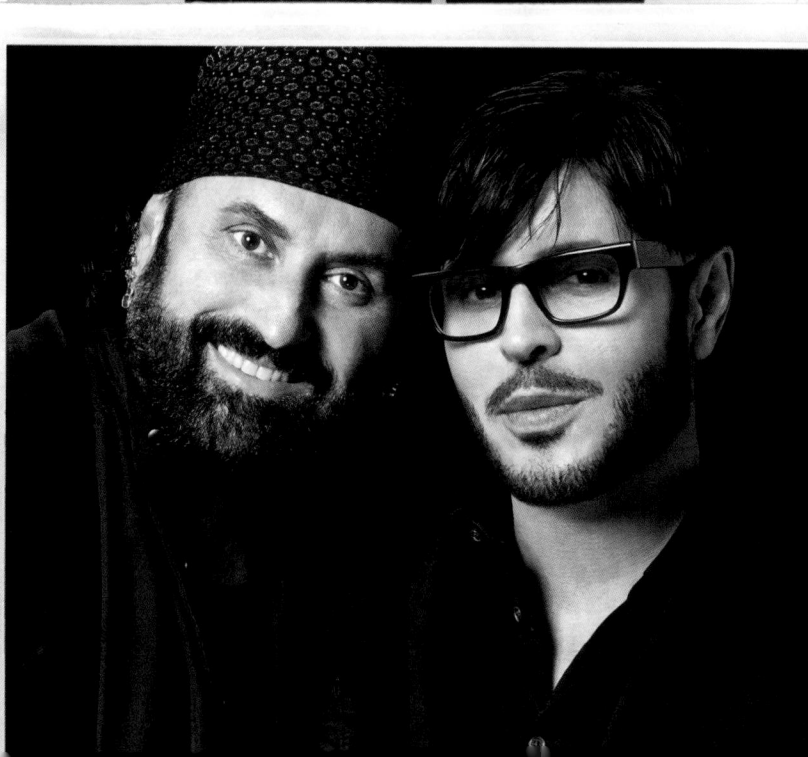

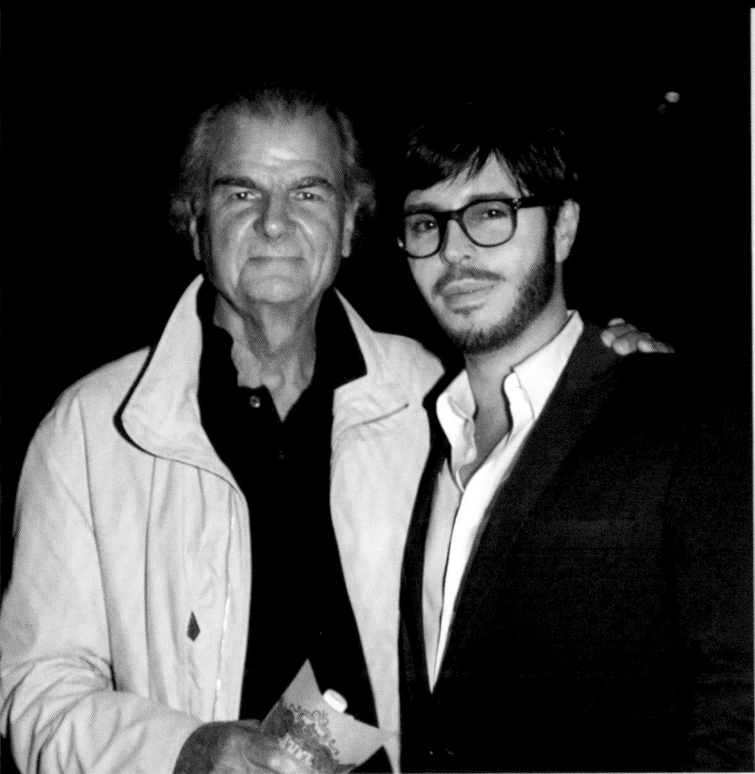

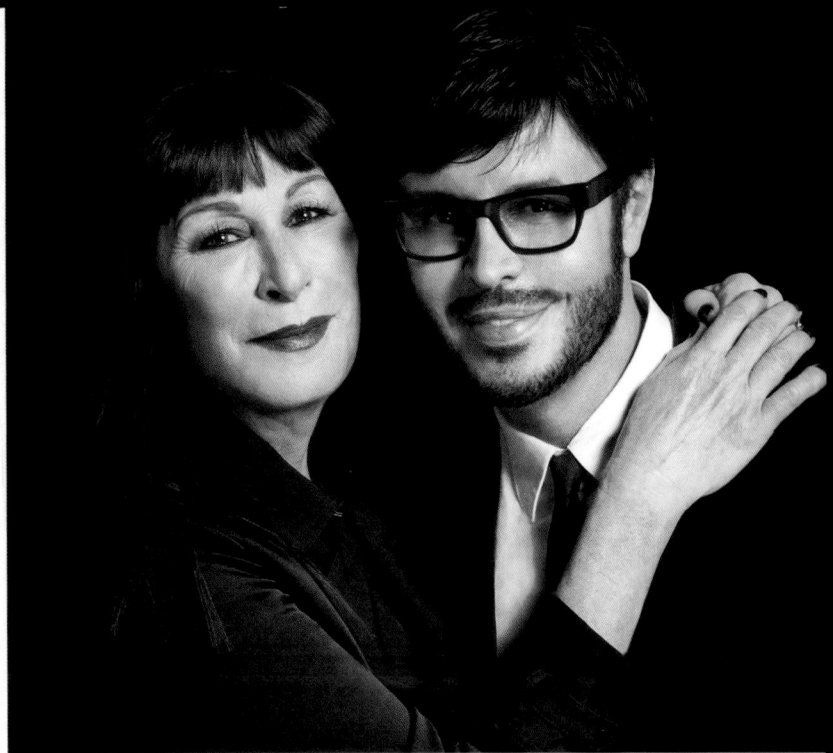

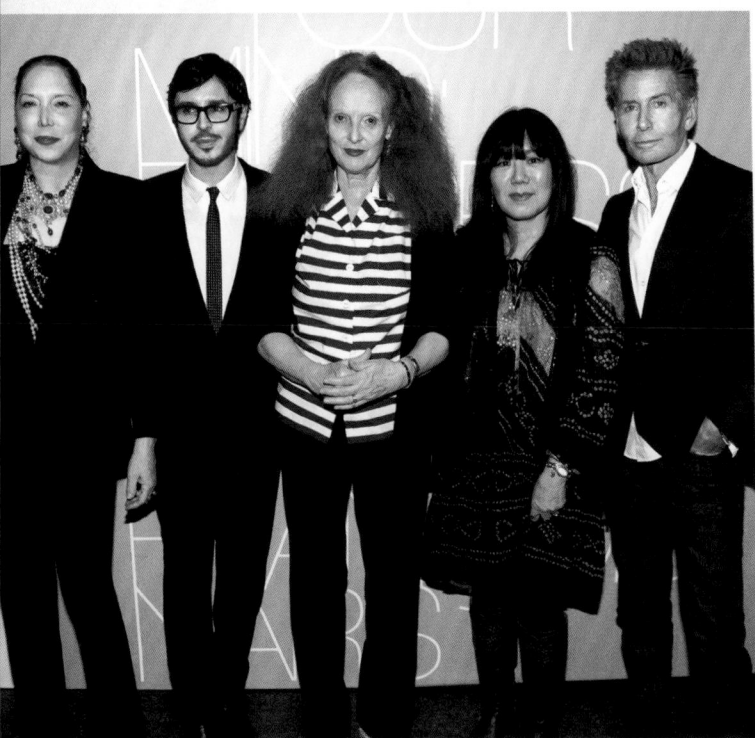

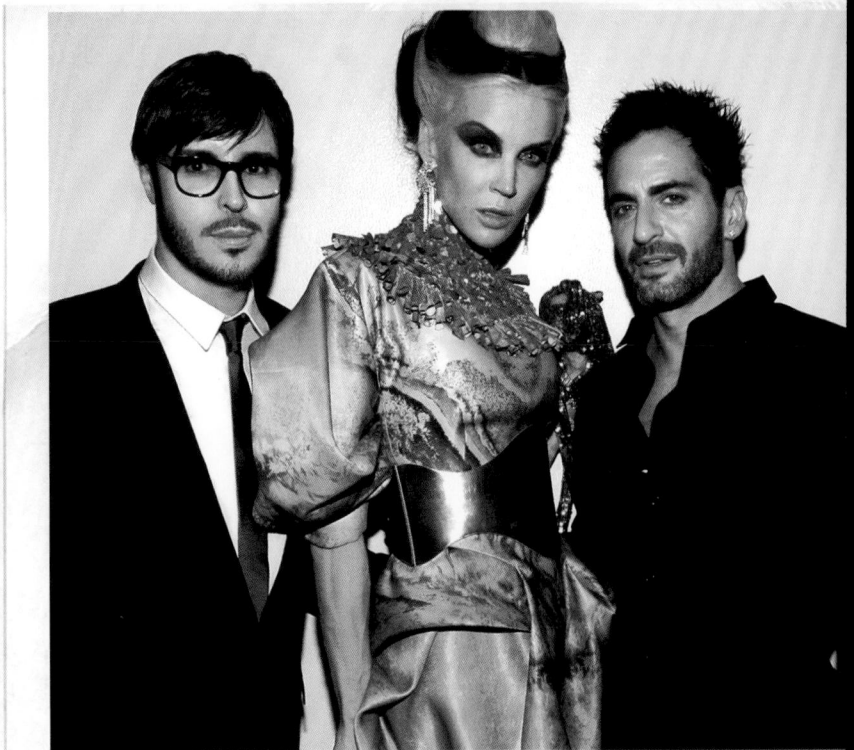

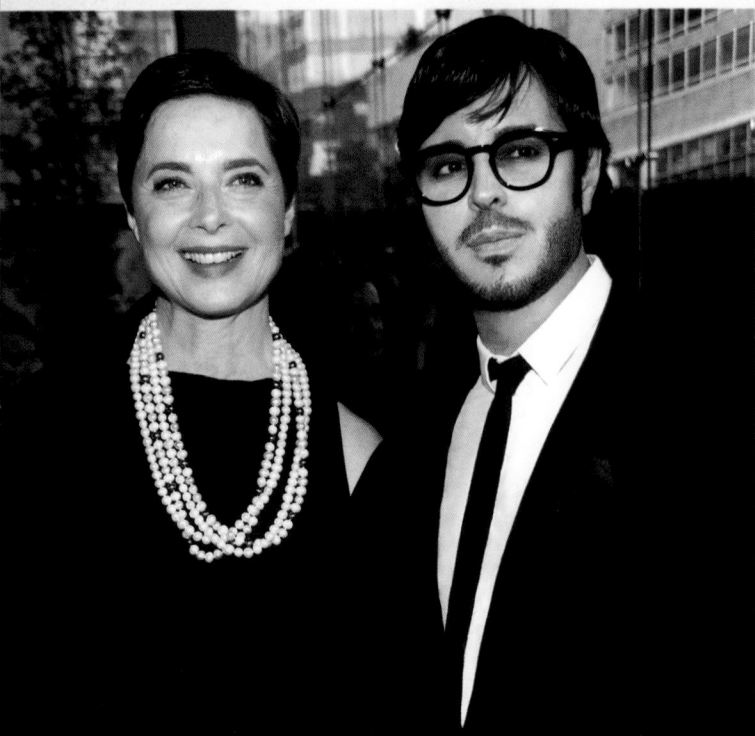

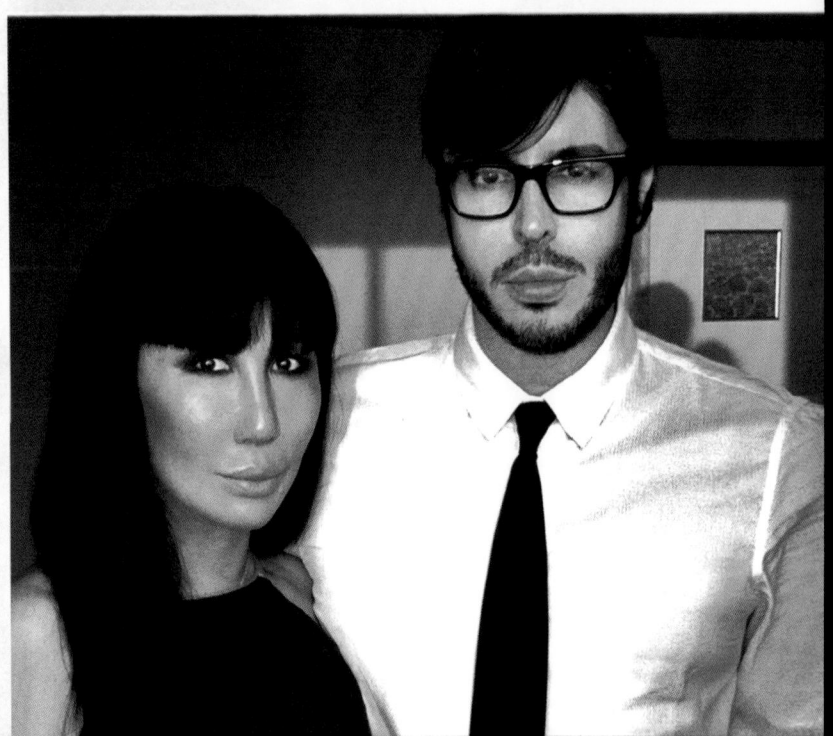

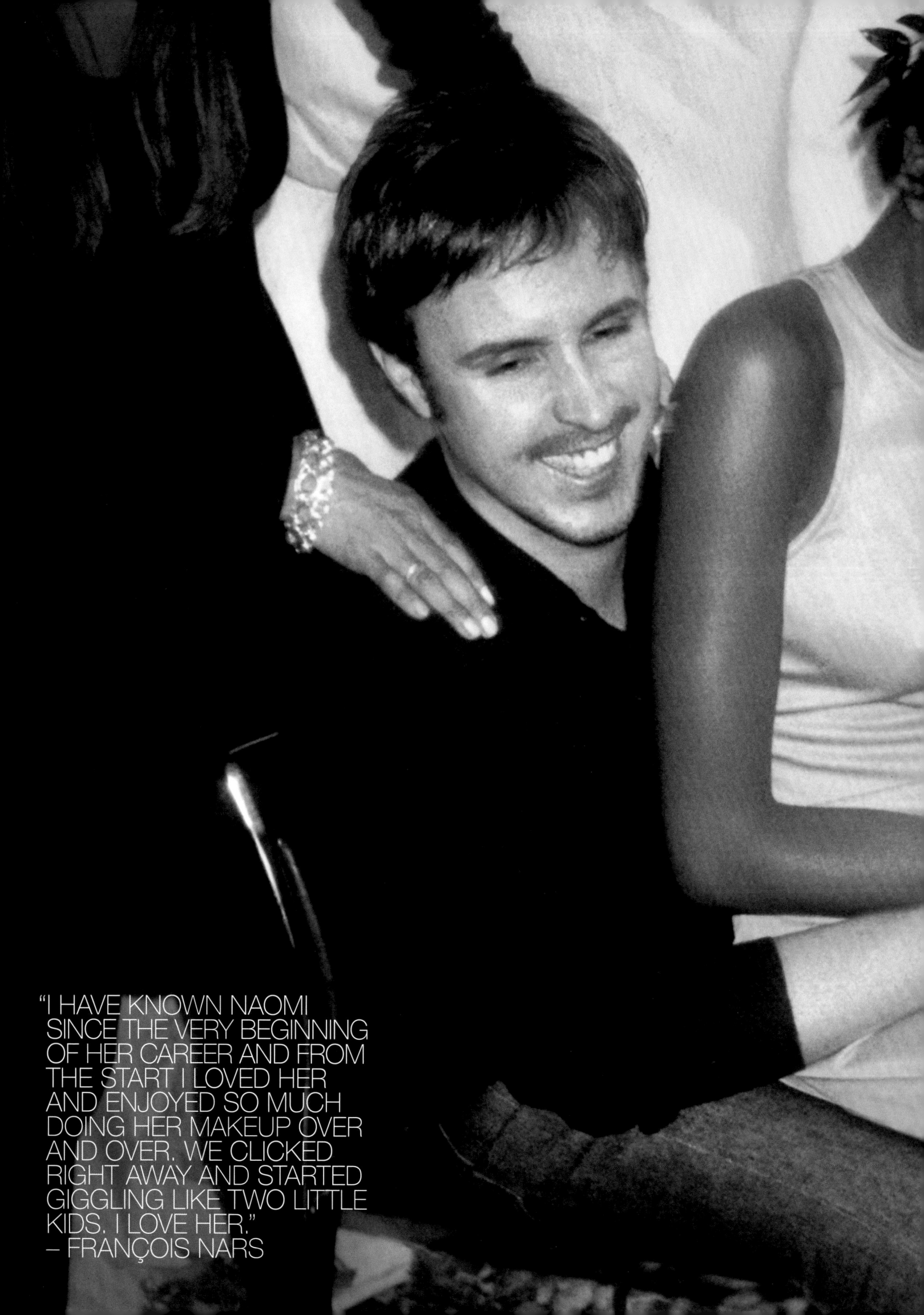

"I HAVE KNOWN NAOMI
SINCE THE VERY BEGINNING
OF HER CAREER AND FROM
THE START I LOVED HER
AND ENJOYED SO MUCH
DOING HER MAKEUP OVER
AND OVER. WE CLICKED
RIGHT AWAY AND STARTED
GIGGLING LIKE TWO LITTLE
KIDS. I LOVE HER."
— FRANÇOIS NARS

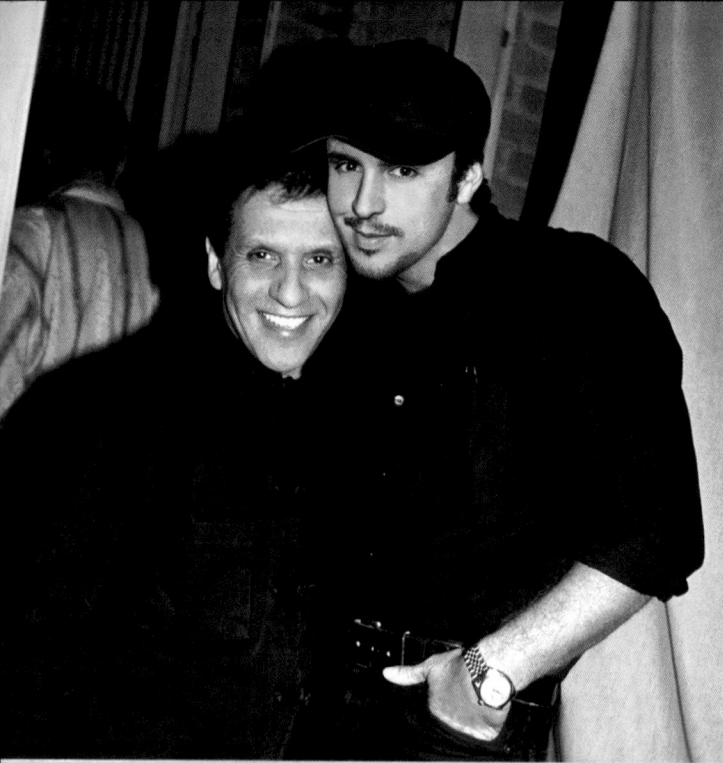

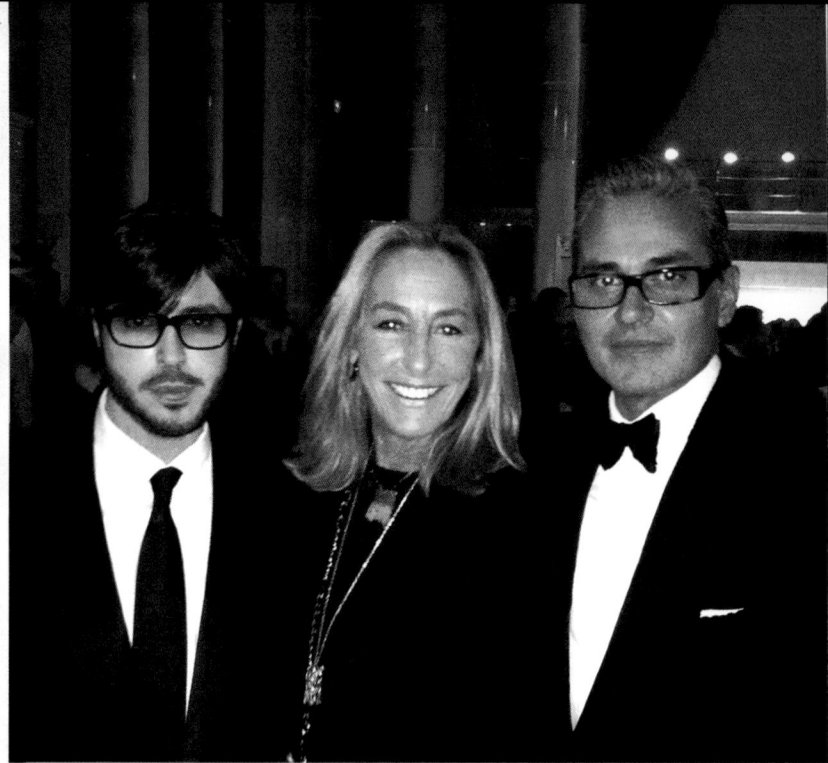

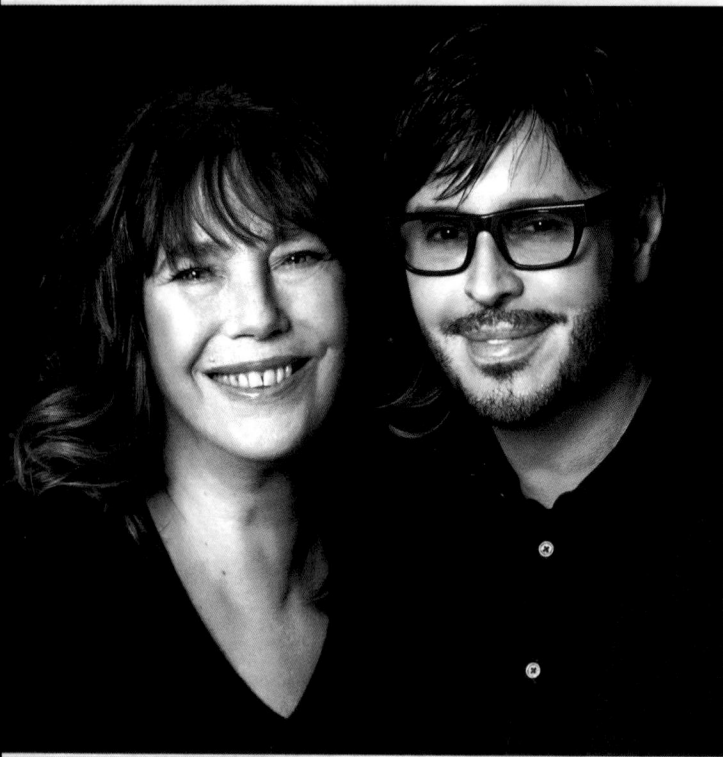

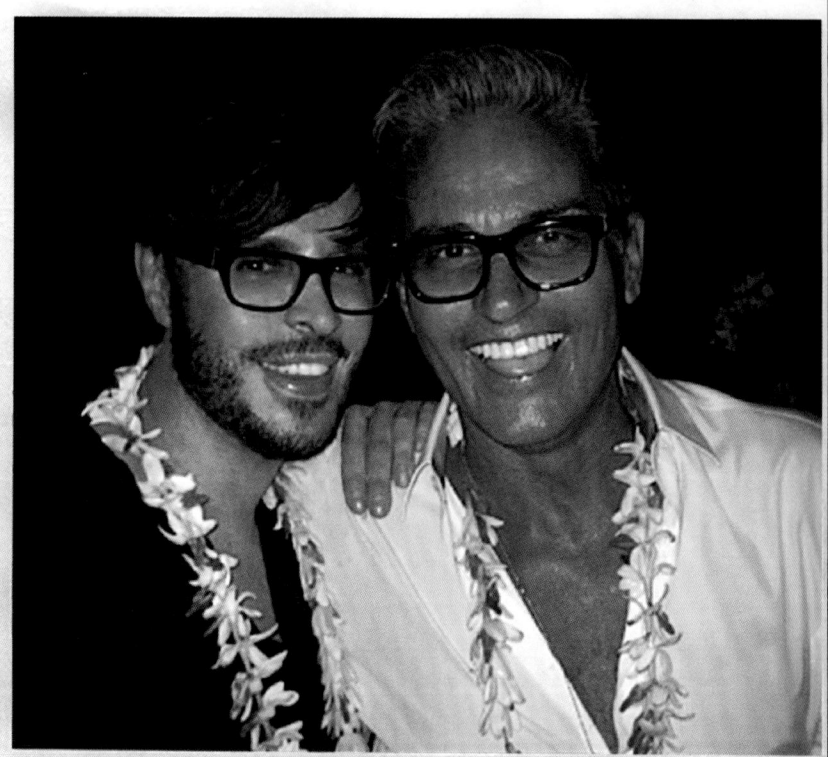

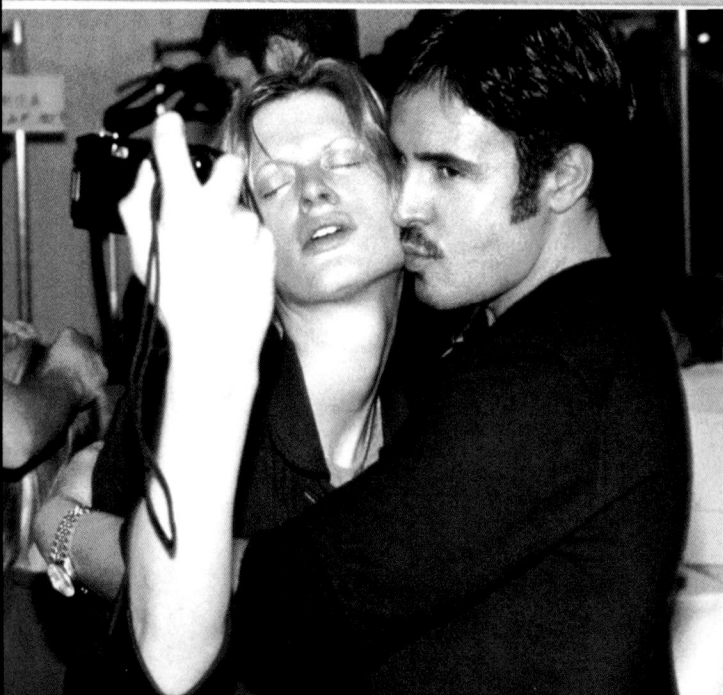

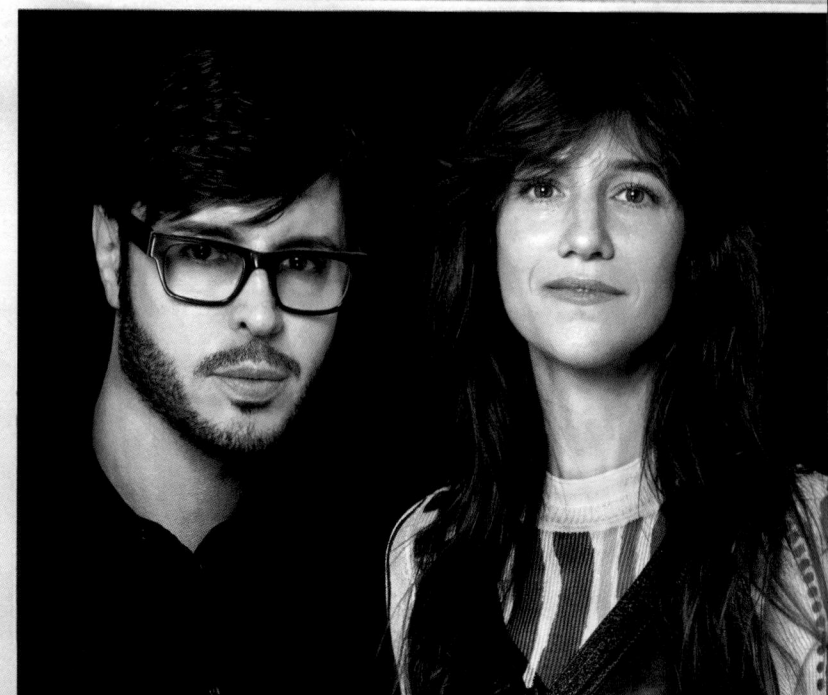

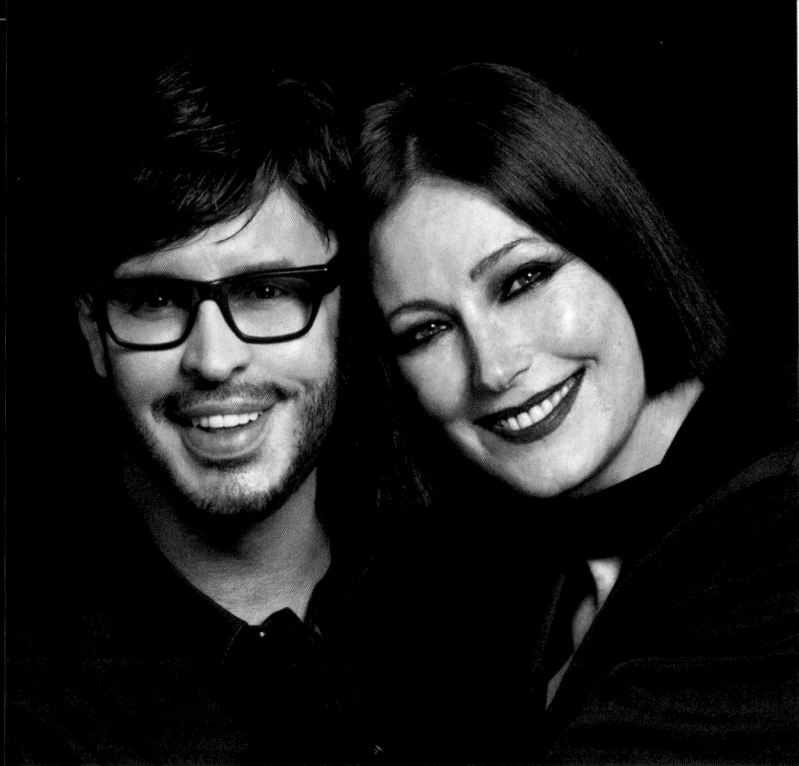

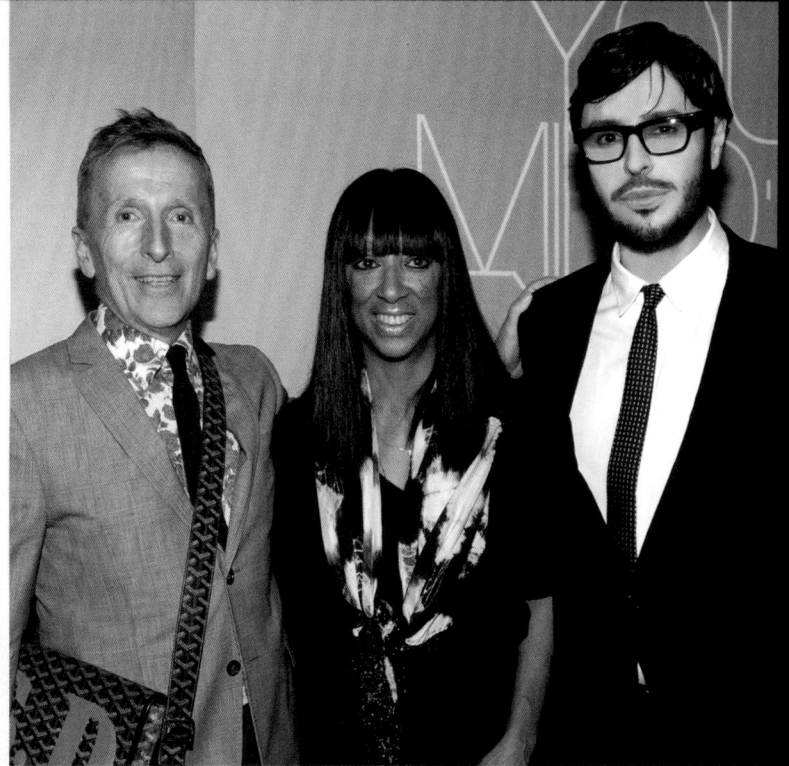

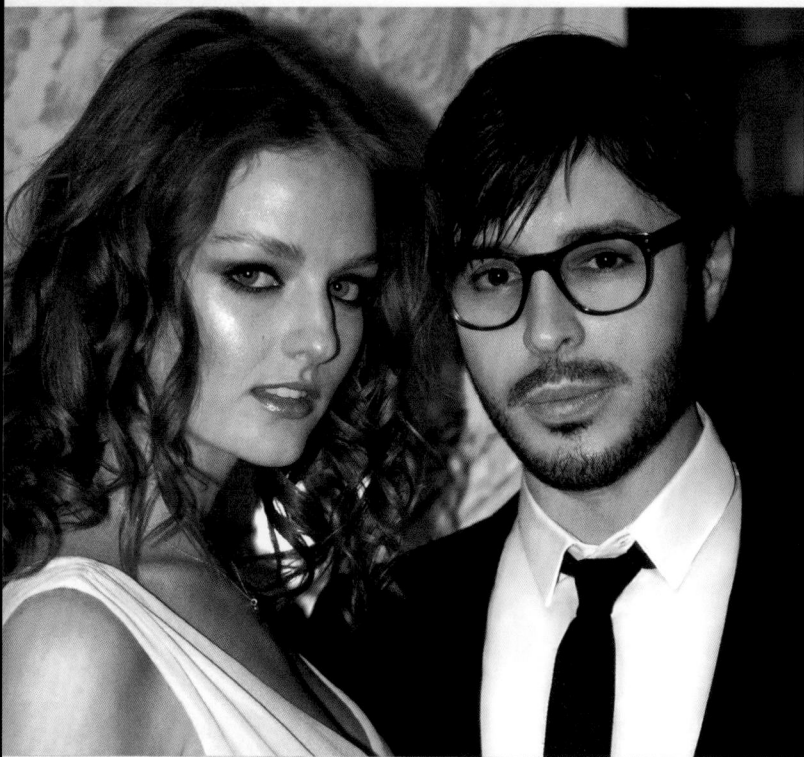

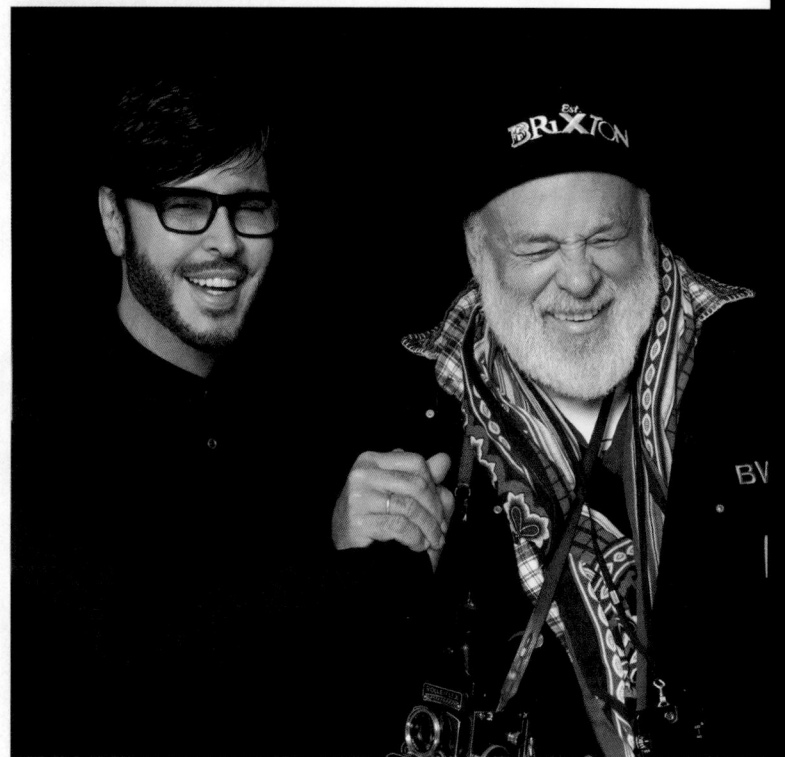

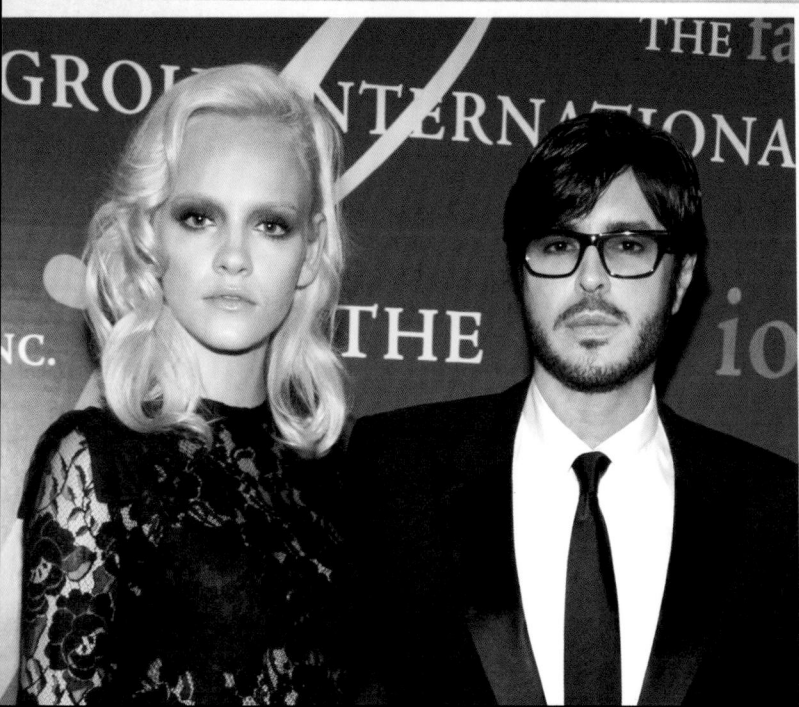

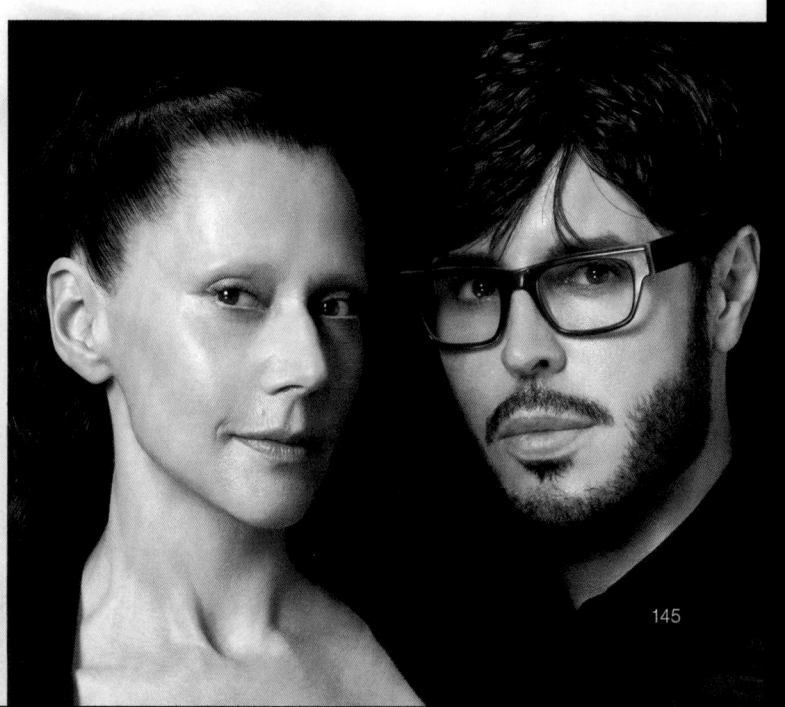

ARTISTRY AND PHOTOGRAPHY ARE INSEPARABLE TO FRANÇOIS NARS—"IT'S REALLY THE SAME APPROACH, MAKING THAT PERSON LOOK BEAUTIFUL." FRANÇOIS FIRST EXPLORED THE CONNECTION BETWEEN CREATING BEAUTY AND CAPTURING IT WITH NARS COSMETICS'S INAUGURAL CAMPAIGN IN 1996. "WE DIDN'T HAVE THE BUDGET TO HIRE SOMEBODY, SO I THOUGHT, 'WHAT THE HELL. GIVE ME A CAMERA.' IT TOOK A LOT OF WORK AND CONCENTRATION, BUT I WAS USED TO WORKING WITH SO MANY PHOTOGRAPHERS—AVEDON, PENN, NEWTON, MEISEL, AND COUNTLESS OTHERS." SO BEGAN FRANÇOIS'S LOVE OF THE LENS.

ALWAYS ALLOWING HIS INTUITIVE, IMAGINATIVE, AND CREATIVE INSTINCTS TO GUIDE HIM, FRANÇOIS'S VISION EXPANDS EVER DEEPER FROM EXERCISES IN LIGHT AND SHADOW, COLOR AND CONTOUR. CHARACTER IS EXALTED. PERSONALITY, PRONOUNCED. THIS NEW DIMENSION FUELS HIS MASTERY WITH A RICHNESS THAT ONLY AN ARTIST UNDERSTANDS, THE RESULTS OF WHICH ALWAYS INFORM HIS MAKEUP FORMULAS. "I KNOW WHAT I LIKE, AND I KNOW WHAT I DON'T LIKE. I'M VERY BLACK-AND-WHITE IN THAT WAY," HE SAYS.

TO FRANÇOIS, PHOTOGRAPHY IS ANOTHER VEHICLE TO EXERCISE HIS CREATIVE VISION. WITH NEARLY TWO DECADES OF NARS SHOOTS BEHIND HIM, HE CONTINUES TO PHOTOGRAPH EVERY ICONIC IMAGE FOR THE BRAND, AS WELL AS REGULARLY CAPTURE FASHION EDITORIALS FOR INTERNATIONAL EDITIONS OF *VOGUE*. HIS PUBLISHED COLLECTIONS INCLUDE *X-RAY*, AN ANTHOLOGY OF RICHLY STYLED PORTRAITS OF TASTEMAKERS AND CELEBRITIES, INCLUDING KATE MOSS, CARINE ROITFELD, ALEXANDER MCQUEEN, AND DONATELLA VERSACE. *MAKEUP YOUR MIND* AND *MAKEUP YOUR MIND: EXPRESS YOURSELF* REINVENT THE BEAUTY MANUAL WITH VIVID BEFORE-AND-AFTERS, WHILE *NARS 15X15* CELEBRATES ICONIC BEAUTY WITH A KALEIDOSCOPIC ALBUM OF CELEBRITY PORTRAITS DONE AS CHARACTERS INSPIRED BY NARS SHADES. EACH IS UNIQUE IN ITS CONCEPT, BUT SHARES FRANÇOIS'S PLAYFUL PERSPECTIVE: "DON'T BE SO SERIOUS; IT'S ONLY MAKEUP."

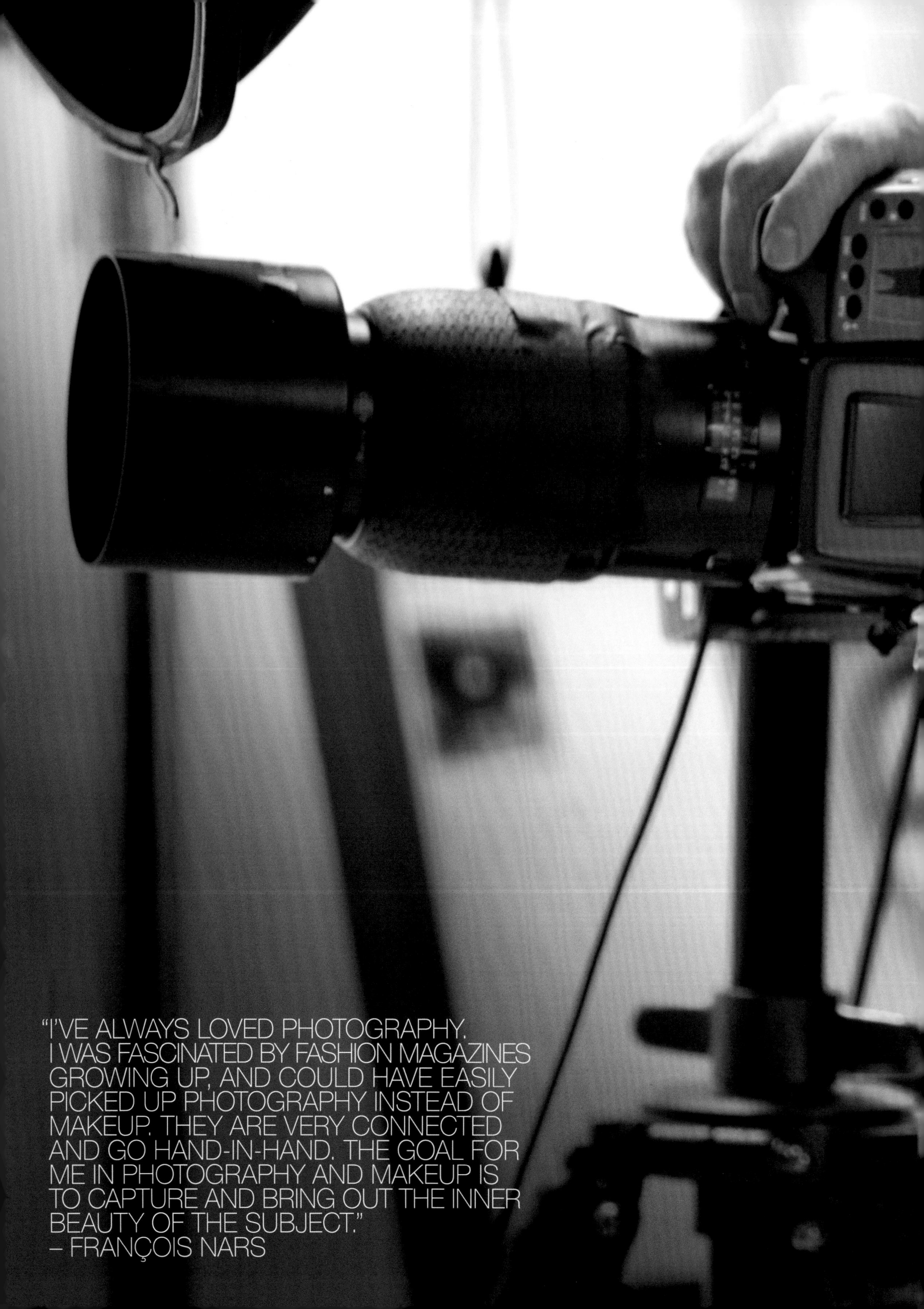

"I'VE ALWAYS LOVED PHOTOGRAPHY.
I WAS FASCINATED BY FASHION MAGAZINES
GROWING UP, AND COULD HAVE EASILY
PICKED UP PHOTOGRAPHY INSTEAD OF
MAKEUP. THEY ARE VERY CONNECTED
AND GO HAND-IN-HAND. THE GOAL FOR
ME IN PHOTOGRAPHY AND MAKEUP IS
TO CAPTURE AND BRING OUT THE INNER
BEAUTY OF THE SUBJECT."
– FRANÇOIS NARS

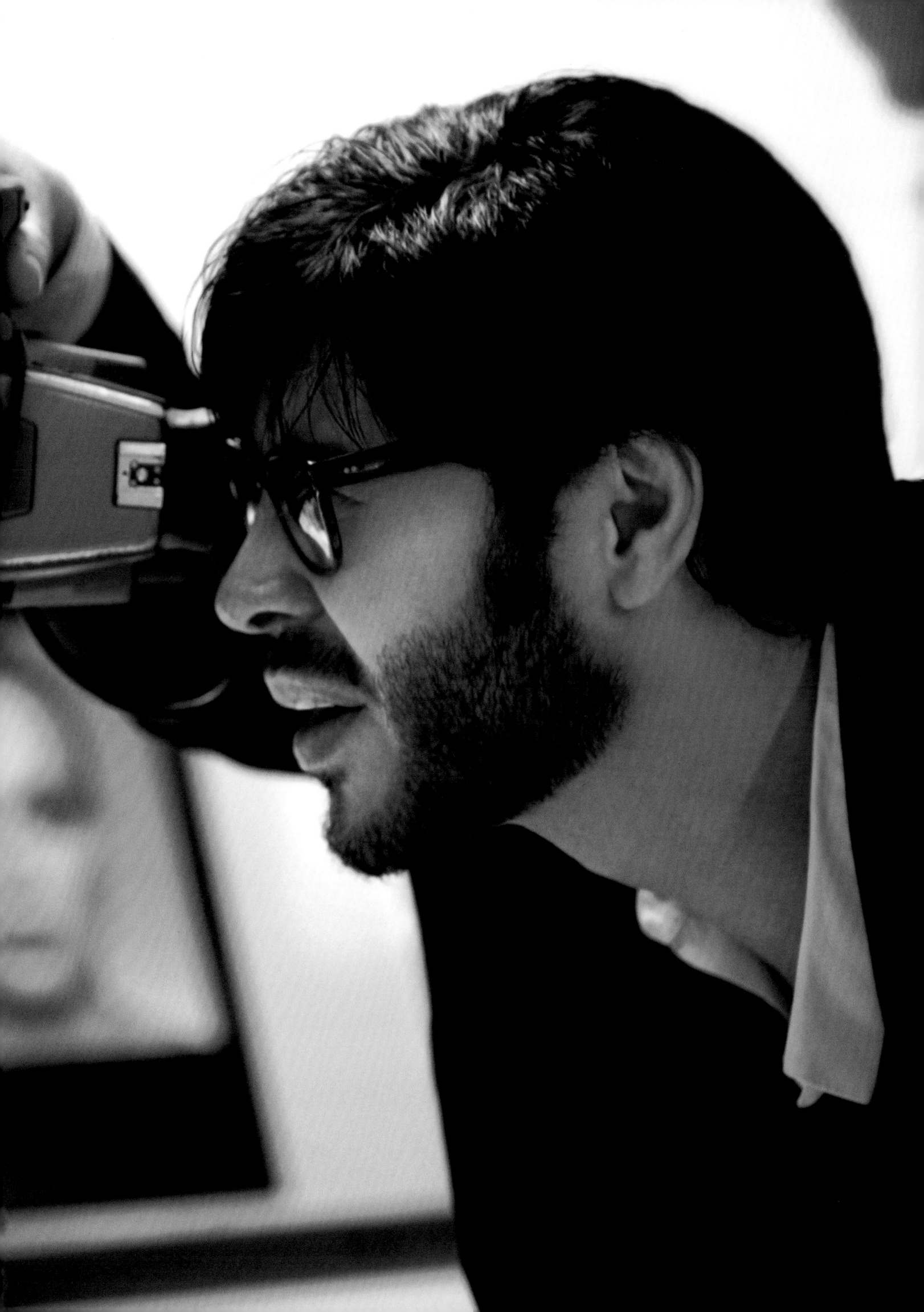

"DISCERNING THE PHOTOGRAPHER,
DEFTLY THE MASTER MAKEUP MAGICIAN,
FRANÇOIS GIVES HIS PERSONAL TOUCH
THROUGH THE COLORS AND SHADES OF
HIS ASTONISHING PALETTE. HE IS TRULY
THE MAN BEHIND HIS MAGIC."
– CHARLOTTE RAMPLING

"I WAS AROUND TWELVE YEARS OLD WHEN I
SAW CHARLOTTE FOR THE FIRST TIME. IT WAS
IN LUCHINO VISCONTI'S MASTERPIECE *THE
DAMNED*. I WAS IMMEDIATELY MESMERIZED BY
HER PRESENCE, HER BEAUTY, HER NATURAL
ELEGANCE. IT WAS LOVE AT FIRST SIGHT.
CHARLOTTE IS UNIQUE, SHE FACINATES ME
ALWAYS. THERE IS NOBODY ELSE LIKE HER."
– FRANÇOIS NARS

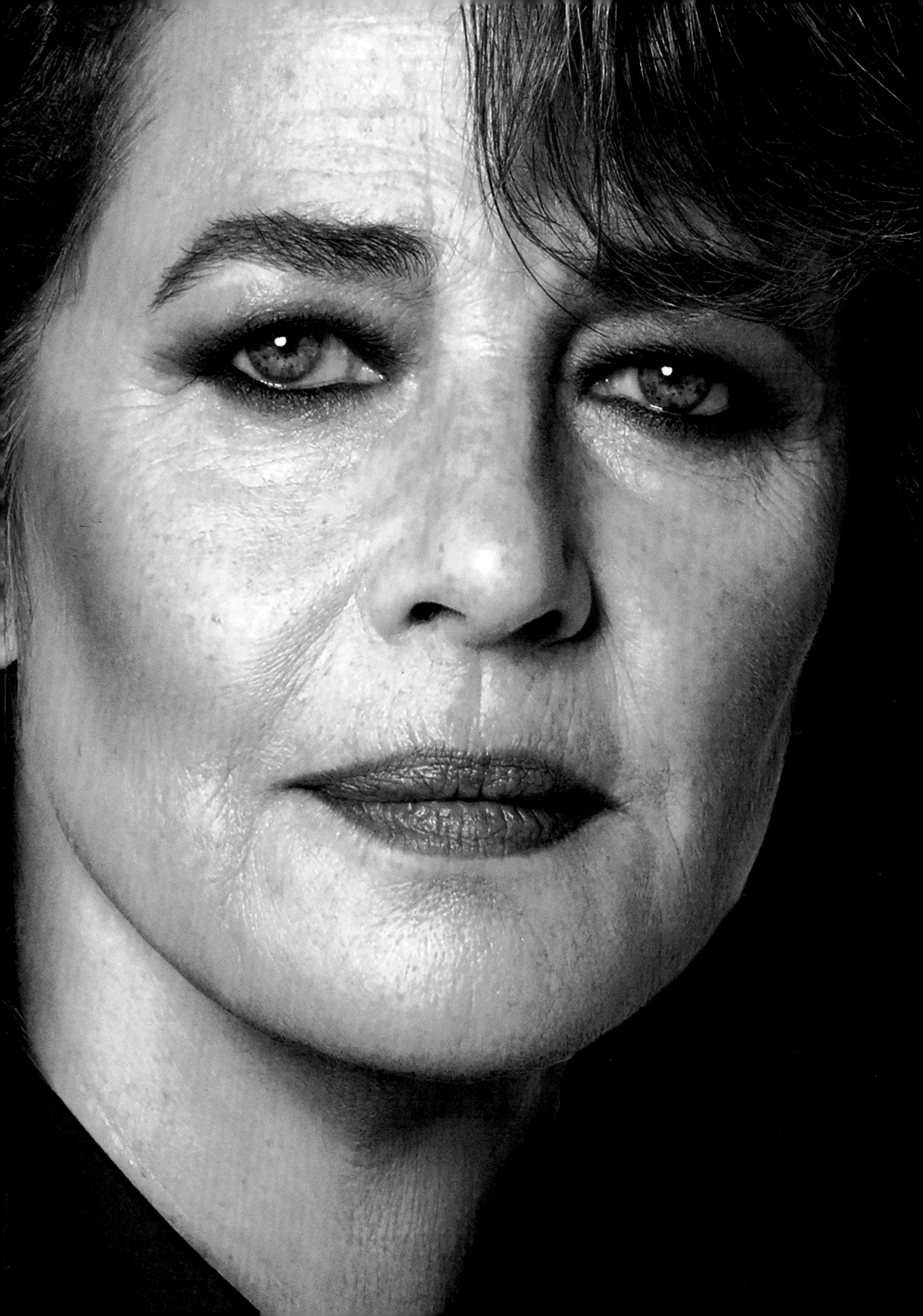

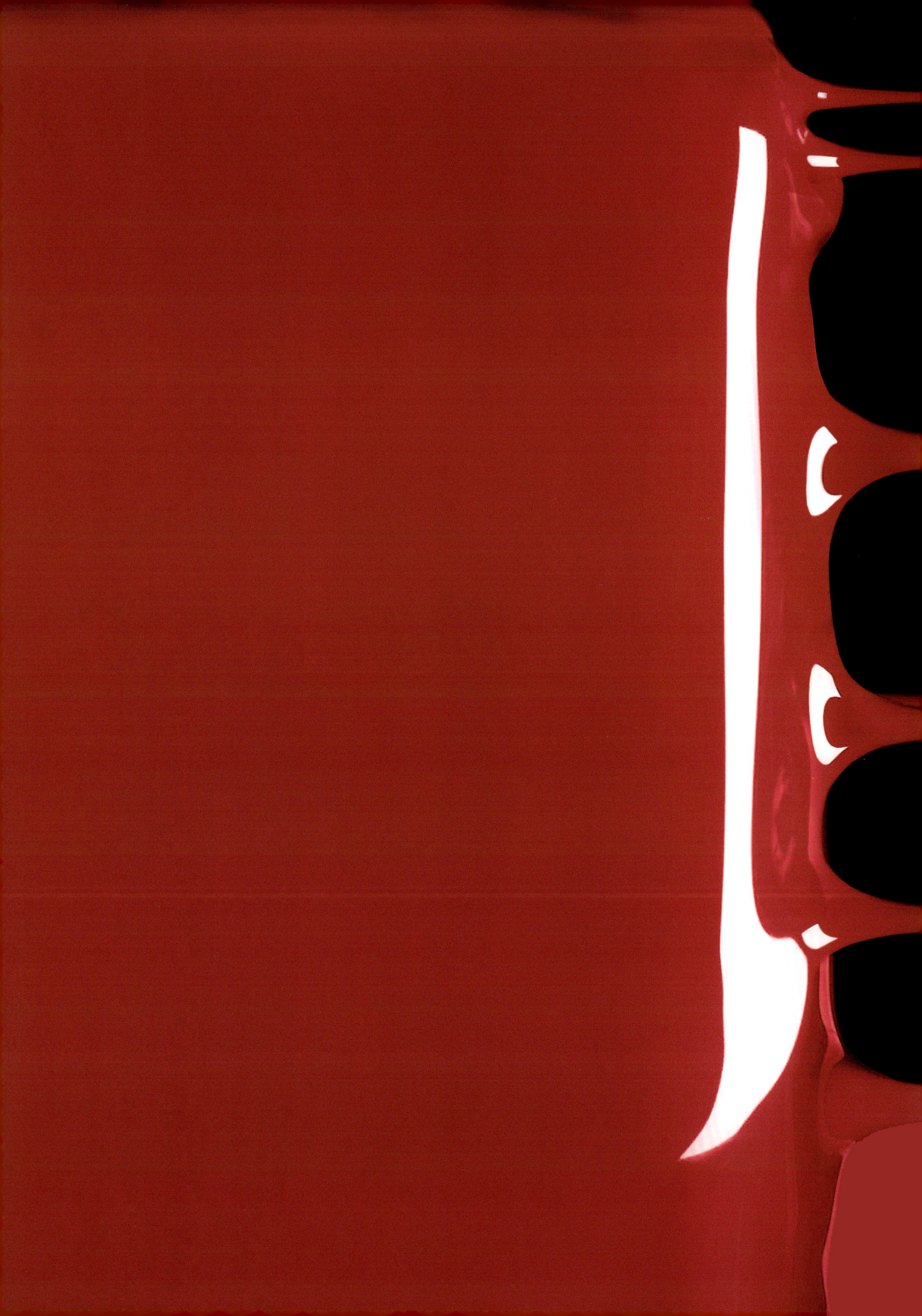

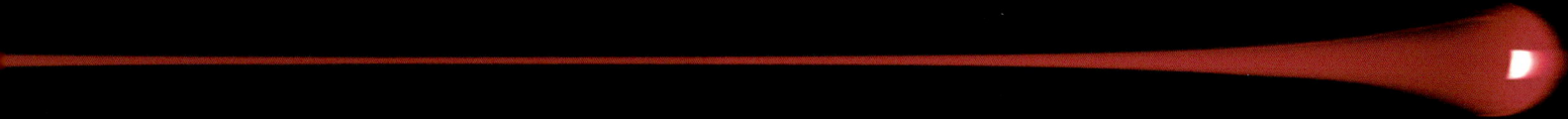

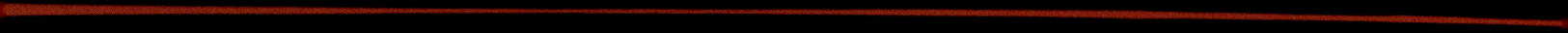

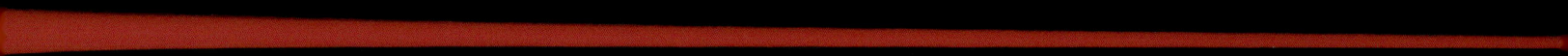

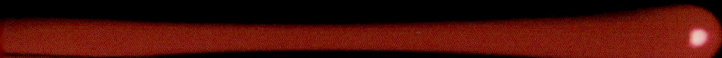

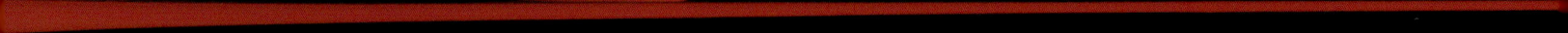

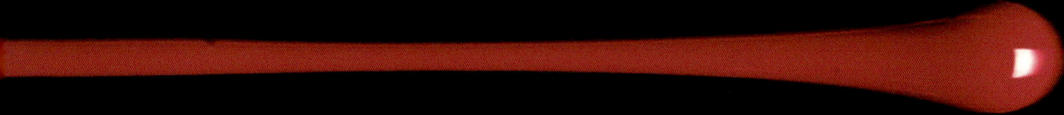

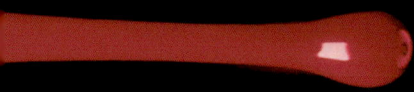

"I LOVE BEING PROVOCATIVE WHEN IT COMES
TO CREATING LOOKS AND SHADES FOR
NARS, BUT I ALSO LOVE CLASSICAL, BASIC
COLORS. THERE ARE TWO SIDES IN ME,
THE SHOCKER AND THE TRADITIONALIST."
– FRANÇOIS NARS

"OVER THE MANY YEARS OF COLLABORATING WITH FRANÇOIS ON CREATING THE BEAUTY LOOKS FOR OUR SHOWS, THE PROCESS IS CONSISTENT. AT THE BEGINNING OF OUR DIALOGUE WE NEVER KNOW EXACTLY WHERE WE ARE GOING, BUT ONE THING IS CERTAIN—THE GIRLS ARE ALWAYS GOING TO LOOK THEIR MOST BEAUTIFUL ONCE FRANÇOIS BRINGS HIS HAND AND VISION TO THE LOOK! WHETHER NO MAKEUP, A FULL FACE OF MAKEUP, OR ANYWHERE IN BETWEEN, HIS WORK IS THE PERFECT FINISH TO THE STORY WE ARE TELLING. FRANÇOIS'S CULTURAL REFERENCES, HIS KNOWLEDGE, HIS SKILL, AND HIS IMAGINATION COUPLED WITH THE INTEGRITY AND PRIDE HE BRINGS TO HIS WORK IS PRECISE AND UNIQUE. FRANÇOIS AND HIS WORK HAVE ALWAYS BEEN AND REMAIN A TRUE INSPIRATION TO ME." — MARC JACOBS

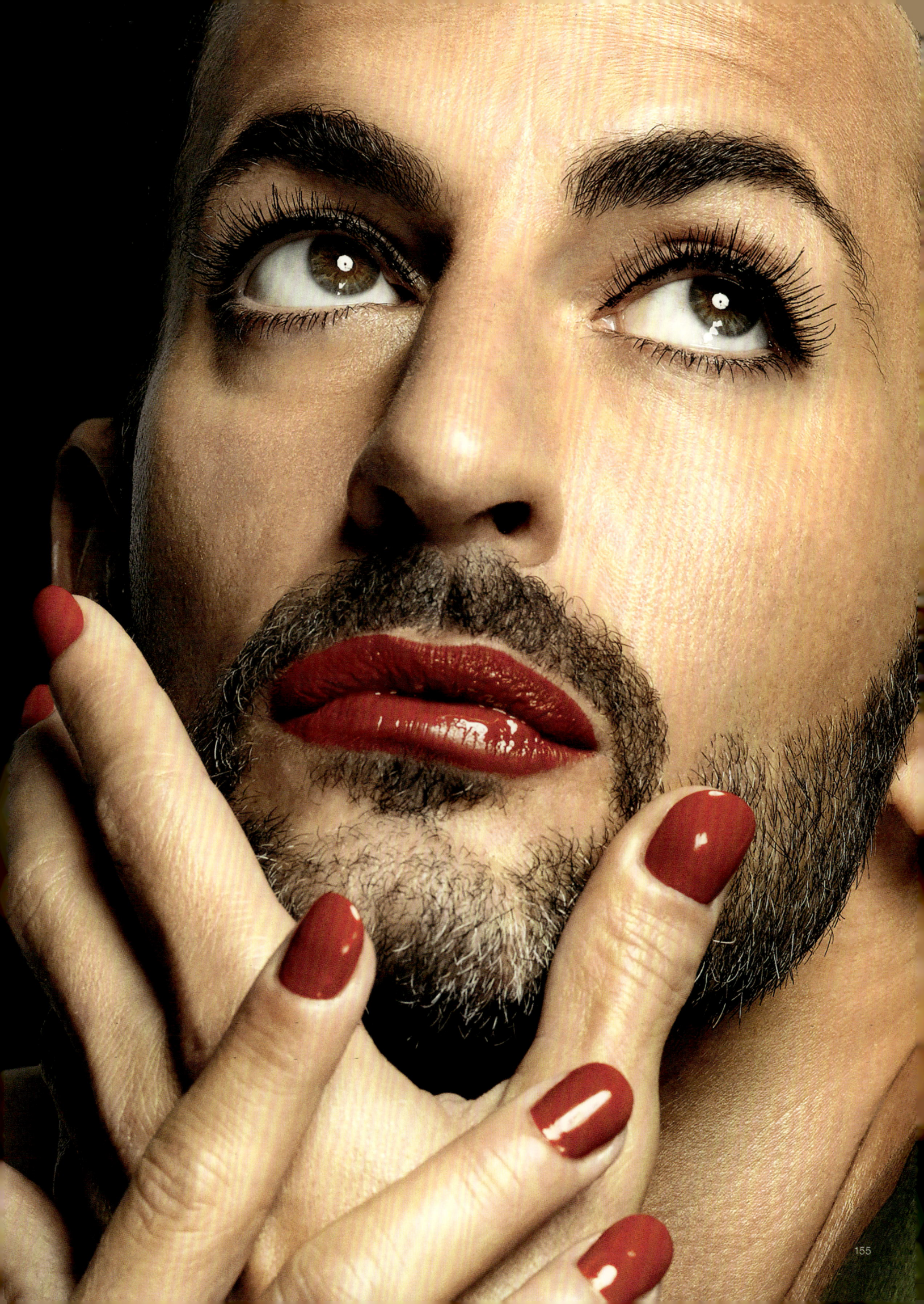

"I'VE ALWAYS LOVED, SINCE THE BEGINNING OF MY CAREER, COLLABORATING WITH DESIGNERS AND CREATING MAKEUP LOOKS FOR THE CATWALK. REUNITING WITH MARC JACOBS IN 2009 WAS EXCITING. IT FELT VERY FRESH AGAIN AND VERY CREATIVE. MARC IS SO MUCH FUN AND SO EXTREMELY TALENTED, A DREAM TO WORK WITH. WE UNDERSTAND EACH OTHER. I USUALLY CLICK VERY QUICKLY AFTER I TALK TO MARC AND SEE THE CLOTHES ABOUT A LOOK FOR THE SHOW. WE'RE ALWAYS ON THE SAME WAVELENGTH." — FRANÇOIS NARS

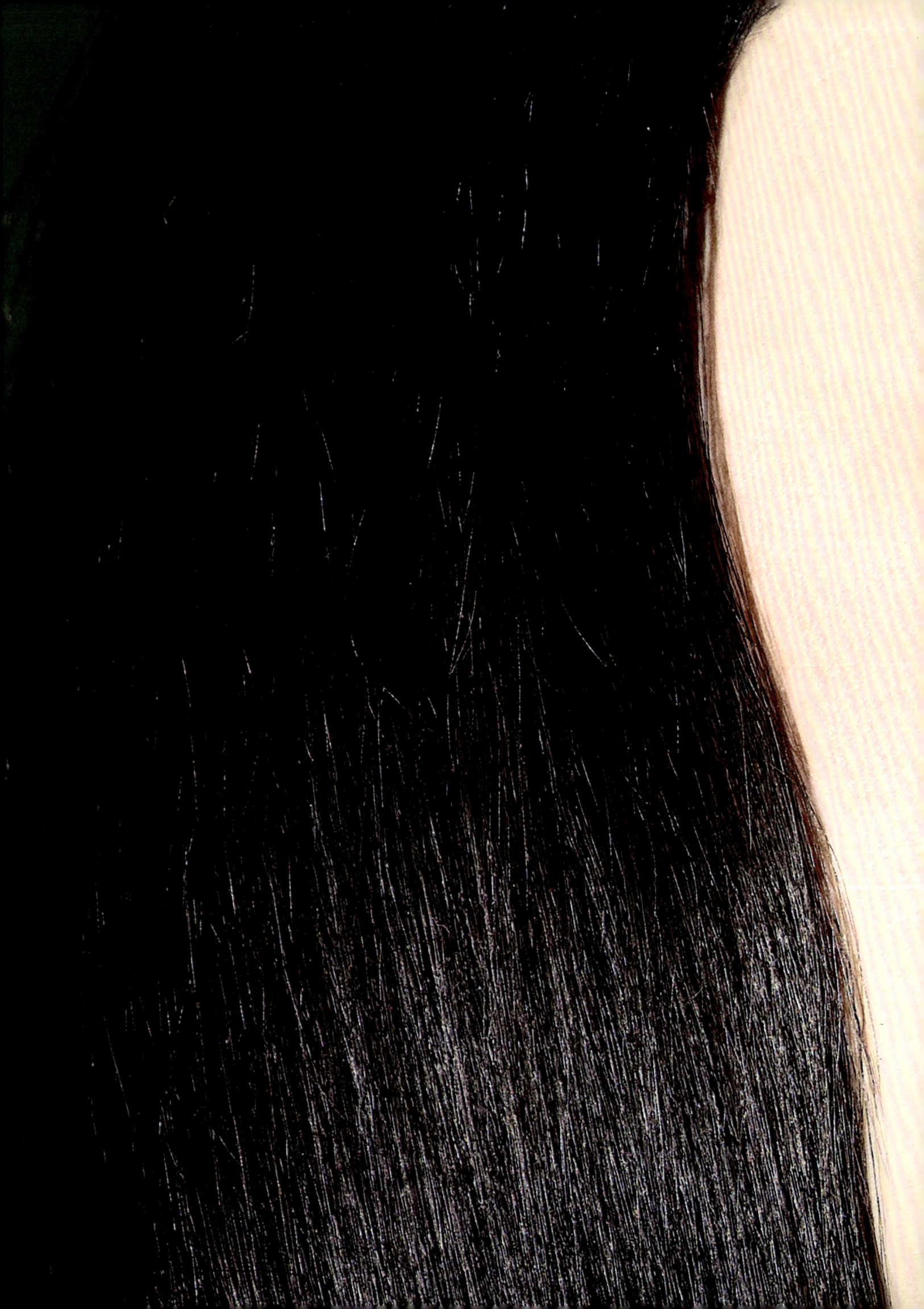

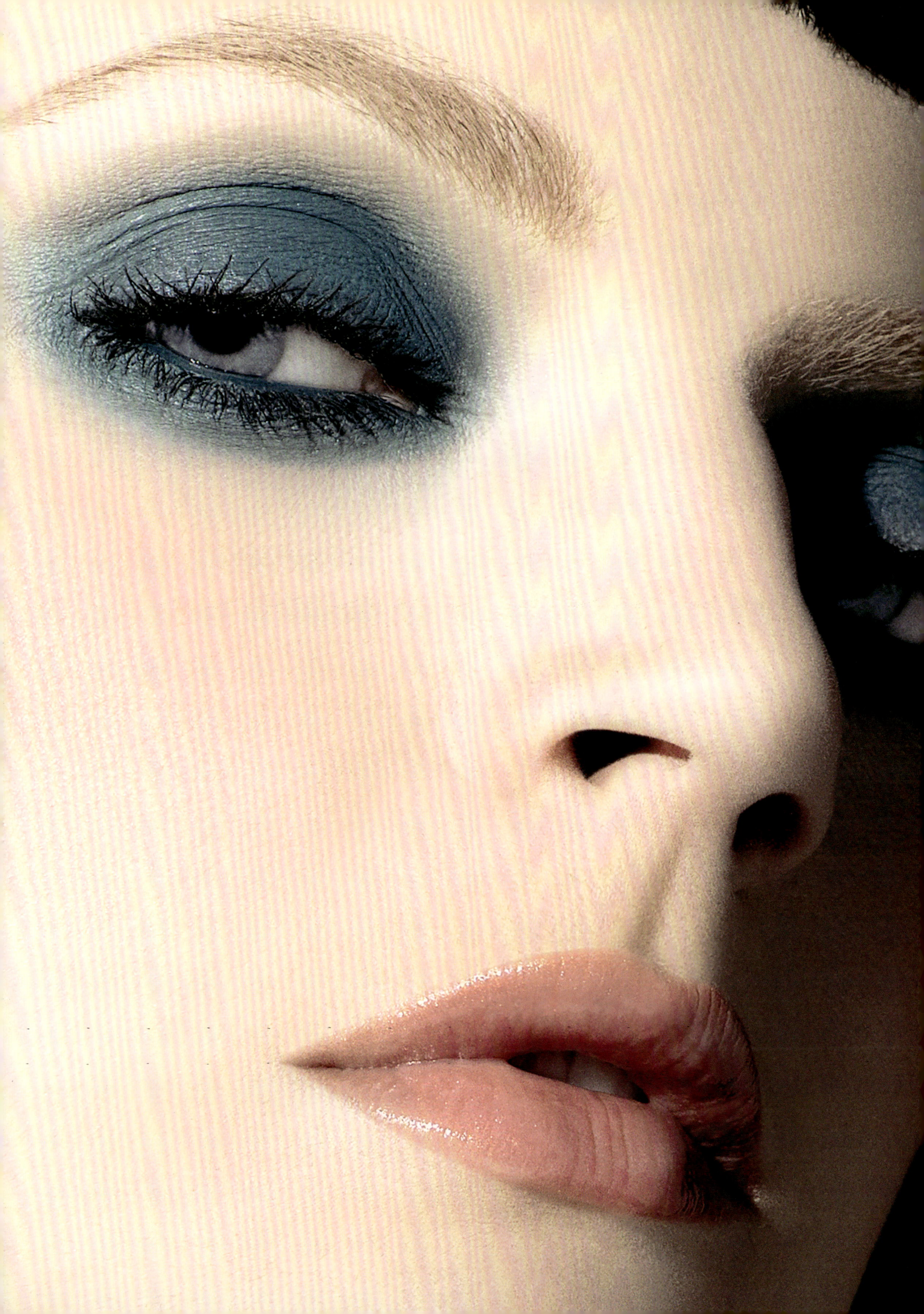

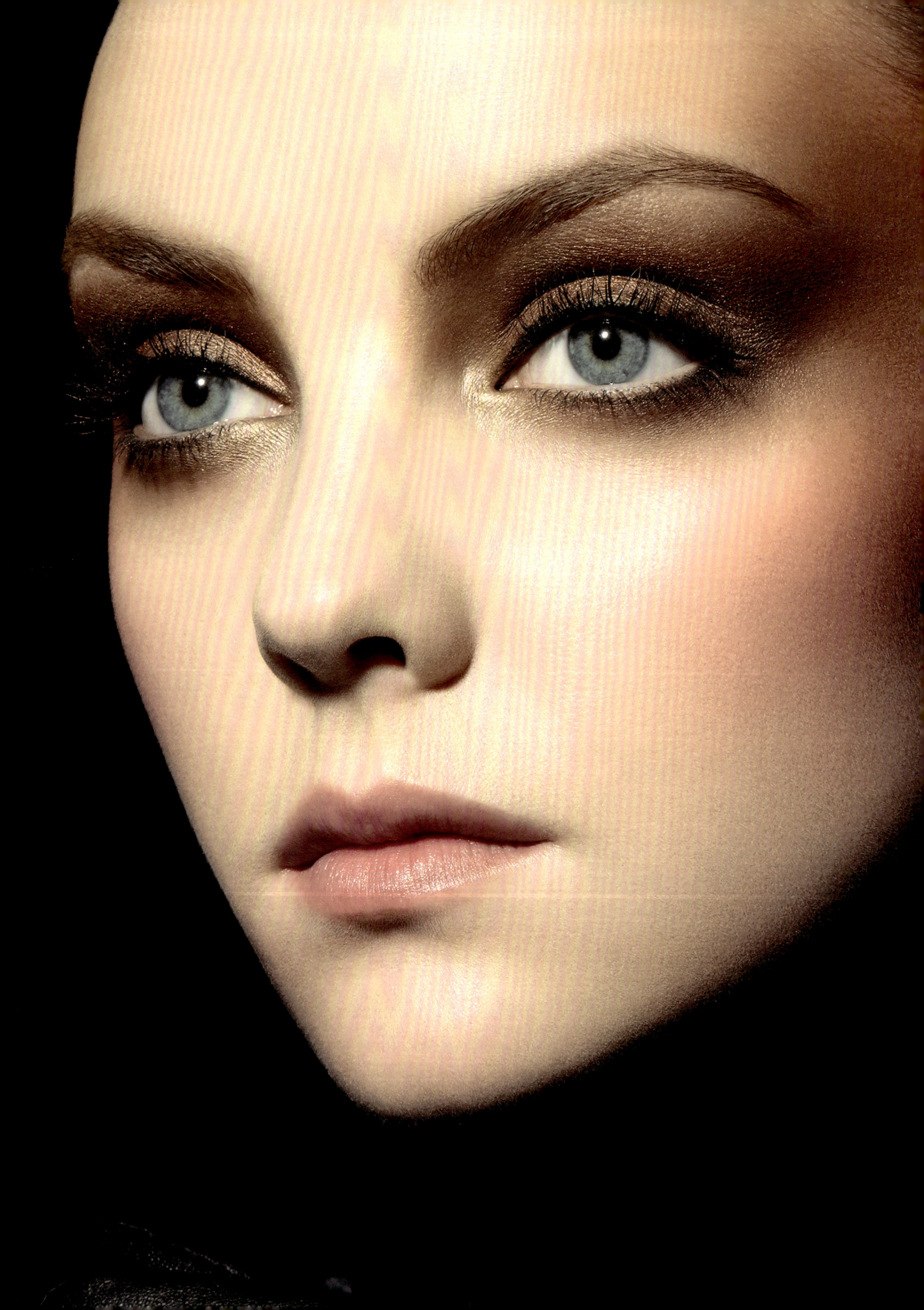

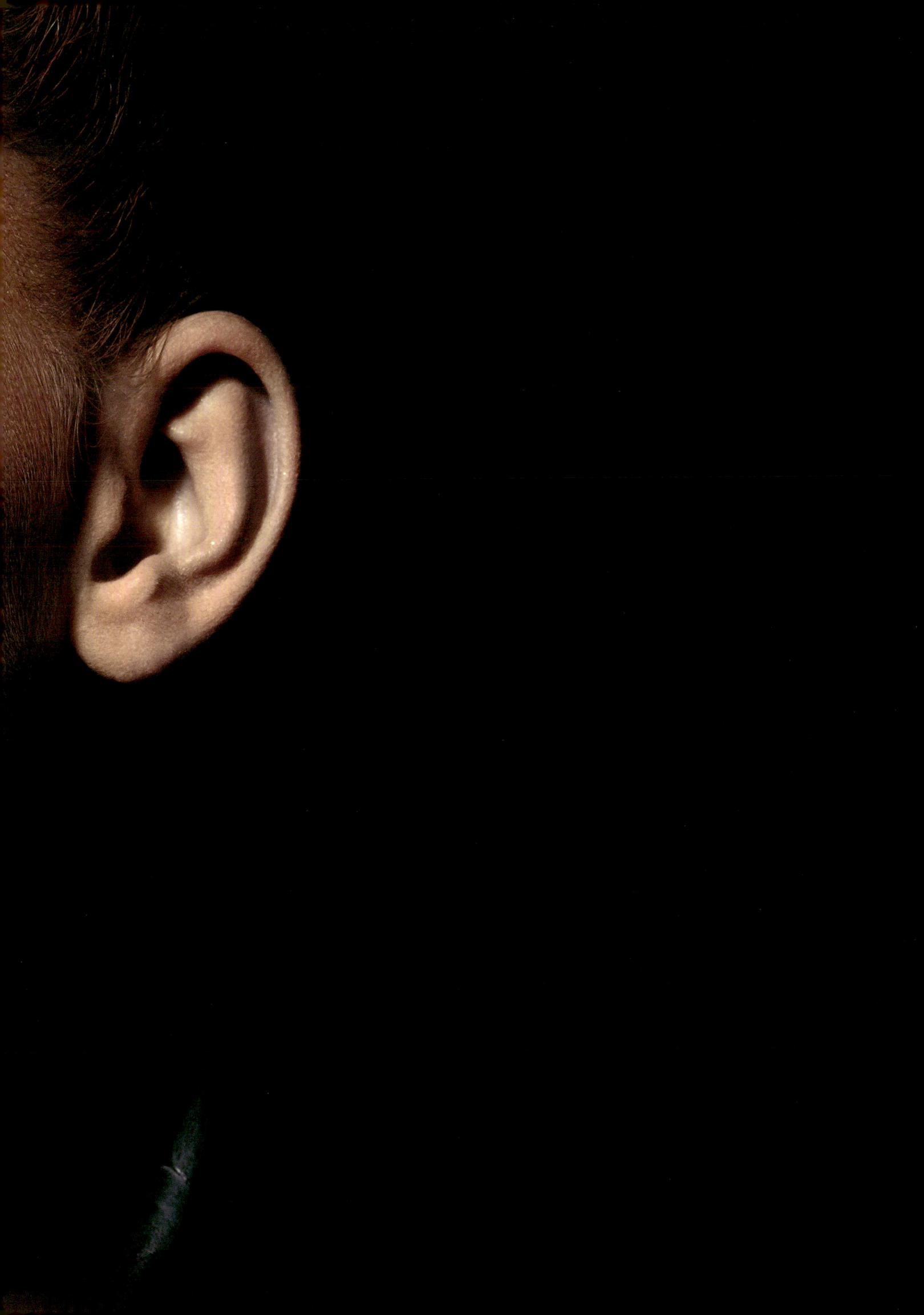

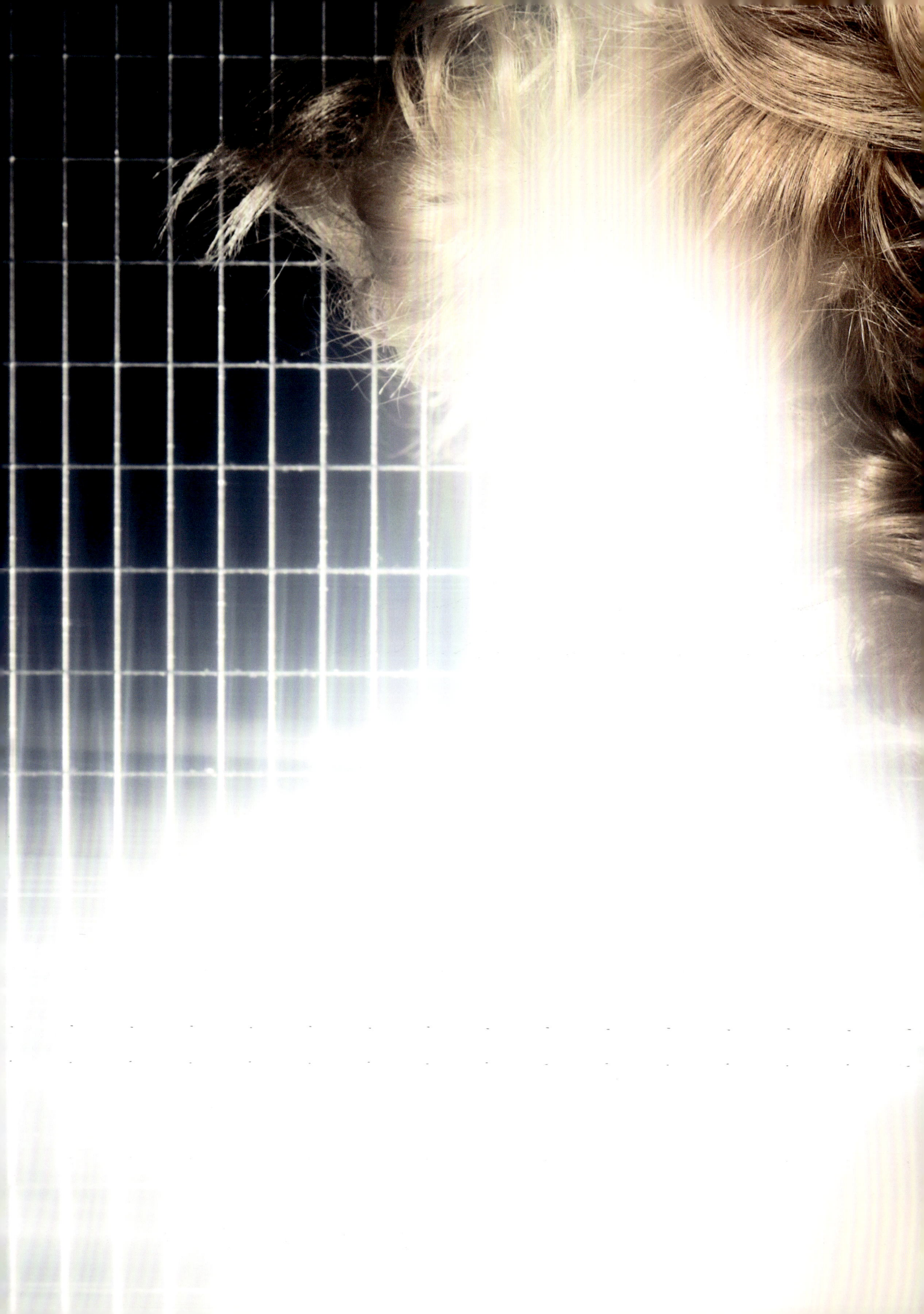

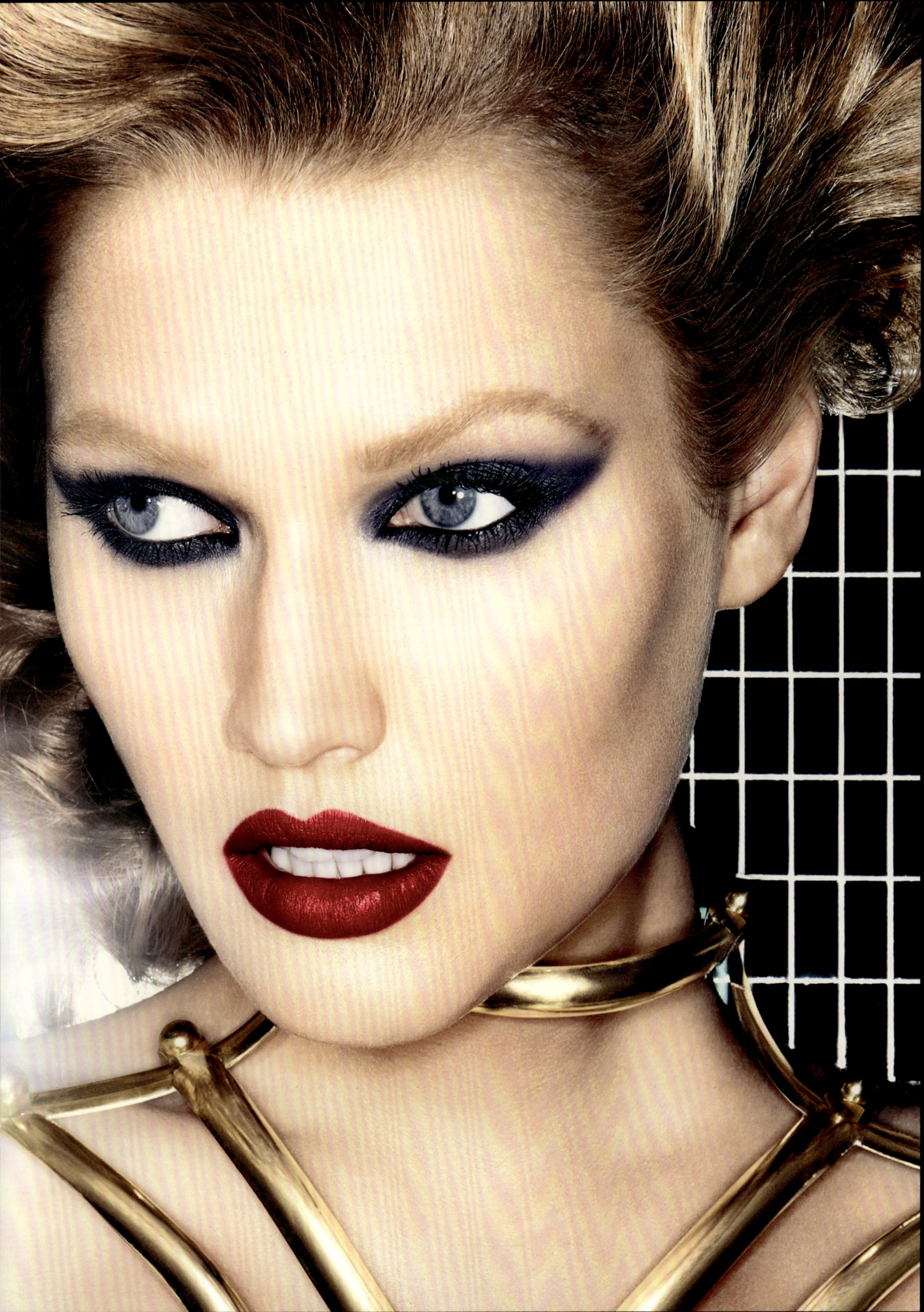

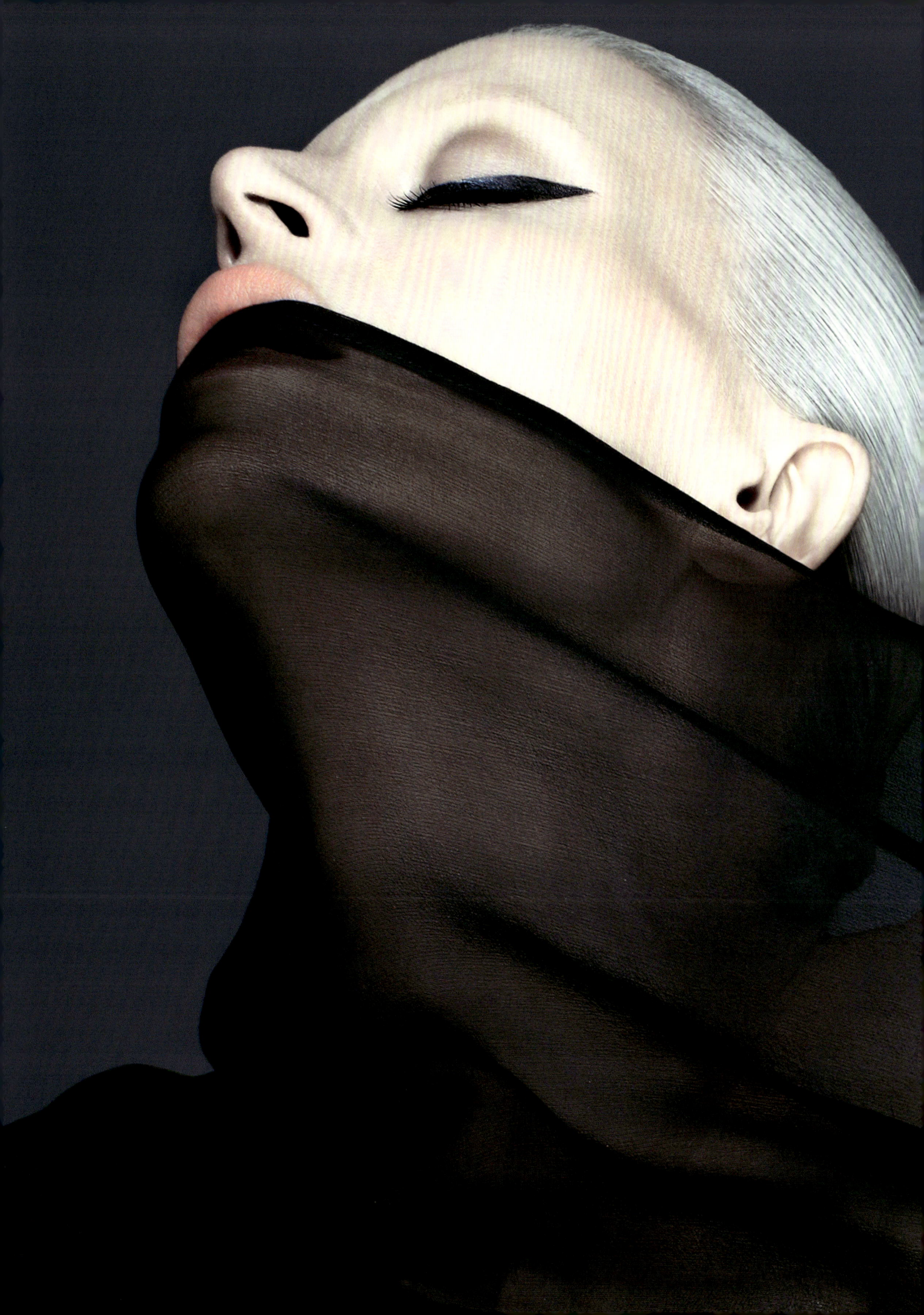

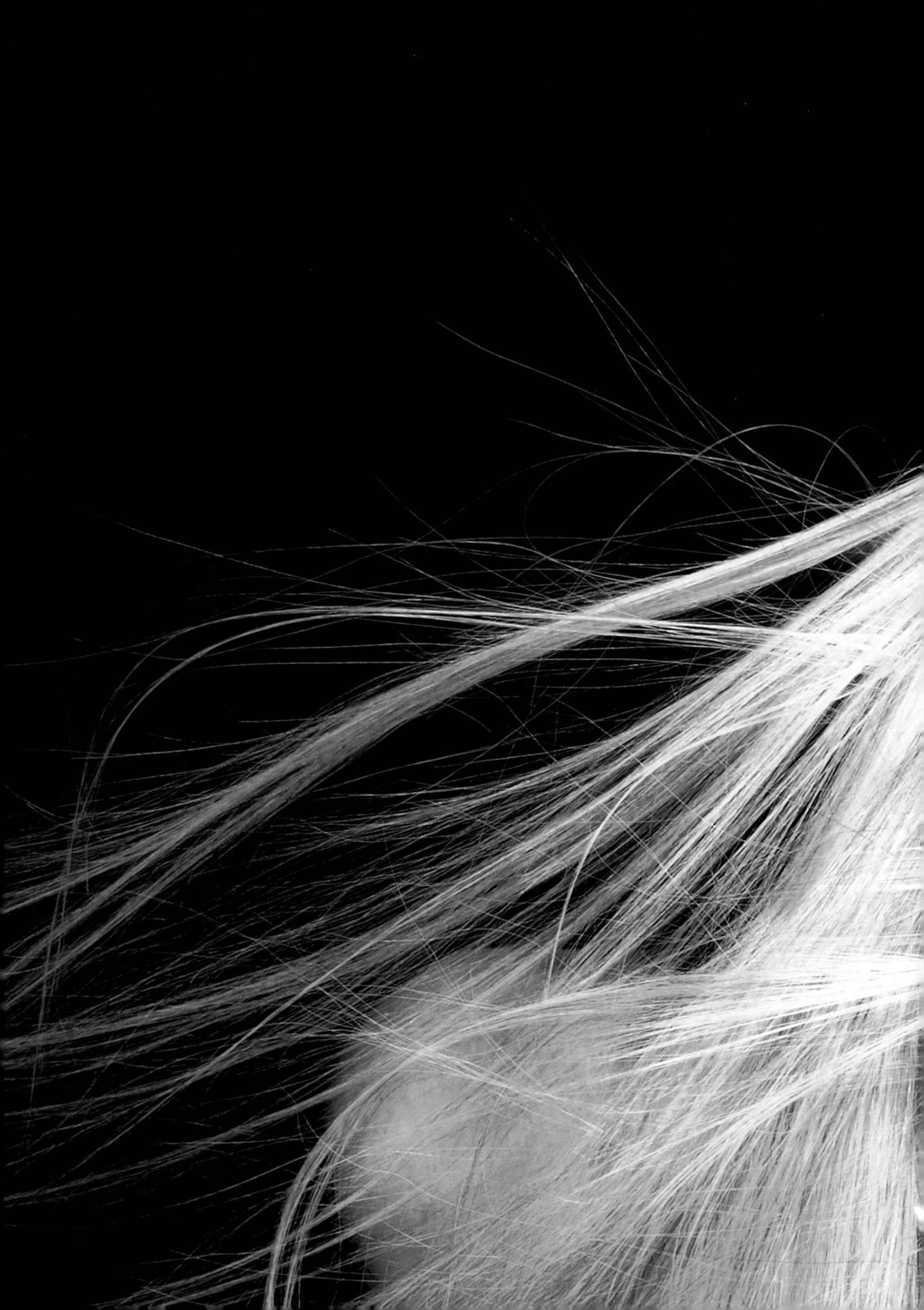

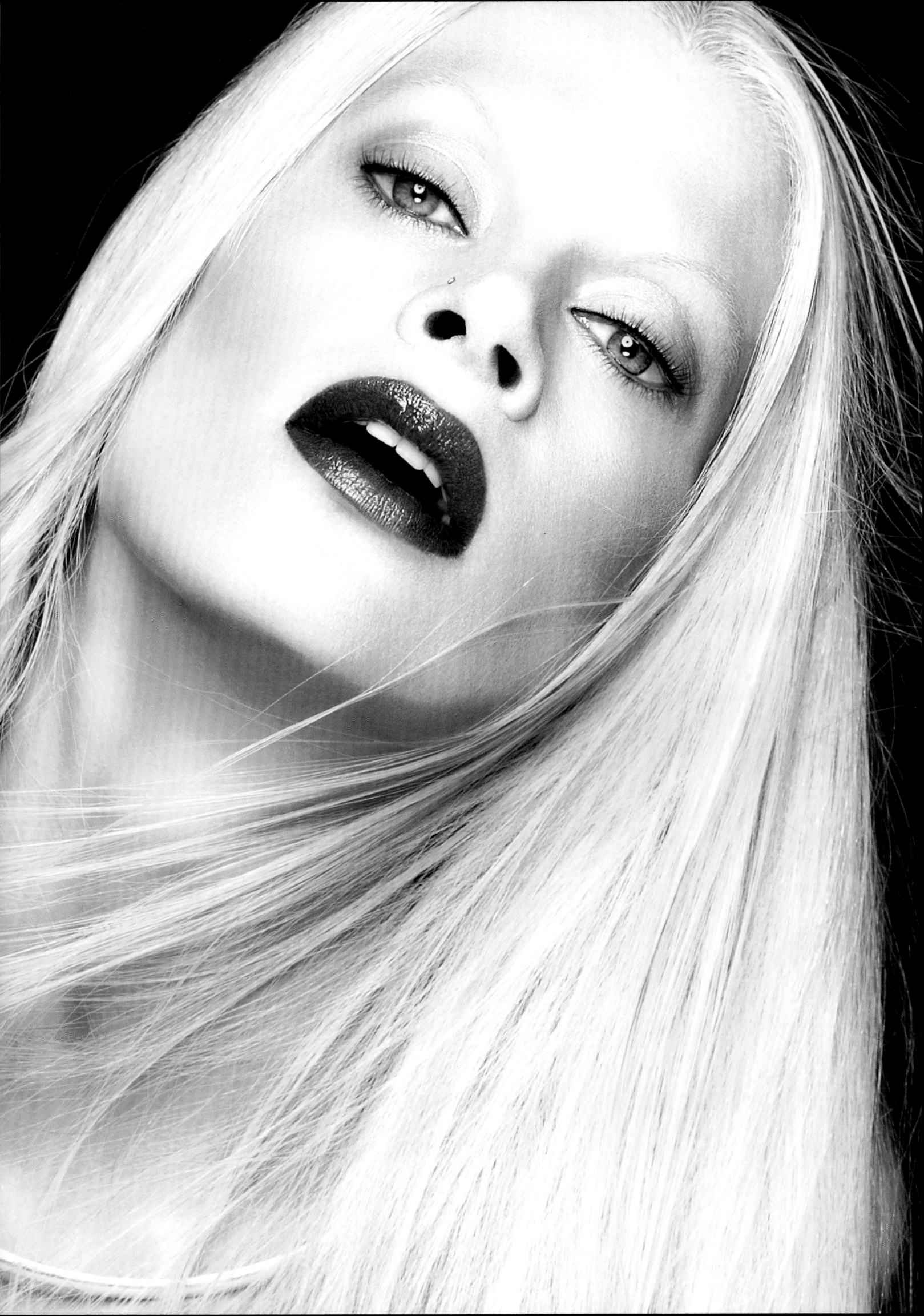

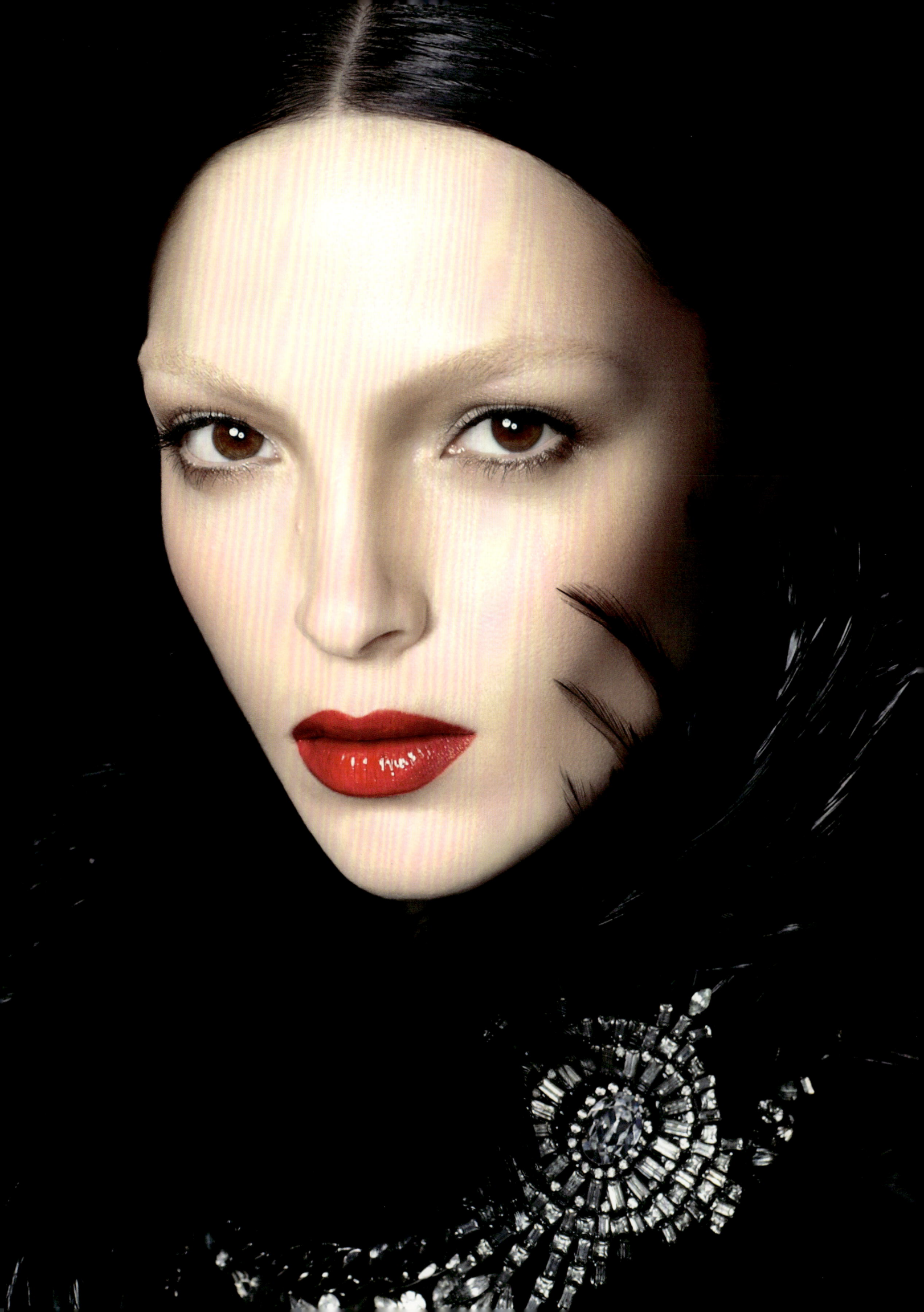

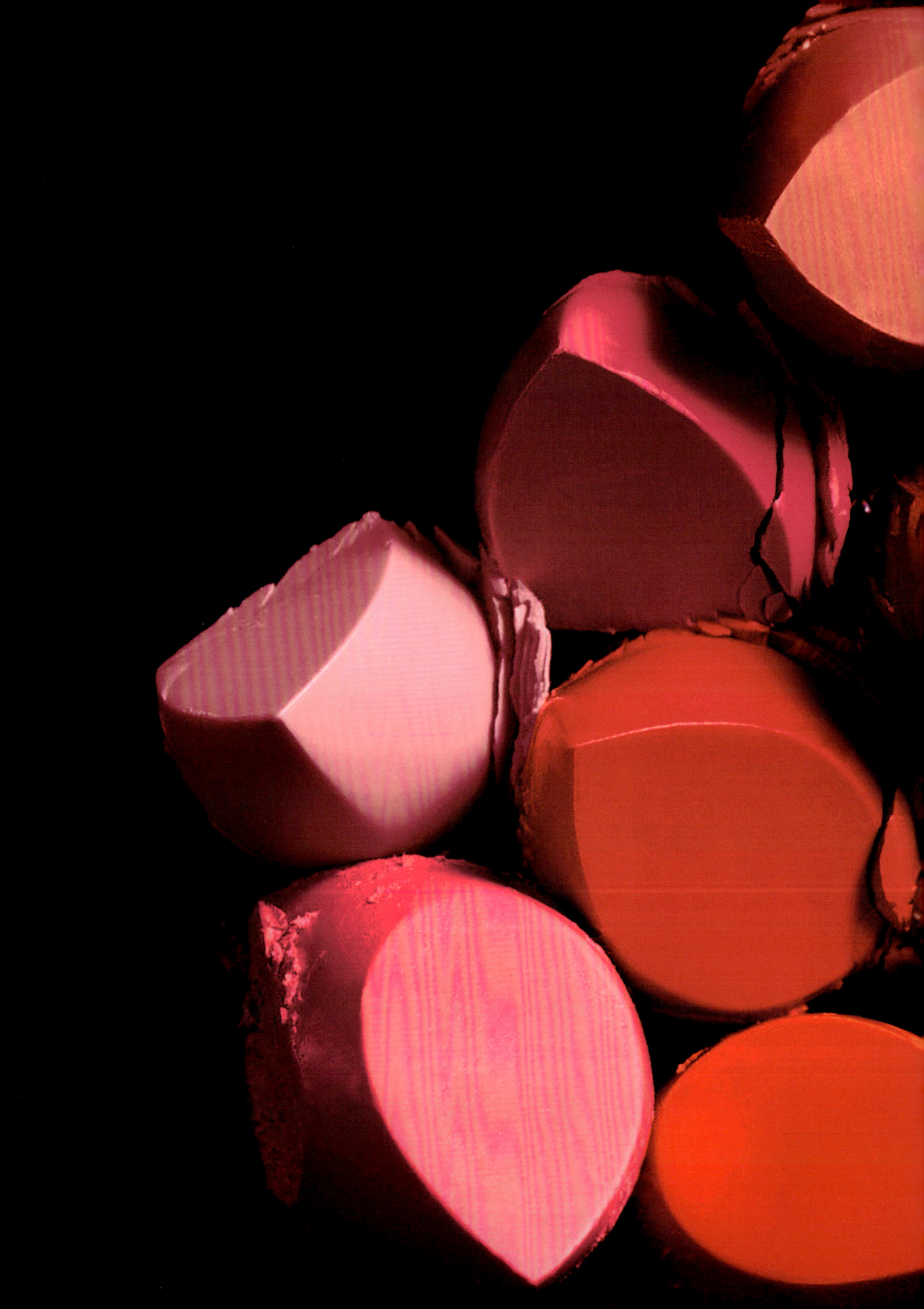

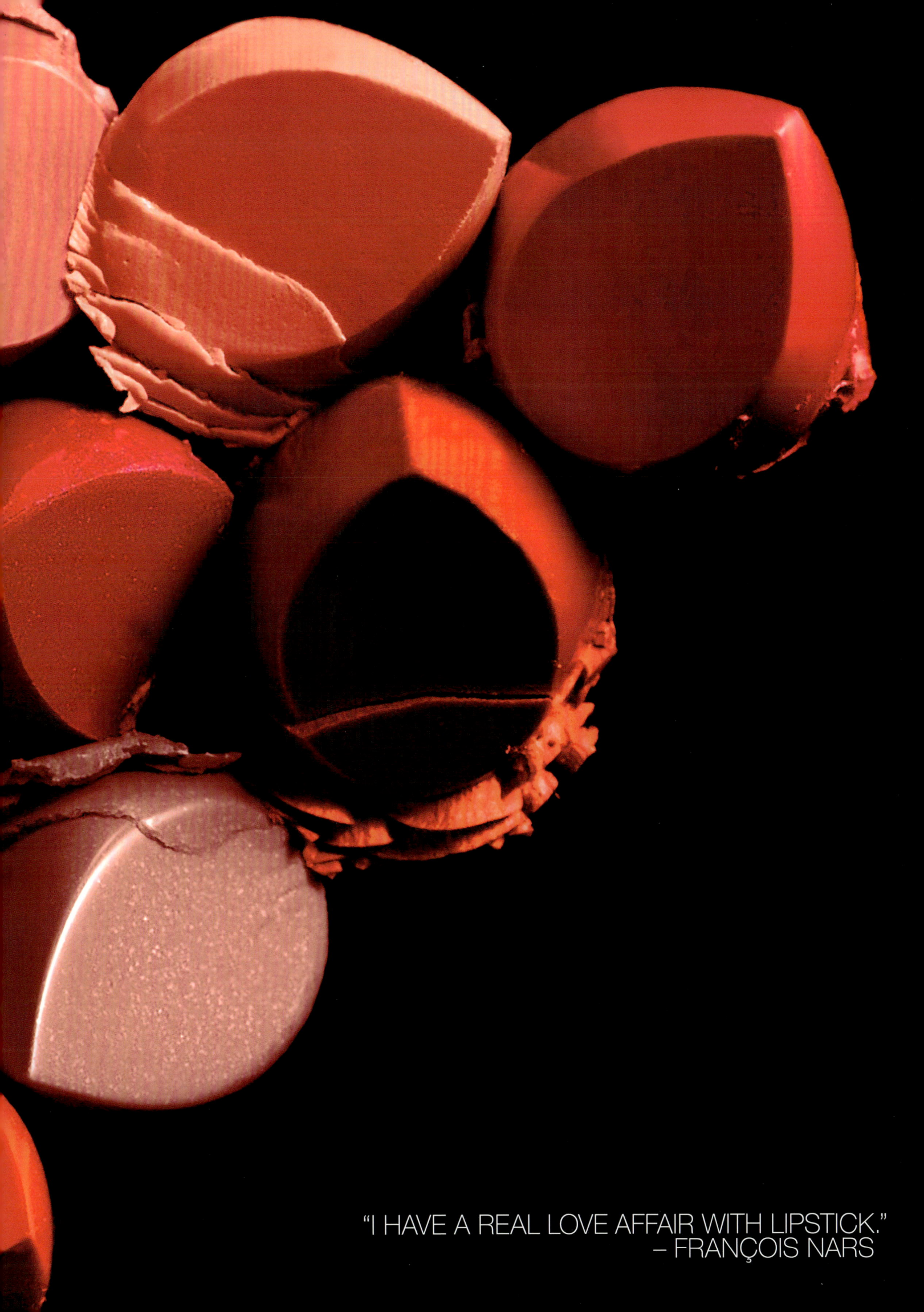

"I HAVE A REAL LOVE AFFAIR WITH LIPSTICK."
– FRANÇOIS NARS

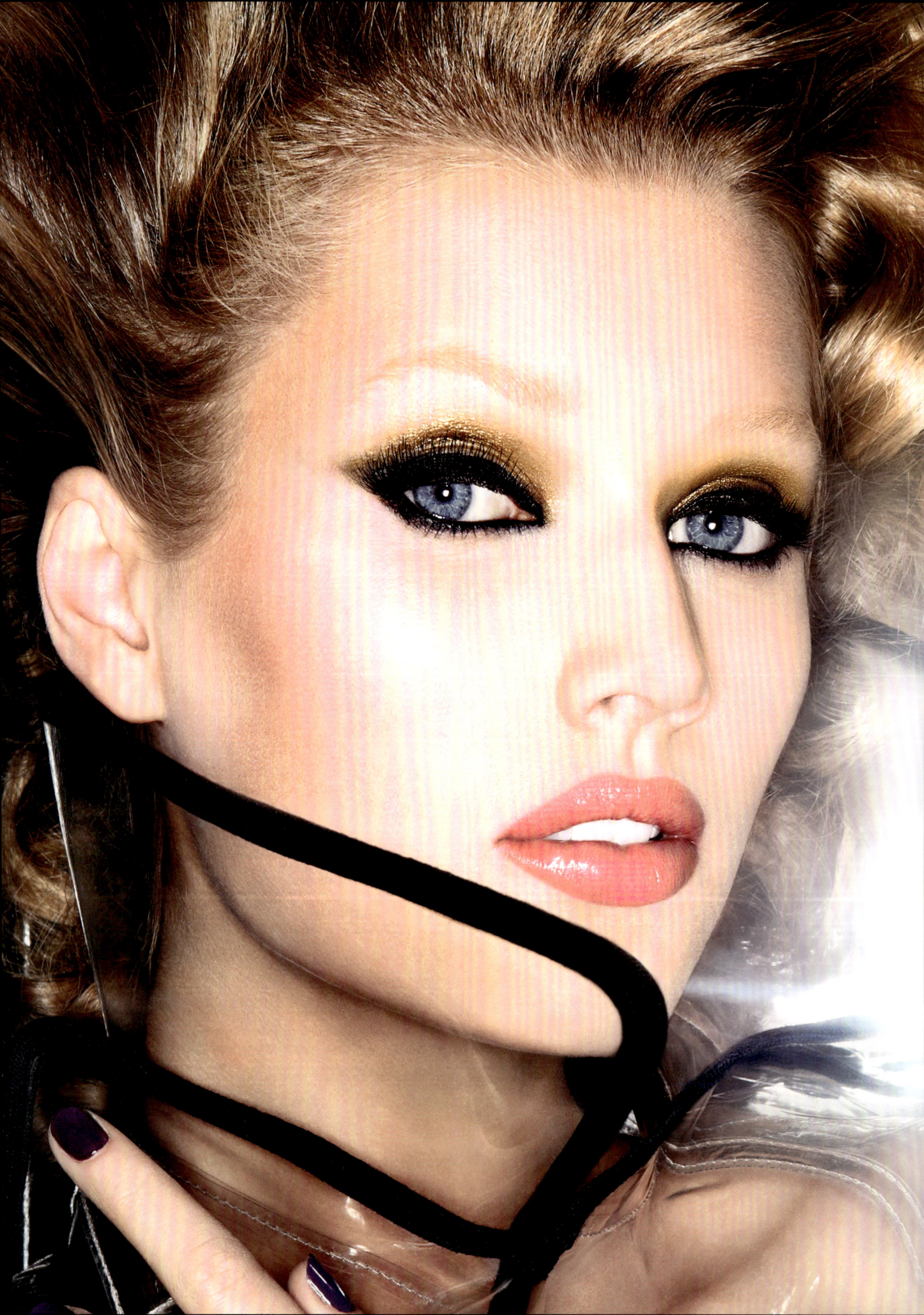

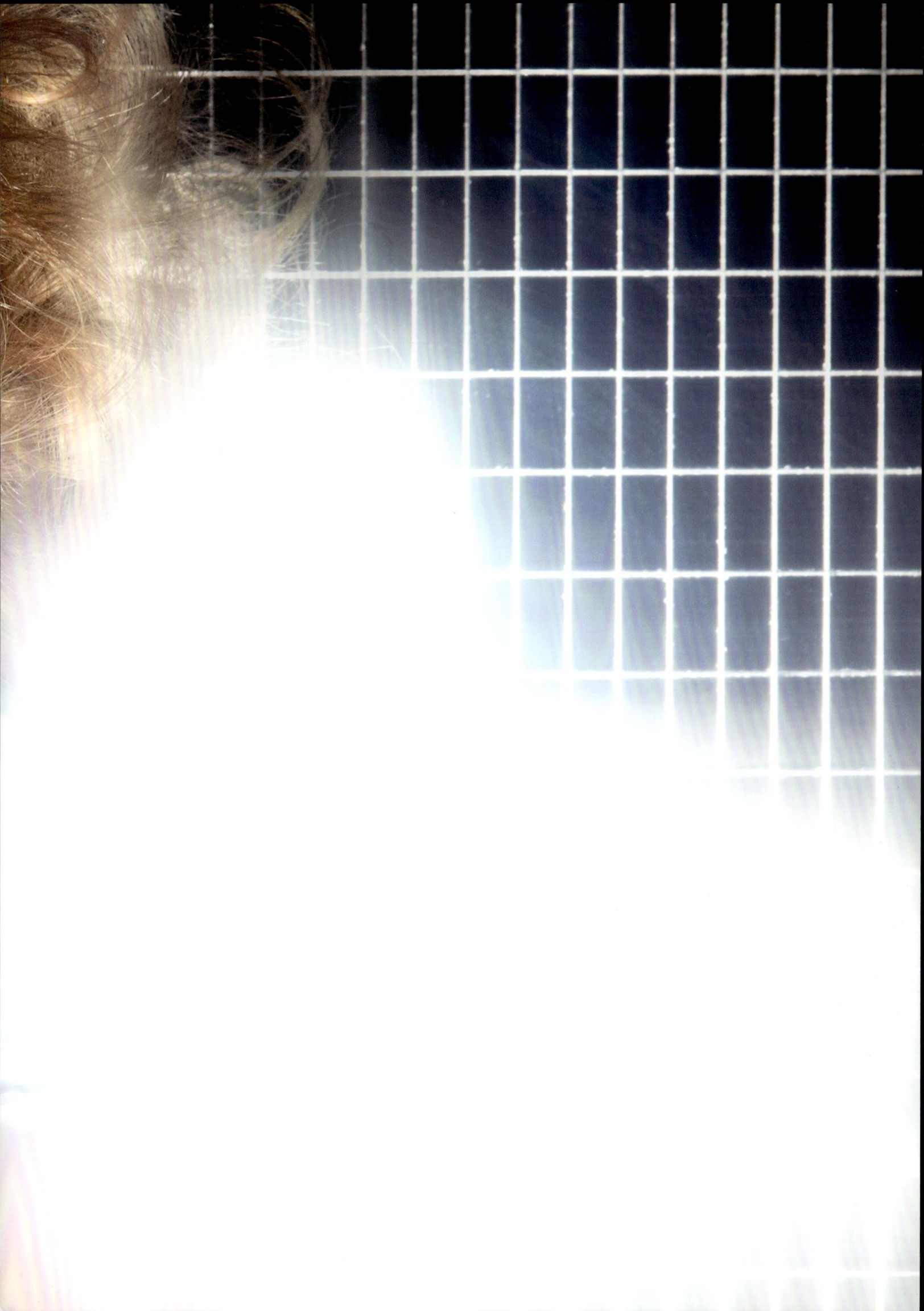

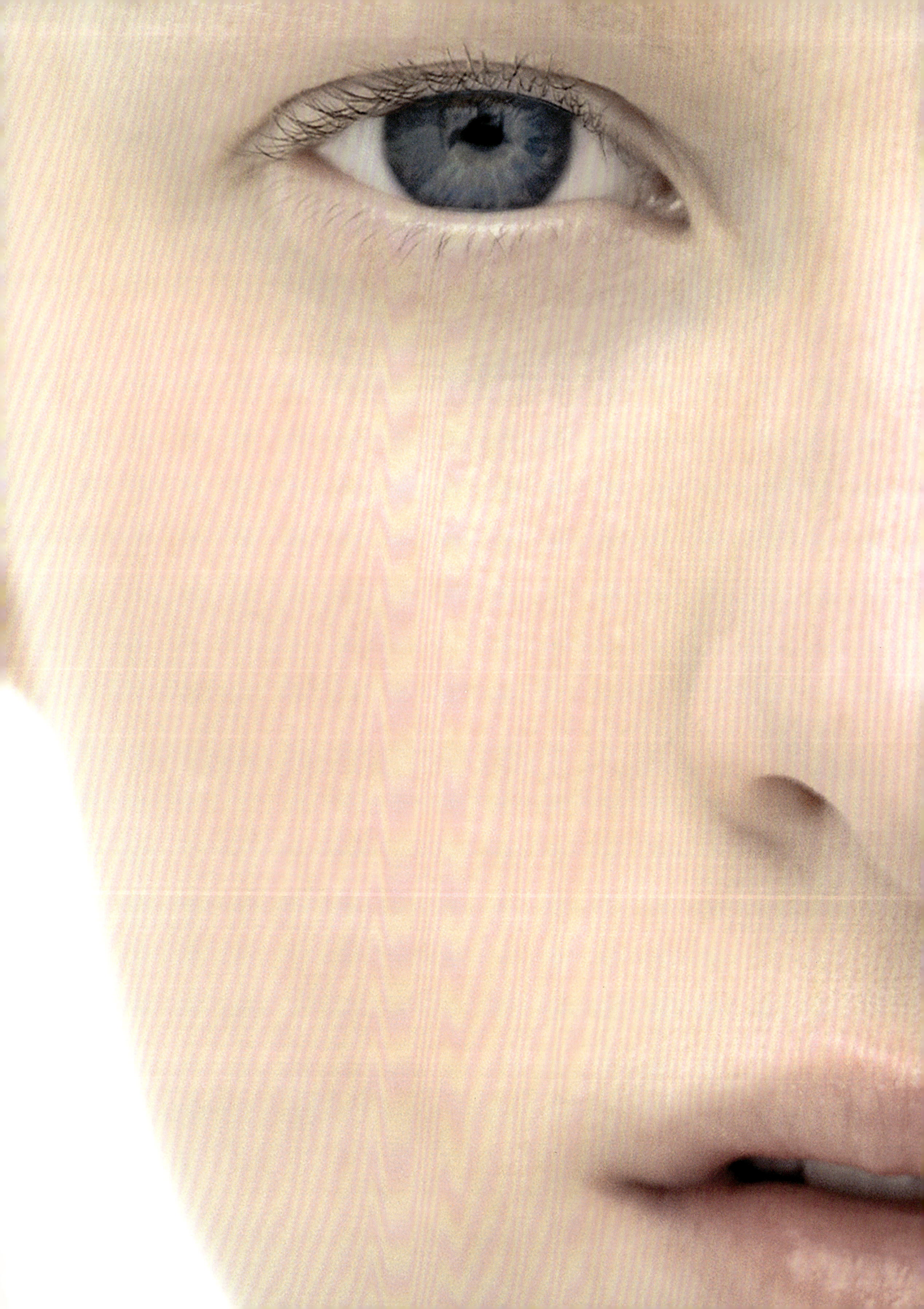

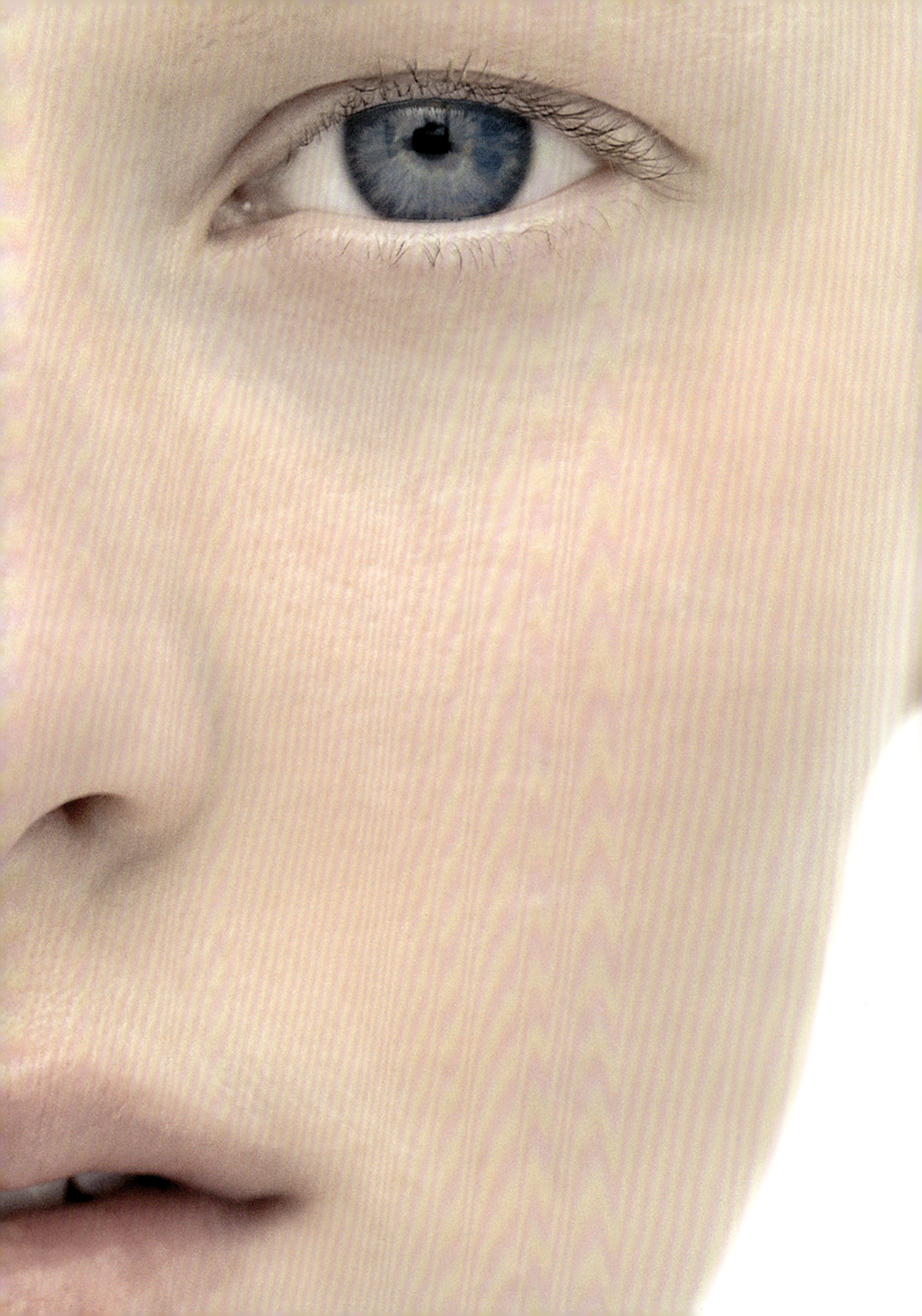

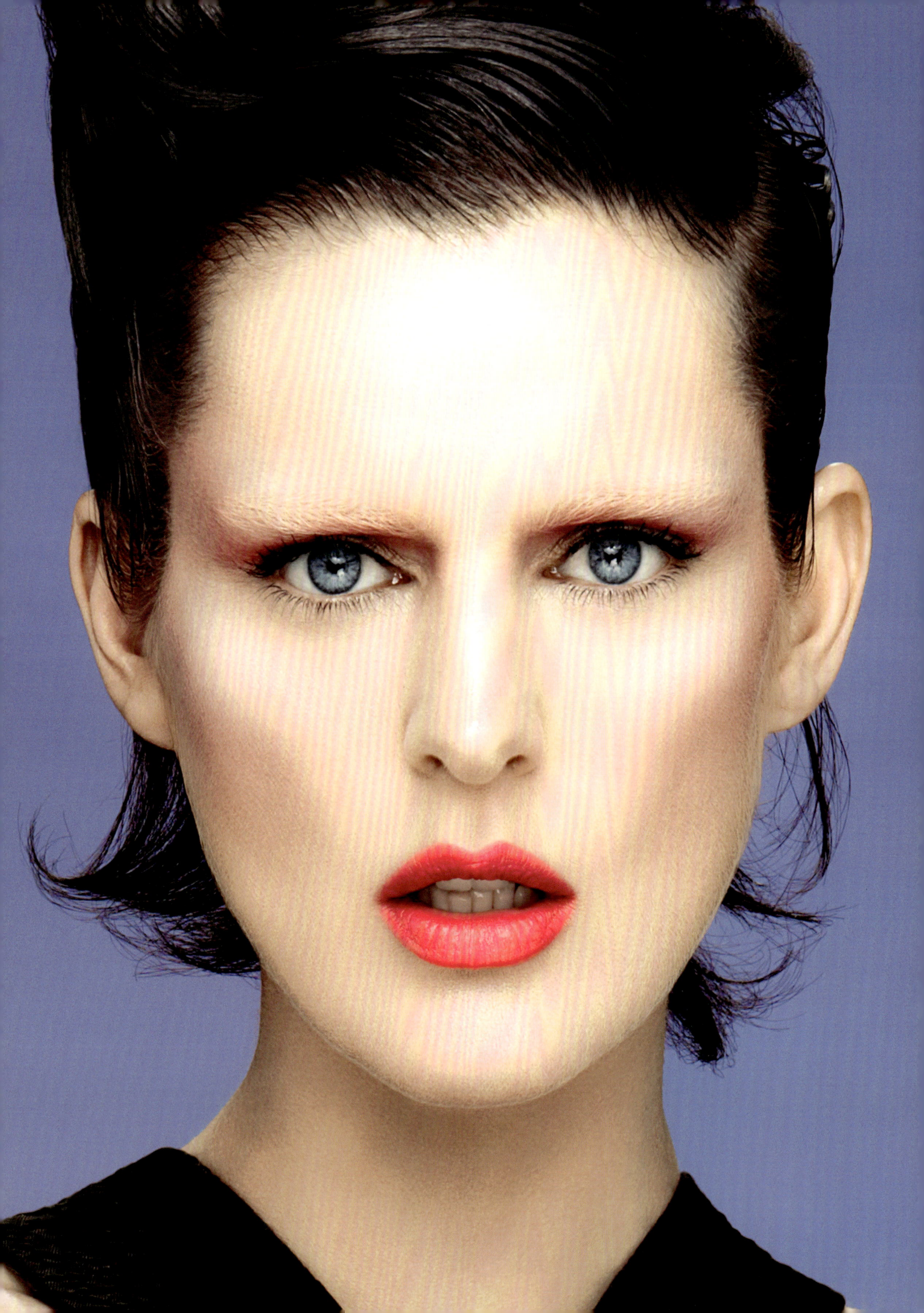

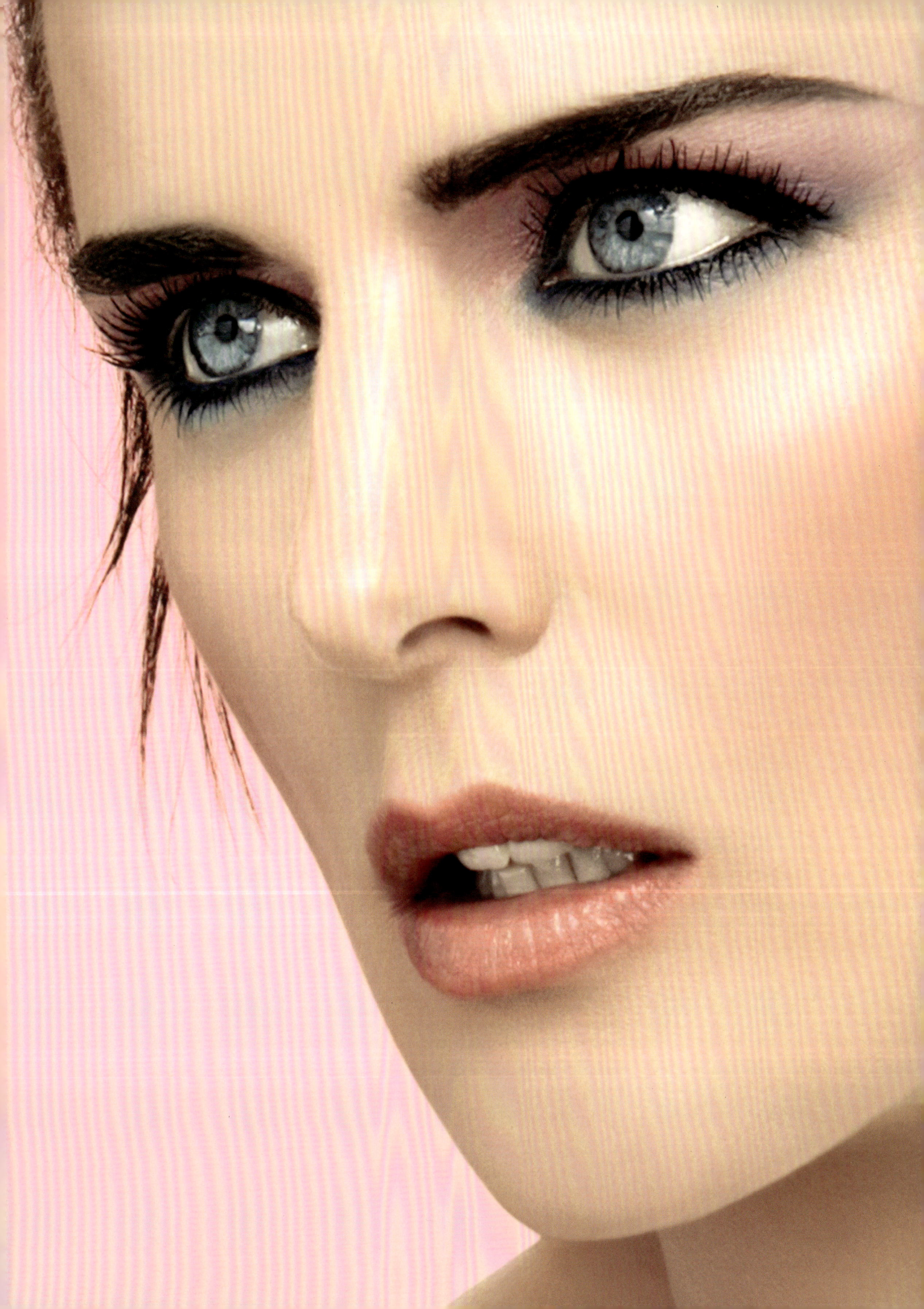

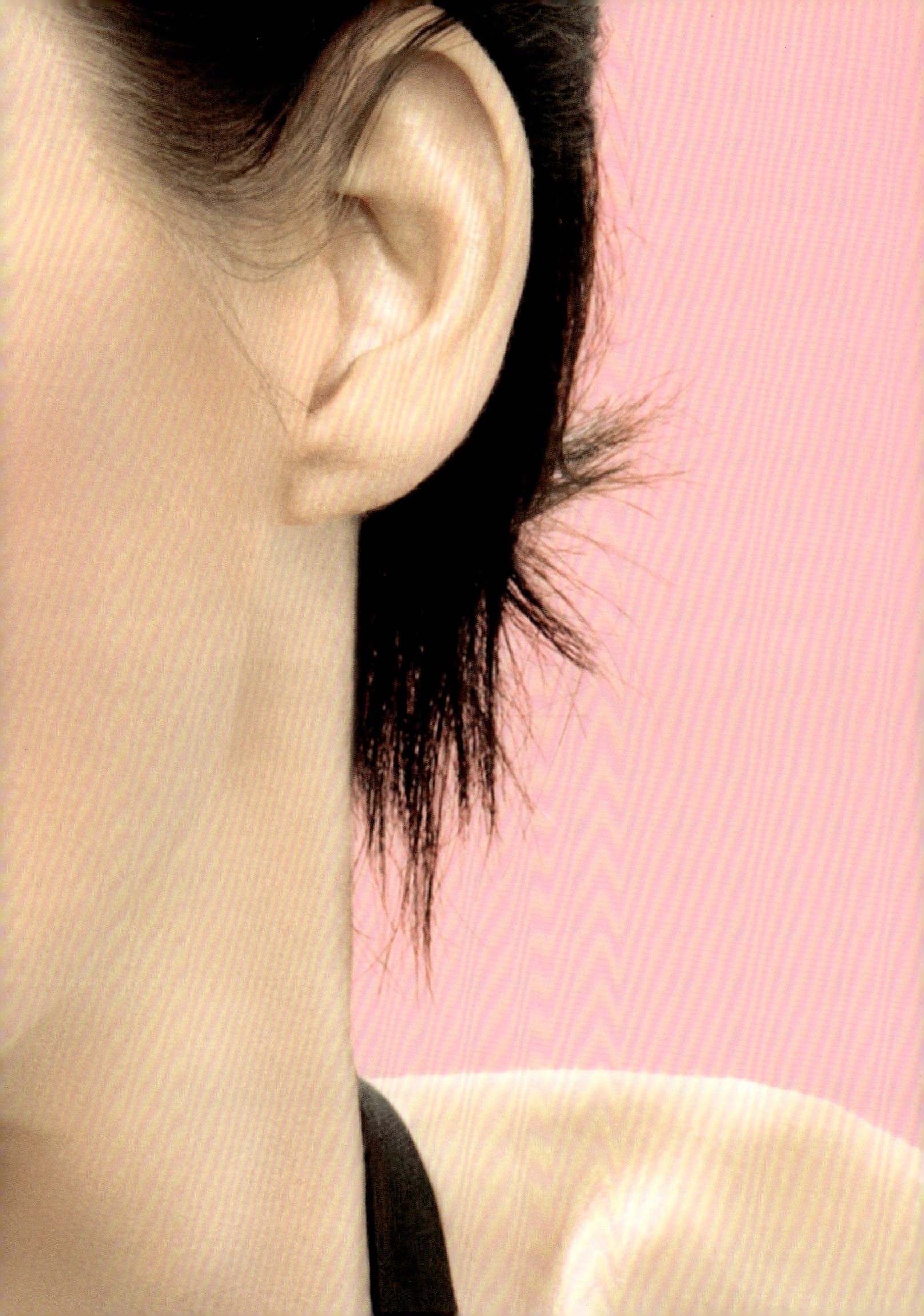

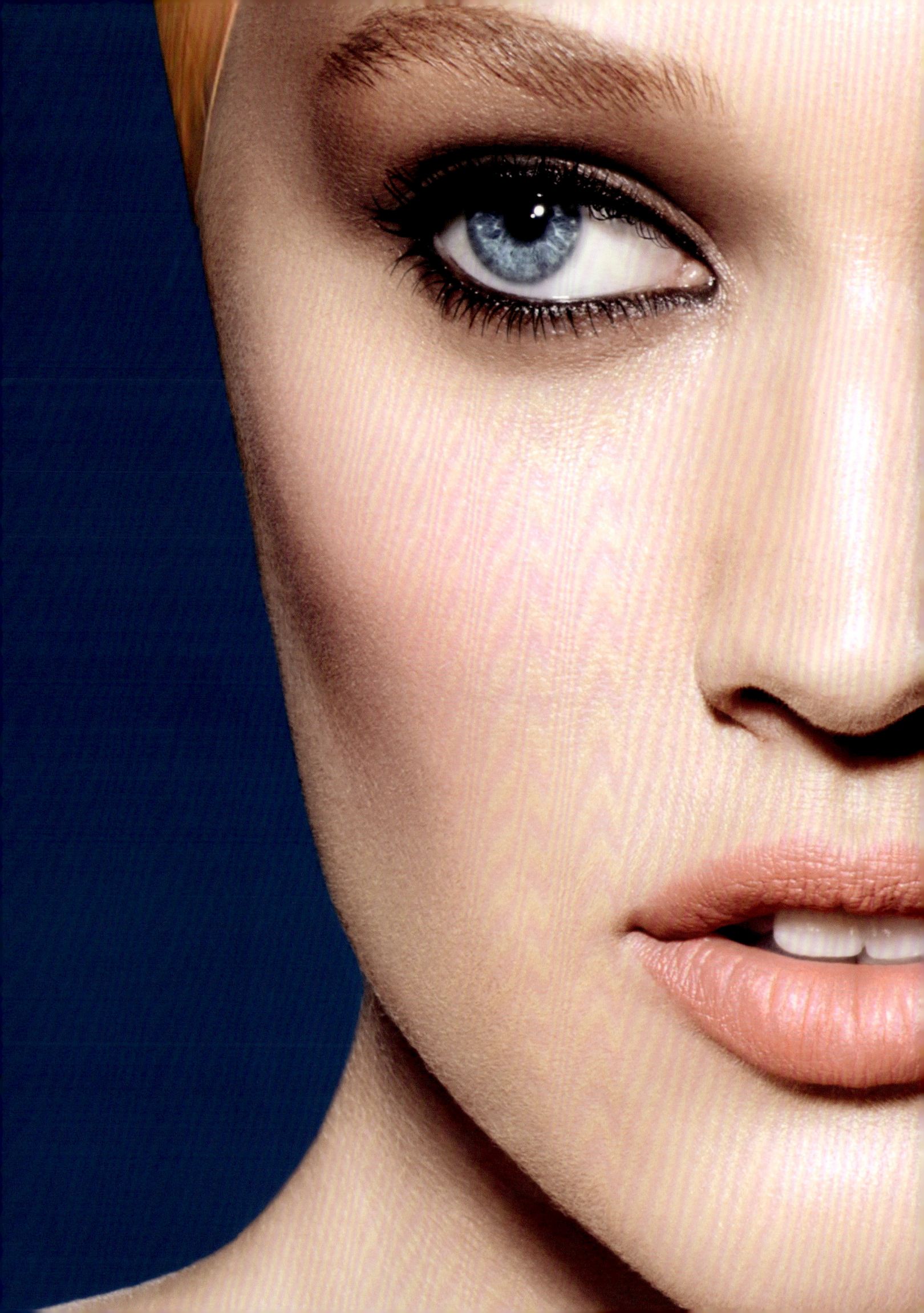

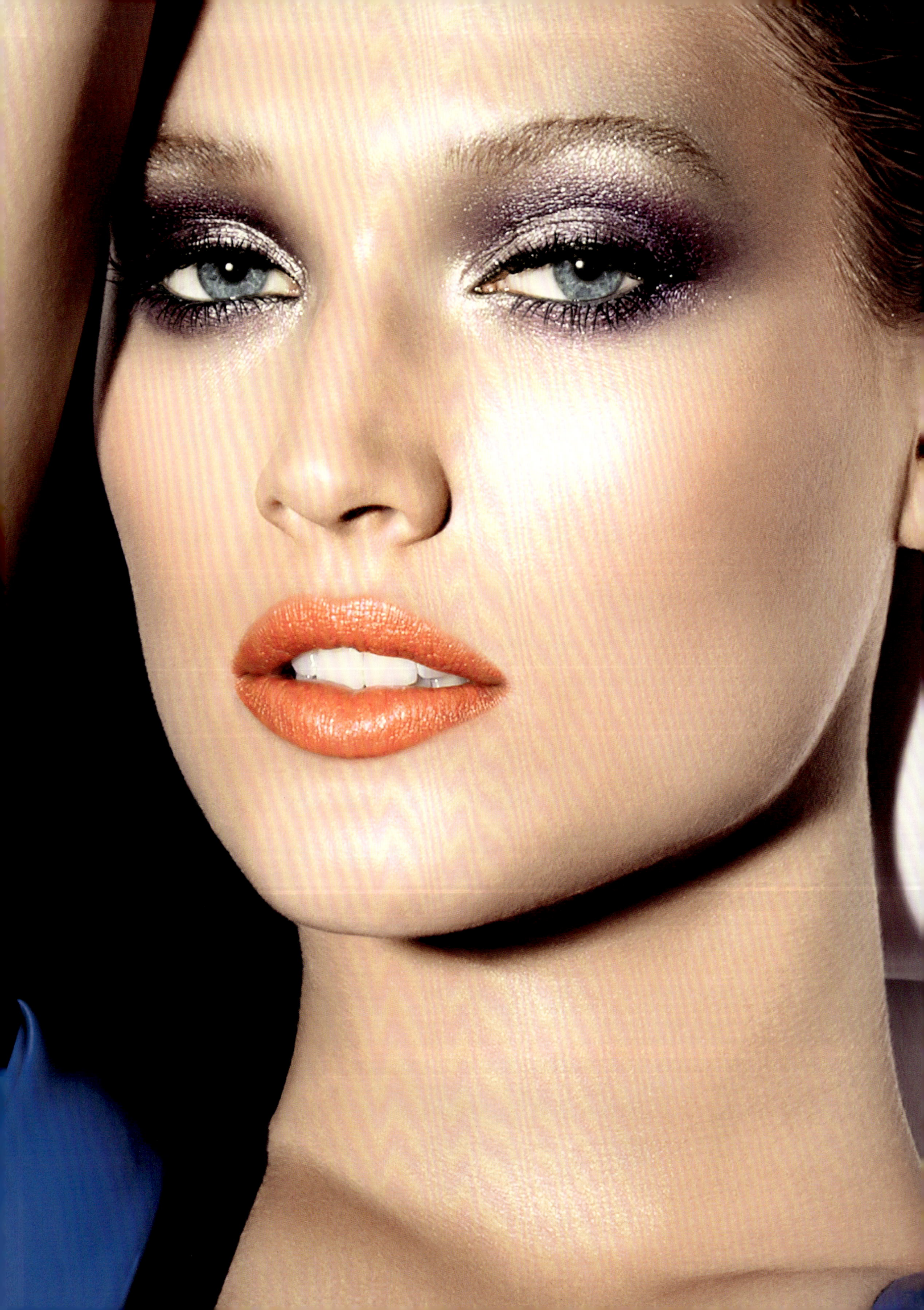

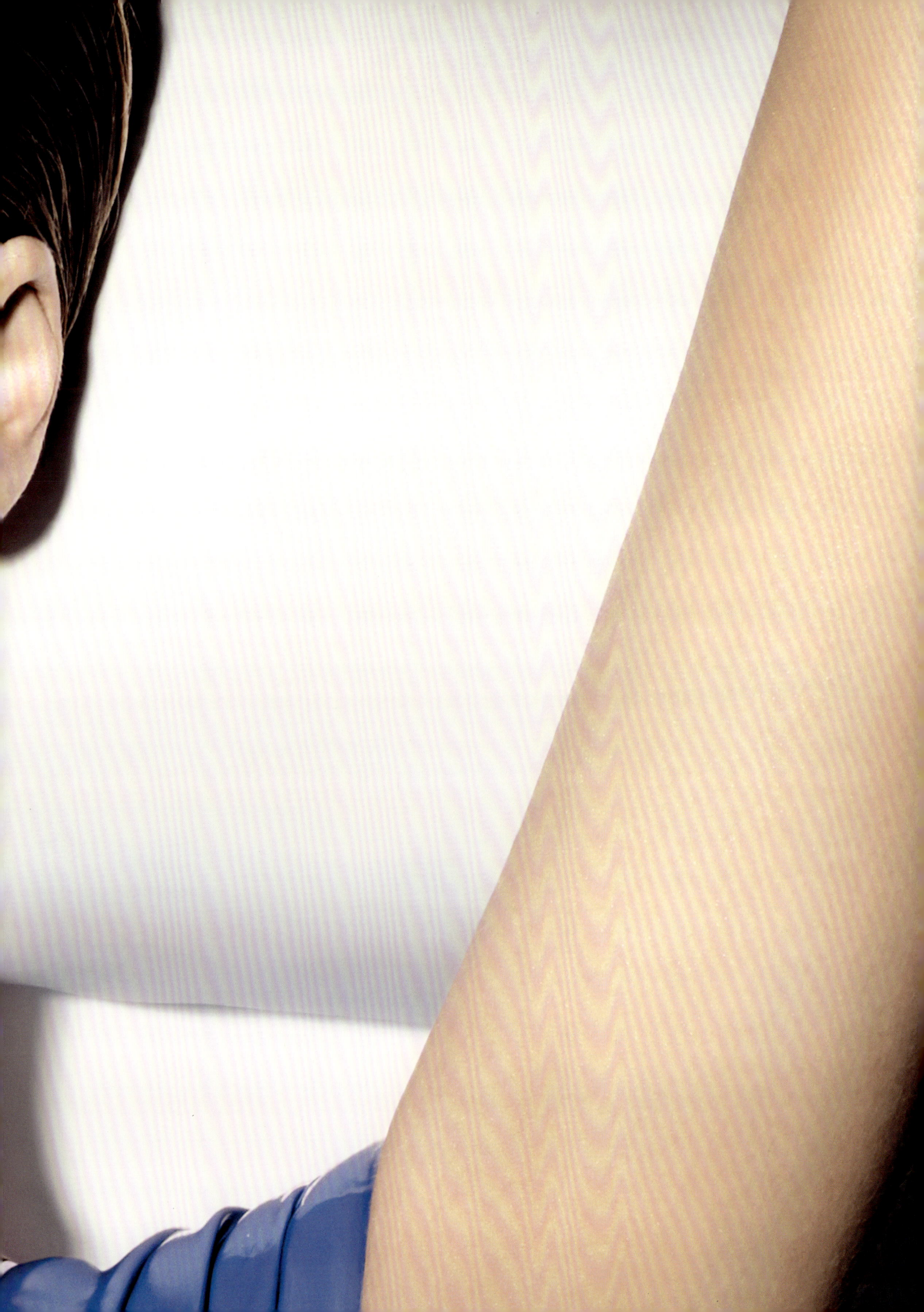

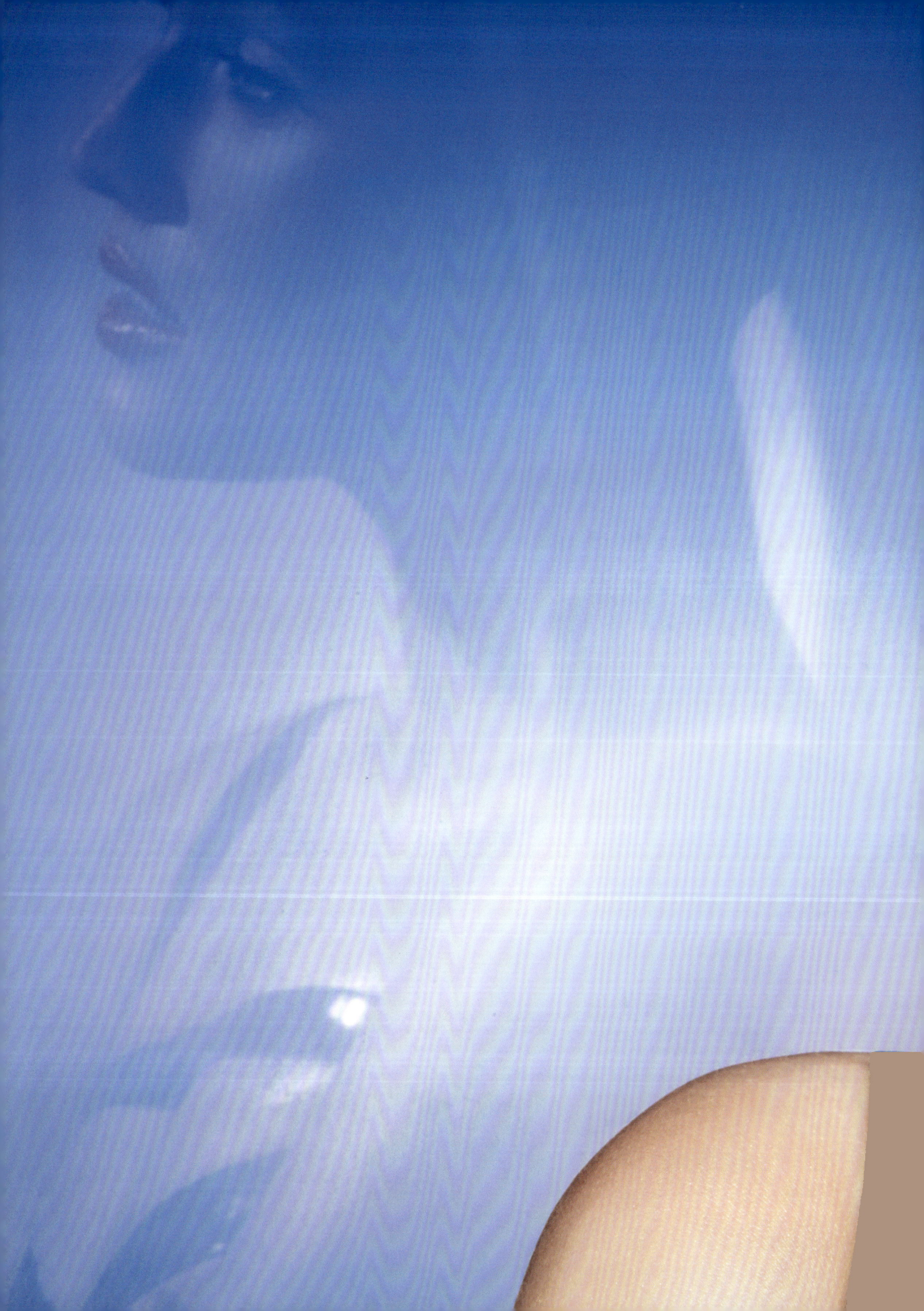

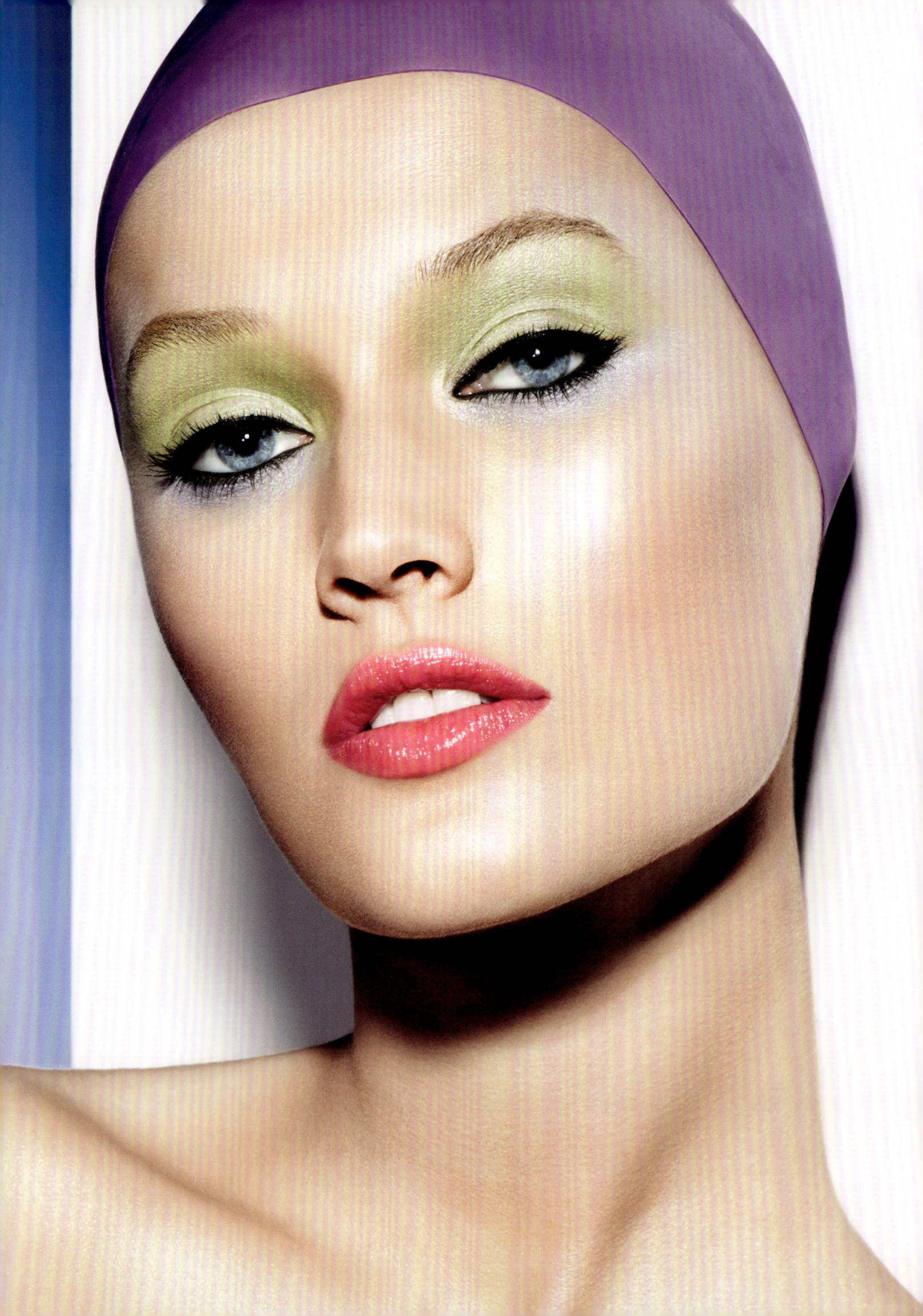

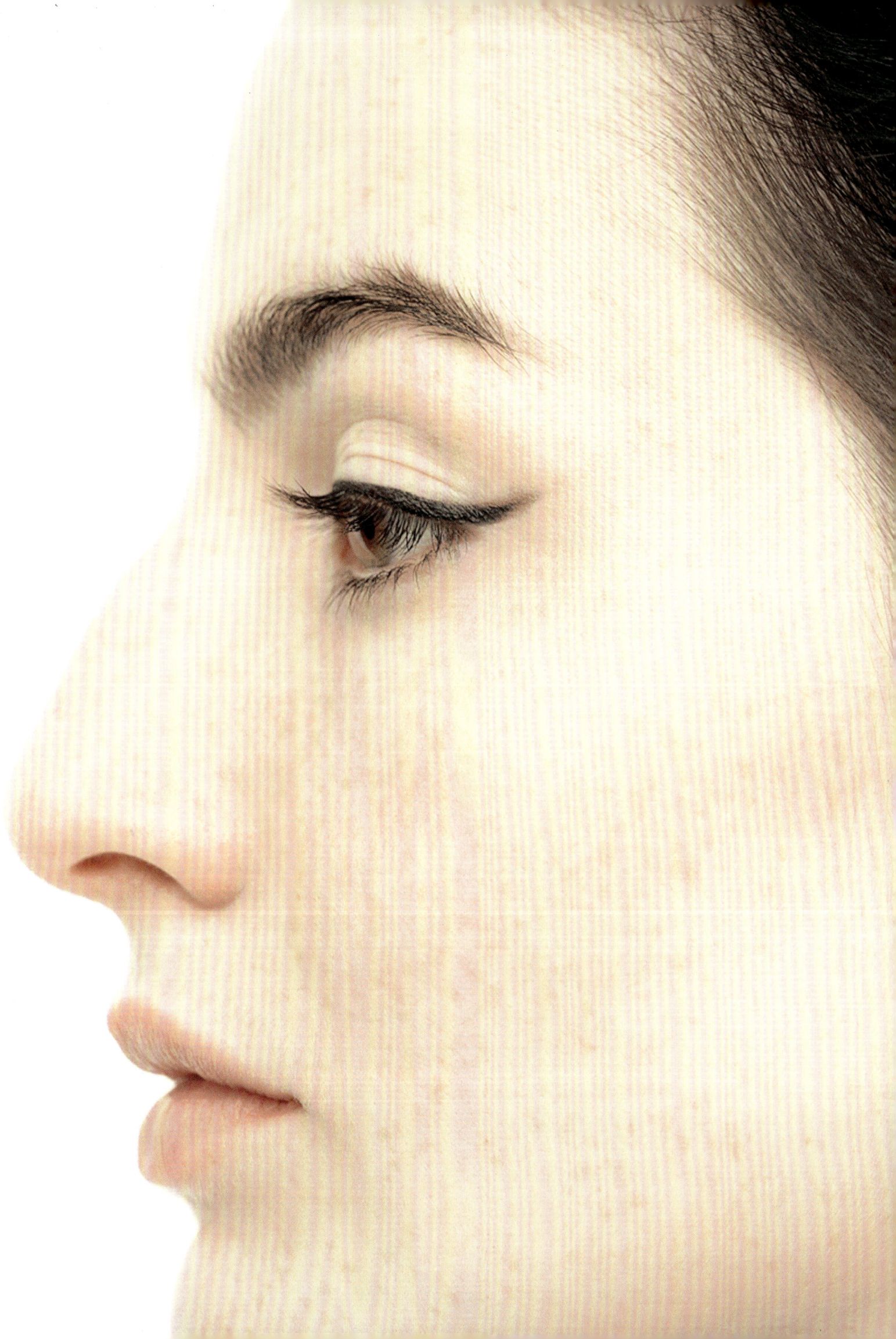

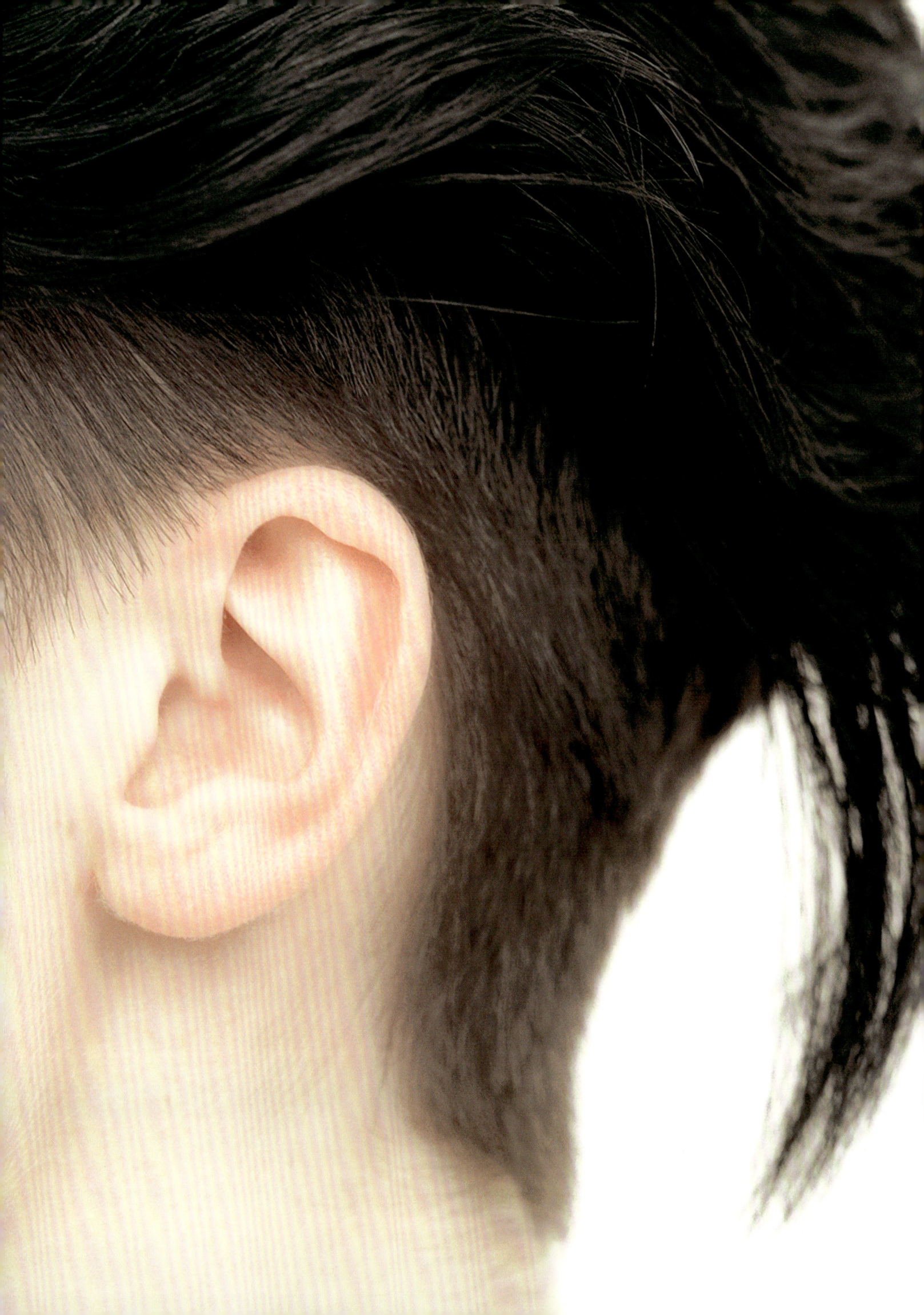

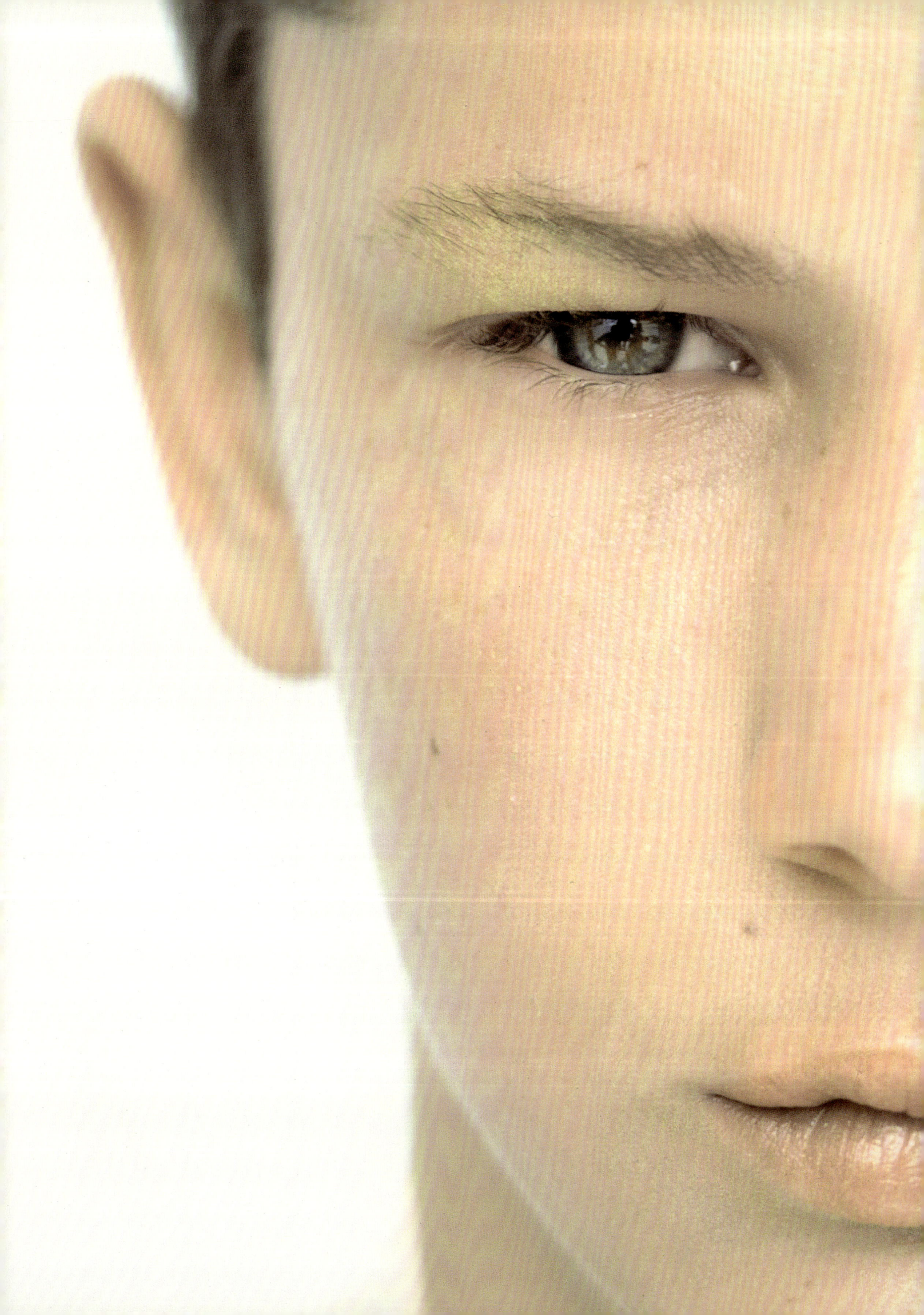

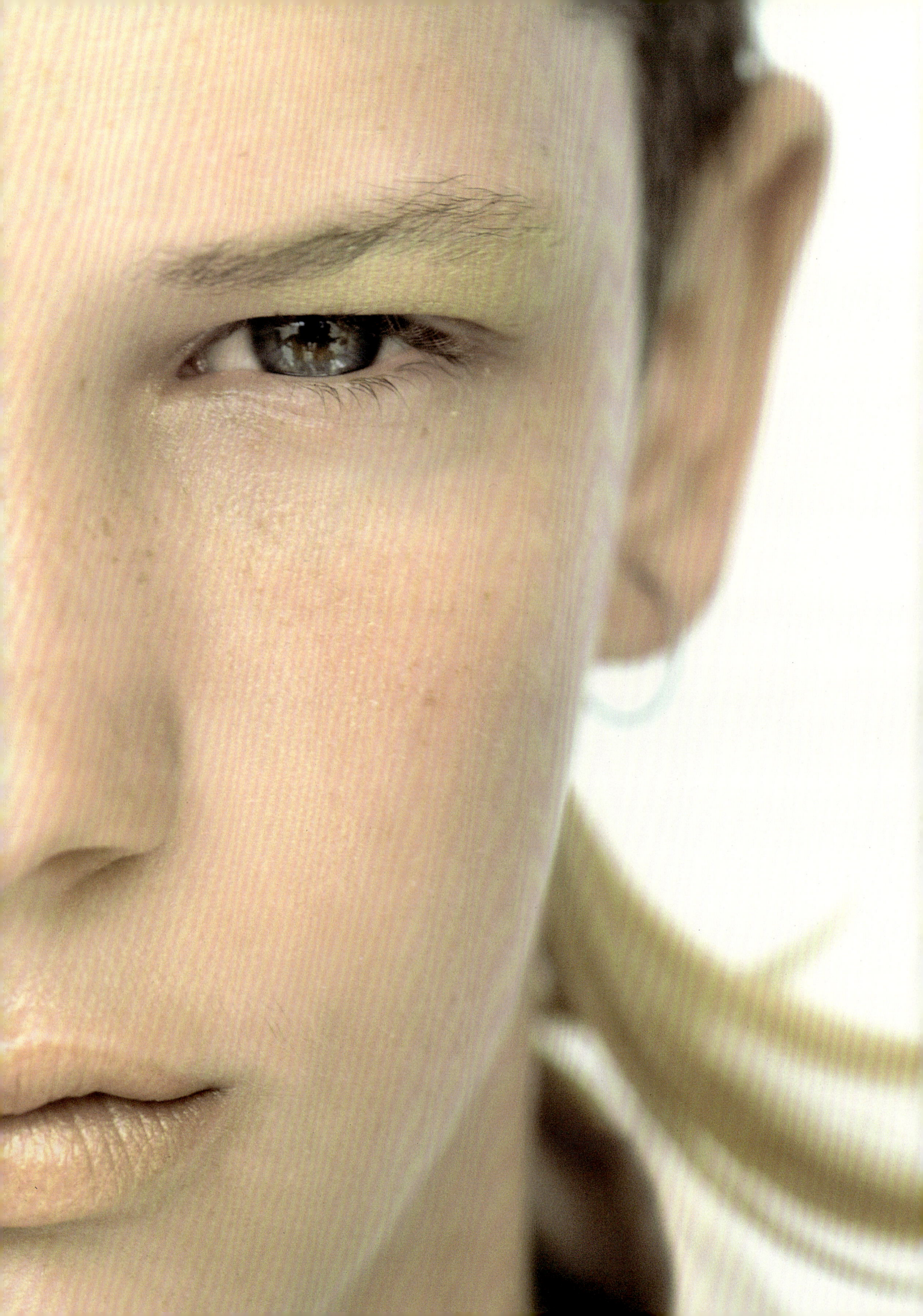

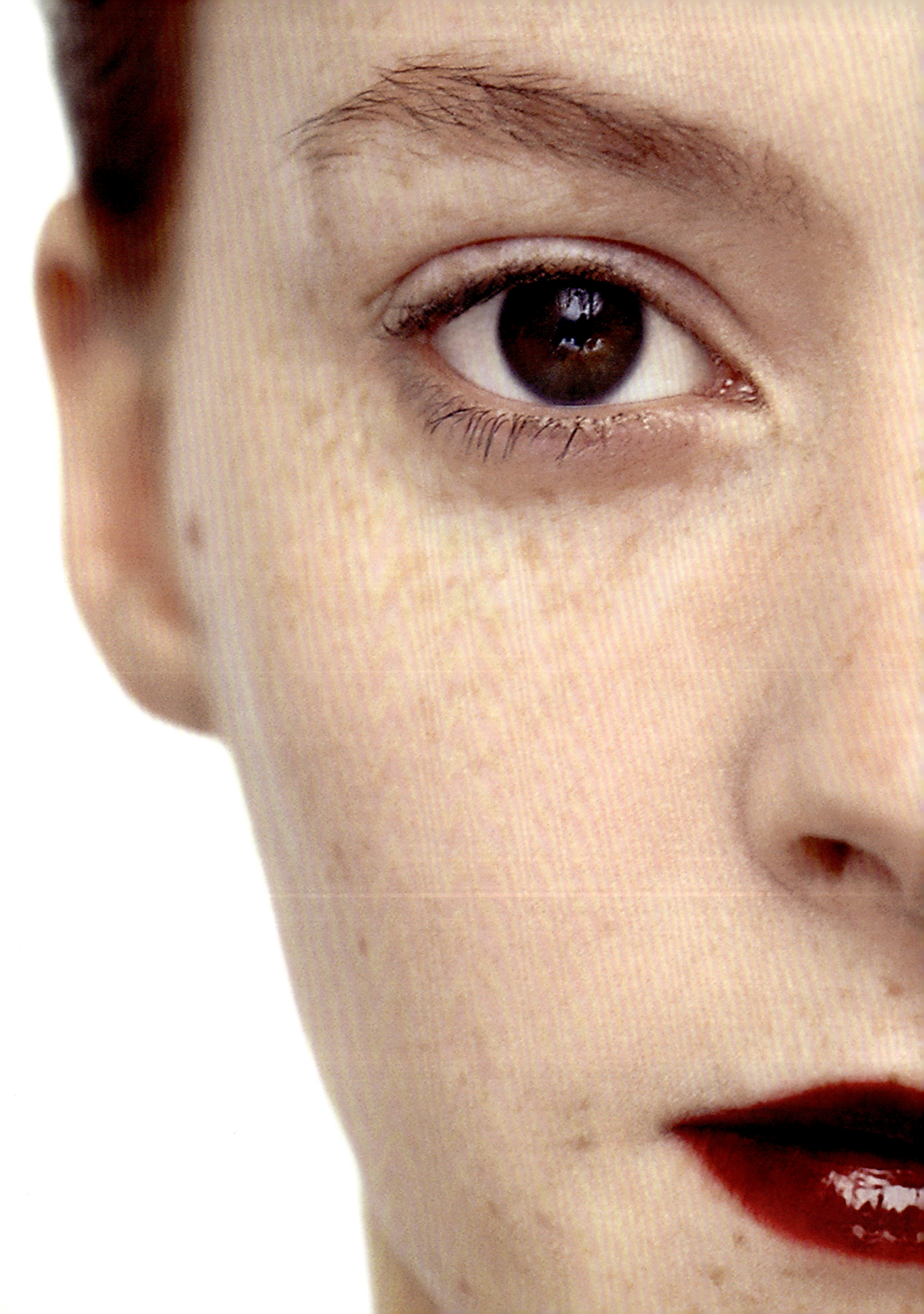

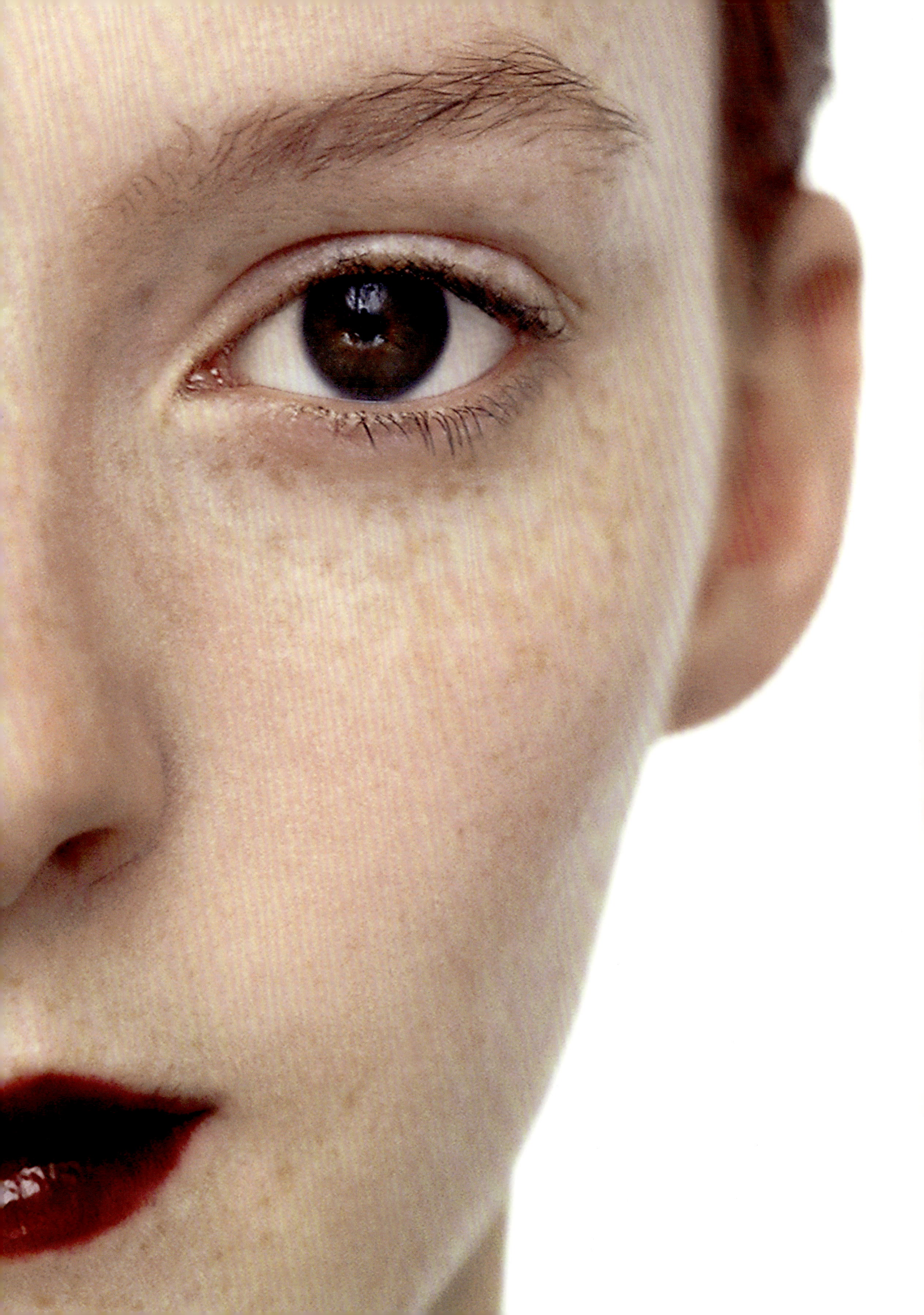

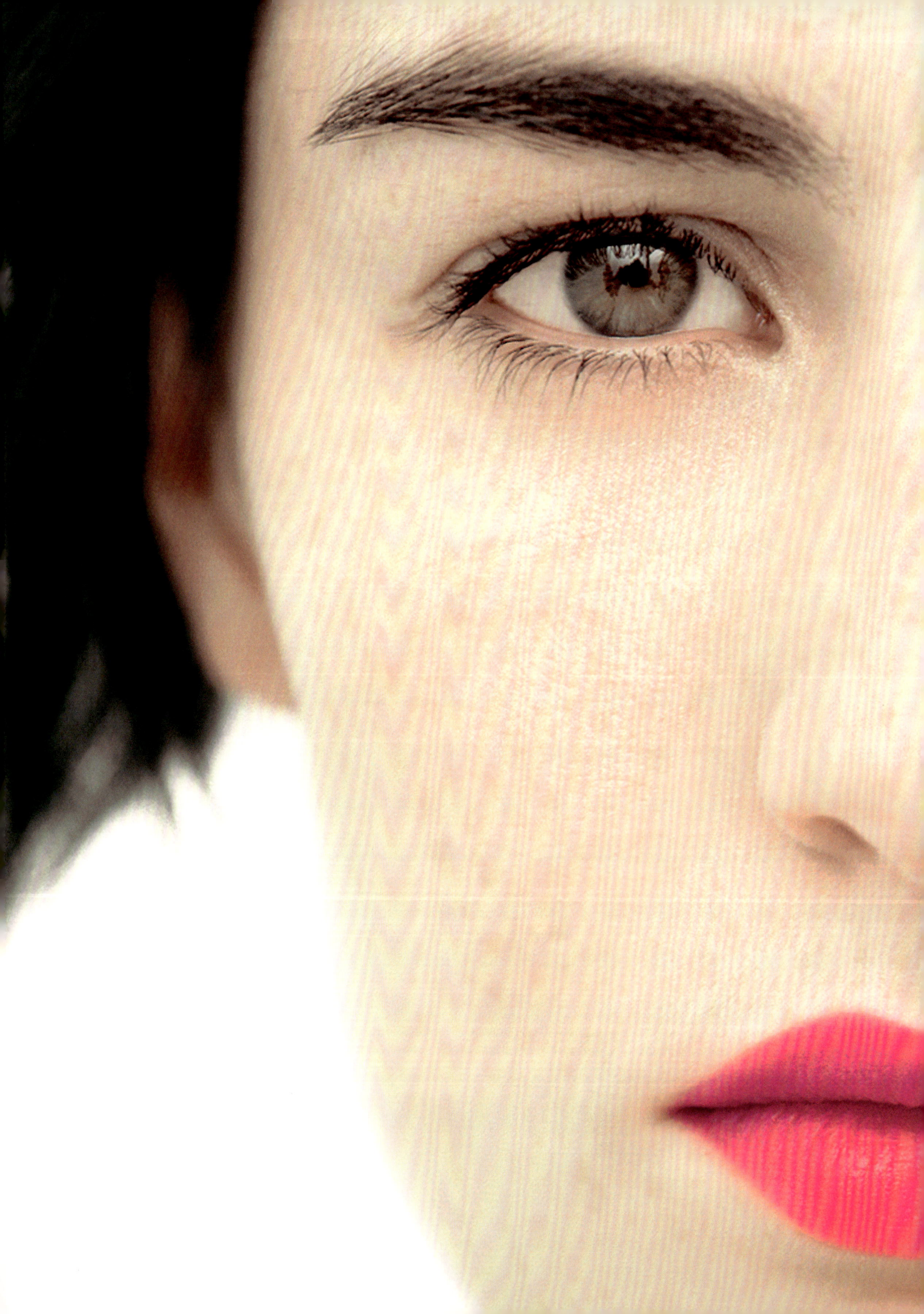

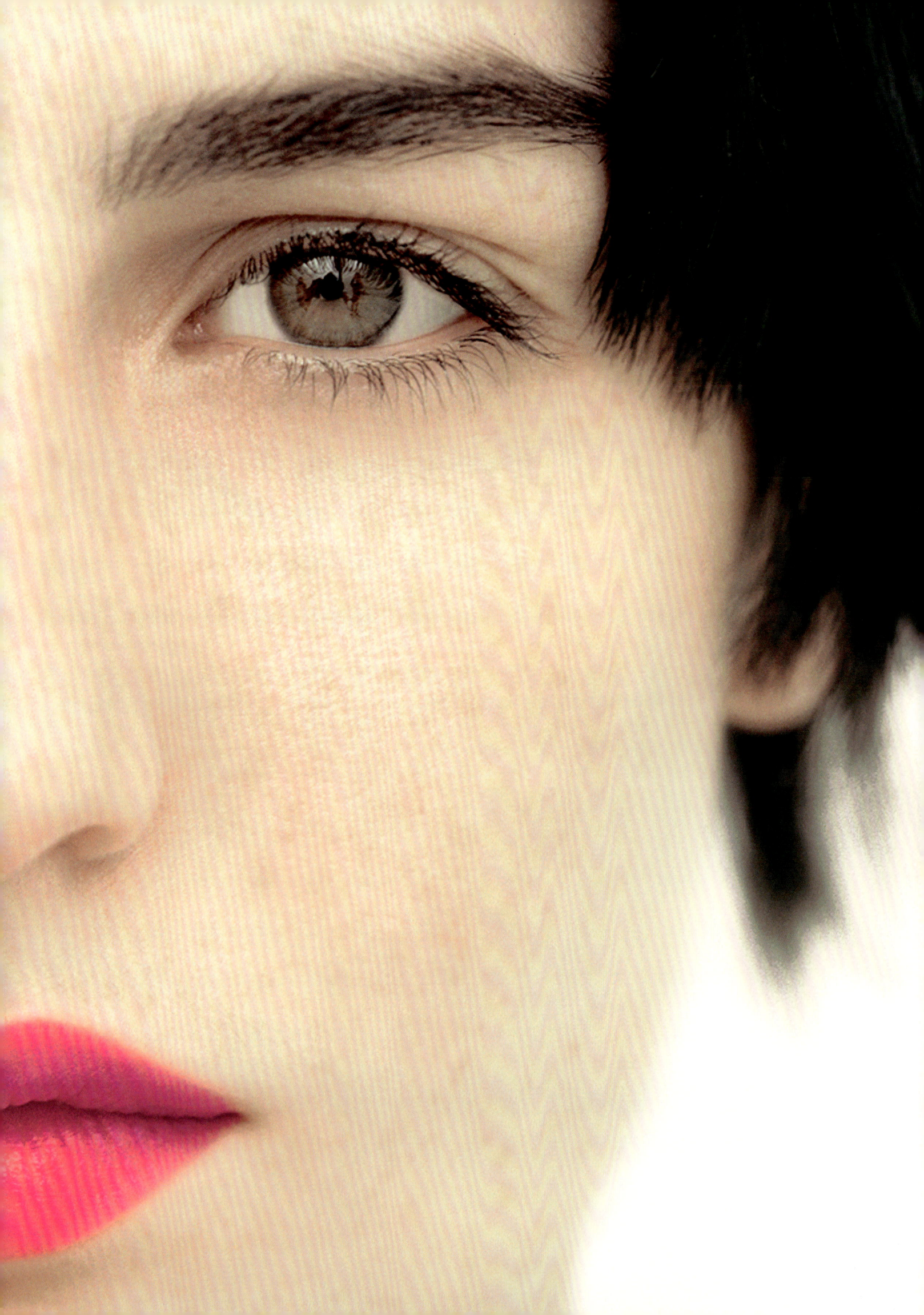

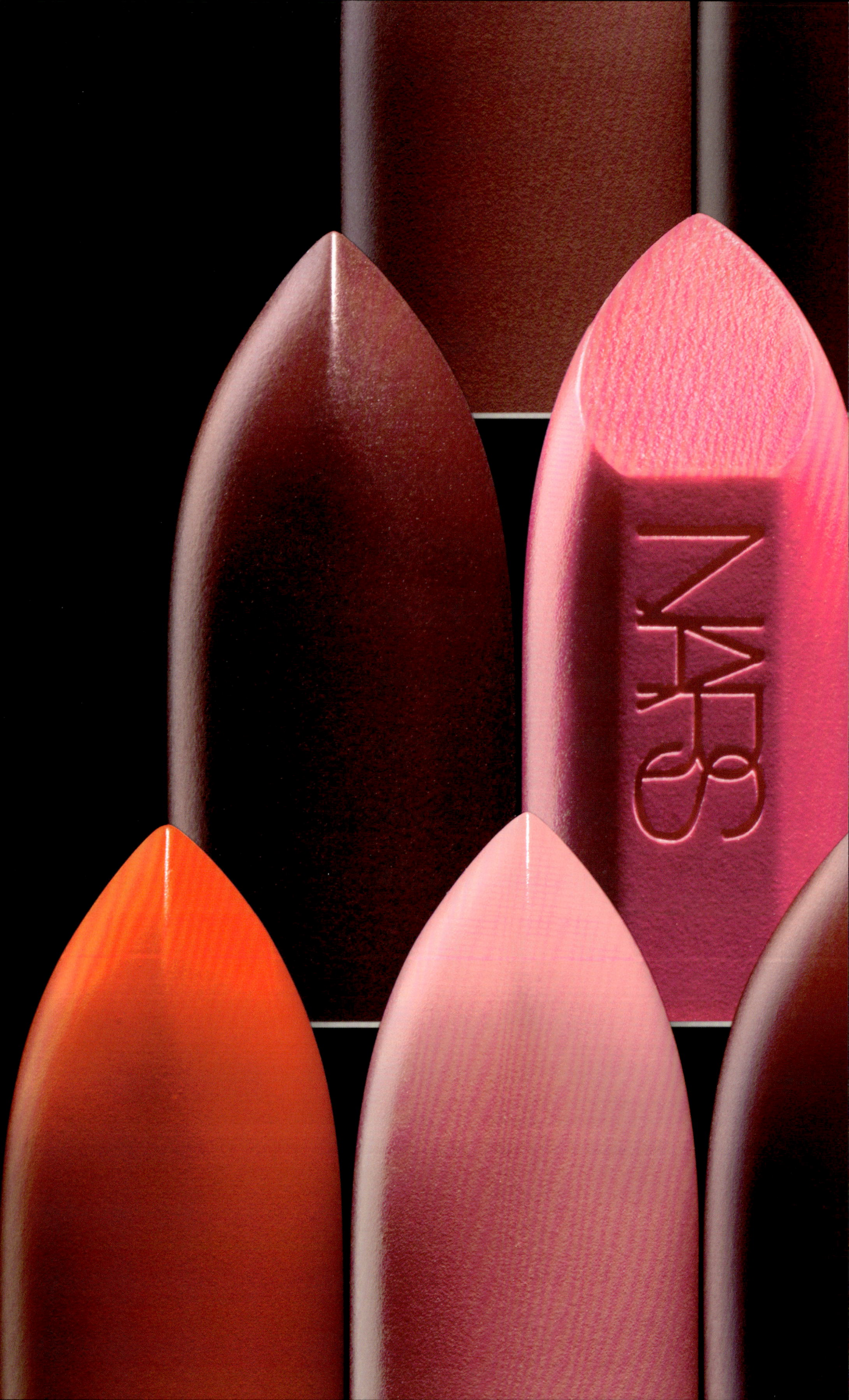

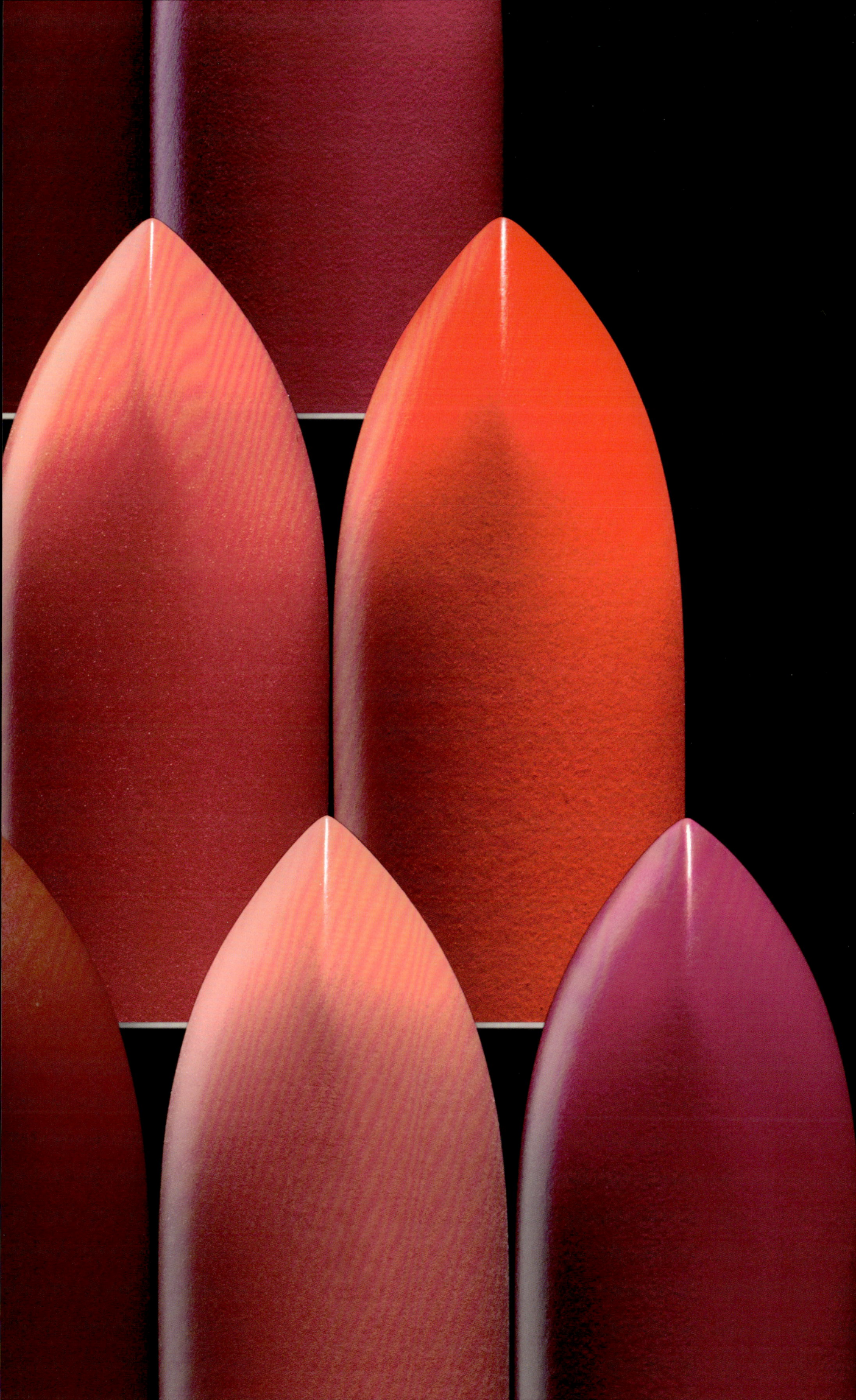

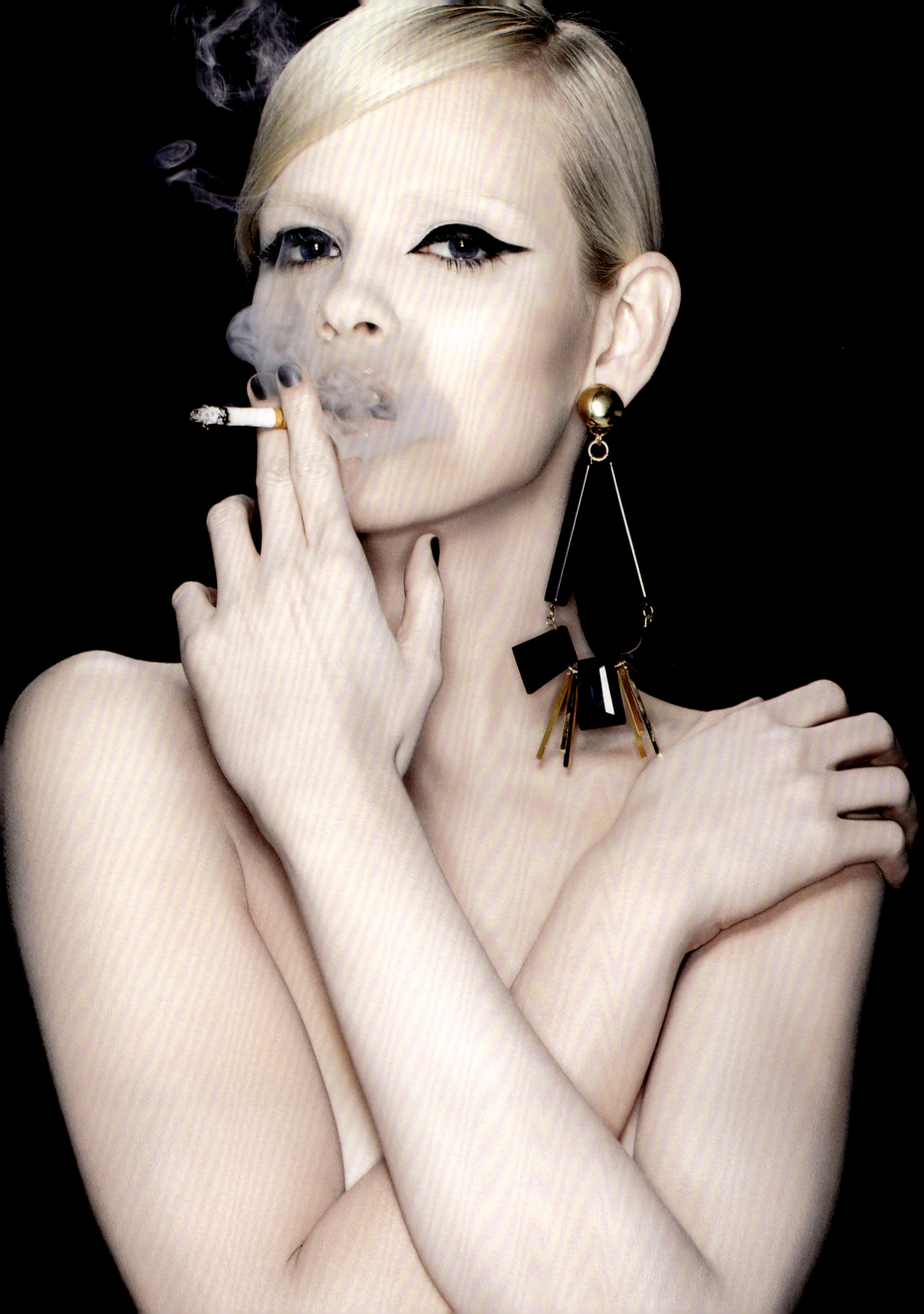

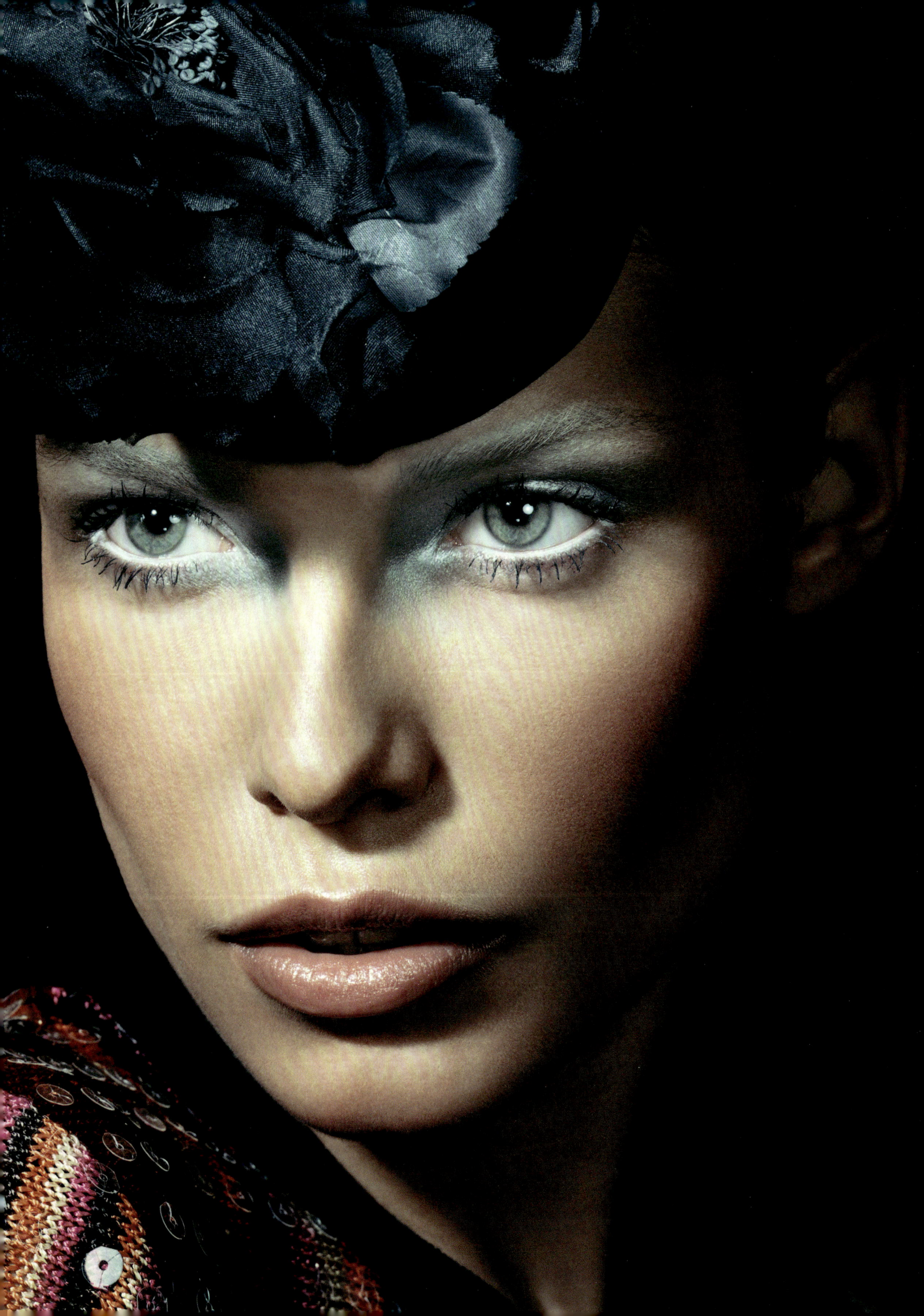

"AYA JONES, KATE MOSS, NAOMI CAMPBELL, KYLIE BAX, KAREN PARK, ALEC WEK, CLARA AKER BENJAMIN, KAREN ELSON, ERIN O'CONNOR, SUNNIVA STORDAL, MICHELLE FERERRA, COLETTE PECHEKHONOVA, ELEONORA BOSE, ALYSSA SUTHERLAND, JAMIE BOCHERT, LOUISE PEDERSEN, LINDA EVANGELISTA, GUINEVERE VAN SEENUS, LILY COLE, ANNE WATANABE, AMY WESSON, PAMELA BERNIER, LYDIA HEARST, HEATHER MARKS, AMBER VALETTA, DAPHNE GUINNESS, IRIS STRUBEGGER, MARIACARLA BOSCONO, GINTA LAPINA, KRISTEN MCMENAMY, STELLA TENNANT, TONI GARRN, DARIA STROKOUS—I LOVE YOU ALL! THANK YOU FOR BEING SO BEAUTIFUL, AND SO MUCH FUN, AND MAKING MY WORK AND MY LIFE SO EXCITING."
— FRANÇOIS NARS

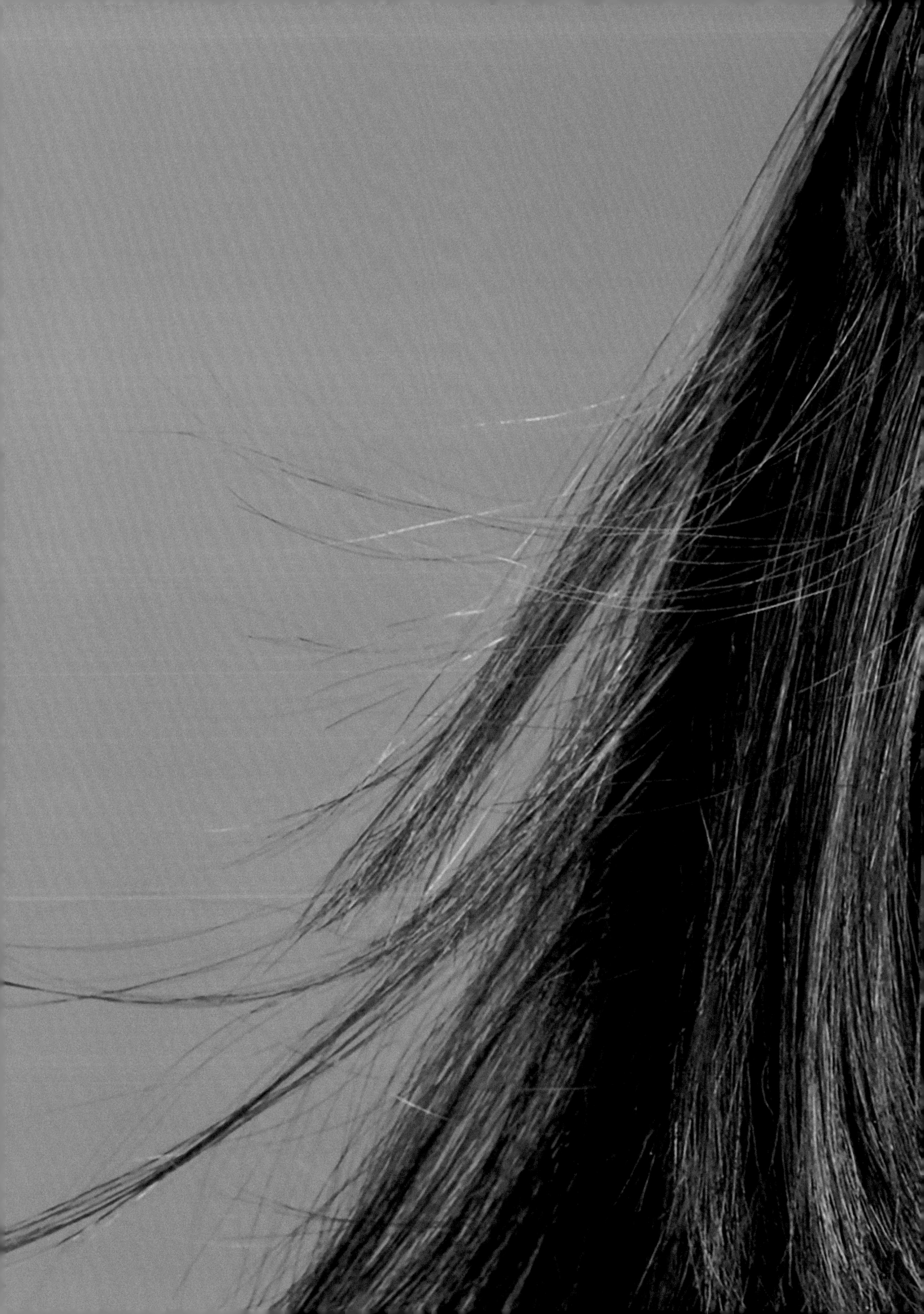

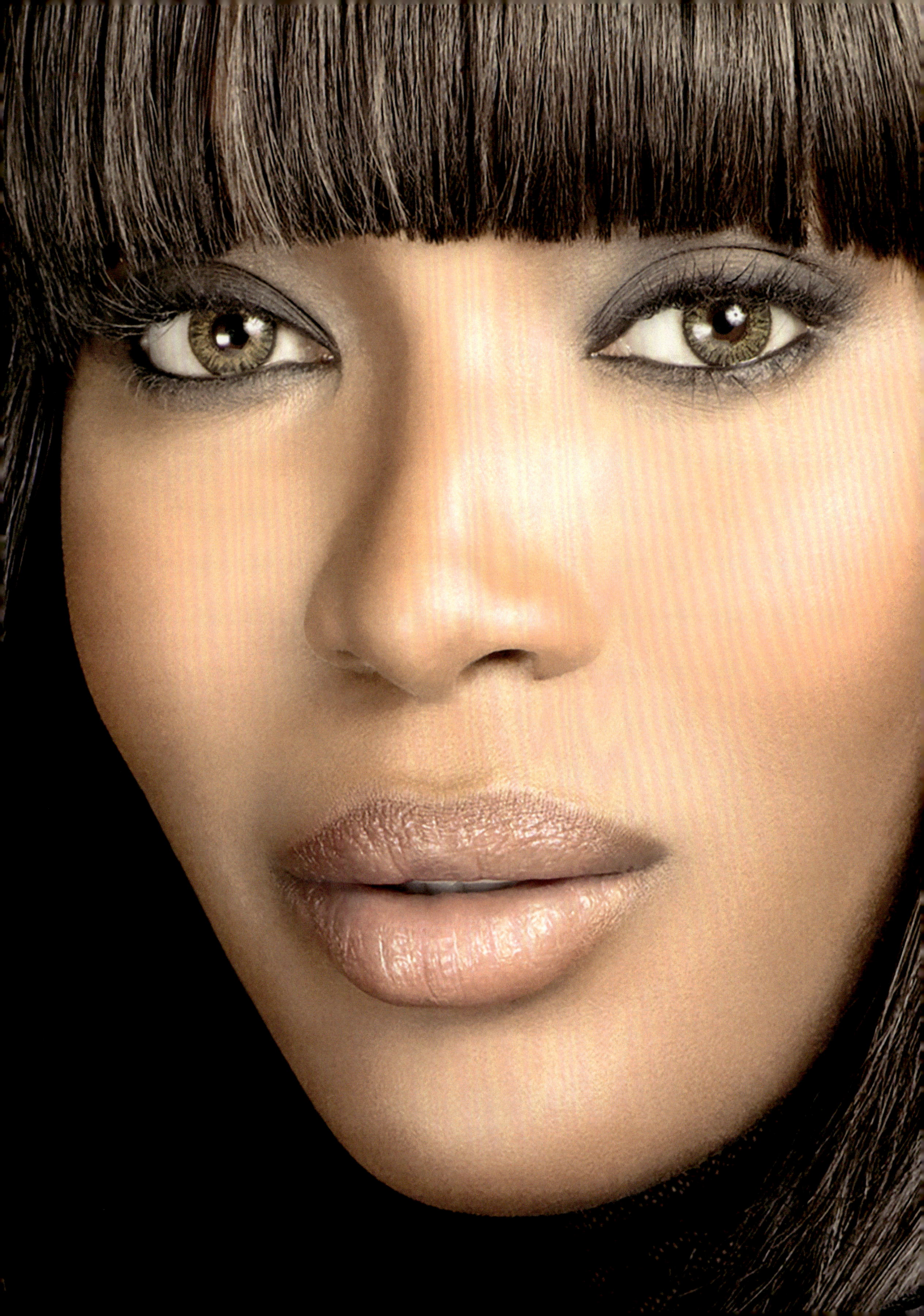

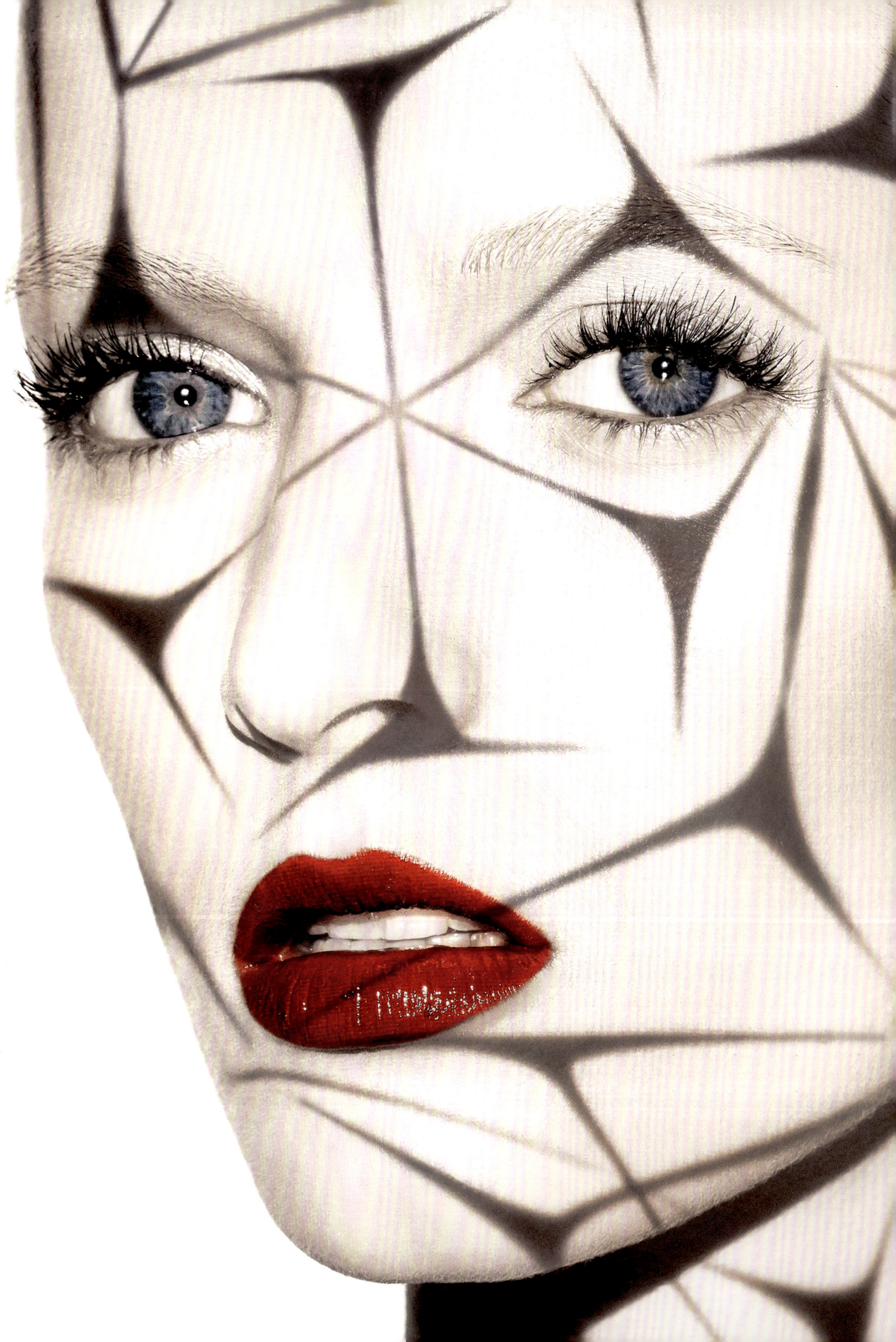

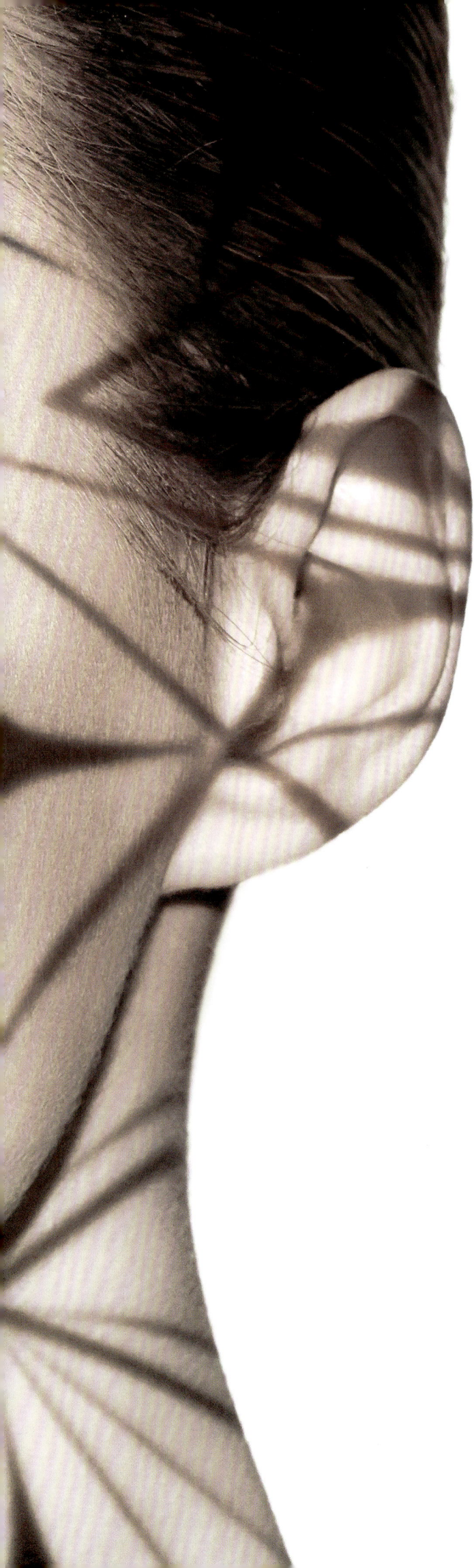

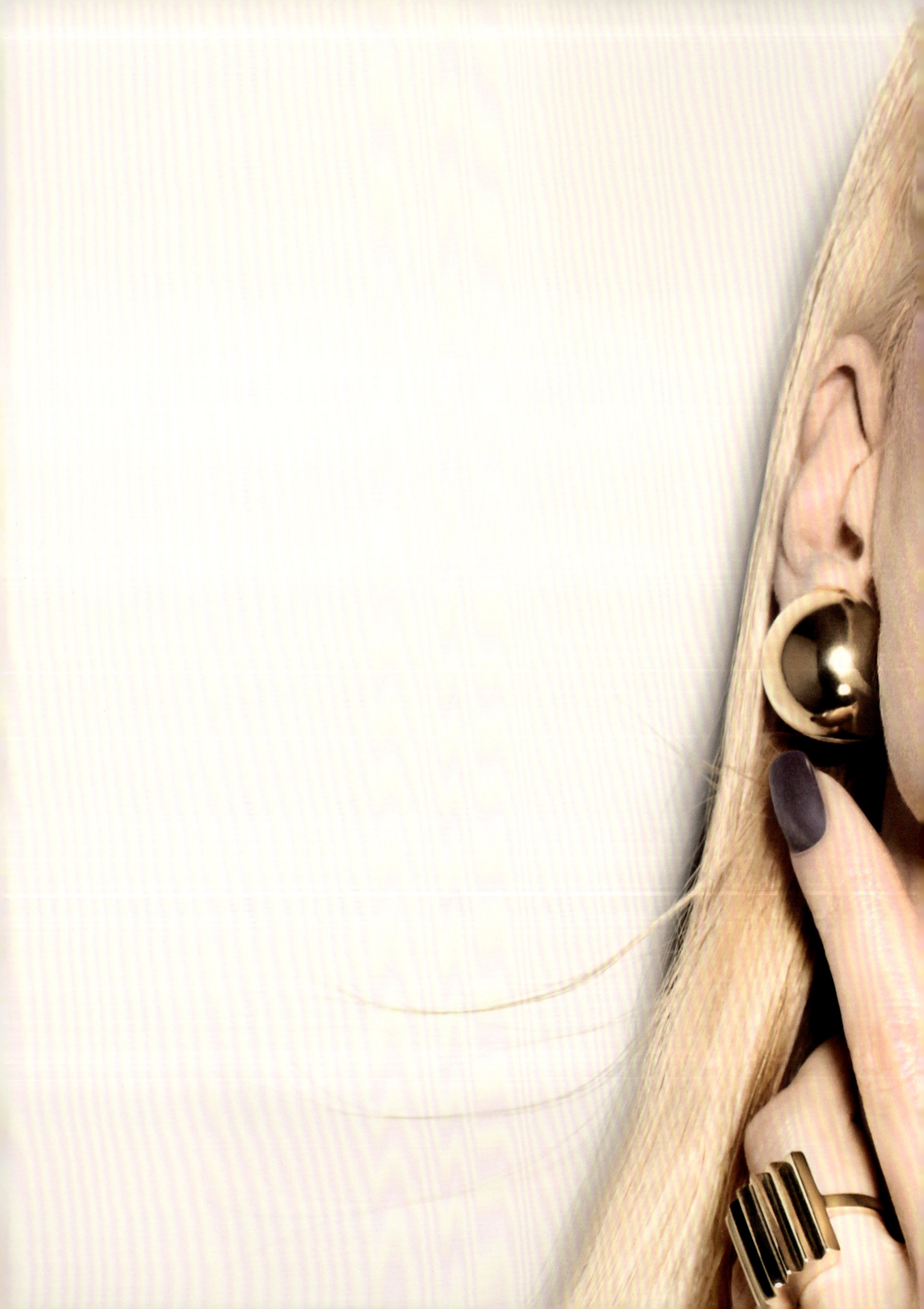

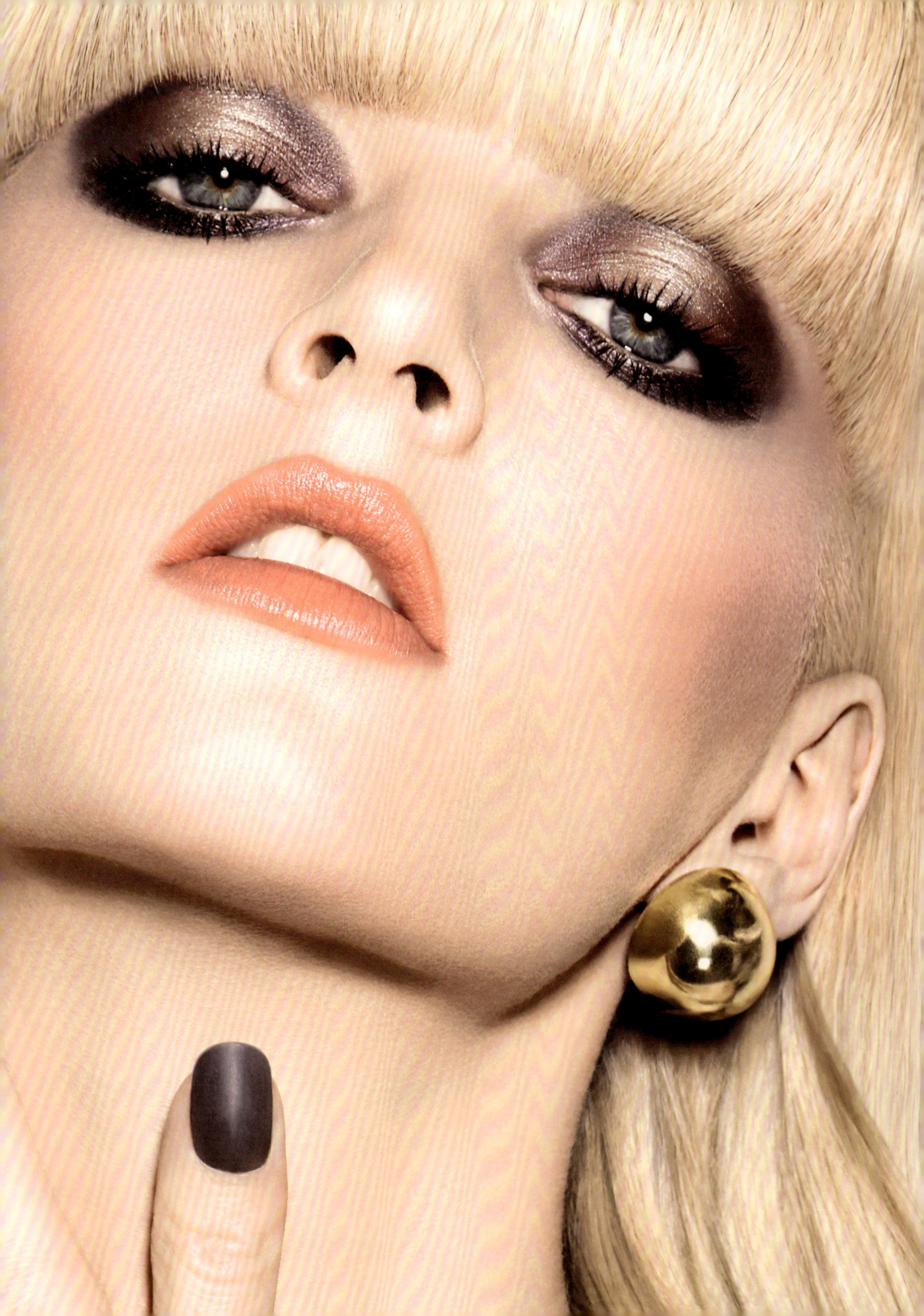

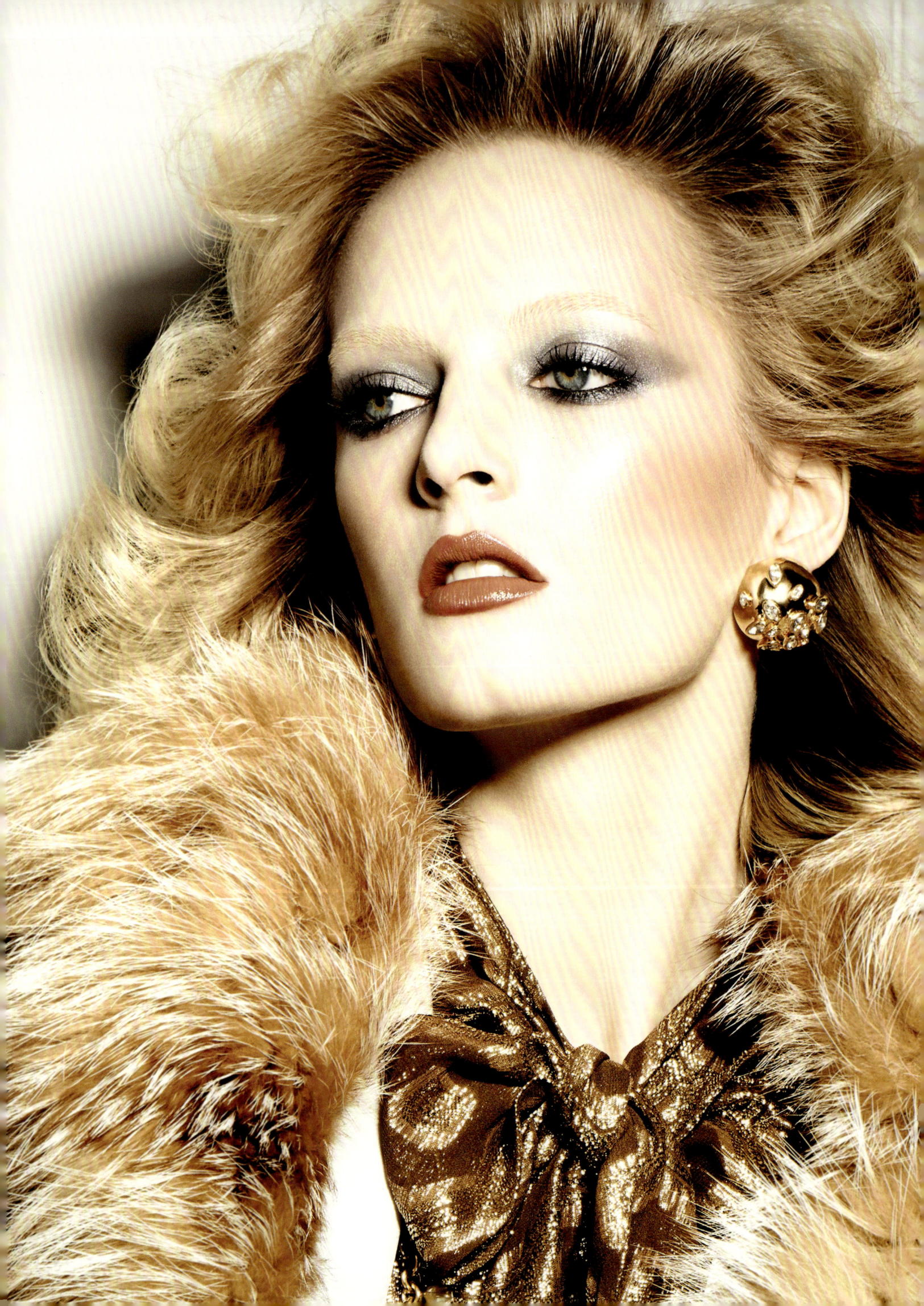

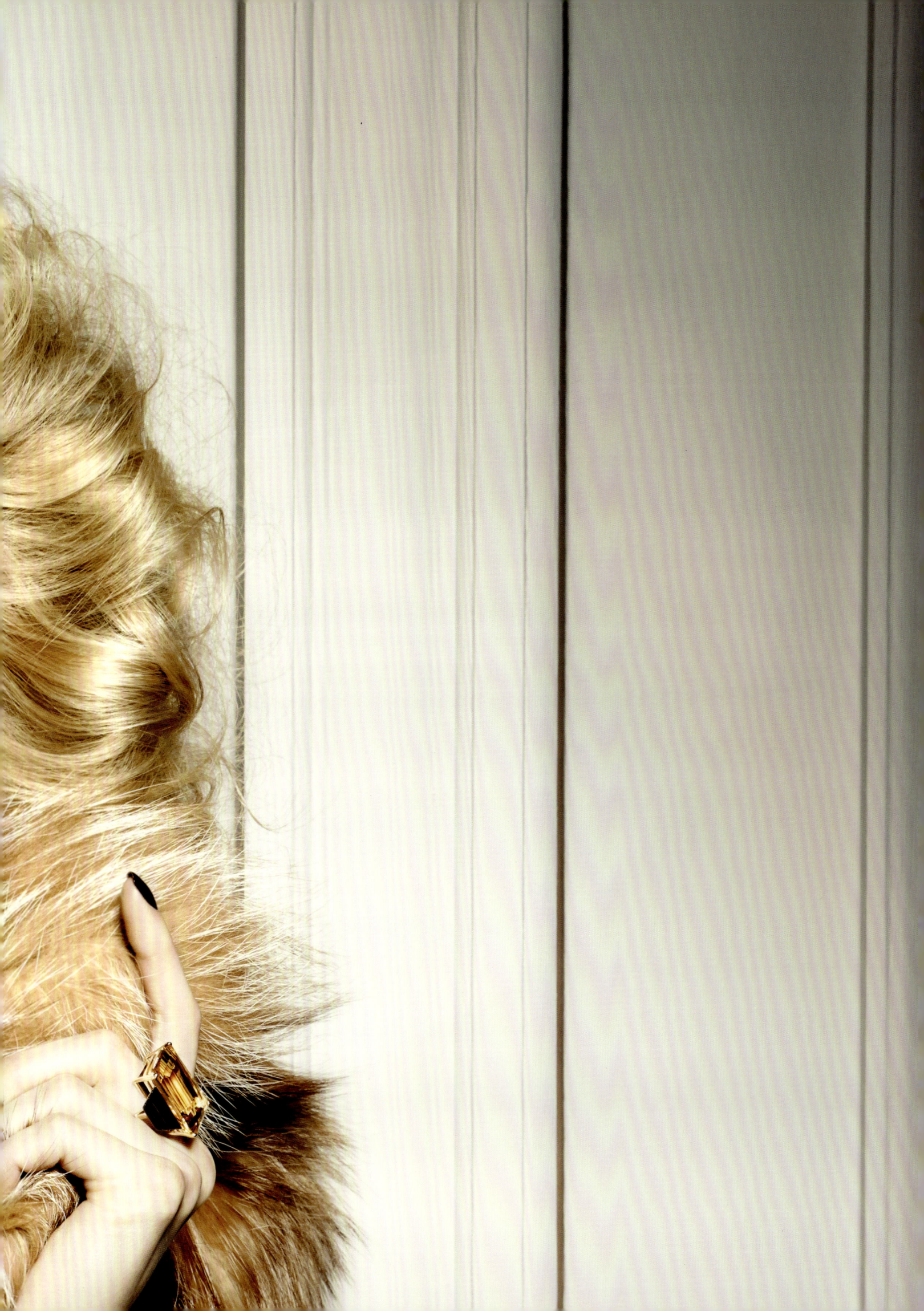

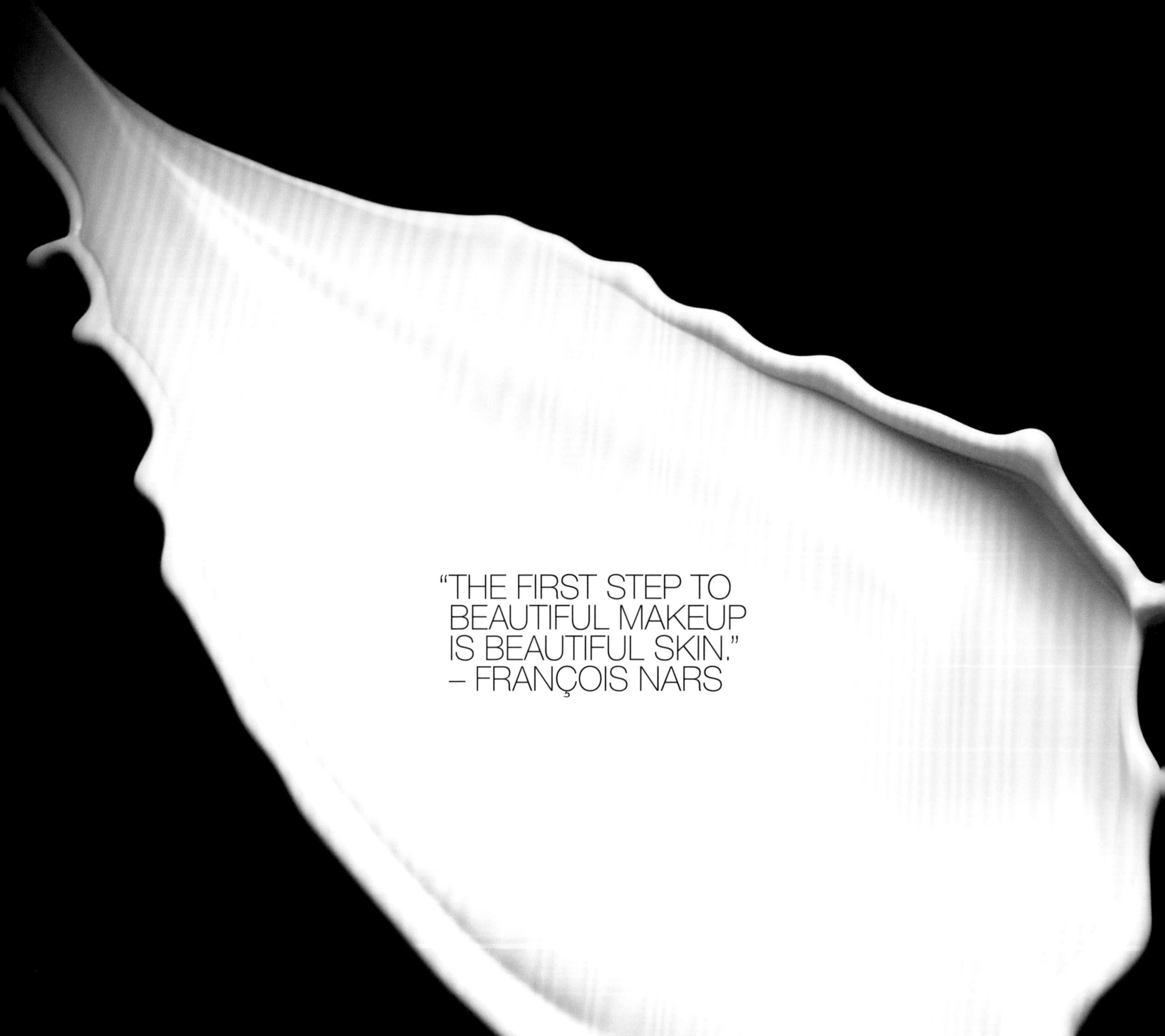

"THE FIRST STEP TO
BEAUTIFUL MAKEUP
IS BEAUTIFUL SKIN."
– FRANÇOIS NARS

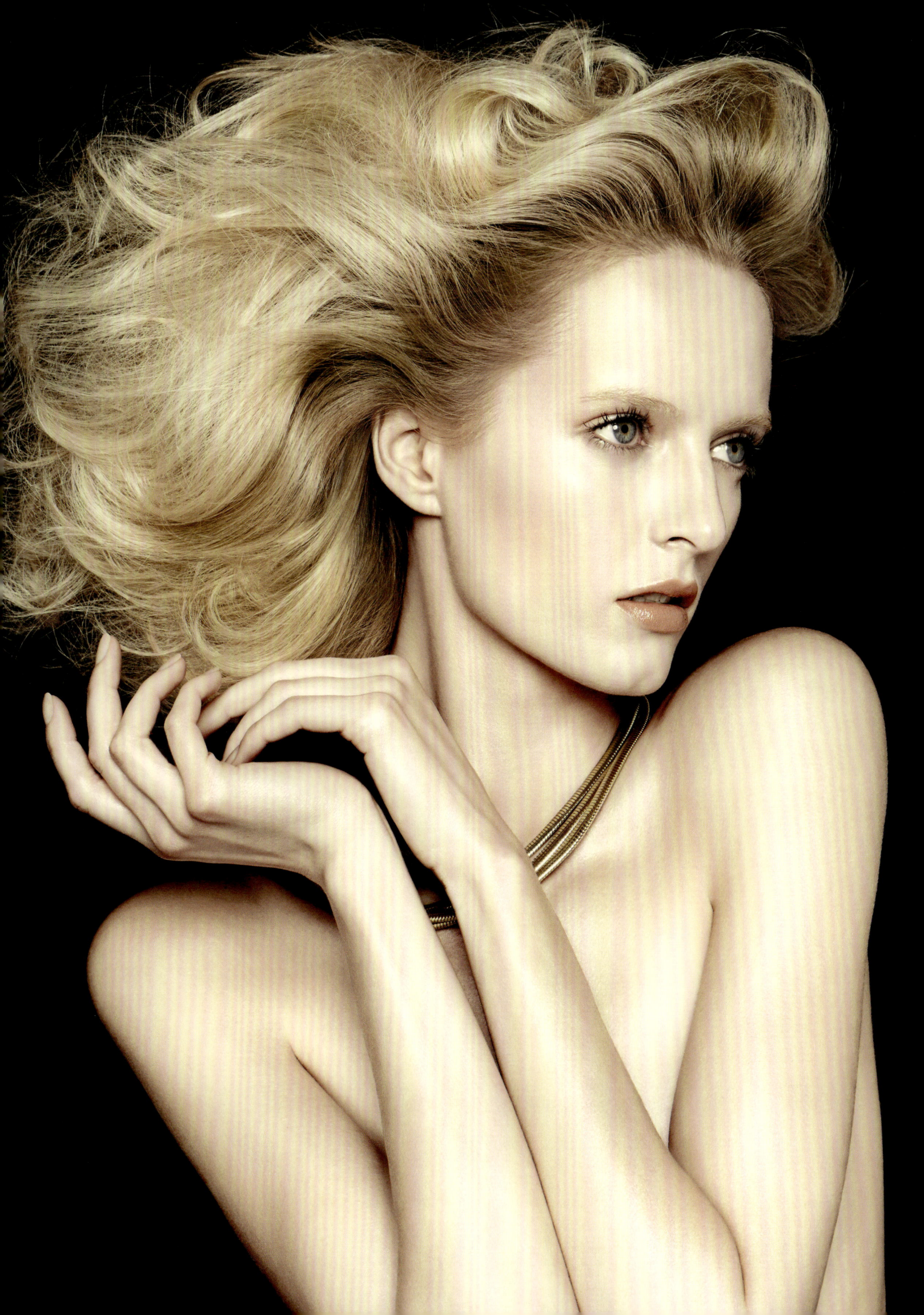

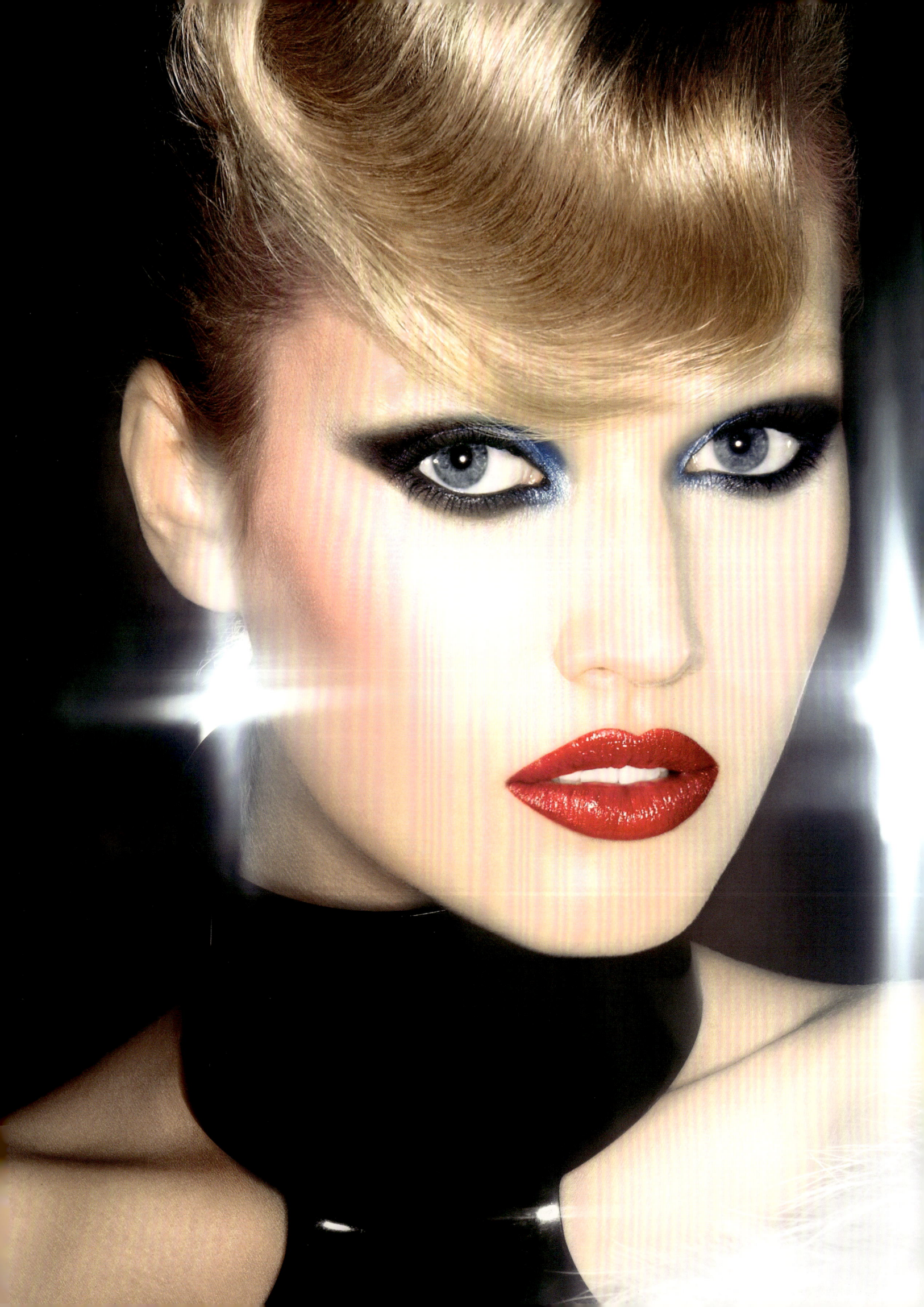

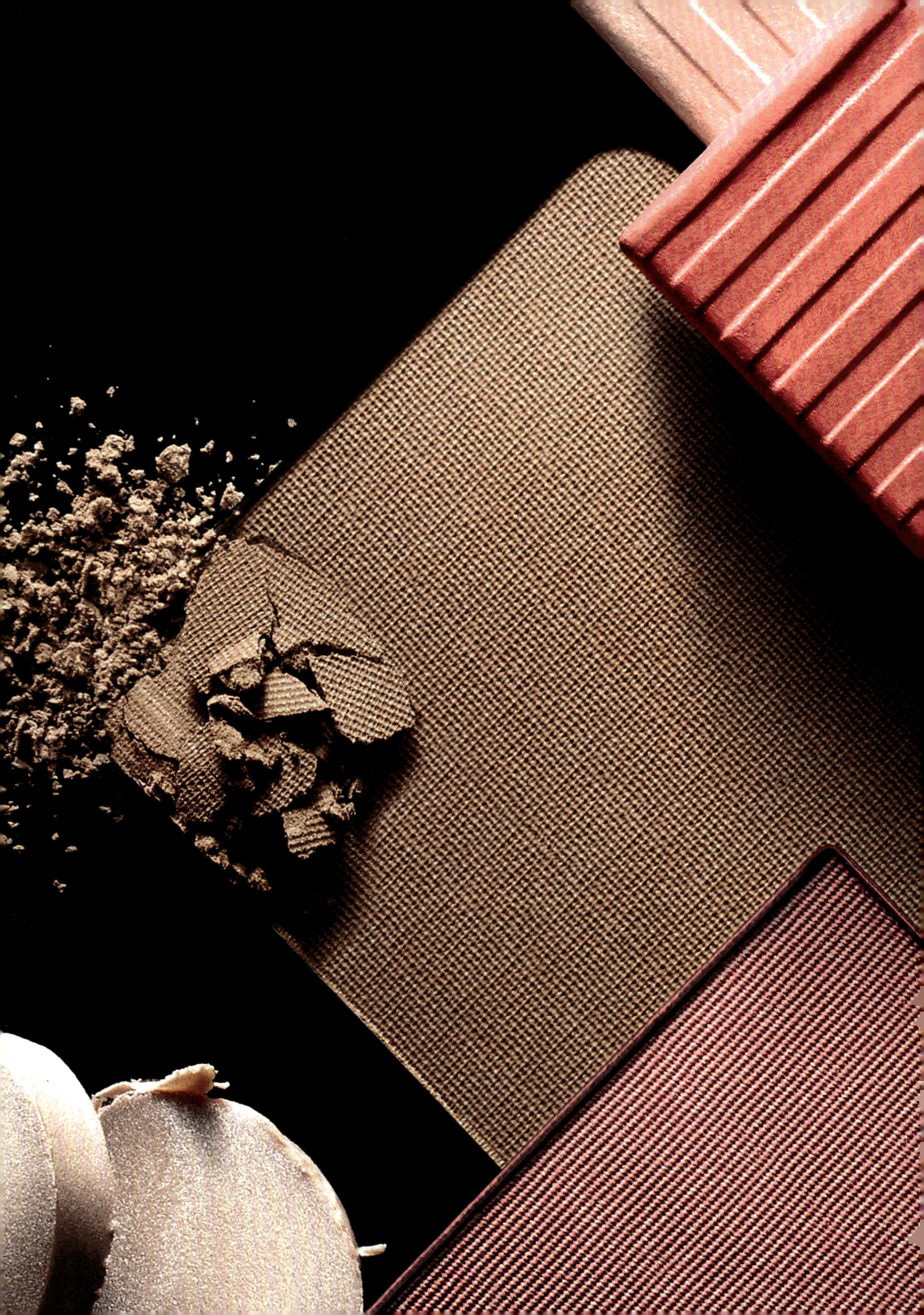

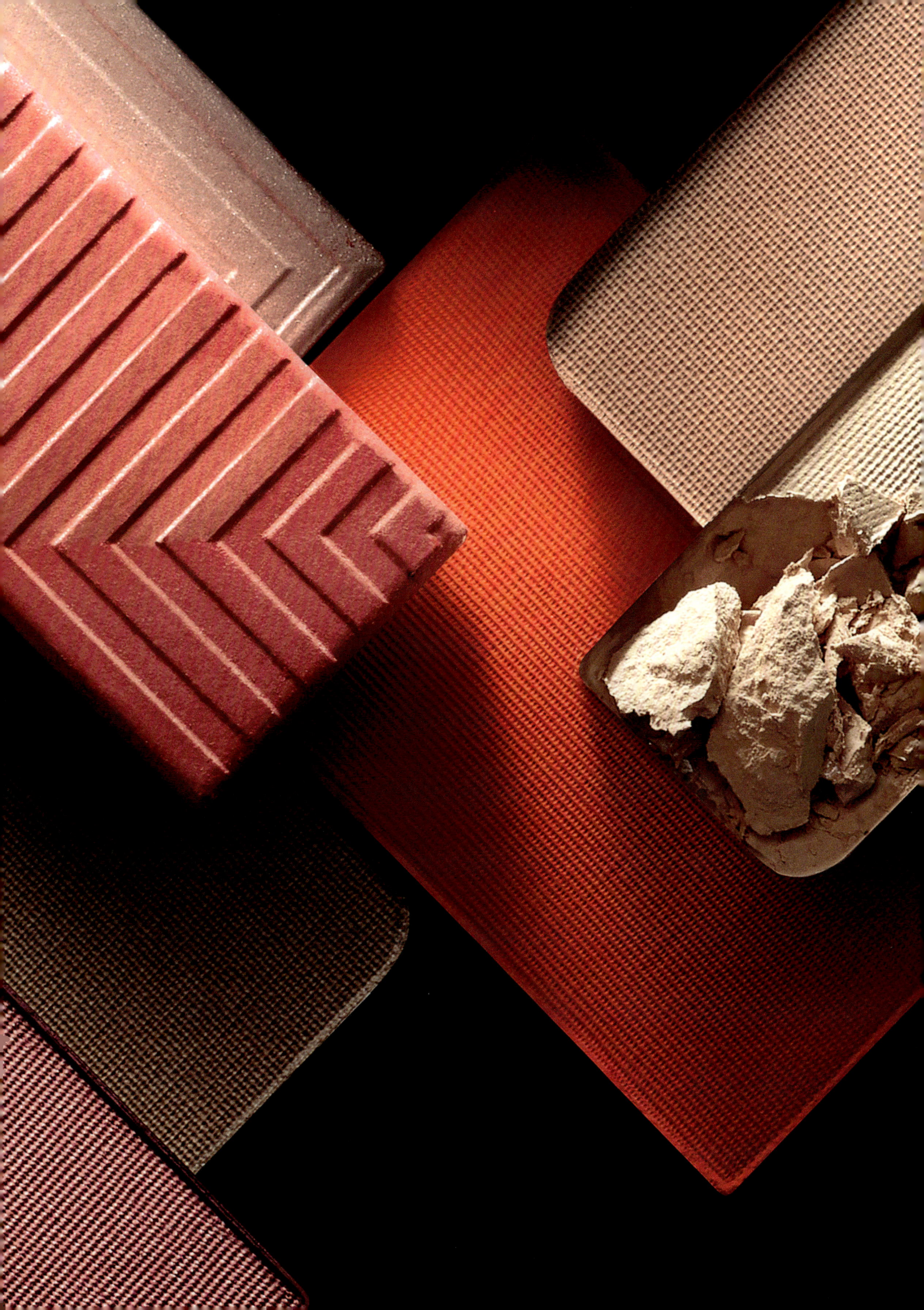

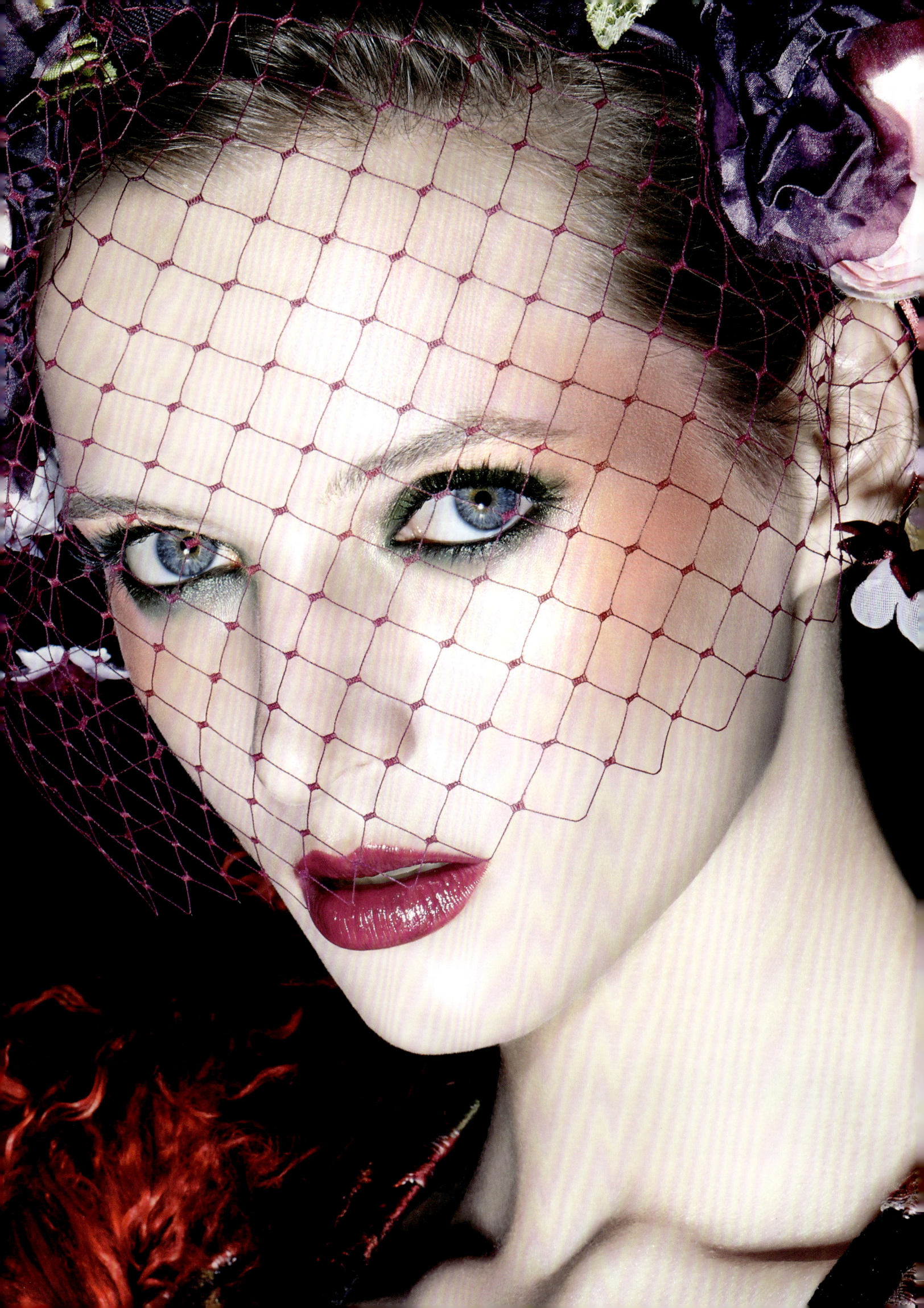

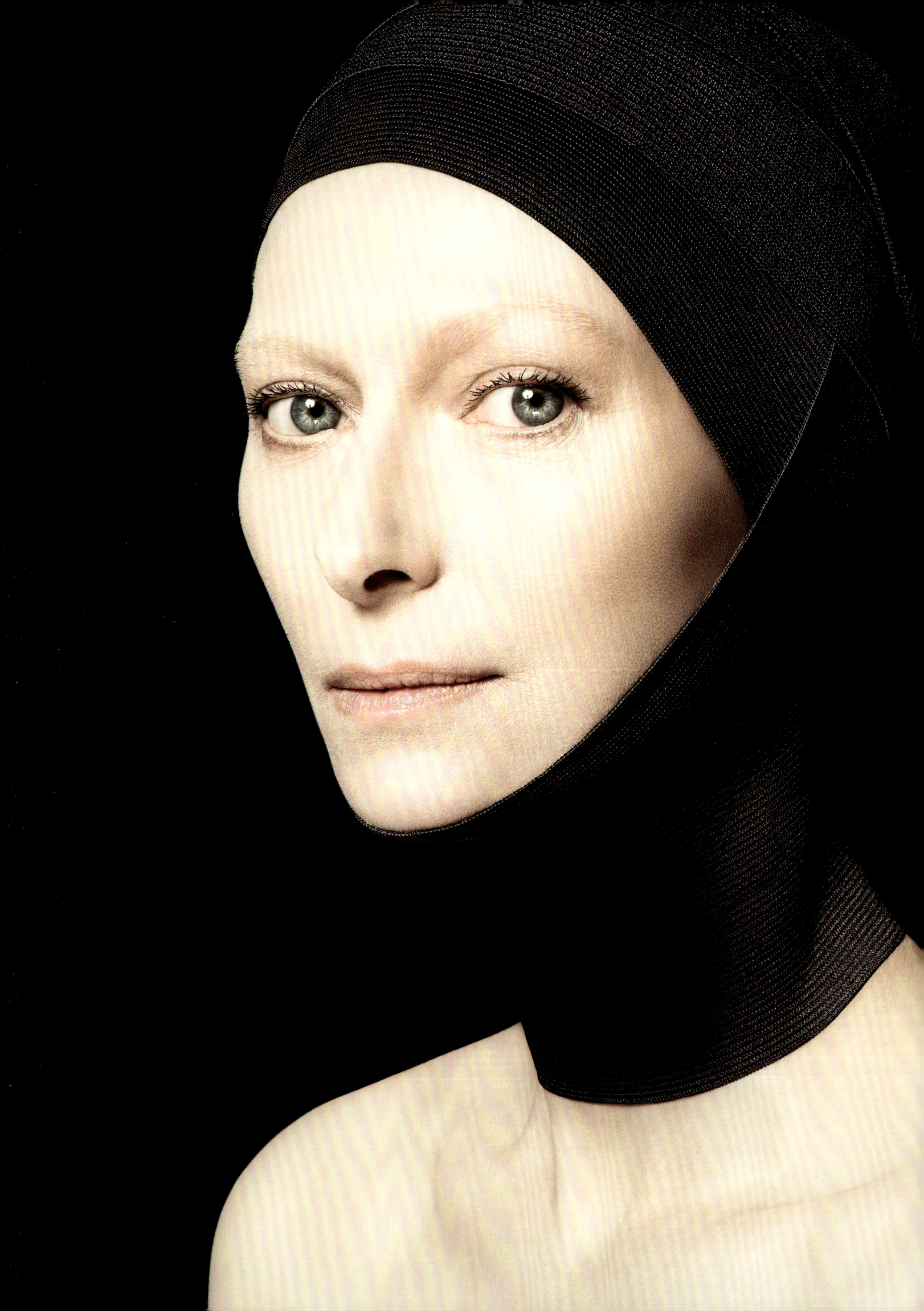

"I MET FRANÇOIS WHEN HE
ASKED TO PHOTOGRAPH
ME FOR HIS BOOK, HAVING
LONG BEEN AN ADMIRER OF
HIS FROM AFAR FOR MANY
YEARS. I LIKED HIM IMMENSELY
AND IMMEDIATELY, AND WE
WERE EAGER FROM THAT
FIRST SESSION TO DO MORE
THINGS TOGETHER. I COULD
NOT BE MORE PROUD TO CALL
HIM MY COLLEAGUE. NOW I
UNDERSTAND WHY HIS WORK
IS SO FRESH AND ORIGINAL:
BECAUSE HE IS SO BRIGHT AND
HAS SUCH A SWEET HEART."
– TILDA SWINTON

"IT WAS SUCH A DREAM
TO WORK WITH TILDA.
SHE IS SO BEAUTIFUL AND
AN INCREDIBLE ARTIST
WHO CAN TRANSFORM
INTO ANY CHARACTER LIKE
A CHAMELEON. I ADORE
PHOTOGRAPHING HER."
– FRANÇOIS NARS

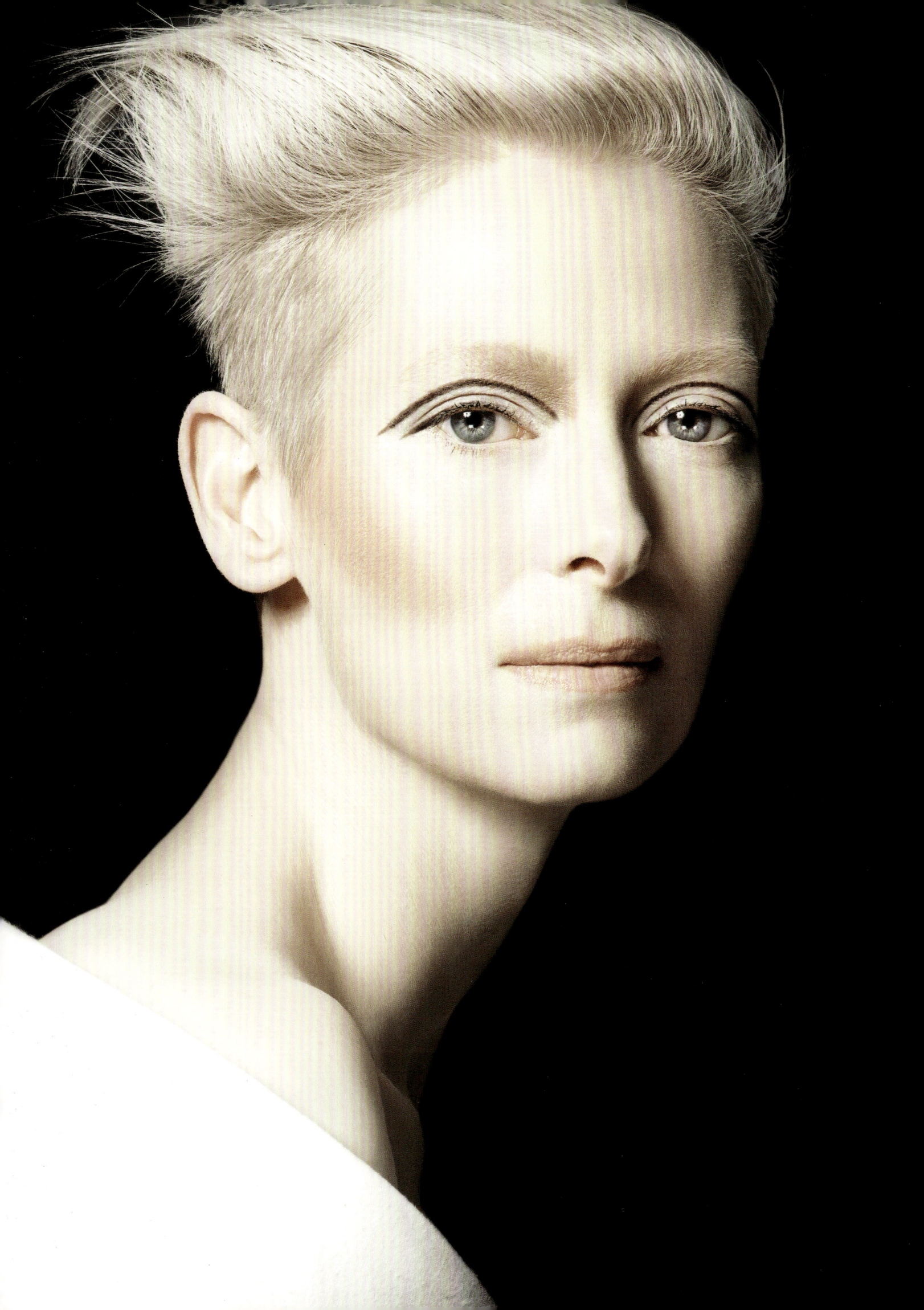

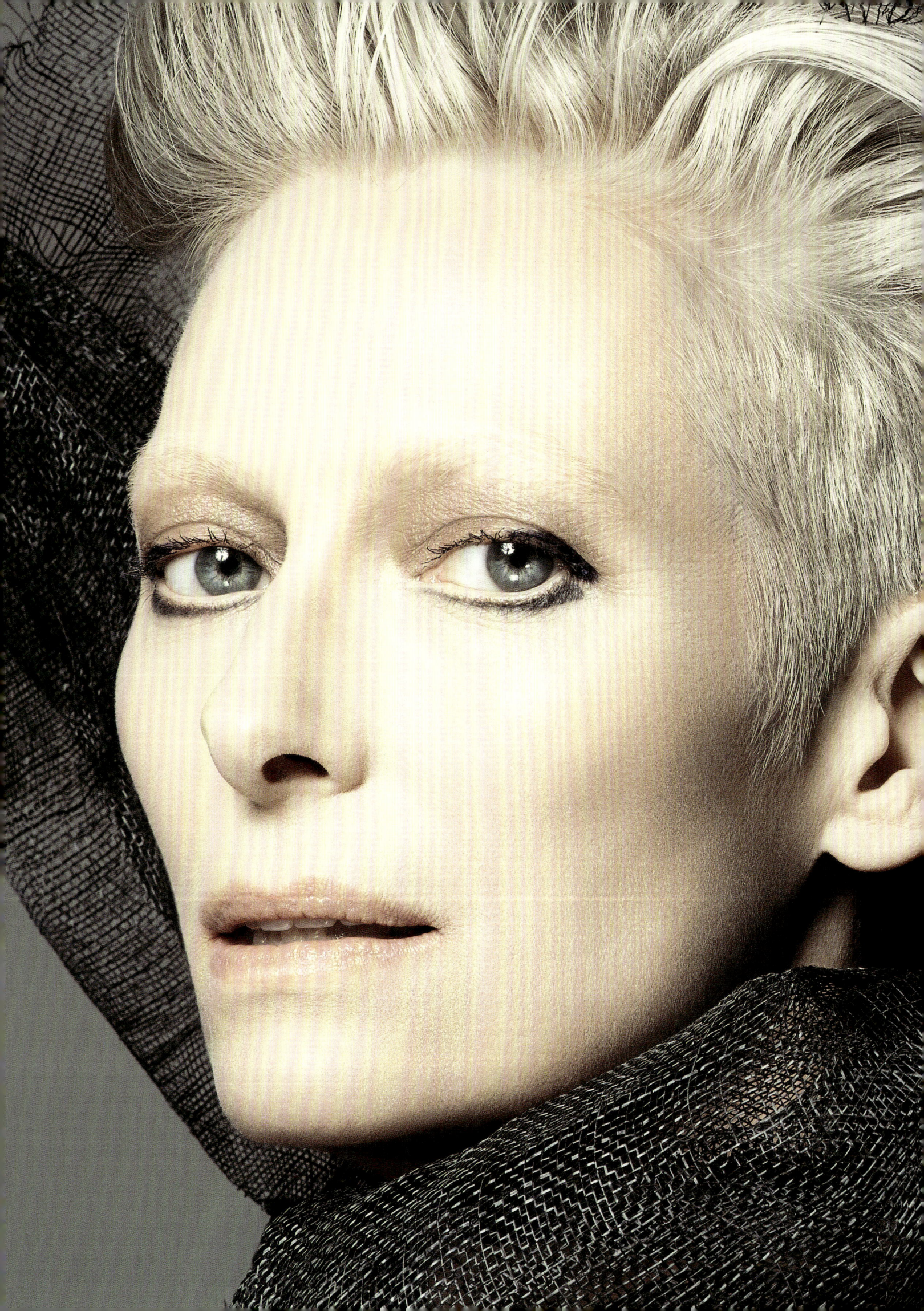

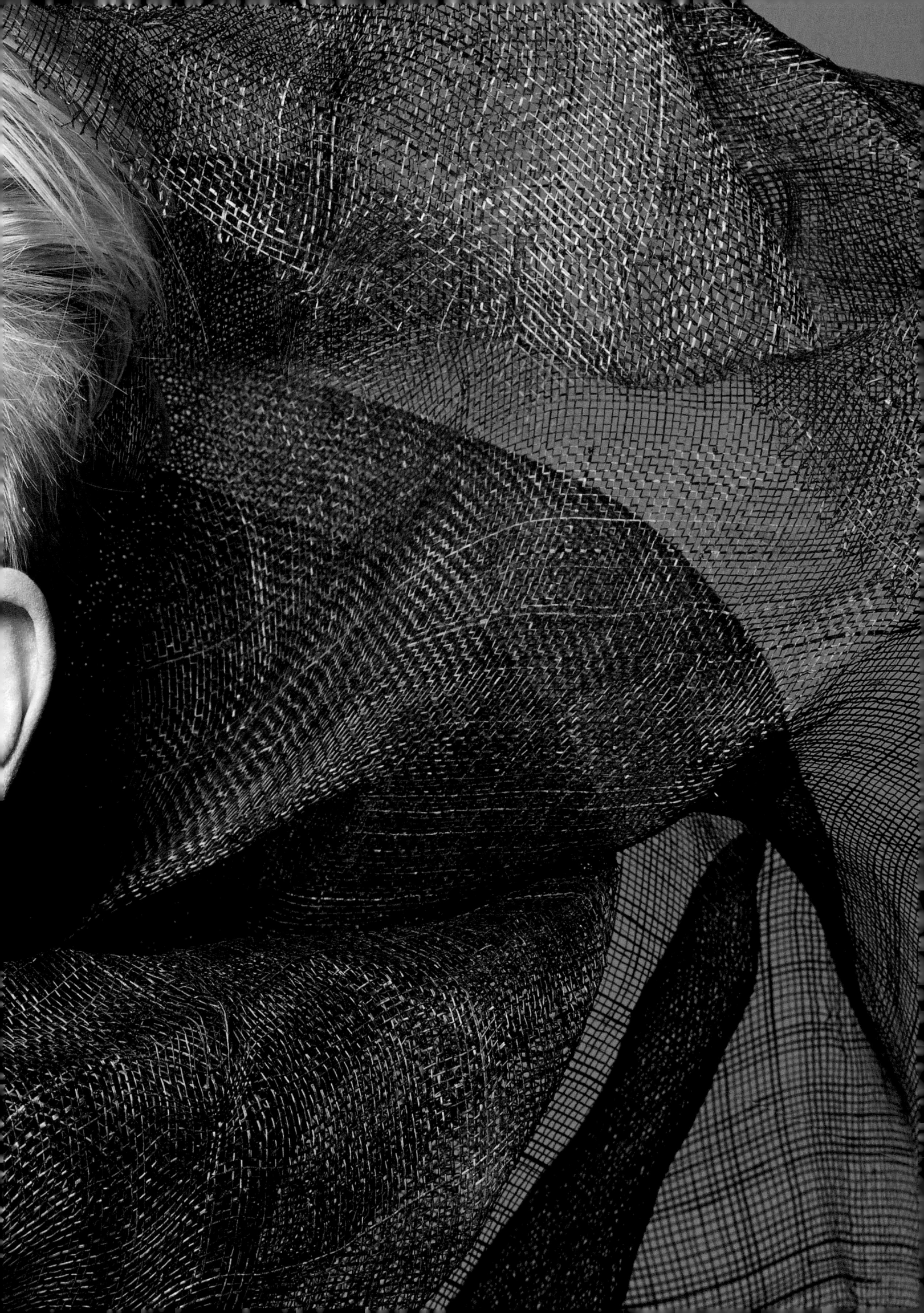

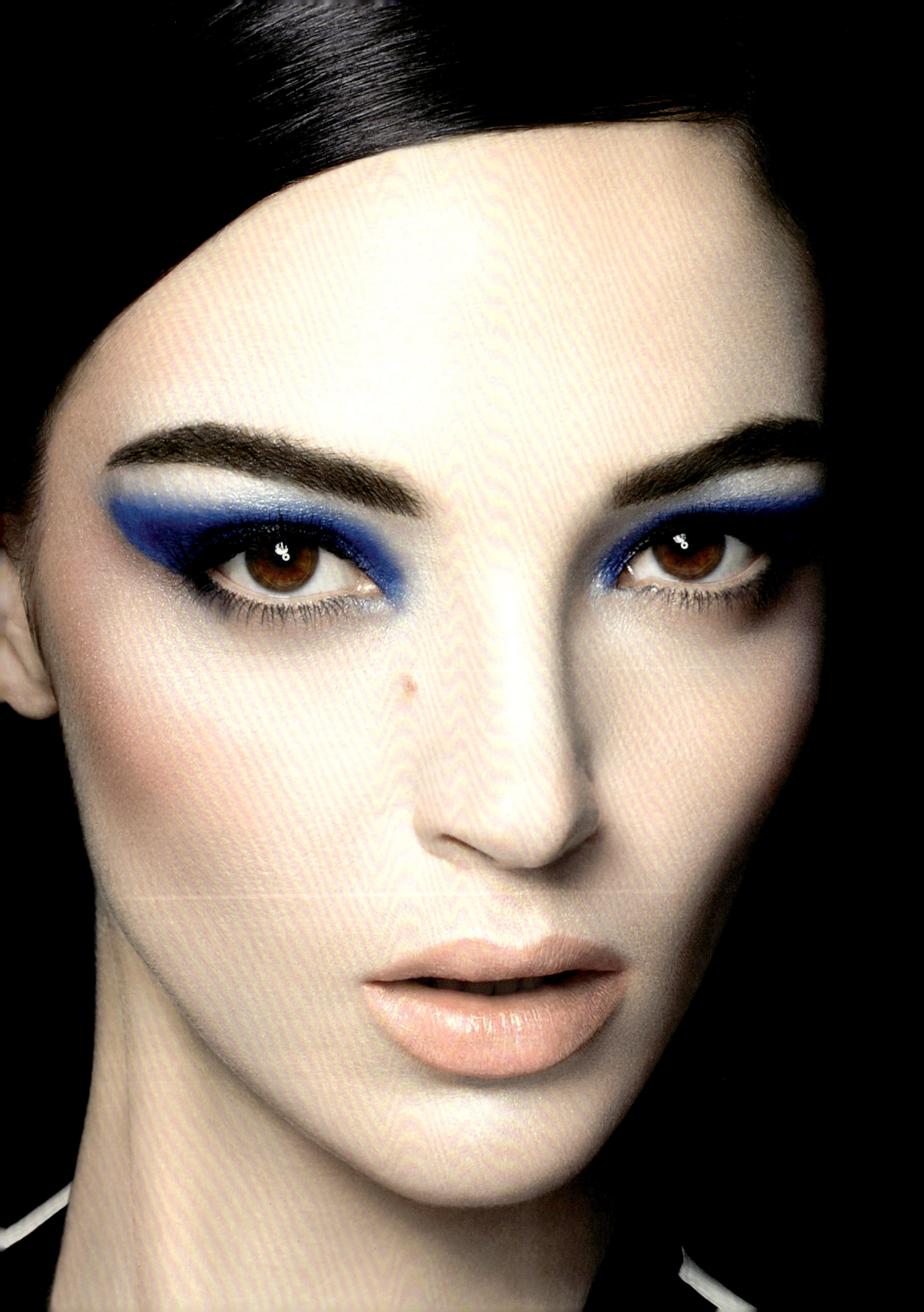

"WHETHER I AM
TAKING PICTURES
FOR CAMPAIGNS
OR FASHION
EDITORIALS OR
EVEN FOR MY OWN
BOOKS, MY GOAL
IS TO MAKE BEAUTY
A STATEMENT AND
BRING OUT WHAT
IS ON THE INSIDE.
I TRULY BELIEVE
THAT TRUE BEAUTY
LIES WITHIN OUR
PERSONALITY
AND SOUL."
— FRANÇOIS NARS

5

"THE MODERNITY AND GENIUS OF GUY'S IMAGES ARE MIND BLOWING. HIS WORK IS TIMELESS. NOBODY COMES CLOSE TO GUY TODAY."
– FRANÇOIS NARS

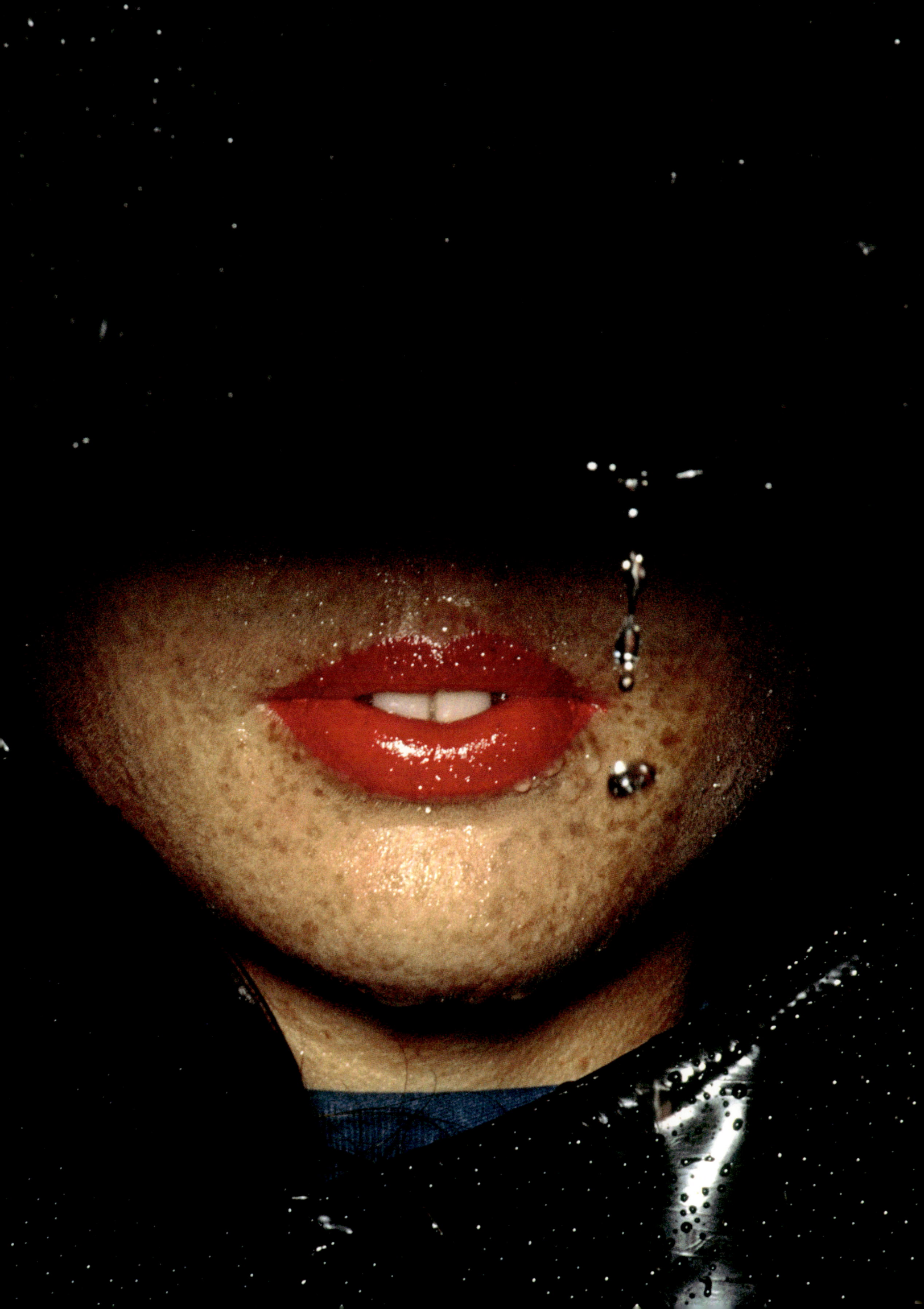

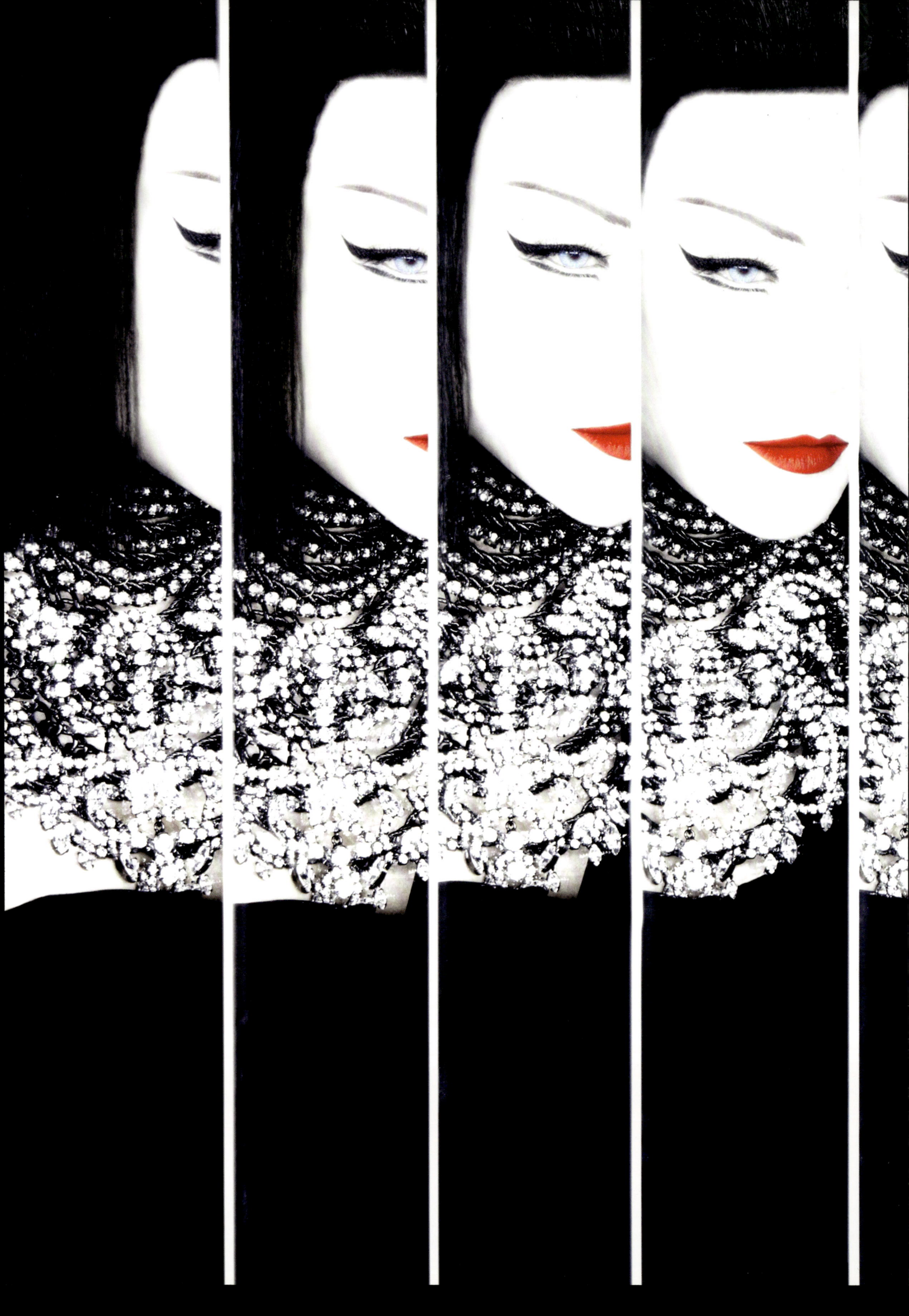

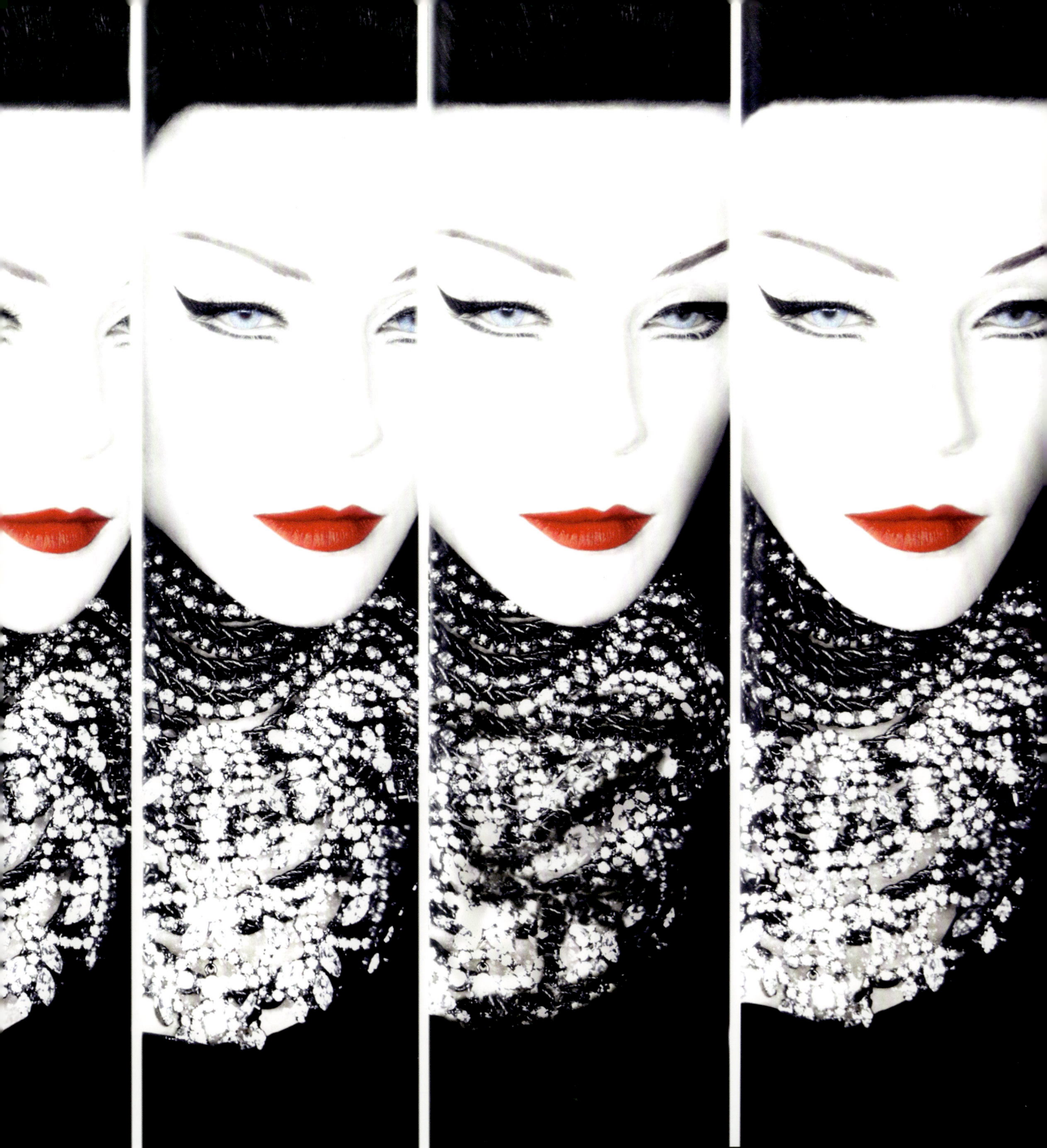

"HOW CAN I DESCRIBE DAPHNE?
A FASHION ICON WITH AN INNATE
SENSE OF STYLE AND ELEGANCE,
A SENSITIVE HUMAN BEING, A VERY
UNIQUE LADY WHO IS DEFINITELY
THE OPPOSITE OF COMMON AND
BORING. SHE IS THE INCARNATION
OF EVERYTHING I LOVE."
– FRANÇOIS NARS

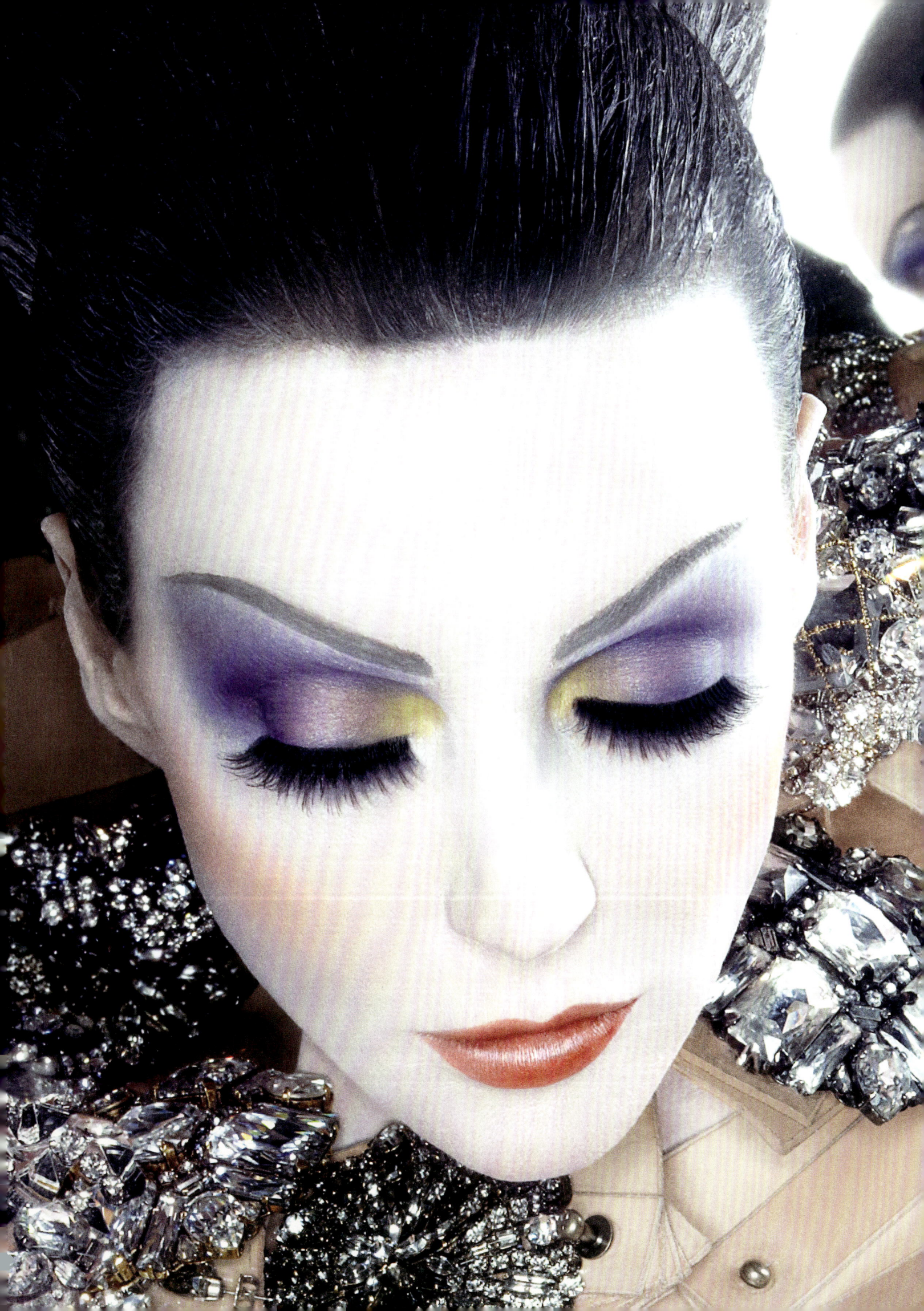

"FRANÇOIS HAS THE ABILITY TO SCOOP YOU OFF THE FLOOR WITH AN ASTOUNDING CREATIVE AND EMOTIONAL ENERGY. HE'S AN ARTIST IN THE TRUE SENSE: WHAT OTHER PEOPLE TAKE HOURS OVER, FRANÇOIS CAN PRODUCE IN SECONDS. HE HAS IMPECCABLE TASTE AND IS A PLEASURE TO WORK WITH, DELIVERING A PRECISE VISION THAT IS AS EFFORTLESS AS IT IS SWIFT." – DAPHNE GUINNESS

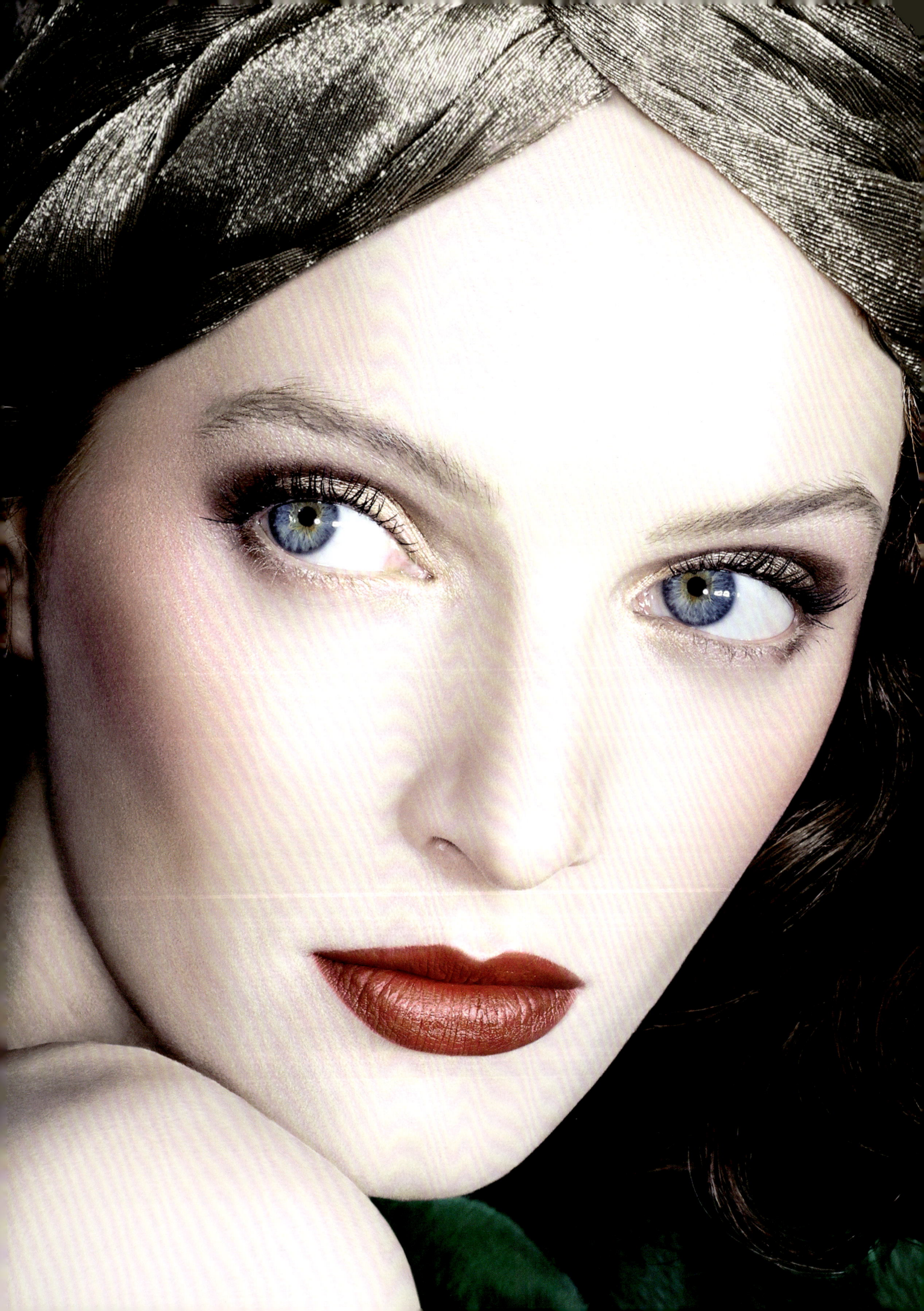

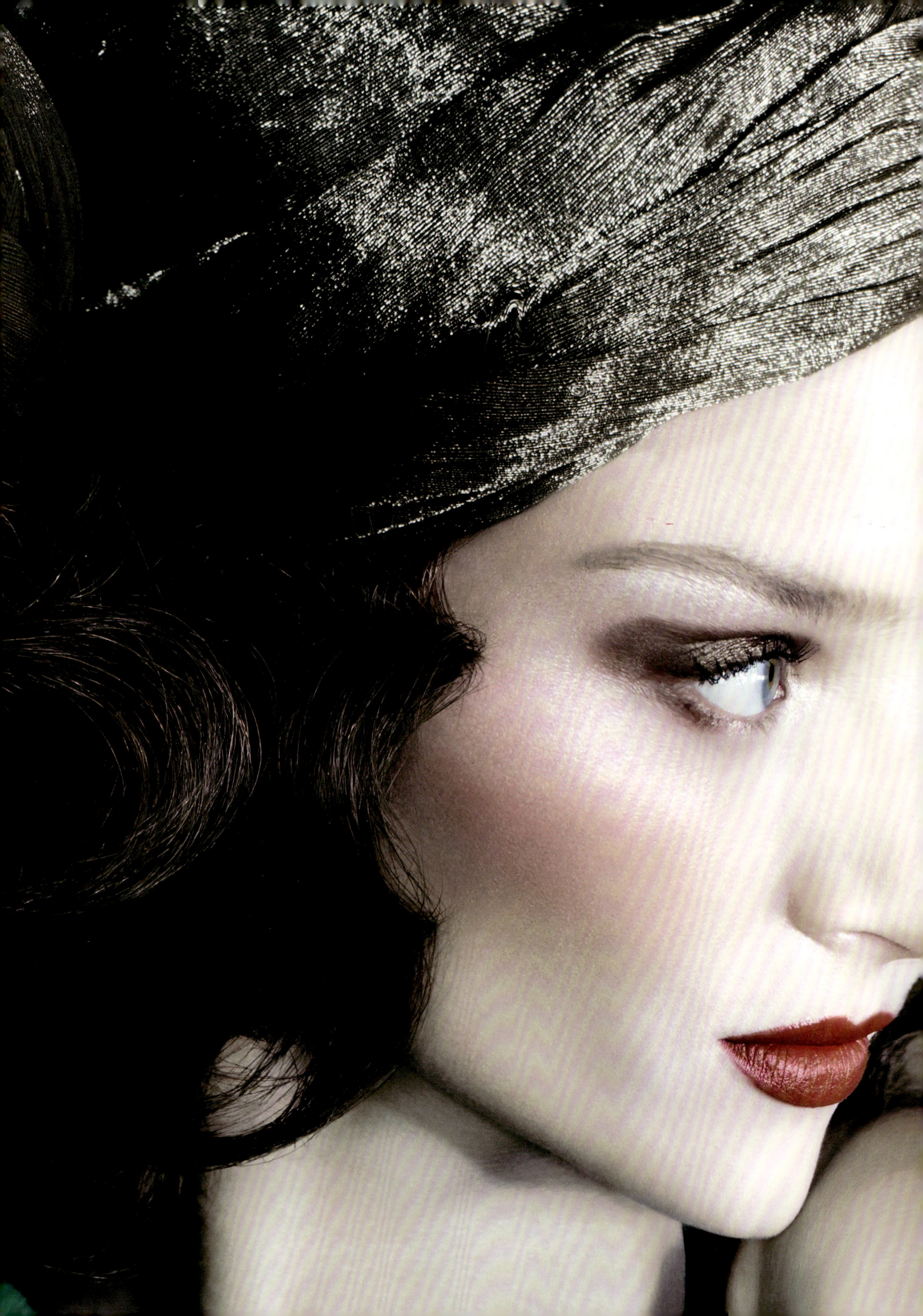

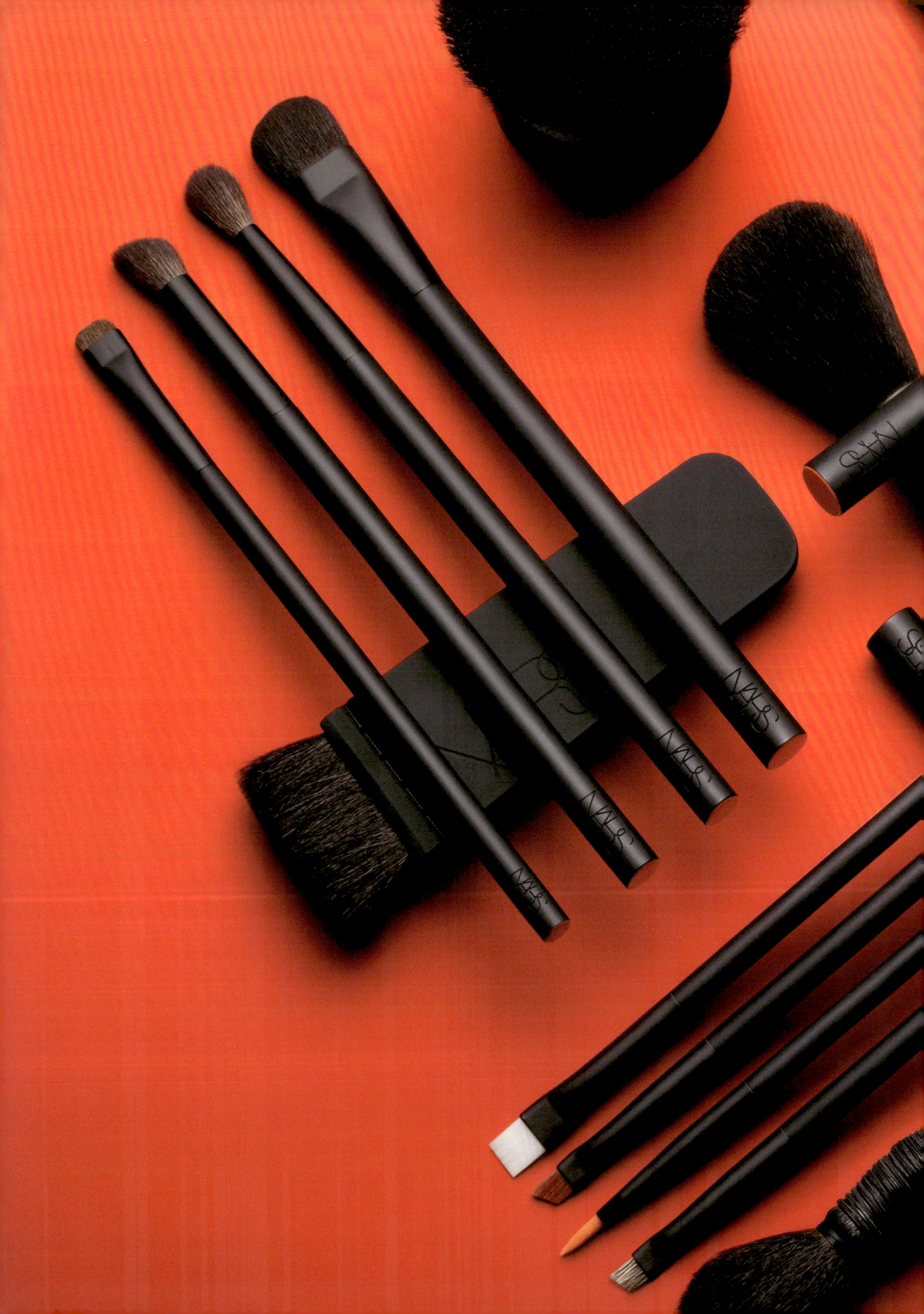

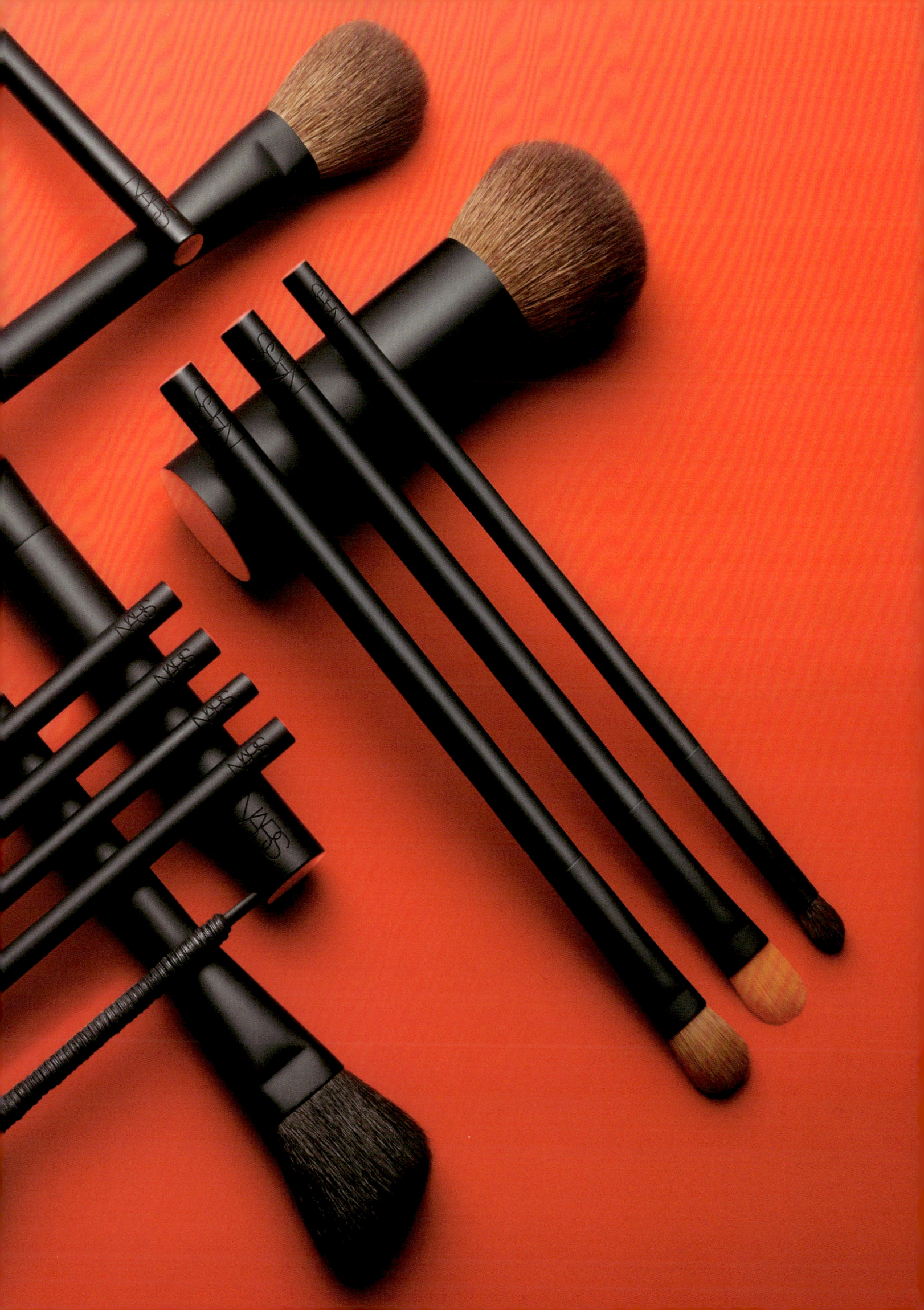

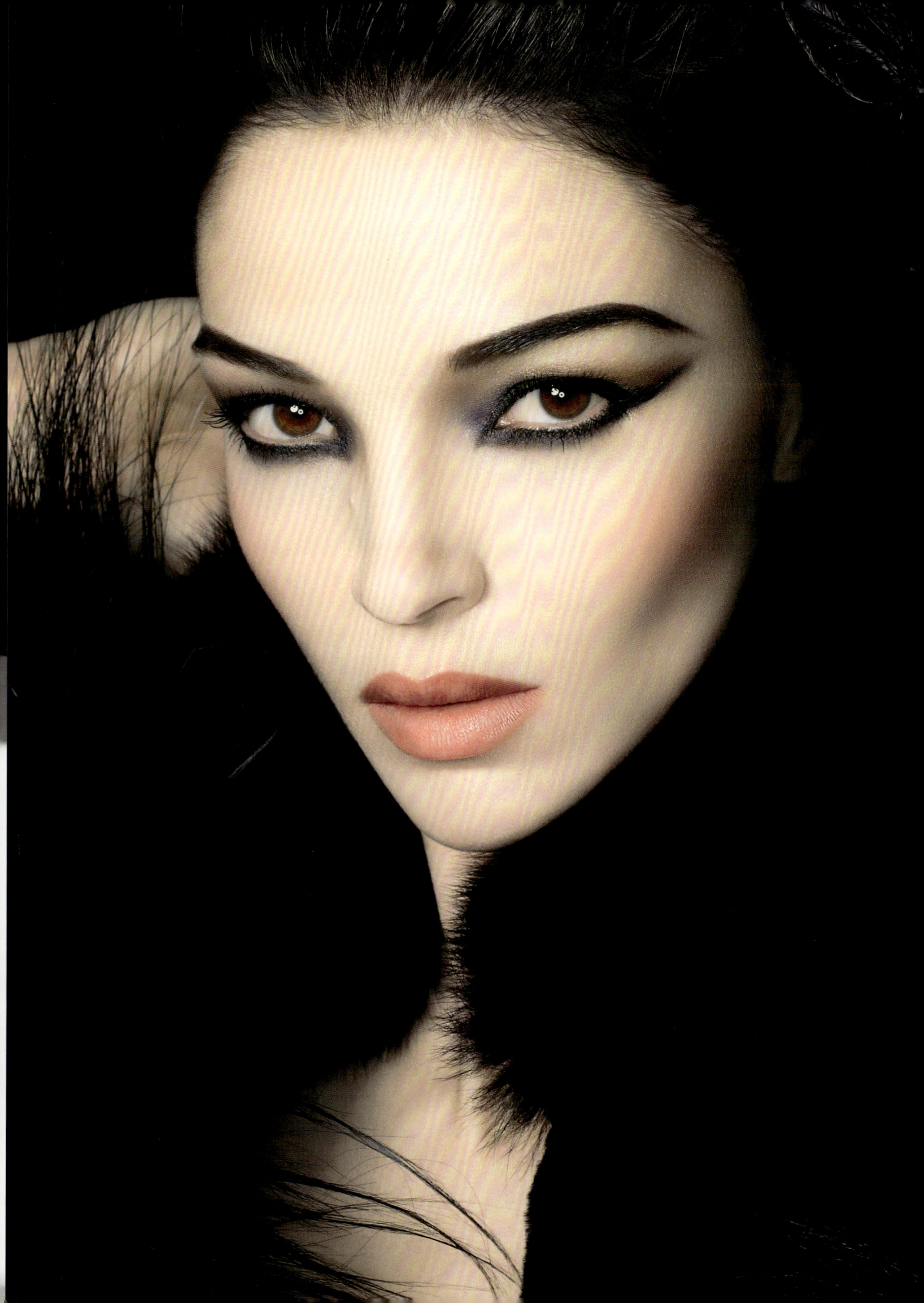

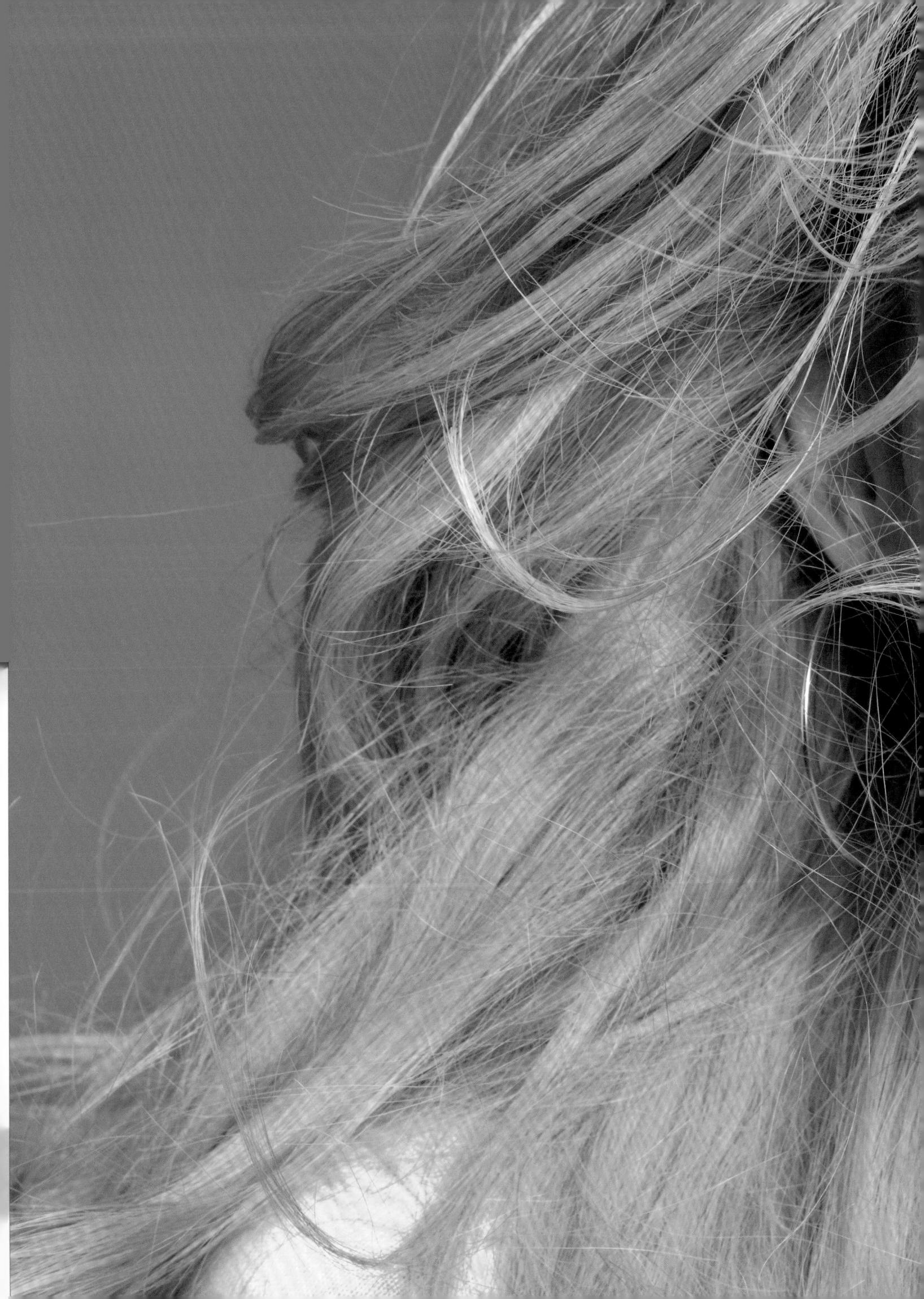

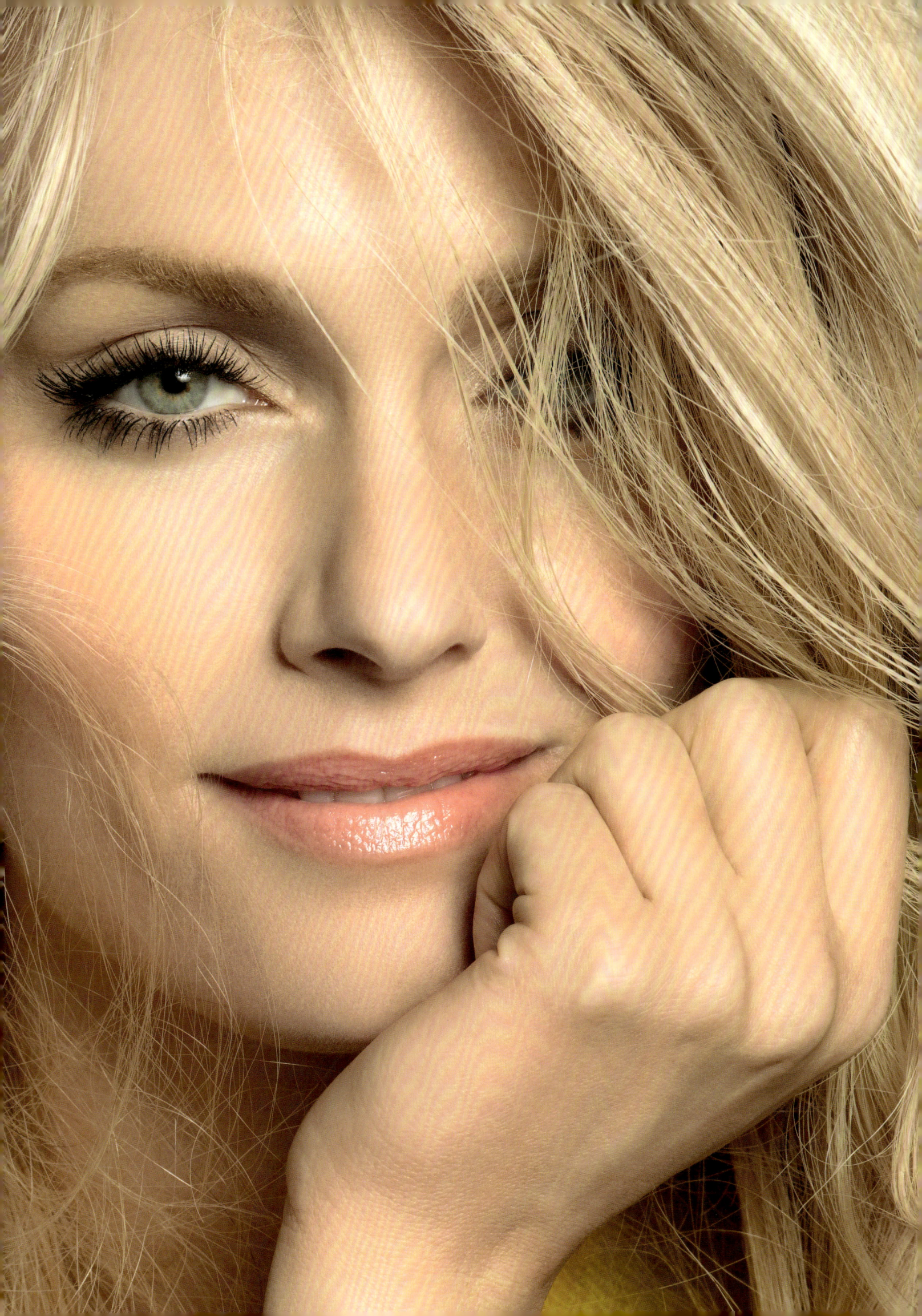

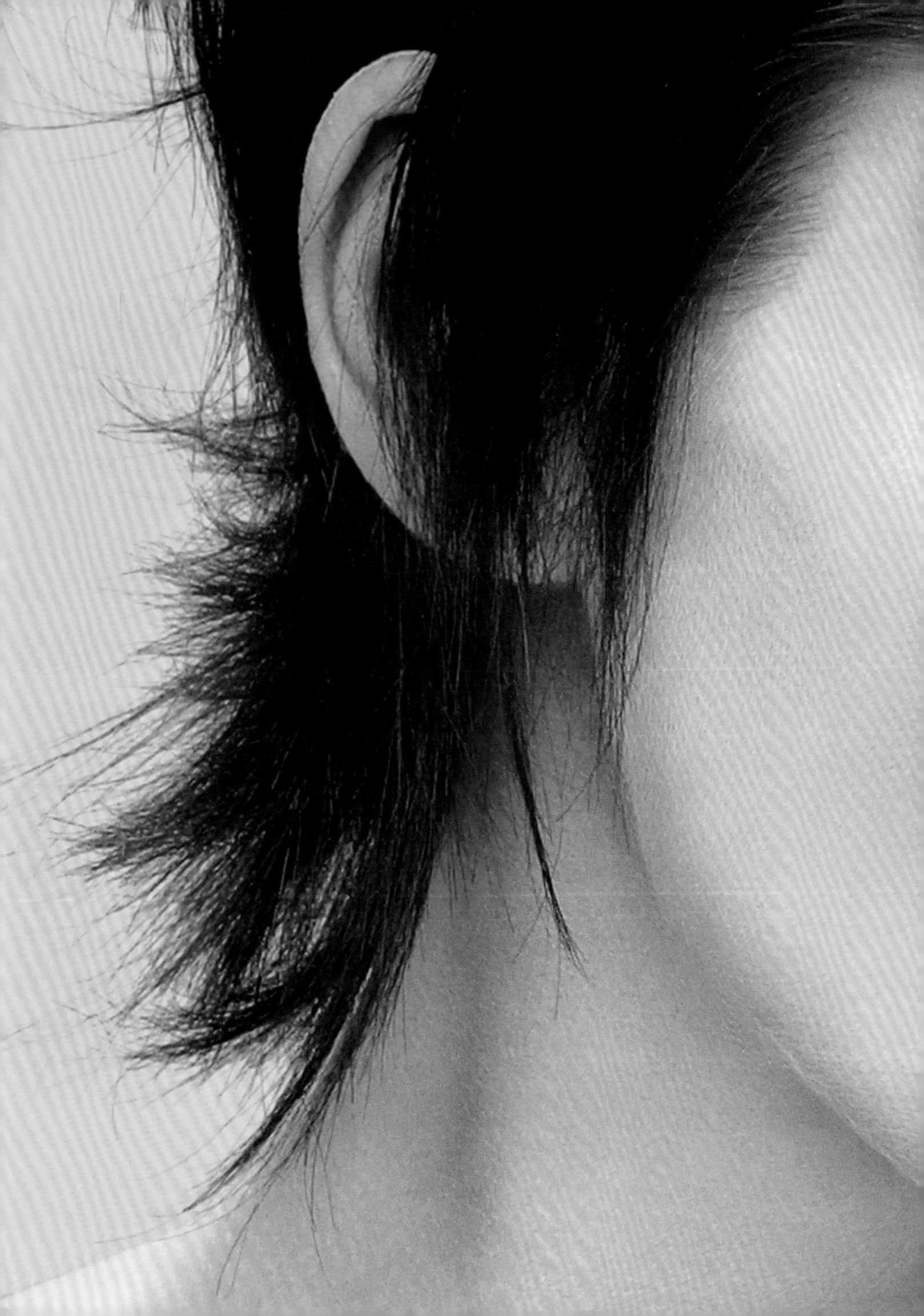

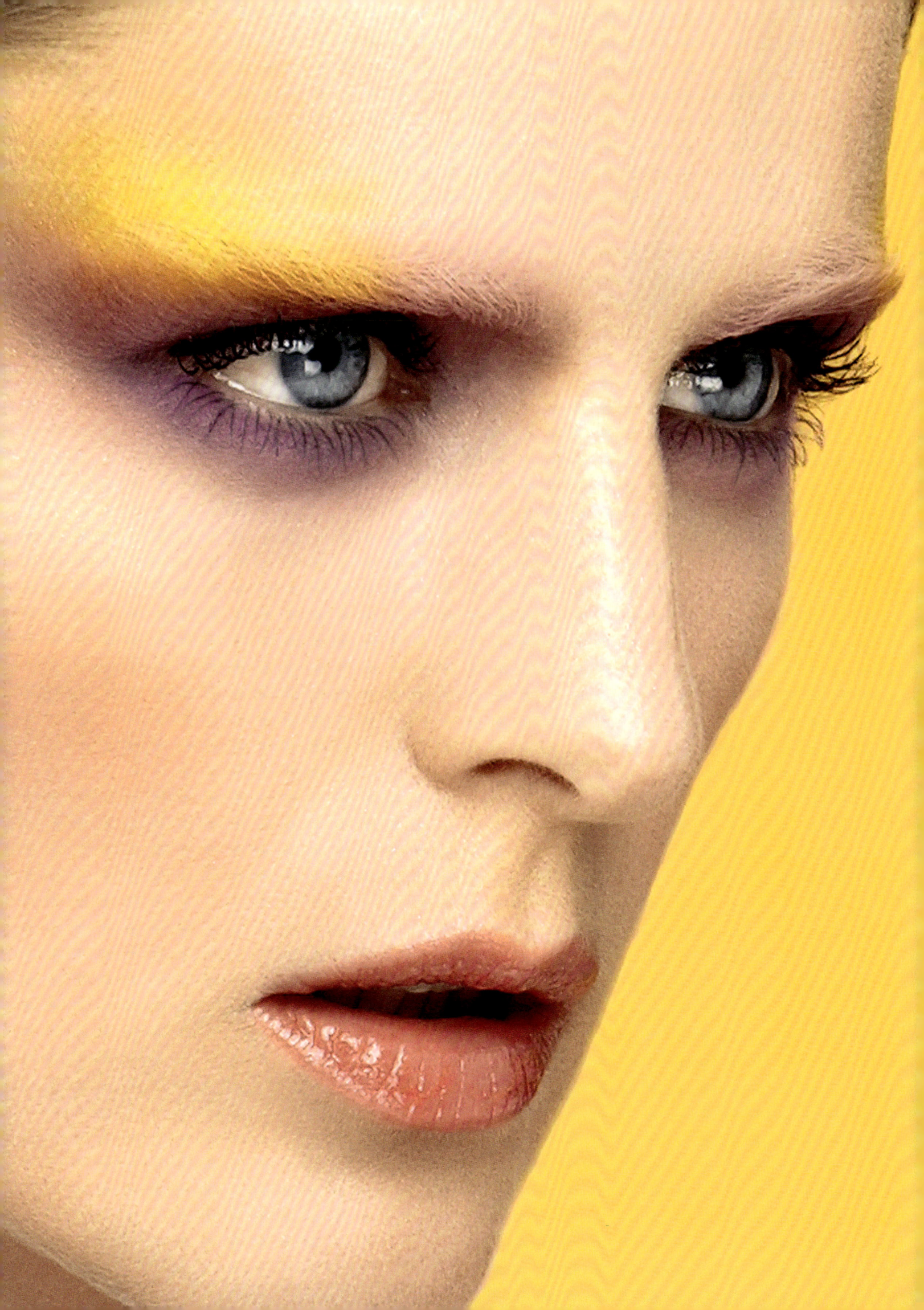

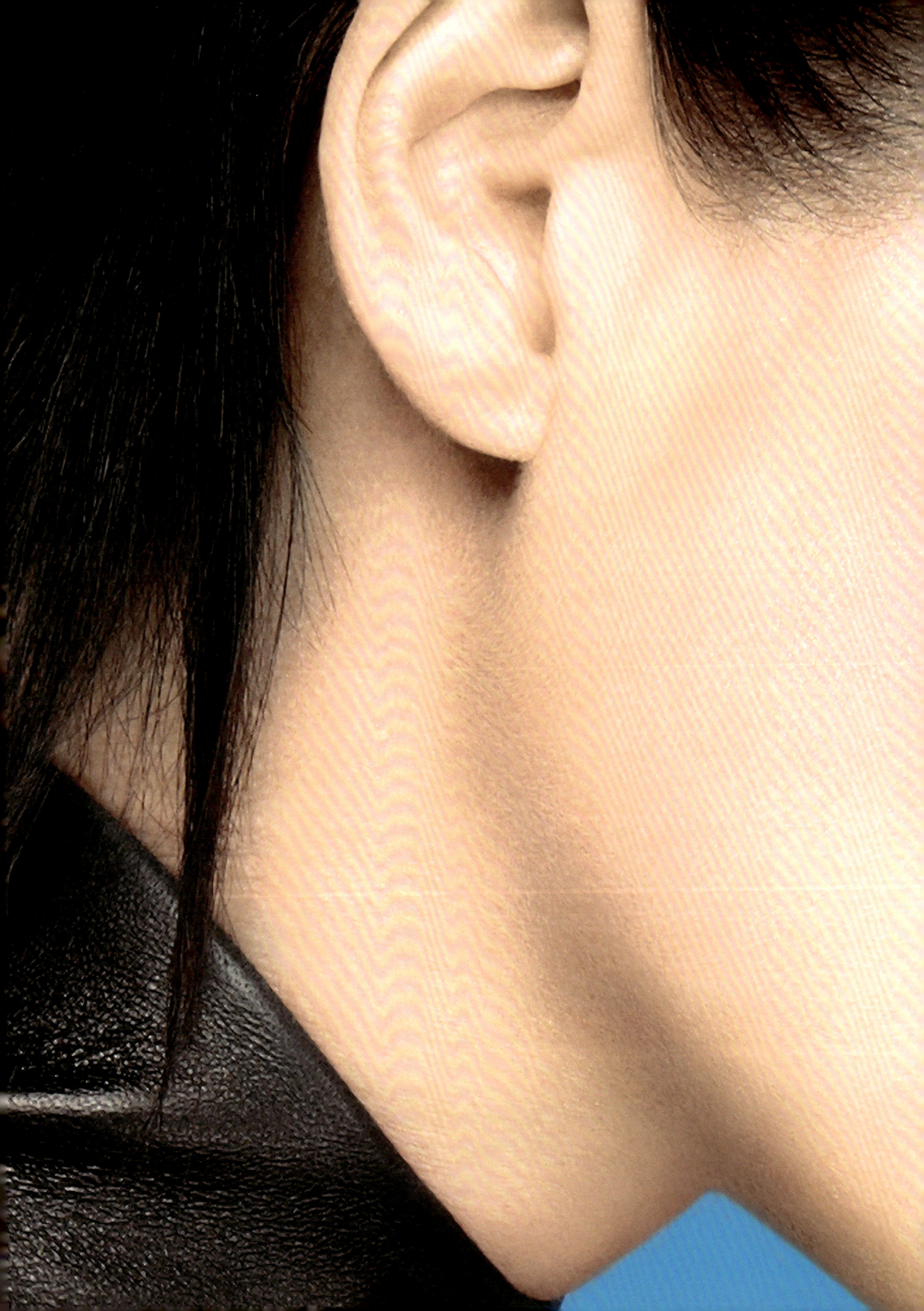

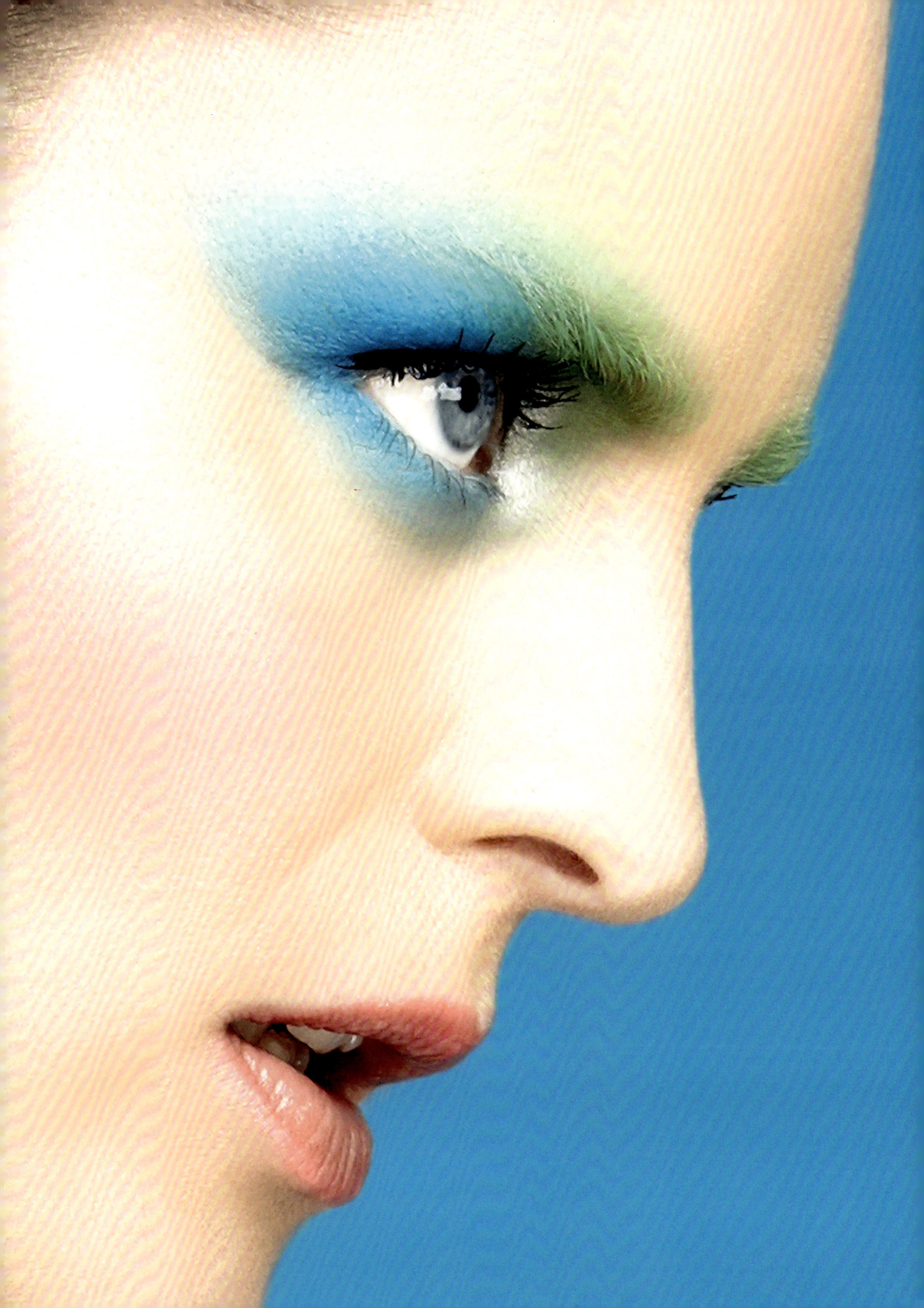

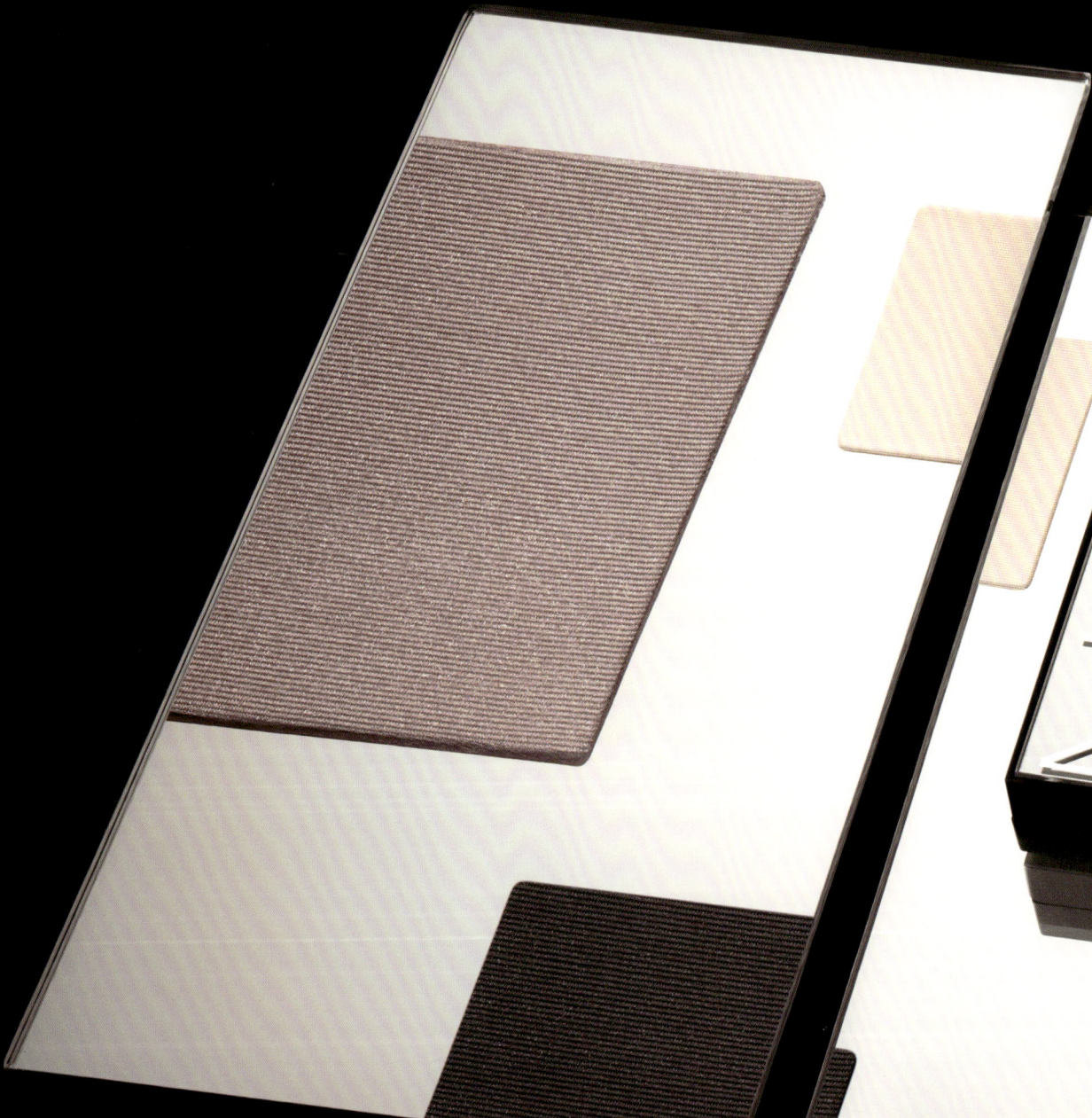
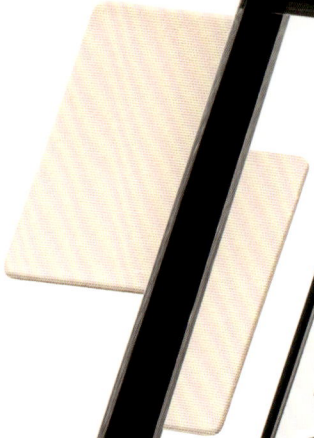
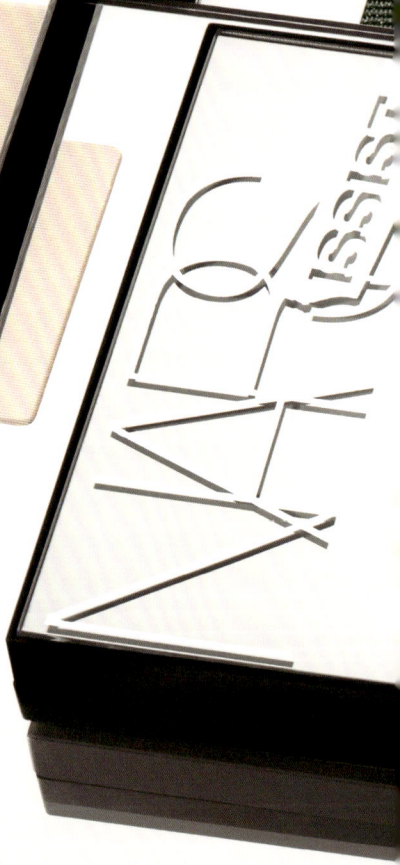
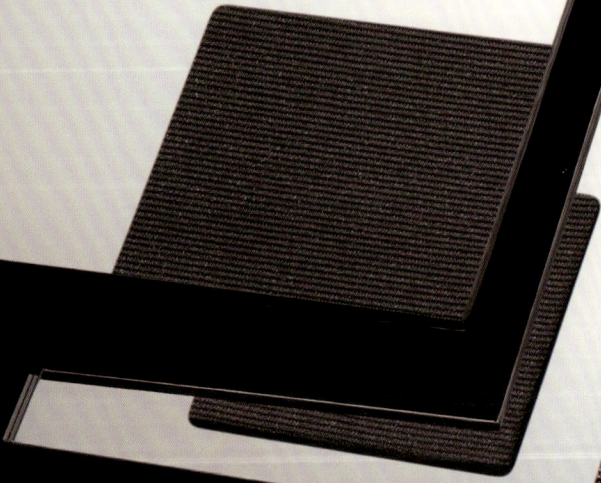

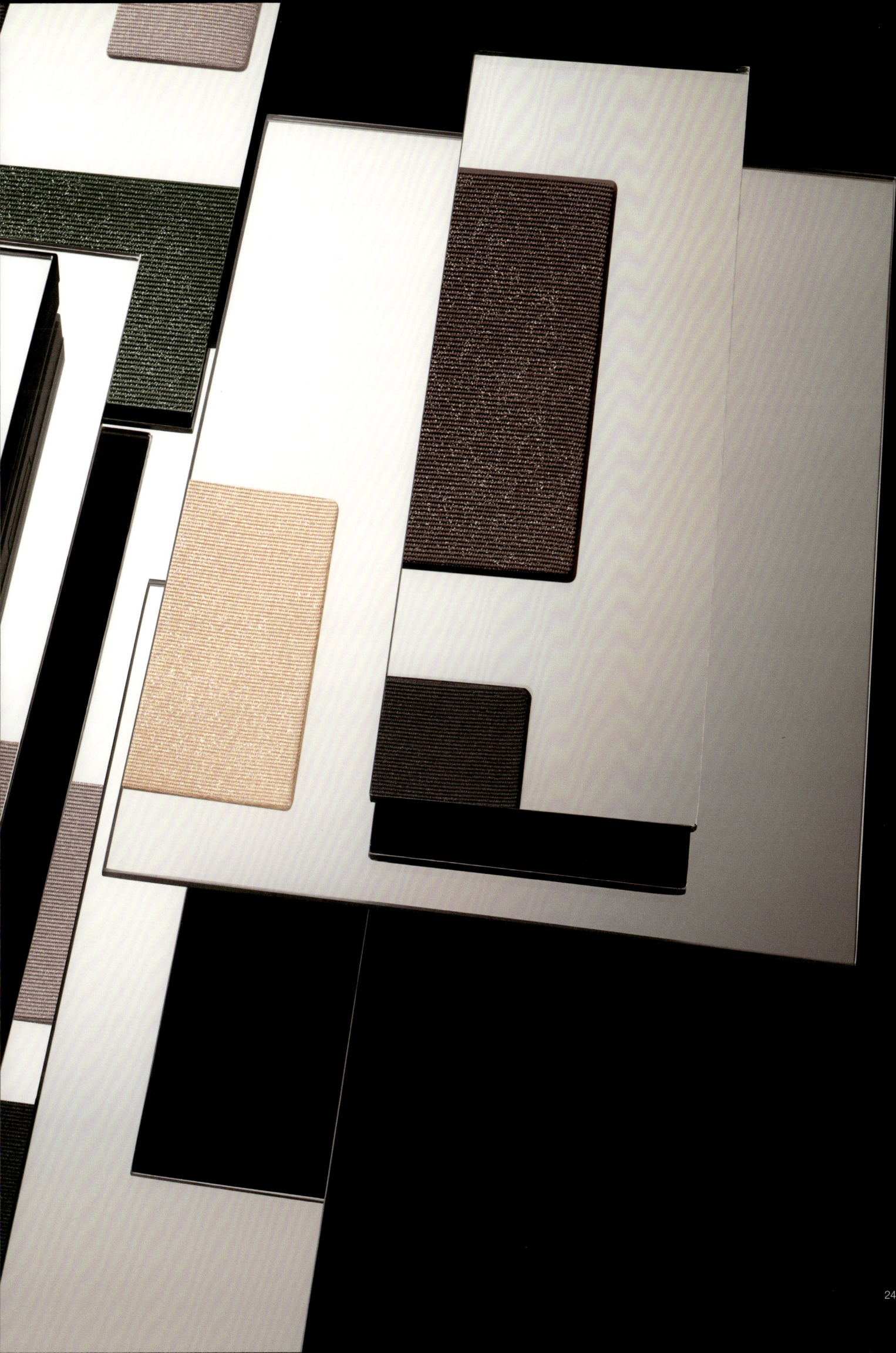

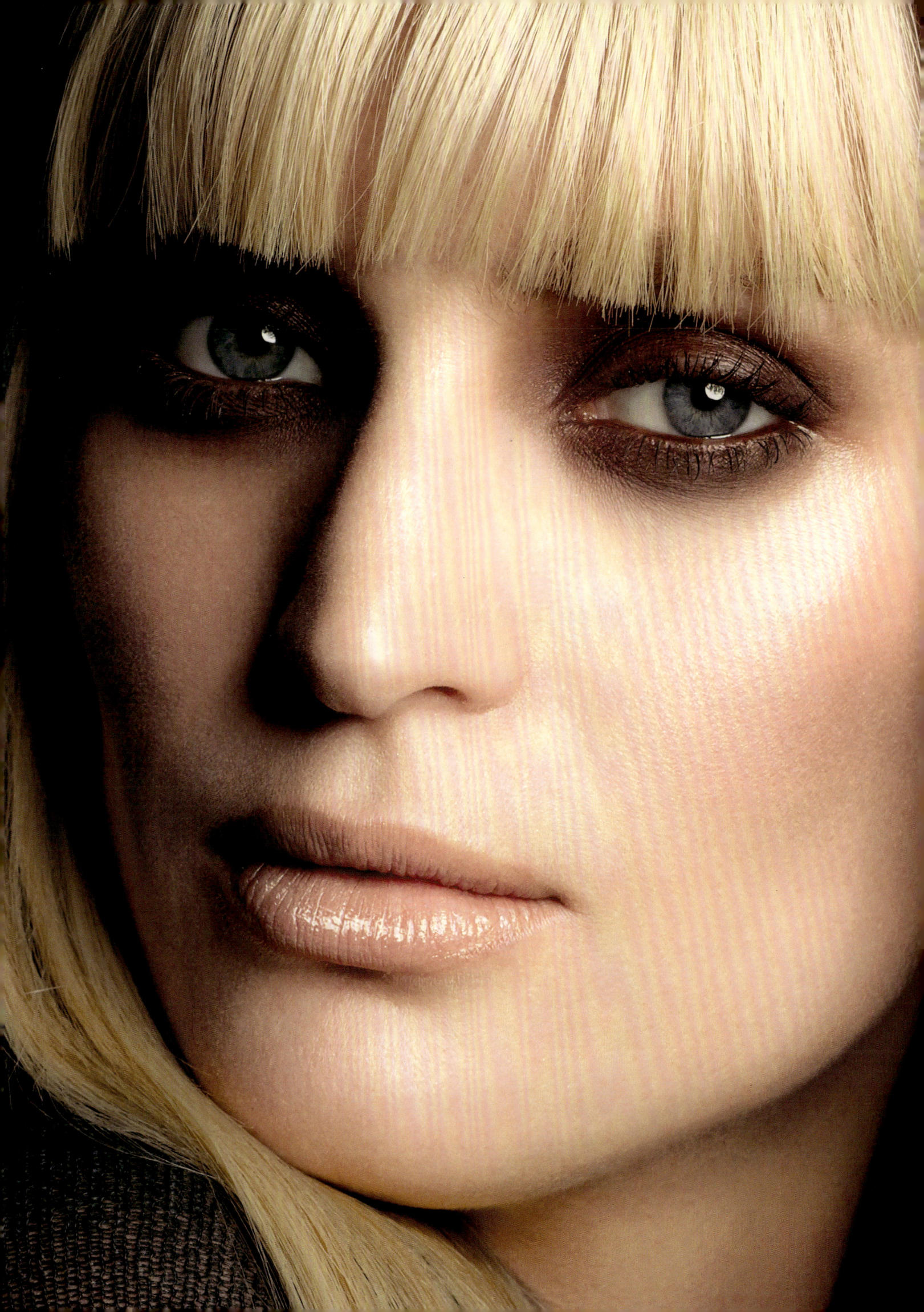

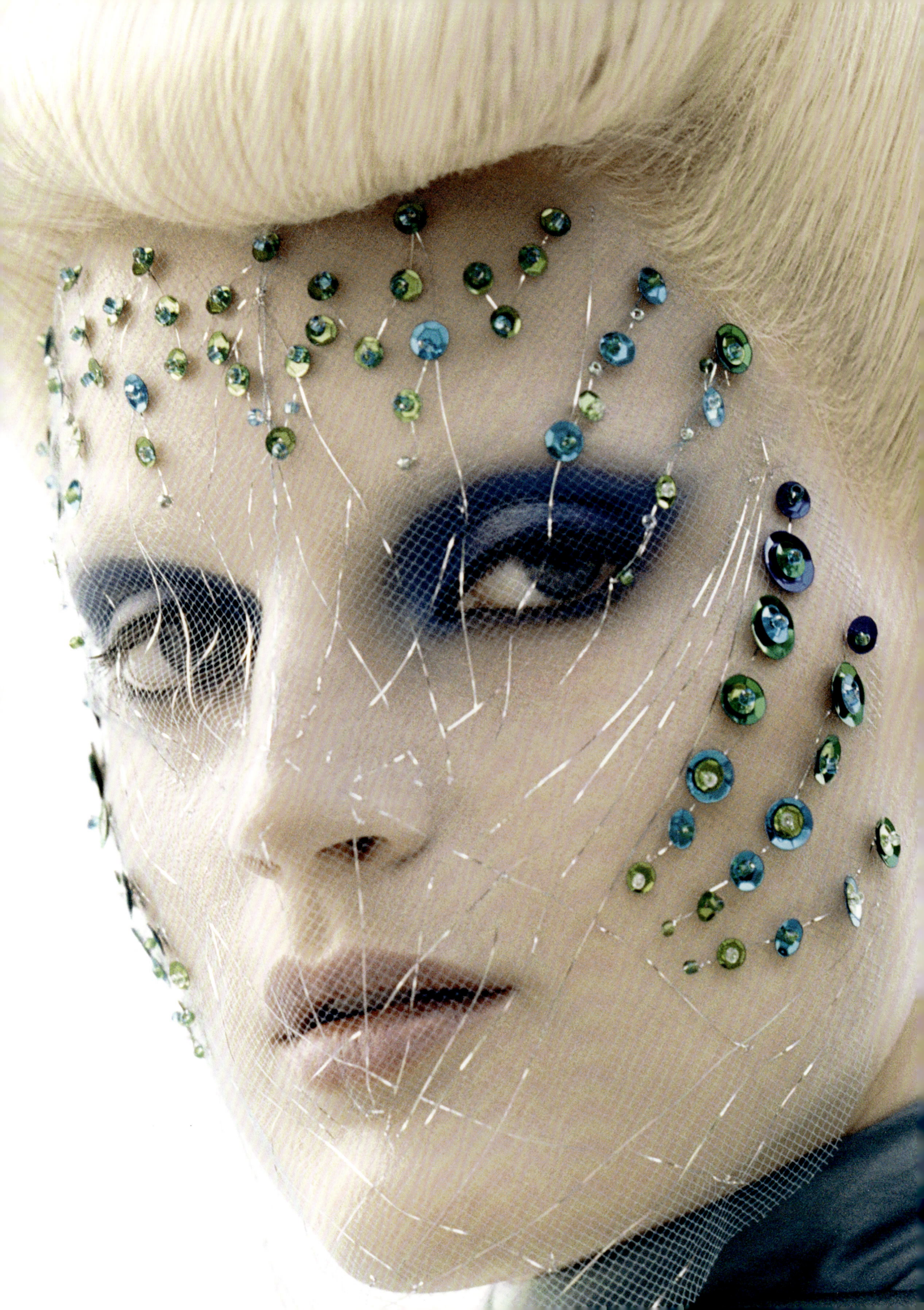

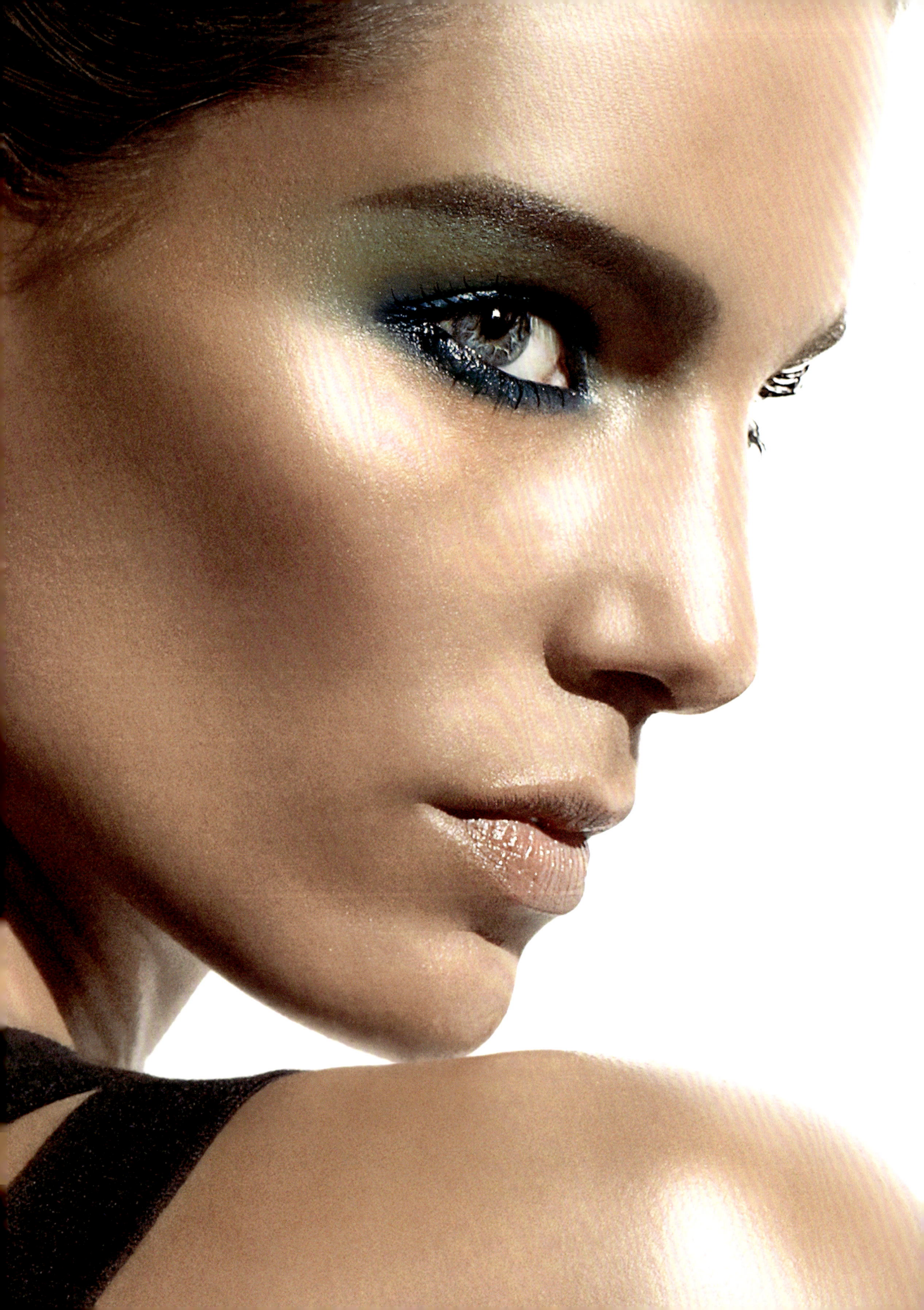

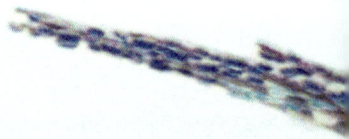

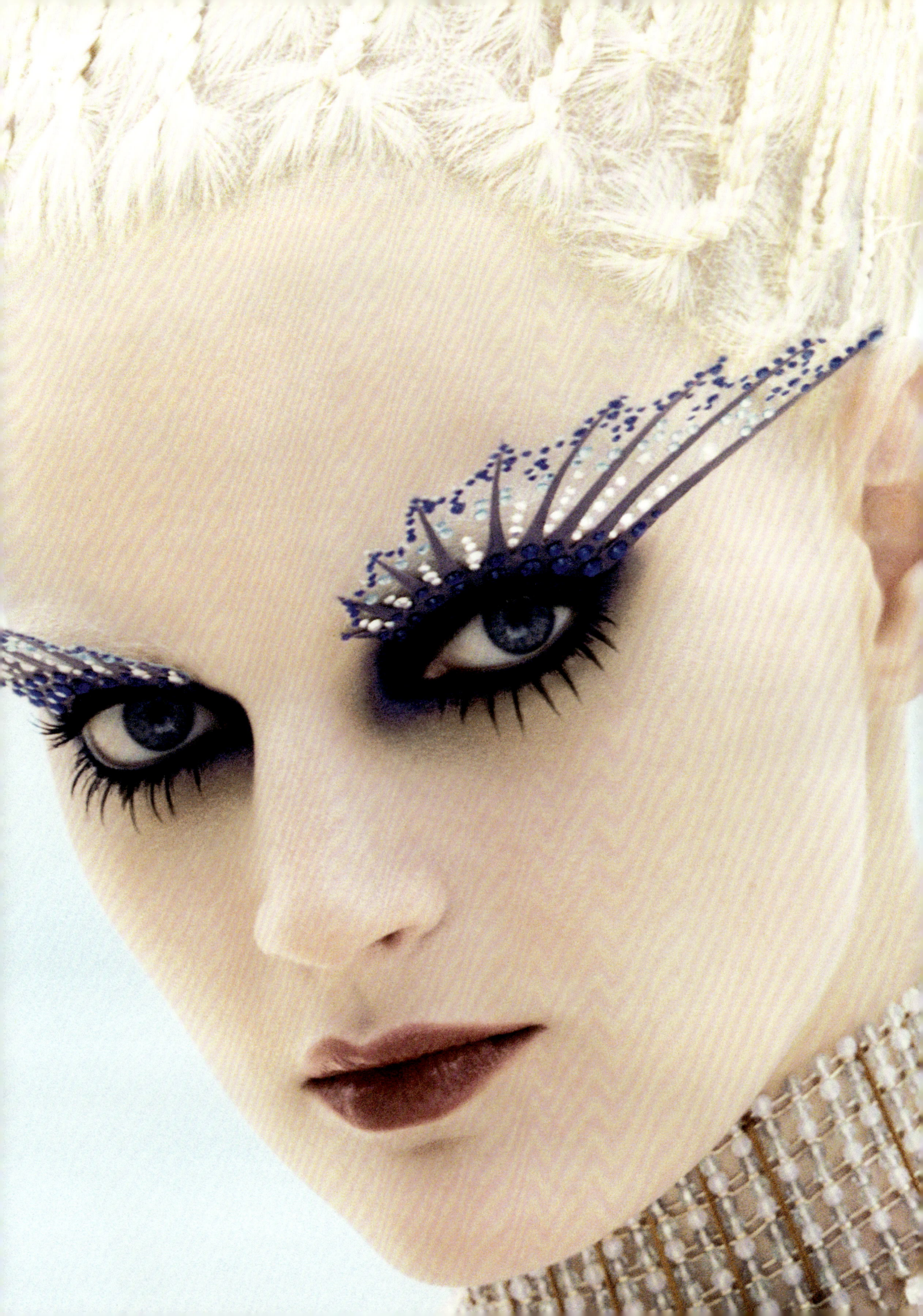

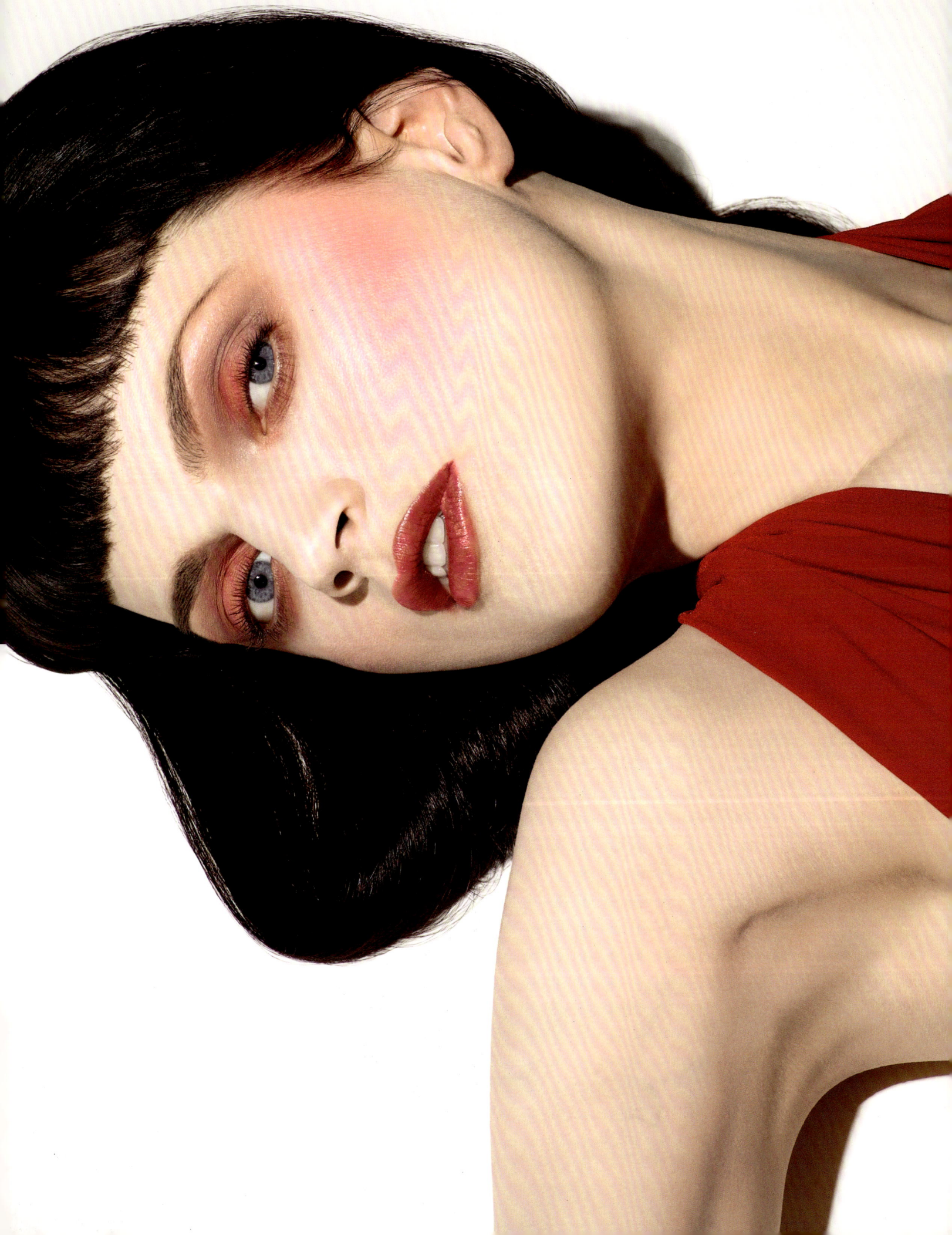

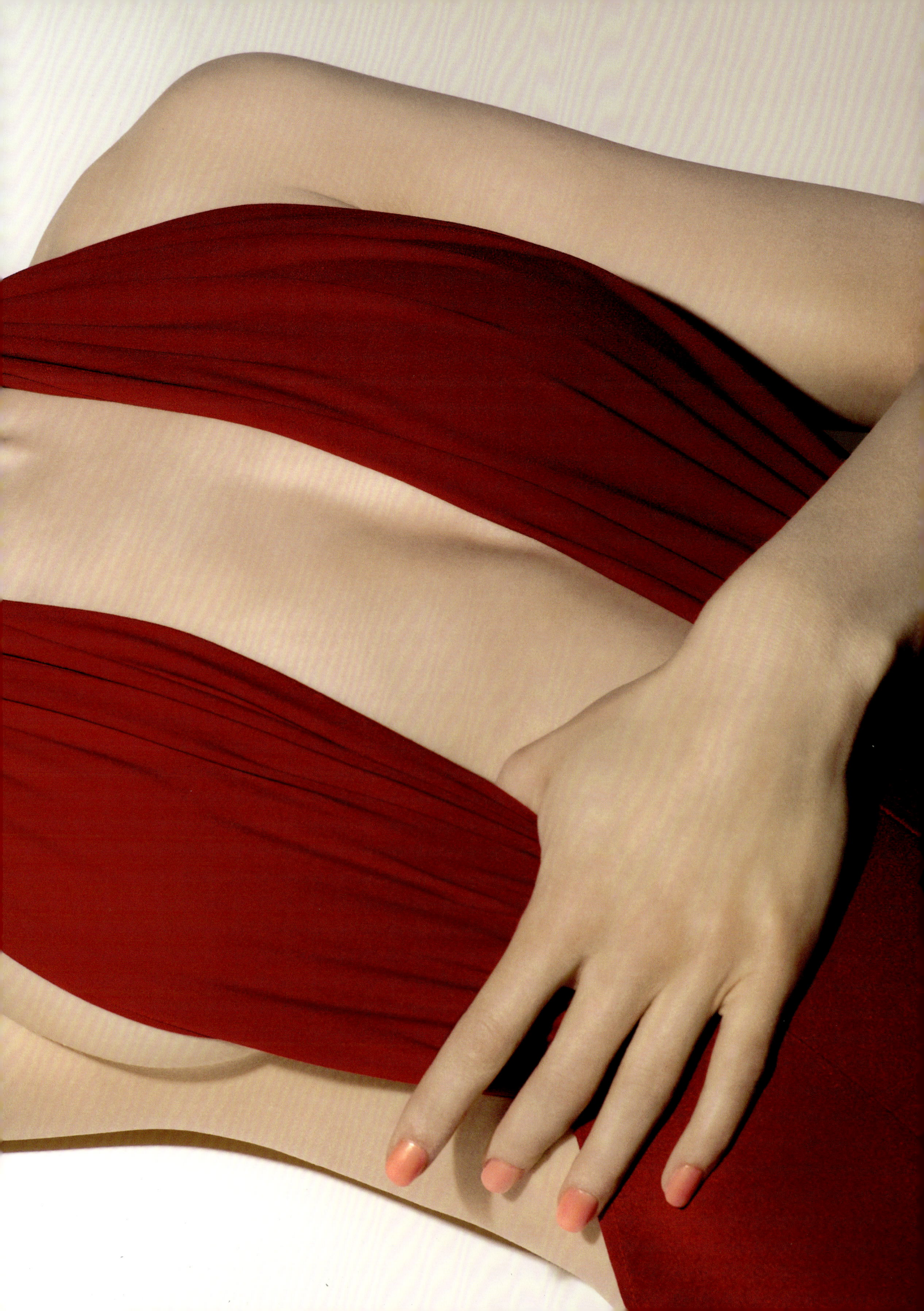

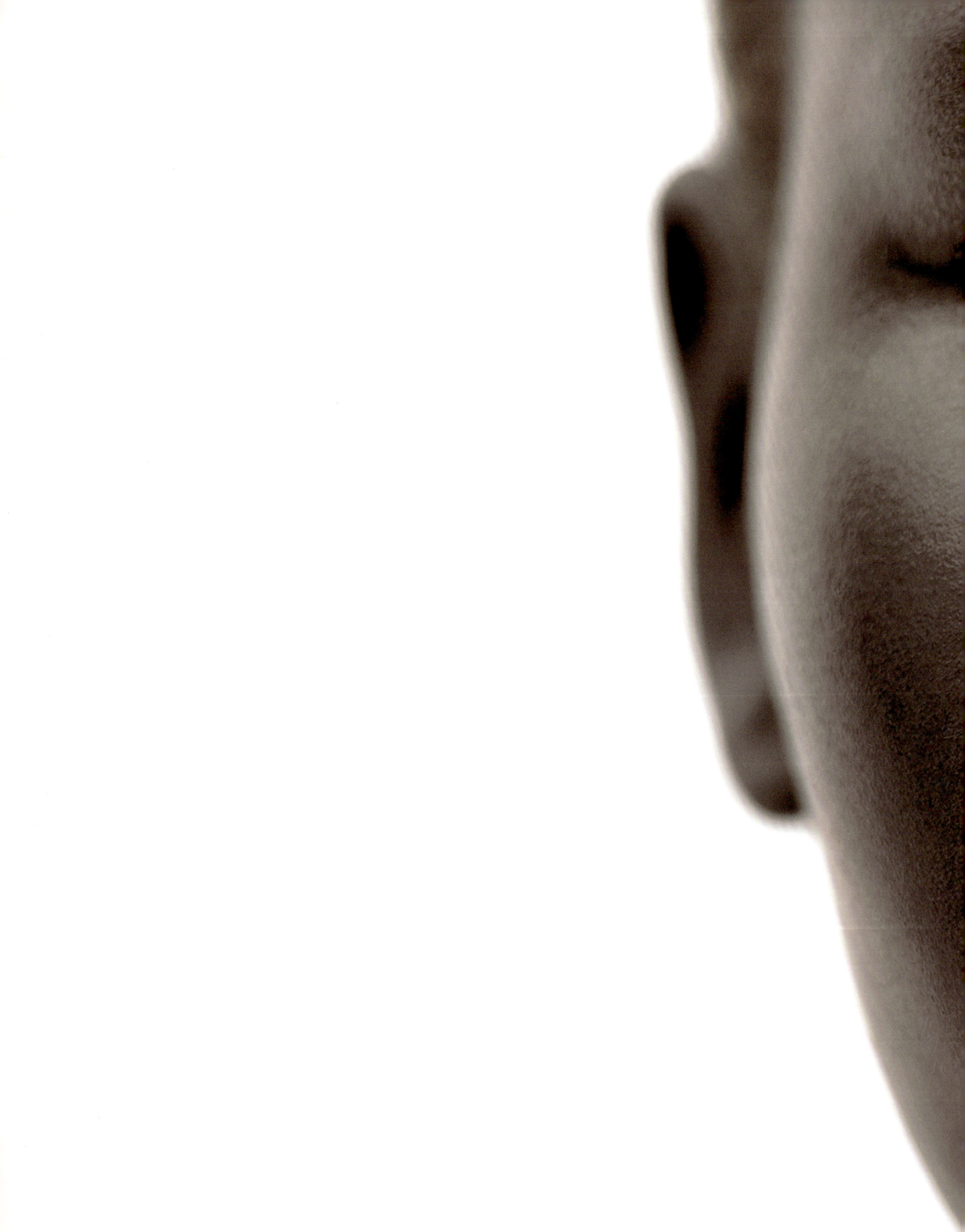

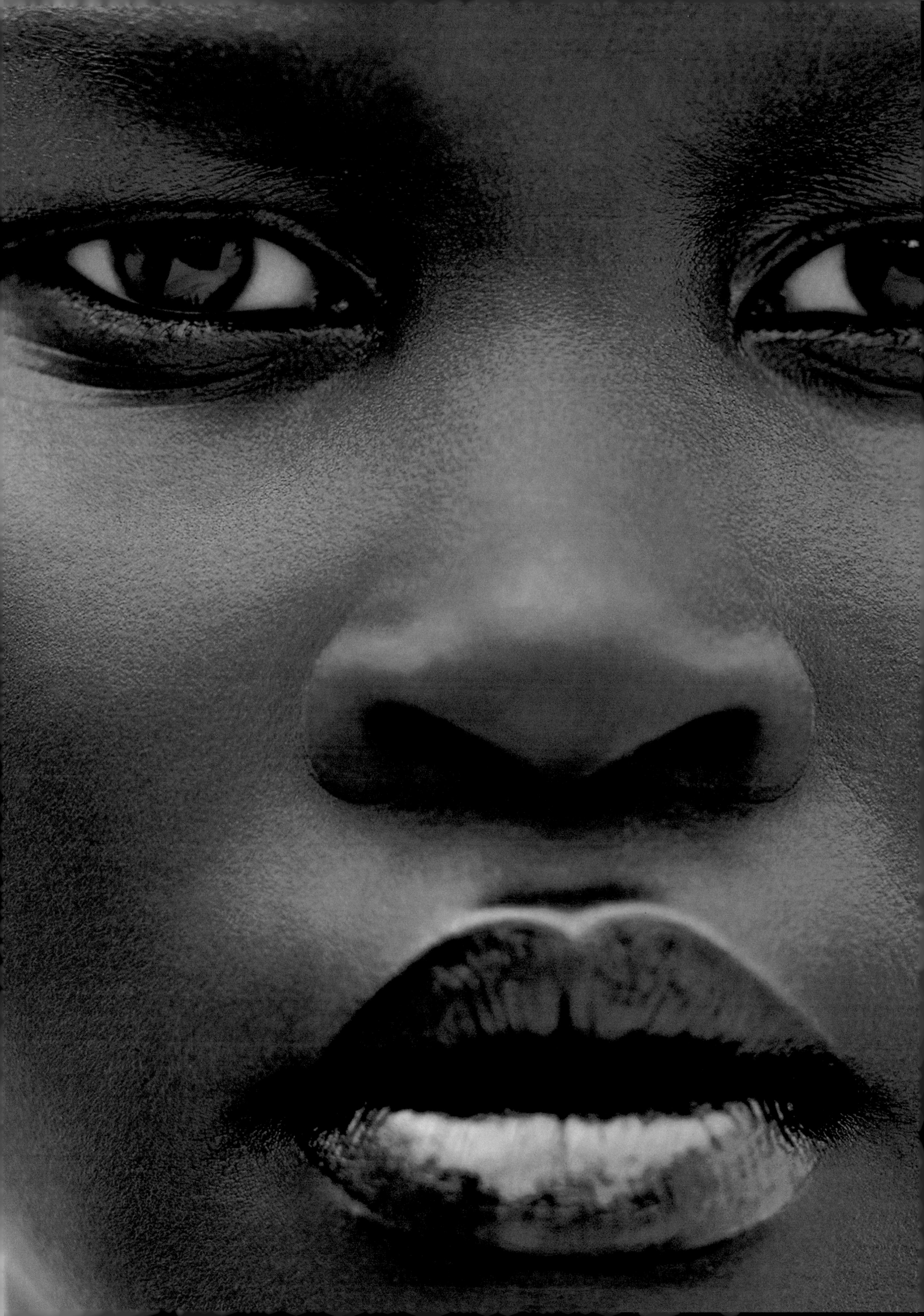

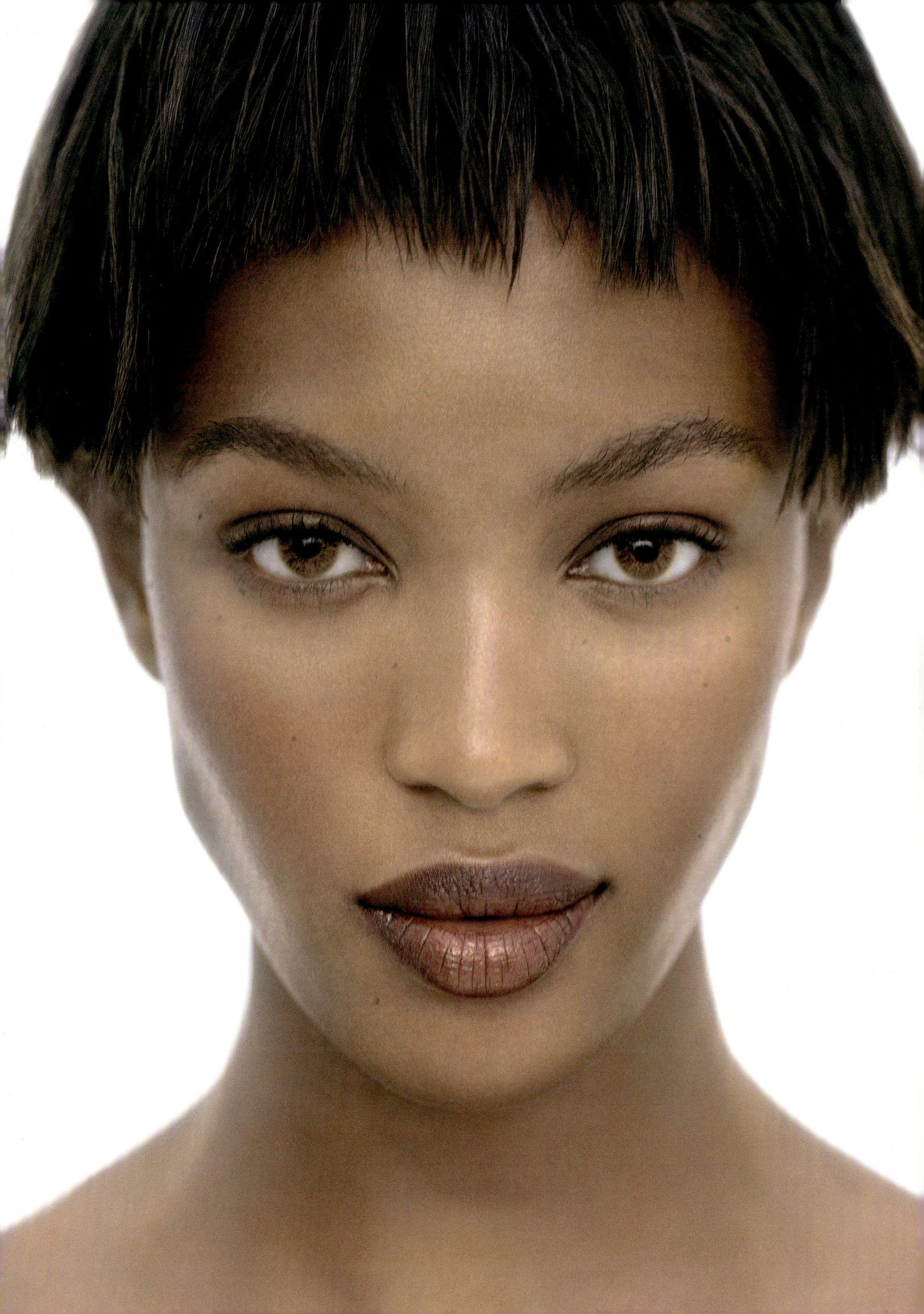

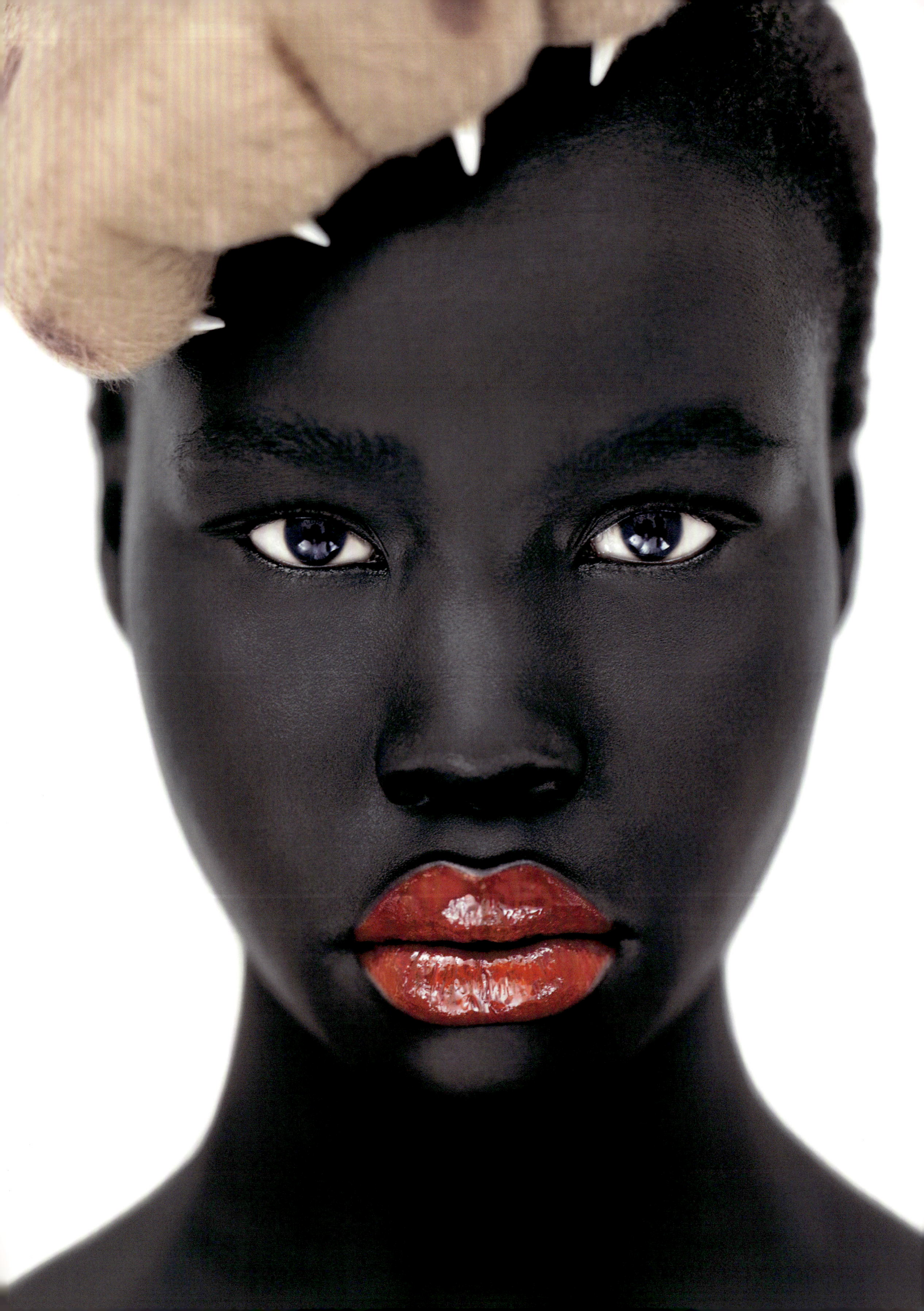

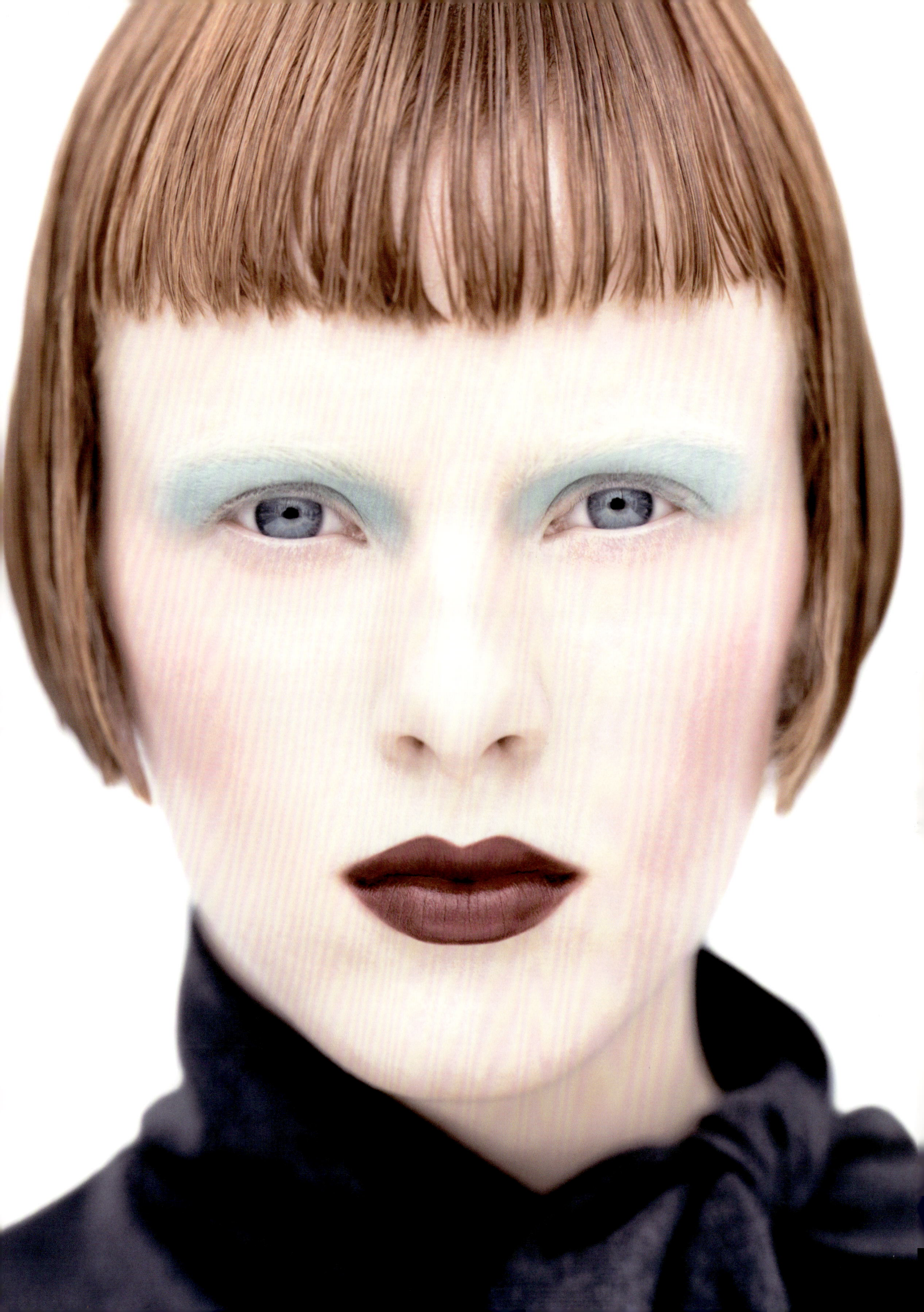

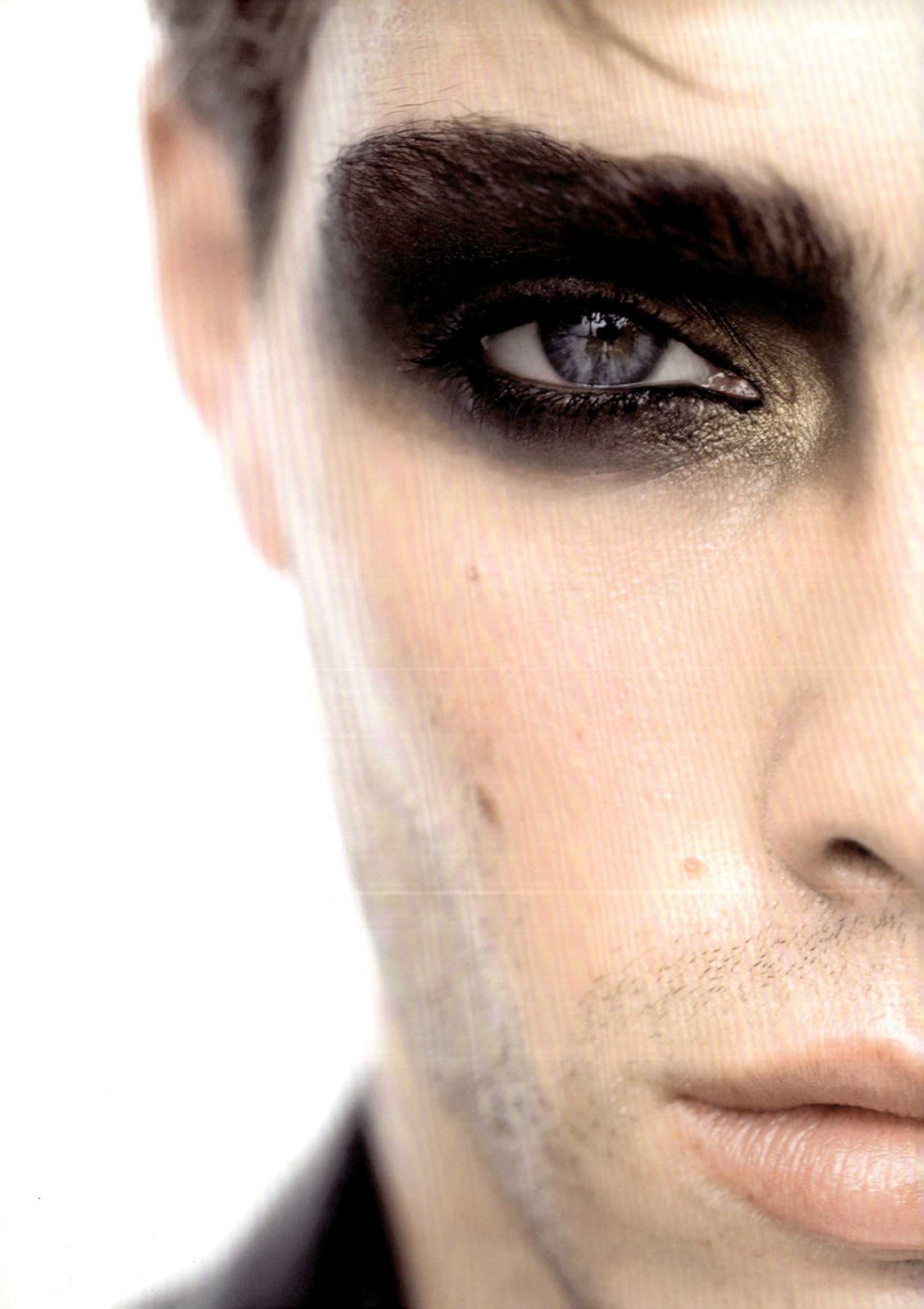

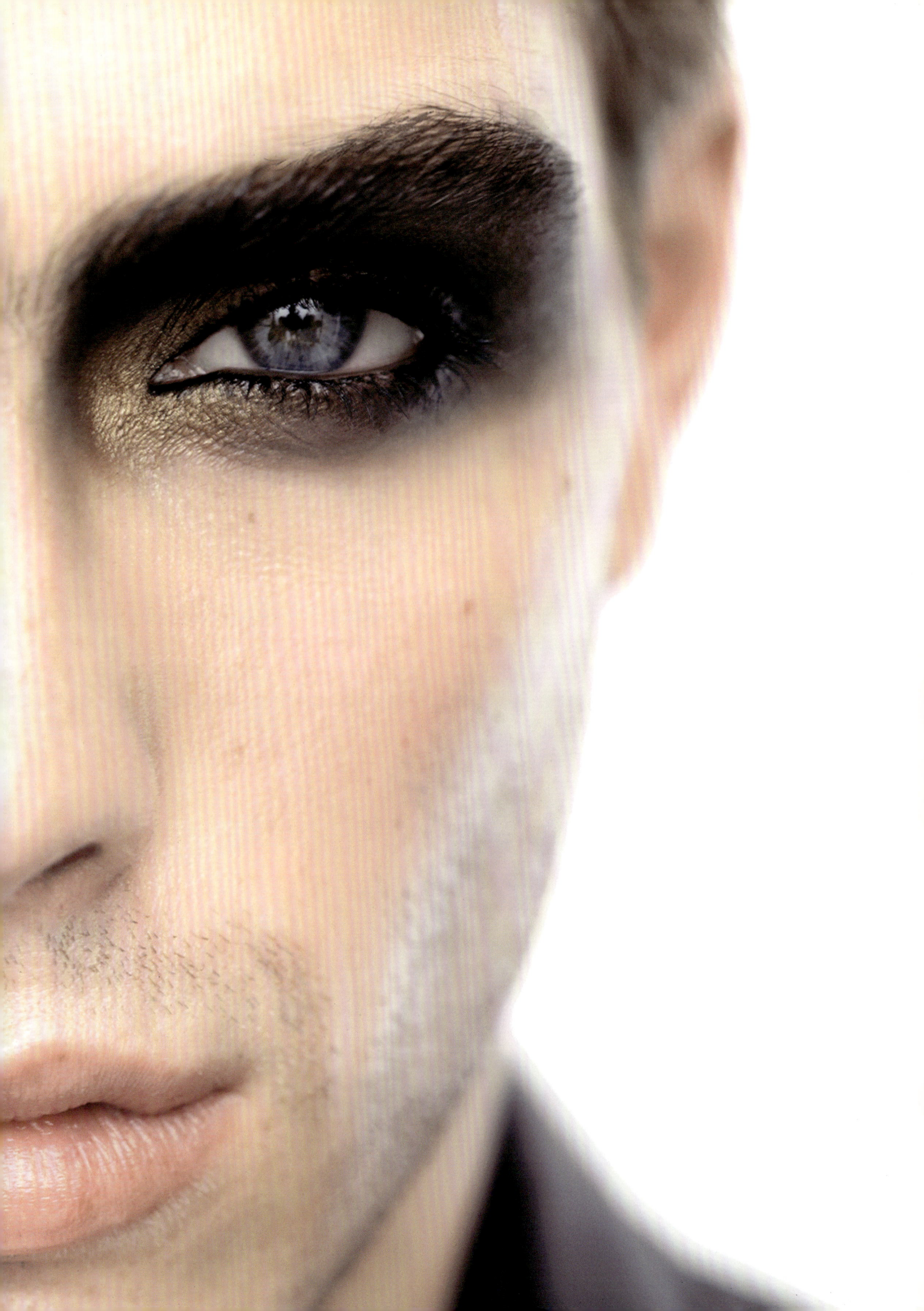

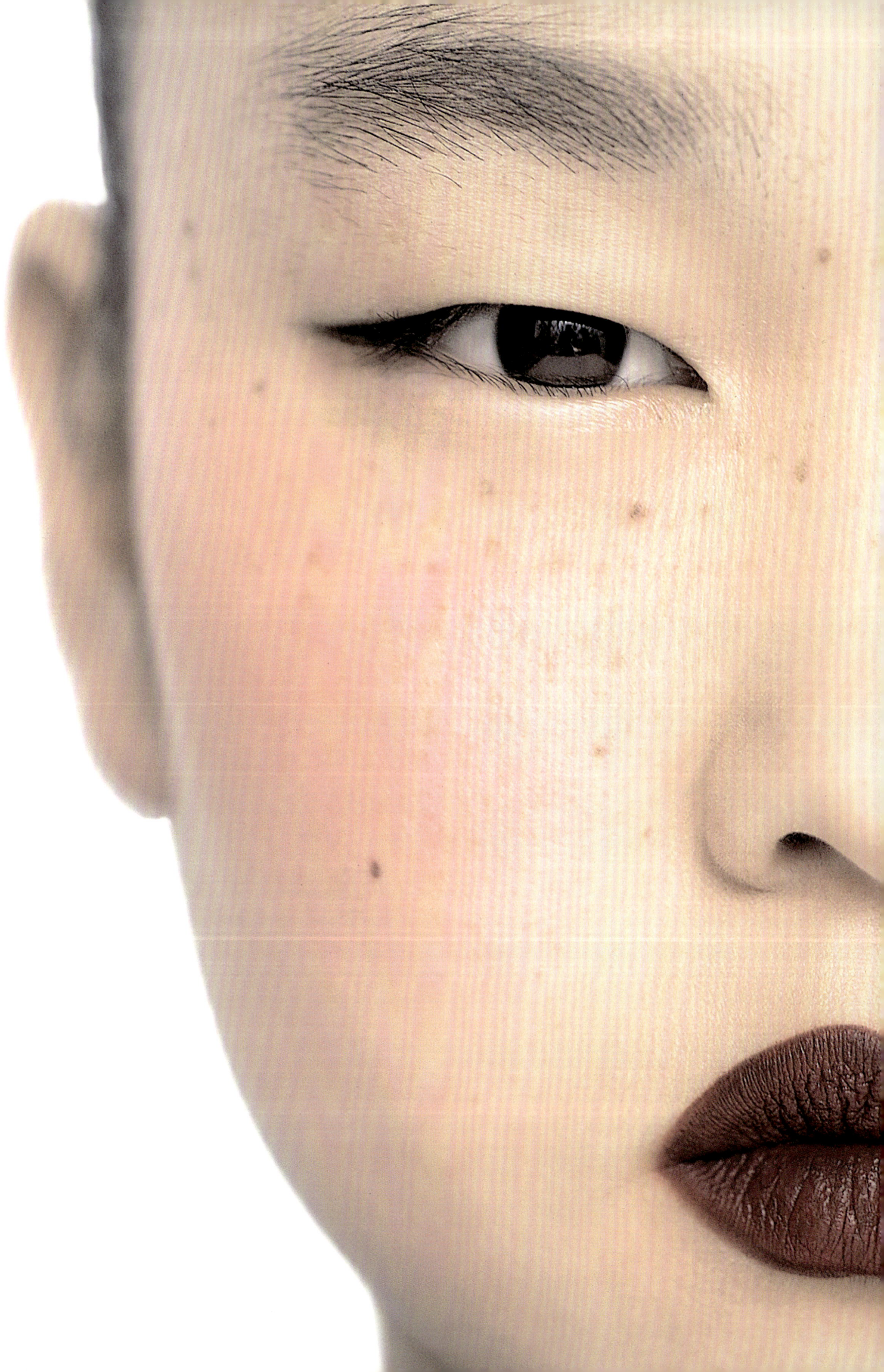

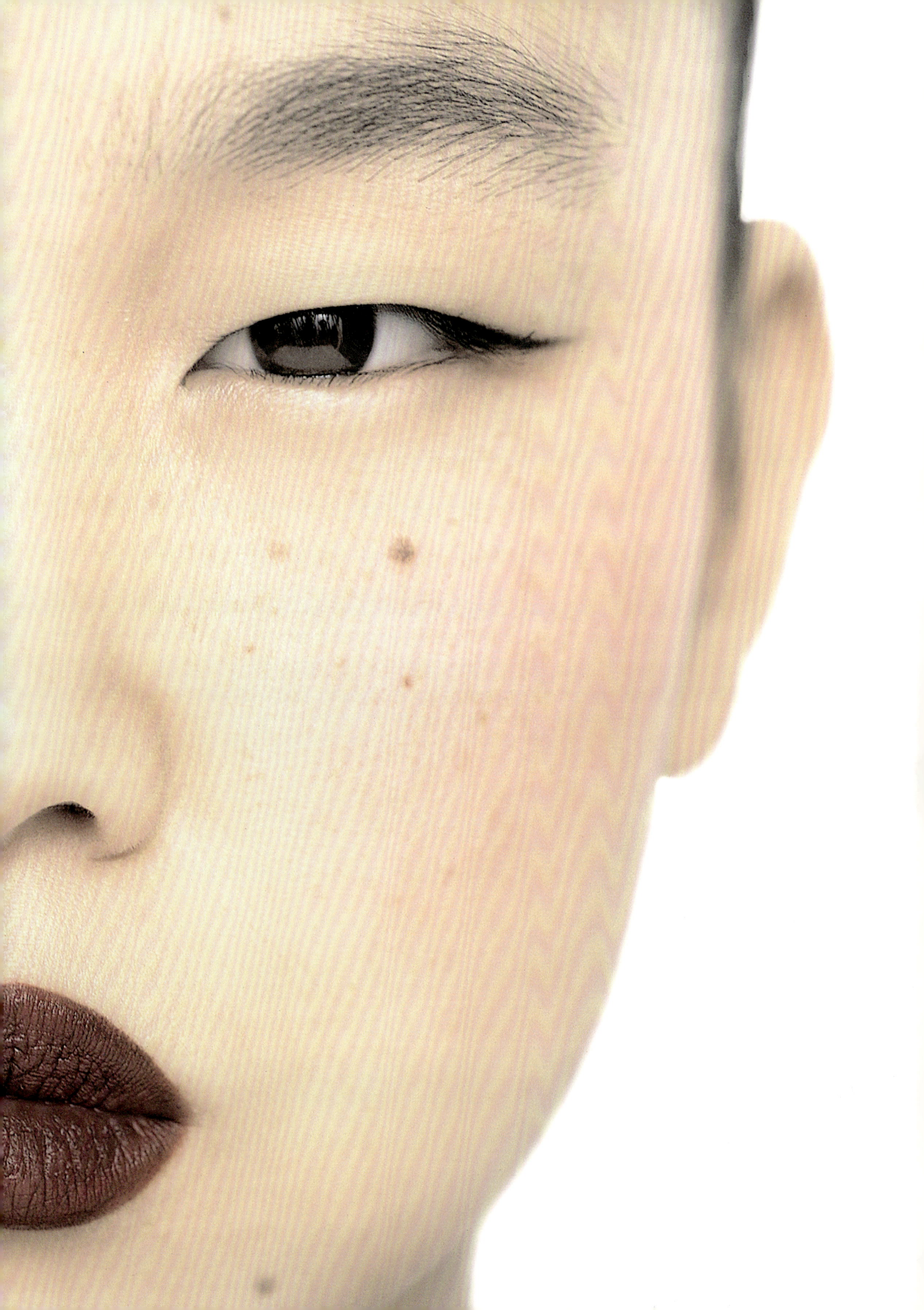

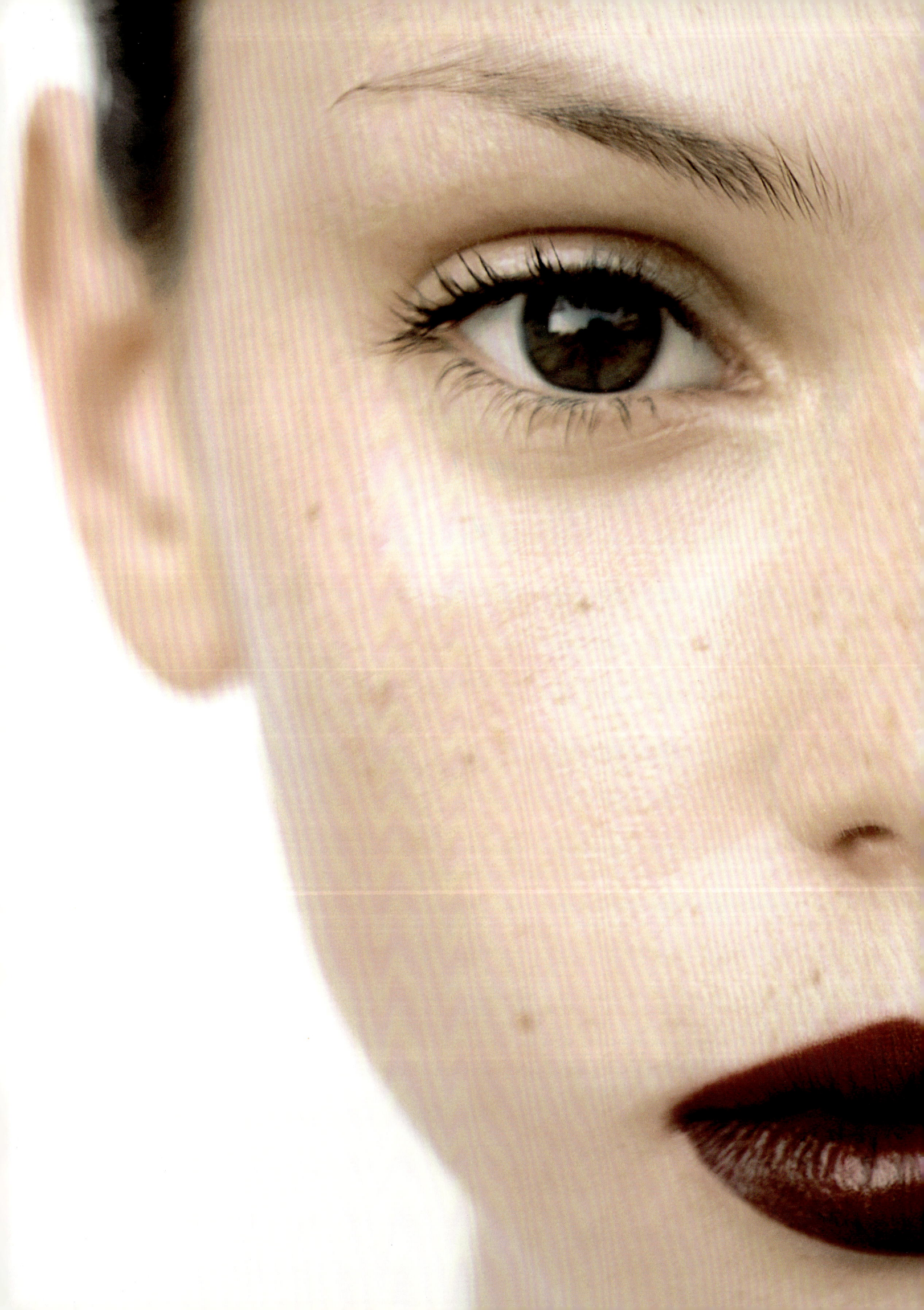

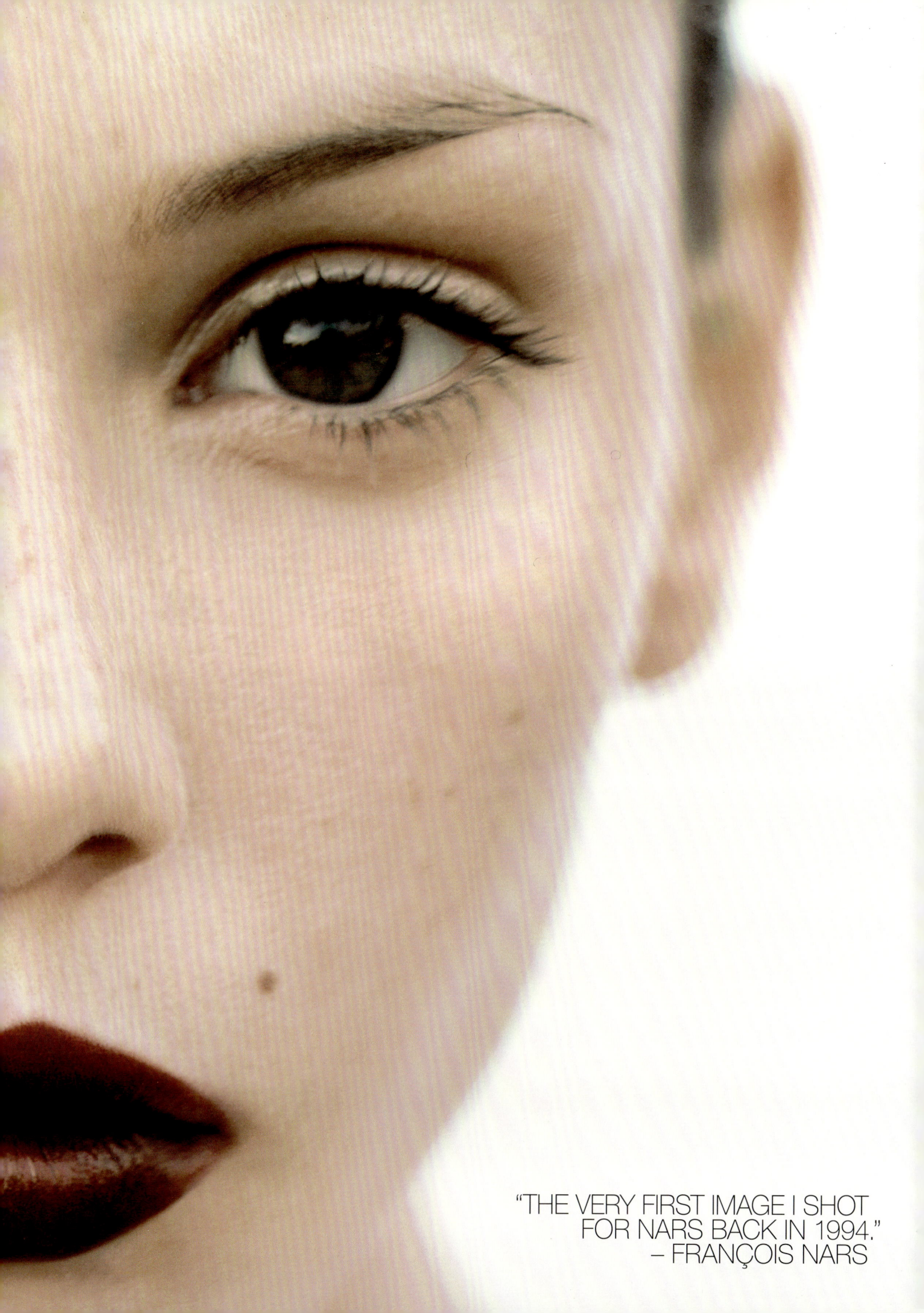

"THE VERY FIRST IMAGE I SHOT
FOR NARS BACK IN 1994."
– FRANÇOIS NARS

"ART IN GENERAL IS VERY INFLUENTIAL TO MY WORK. SOME OF MY FAVORITE PAINTERS ARE MATISSE, PICASSO, DALI, ROTHKO, GAUGUIN, AND MANY MORE. ADMIRING THEIR PAINTINGS JUST TOTALLY FUELS MY CREATIVITY."
– FRANÇOIS NARS

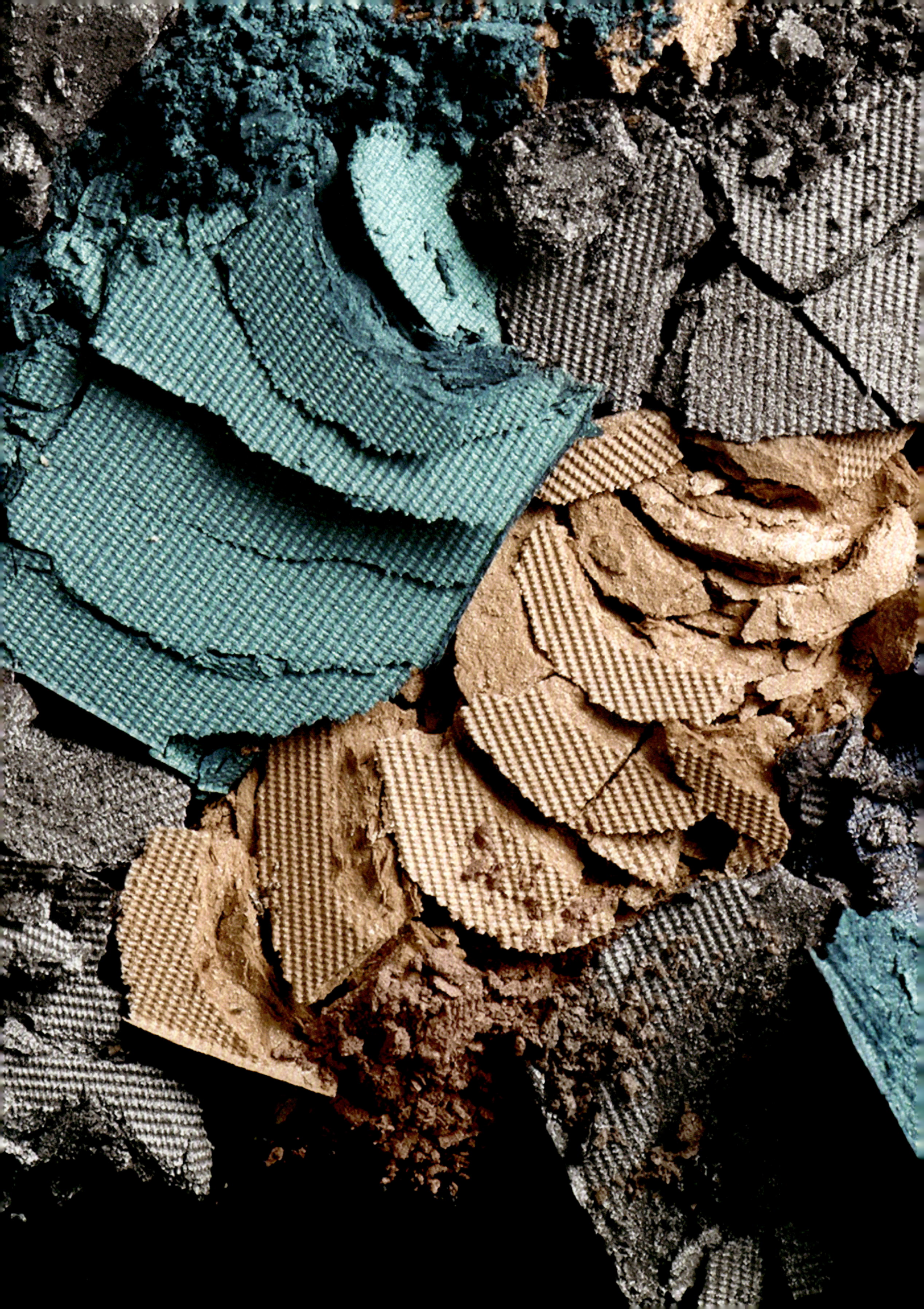

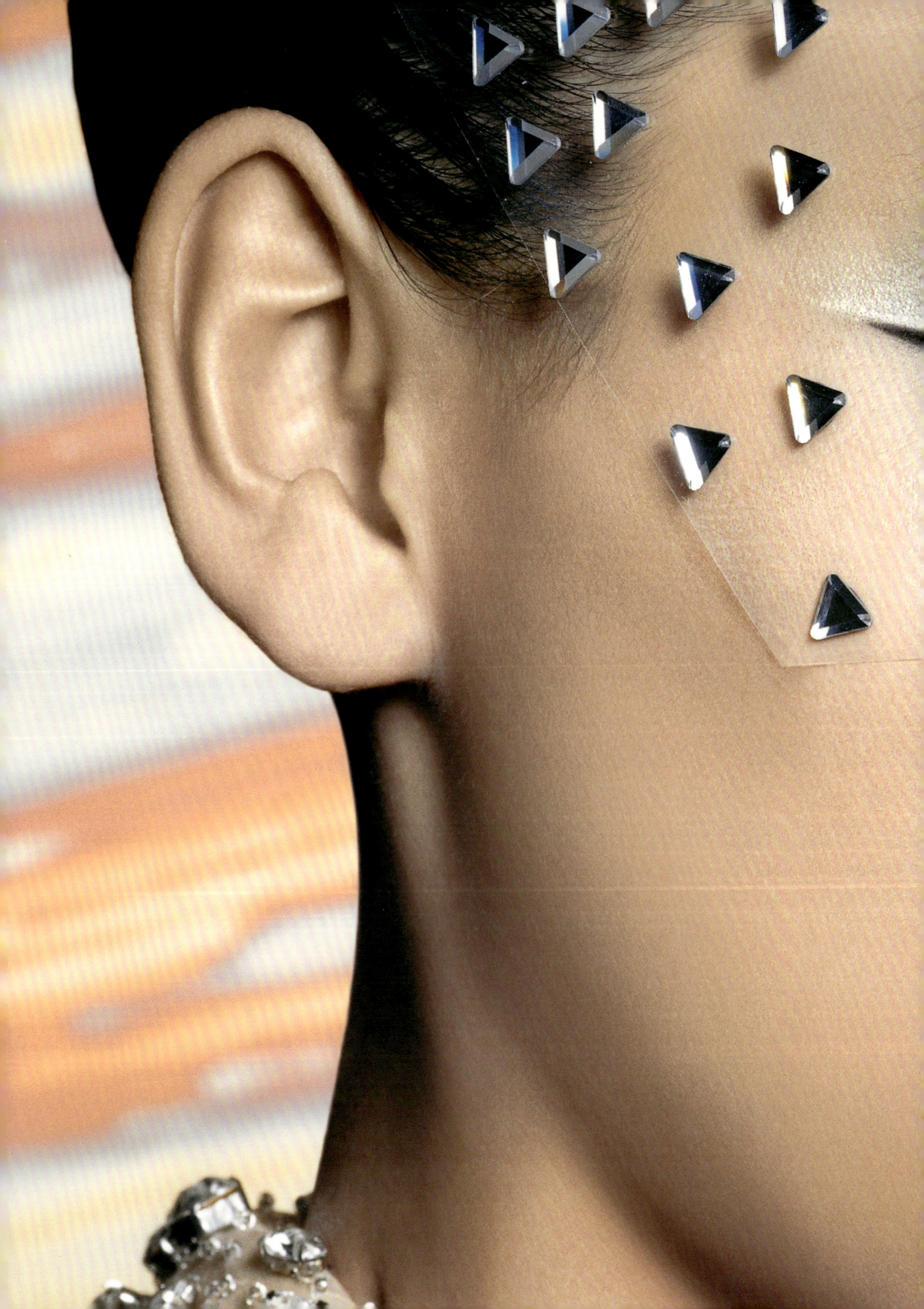

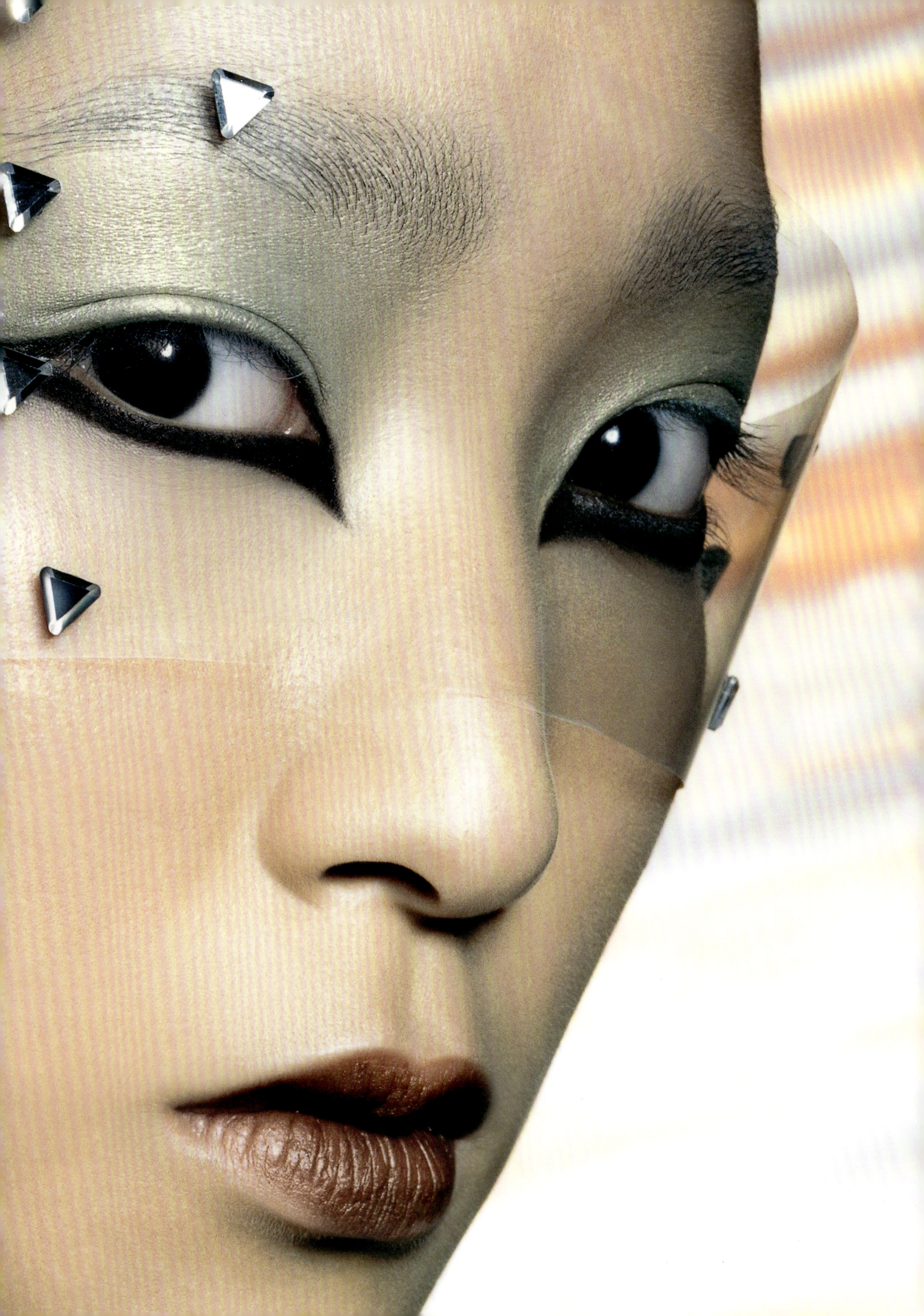

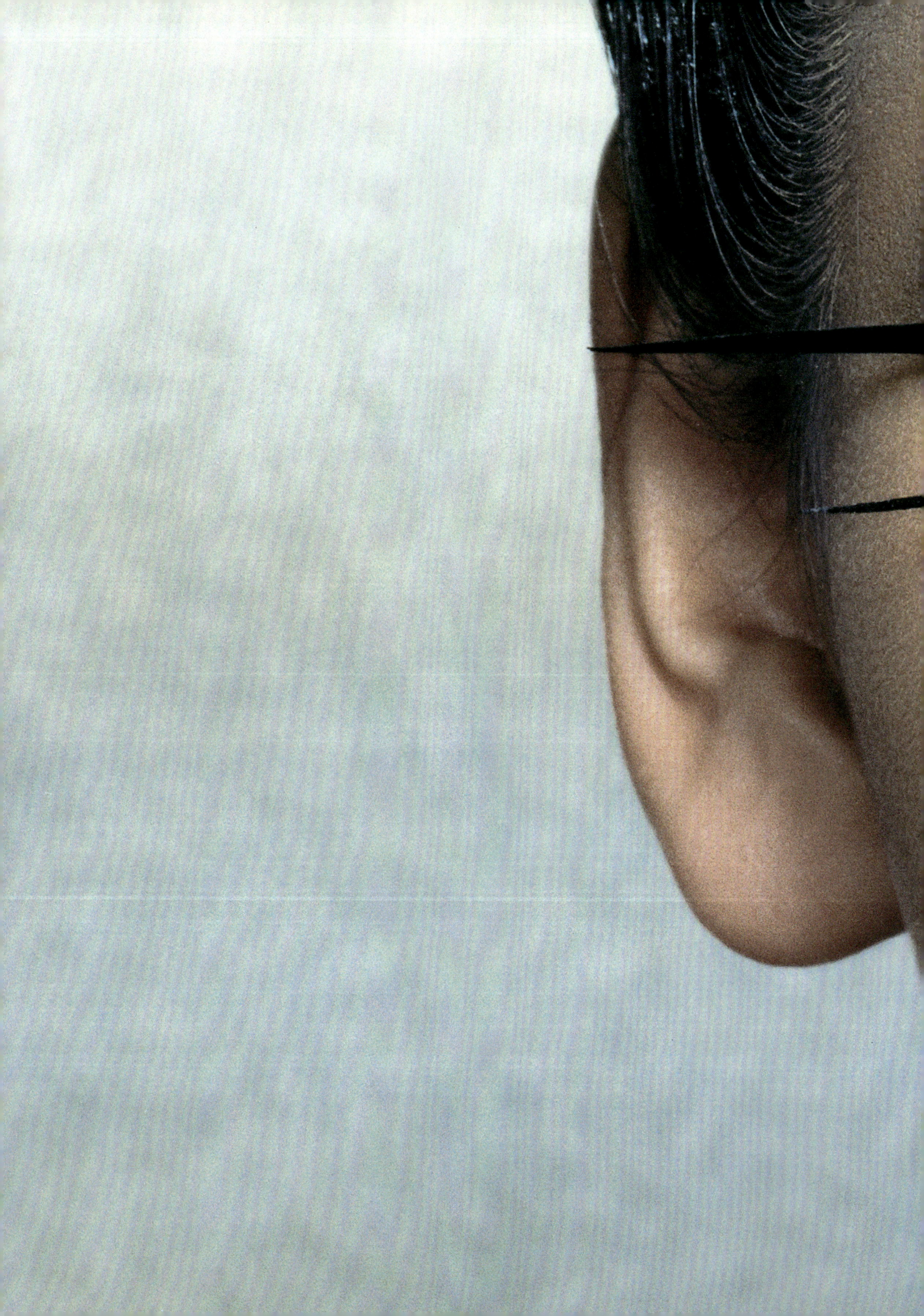

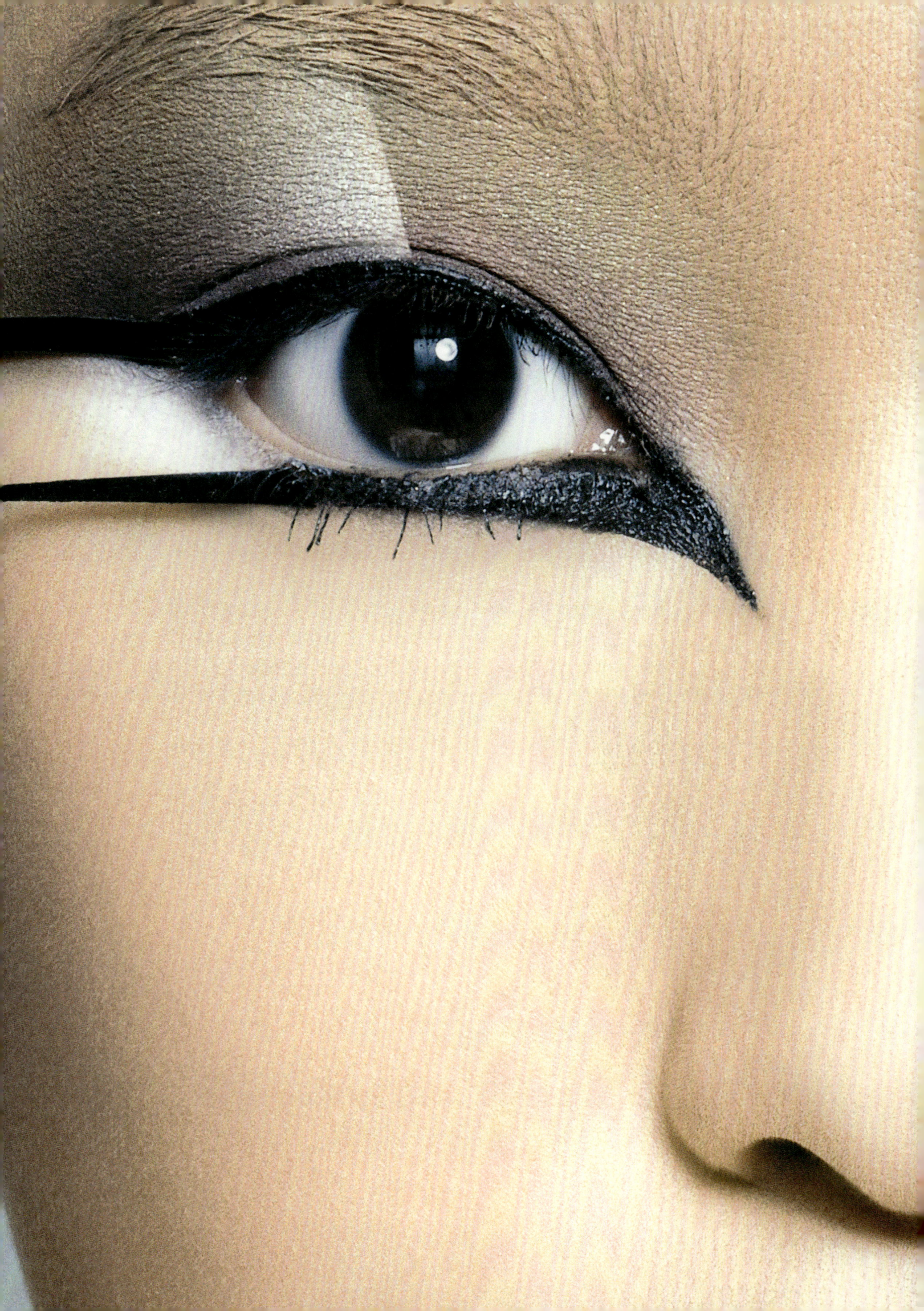

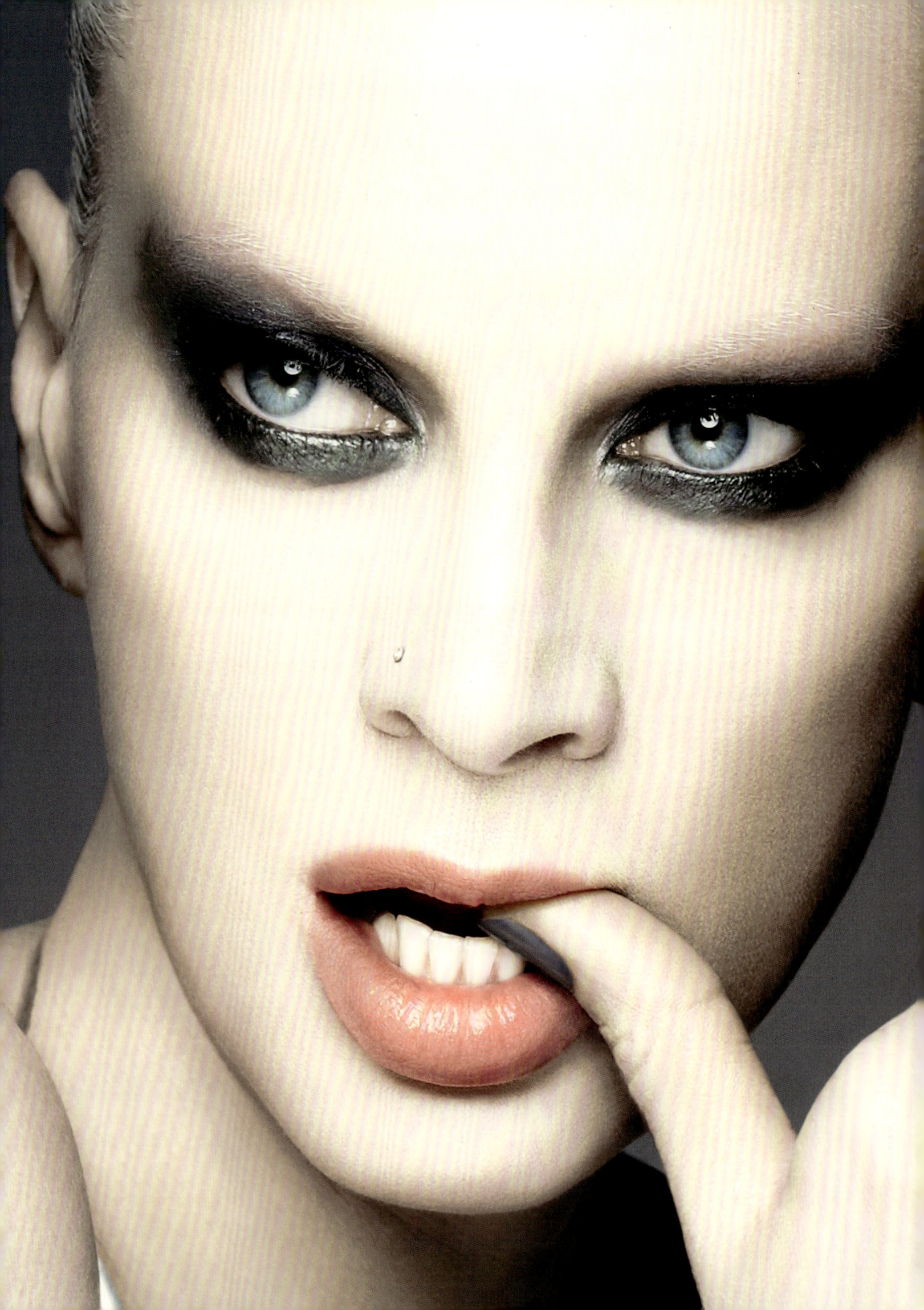

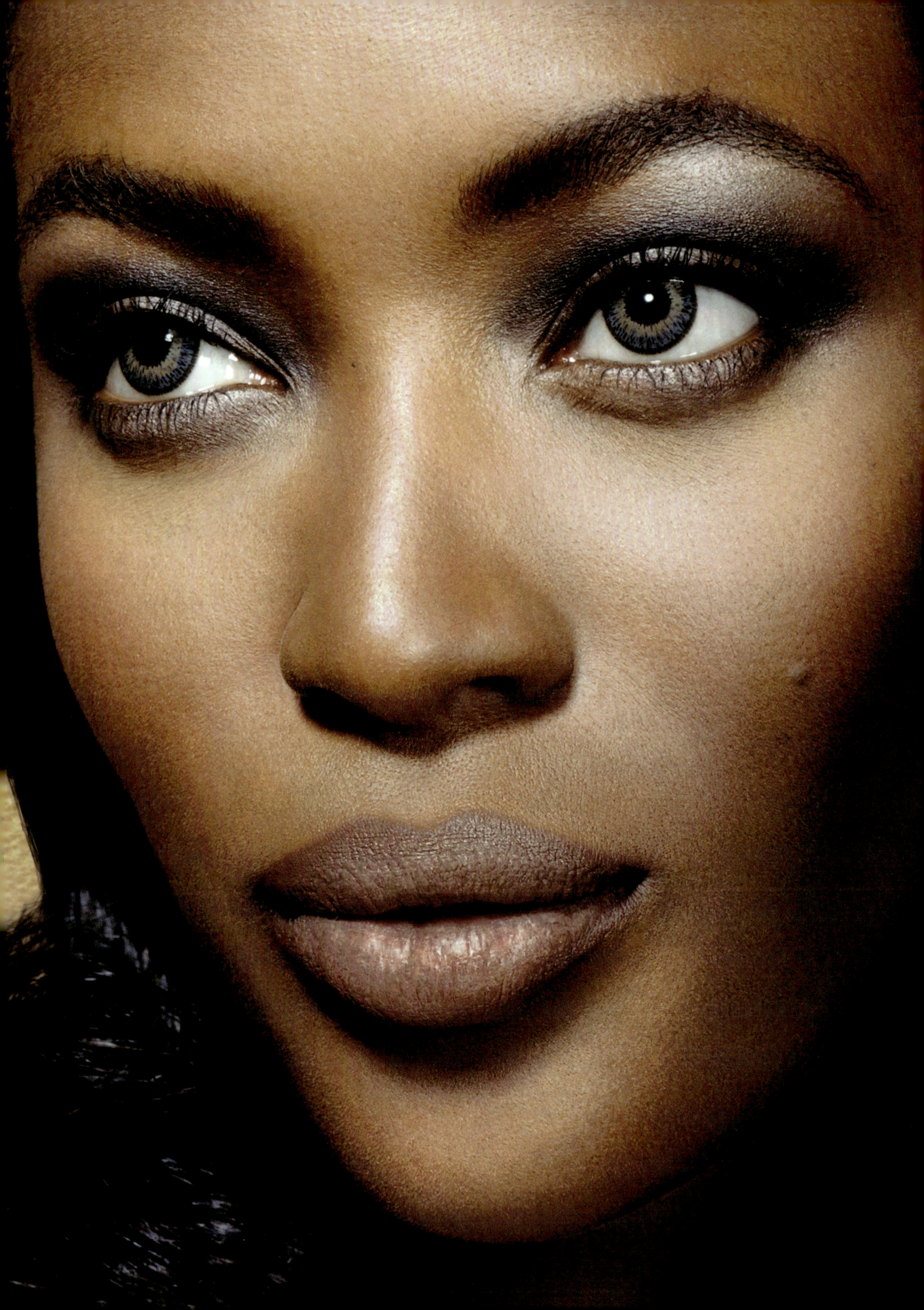

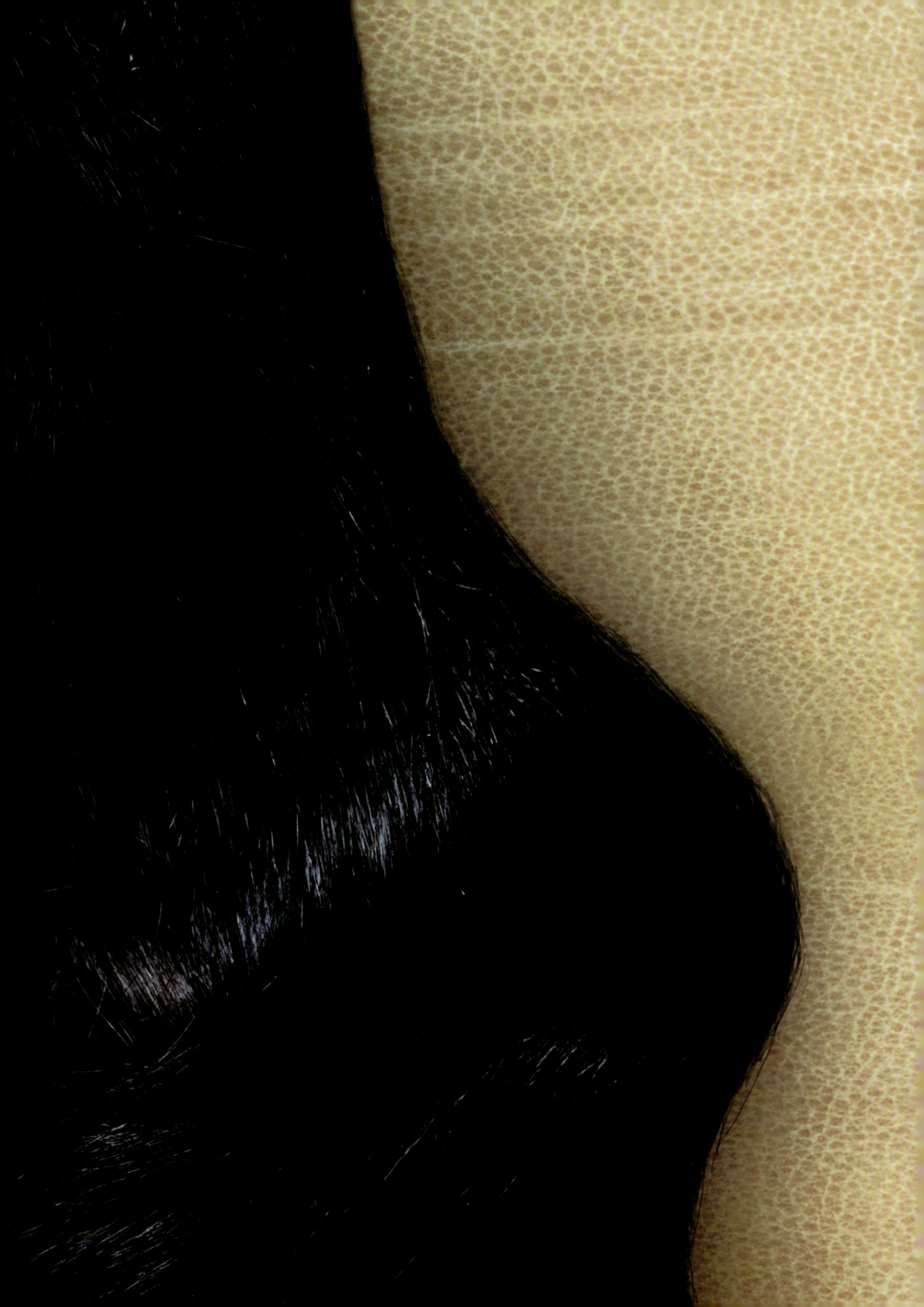

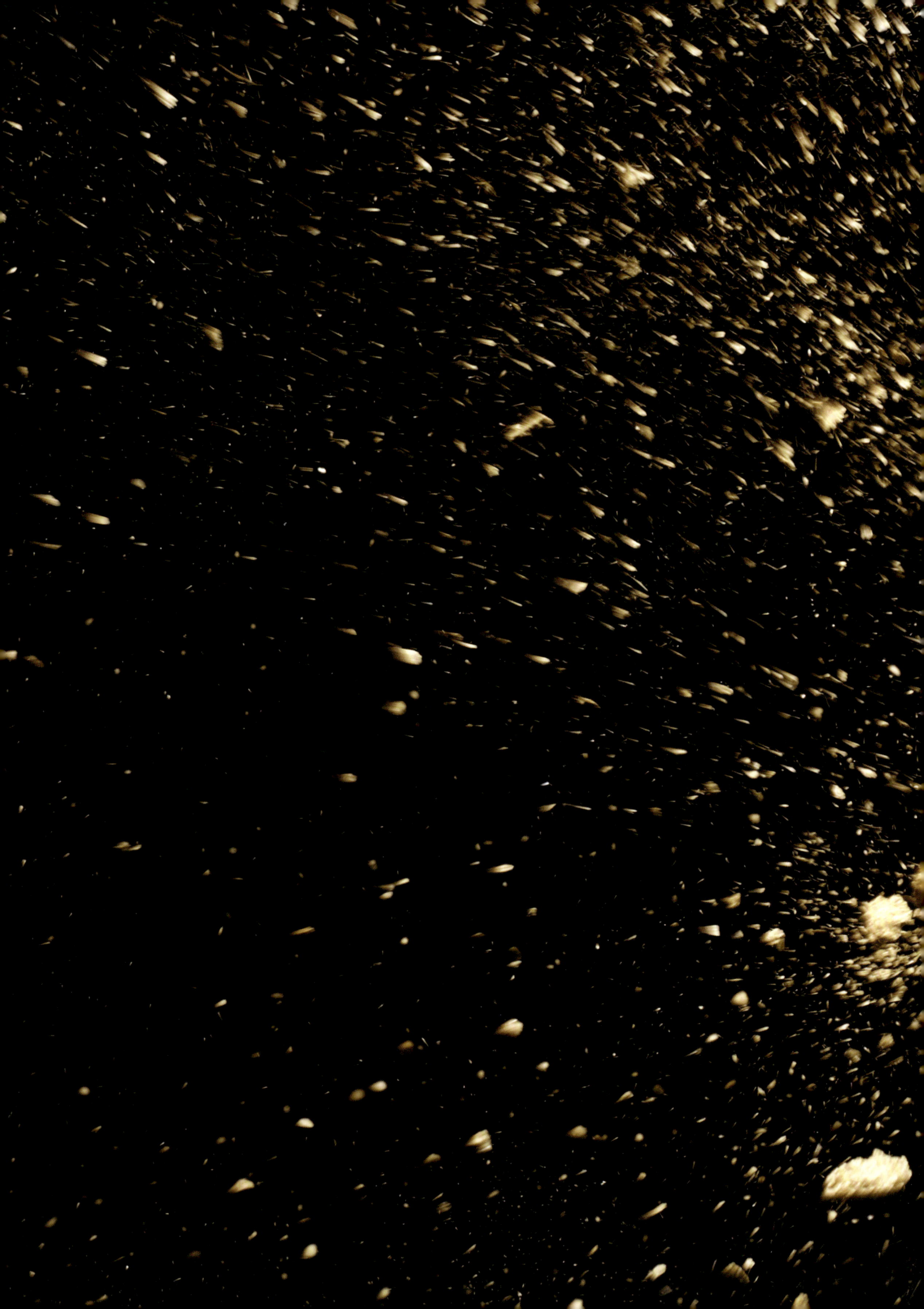

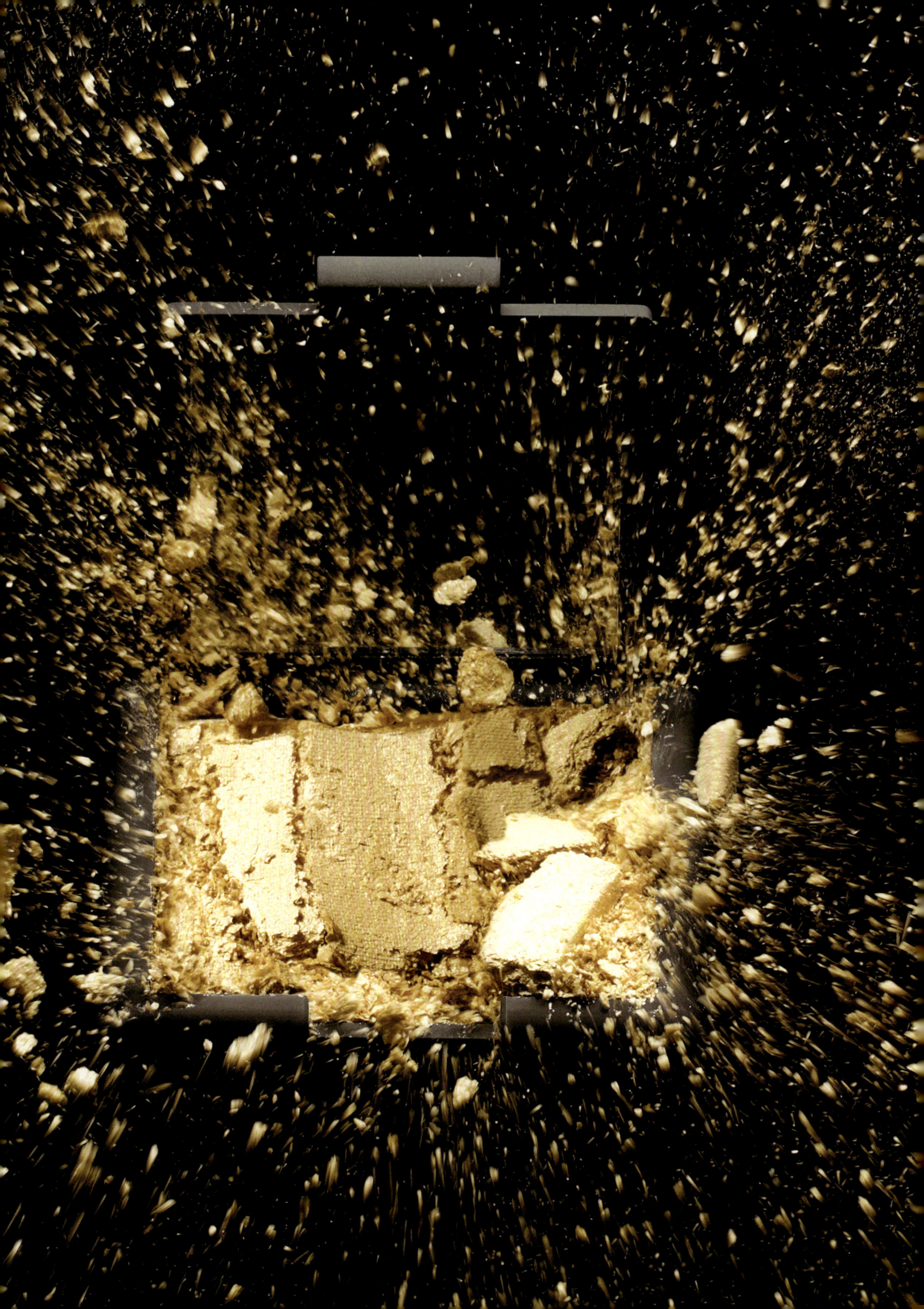

"TO MERELY SAY THAT FRANÇOIS IS A TRUE ARTIST, ISN'T ENOUGH. HE'S A GENIUS WHO CONTINUES TO AMAZE ME WITH HIS TALENT. OVER THE COURSE OF MY CAREER, I HAVE WORKED WITH TRULY THE MOST TALENTED MAKEUP ARTISTS WHO HAVE EVER LIVED, AND NO ONE HAS EVER PAINTED MY FACE LIKE FRANÇOIS."
— LINDA EVANGELISTA

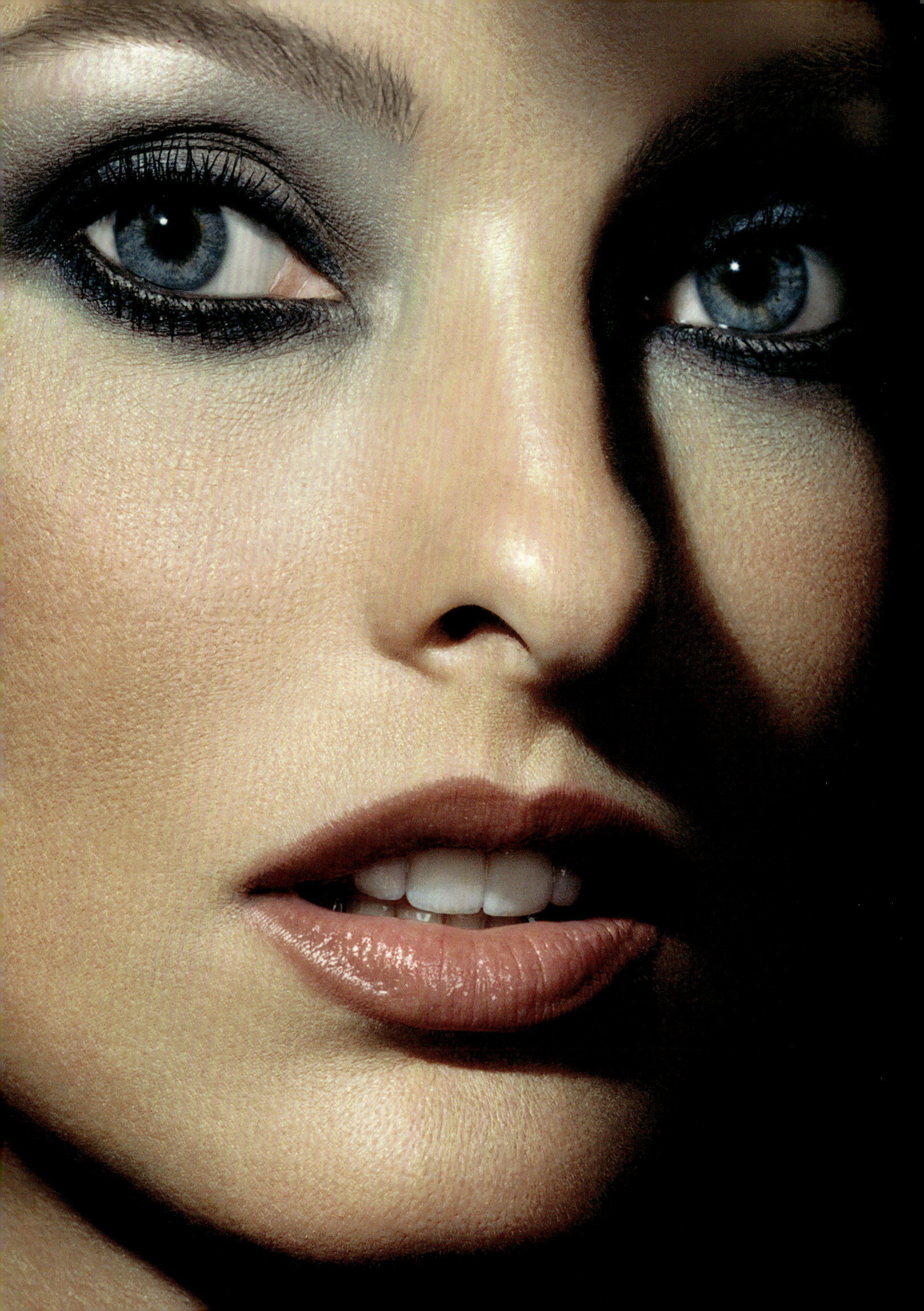

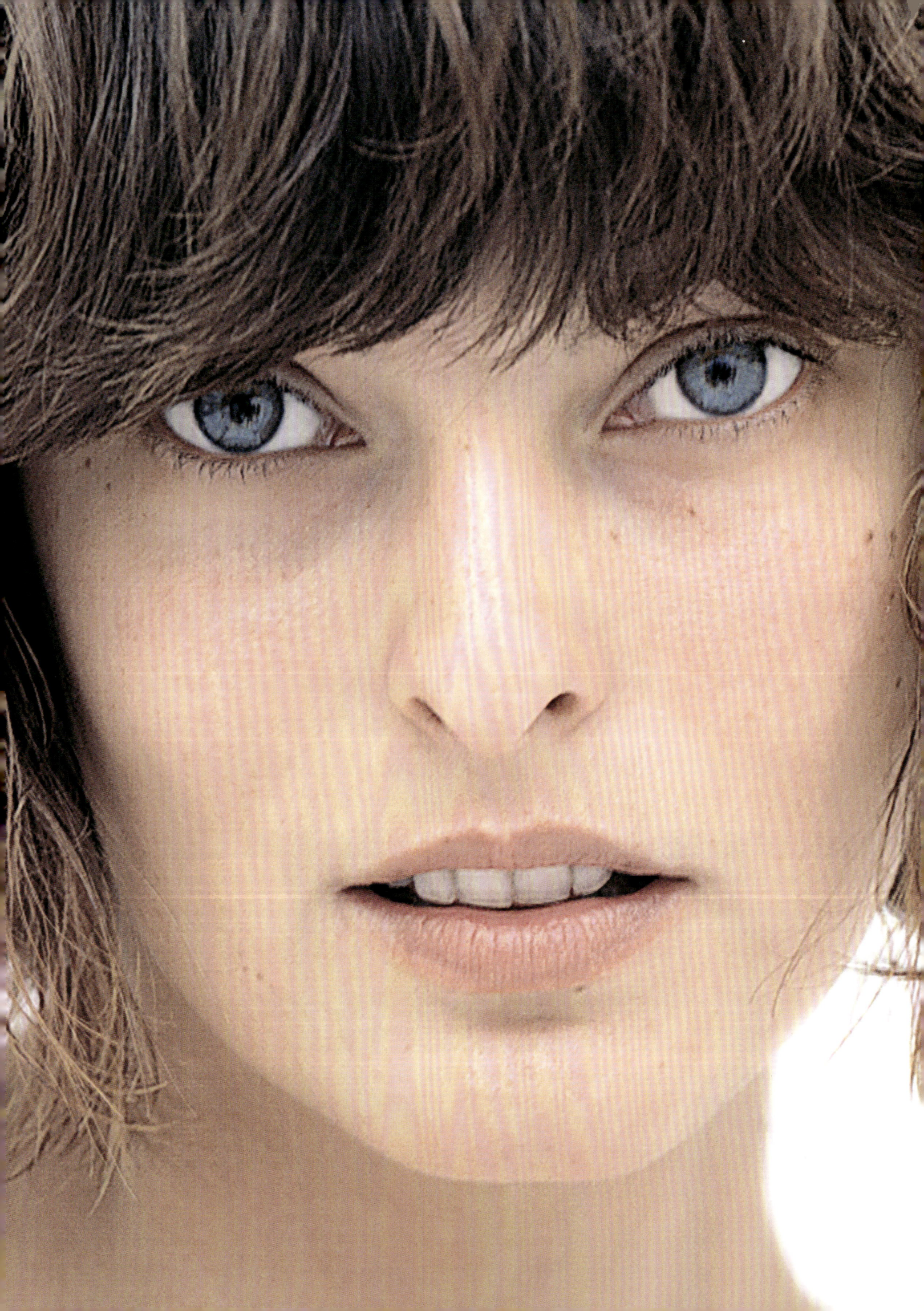

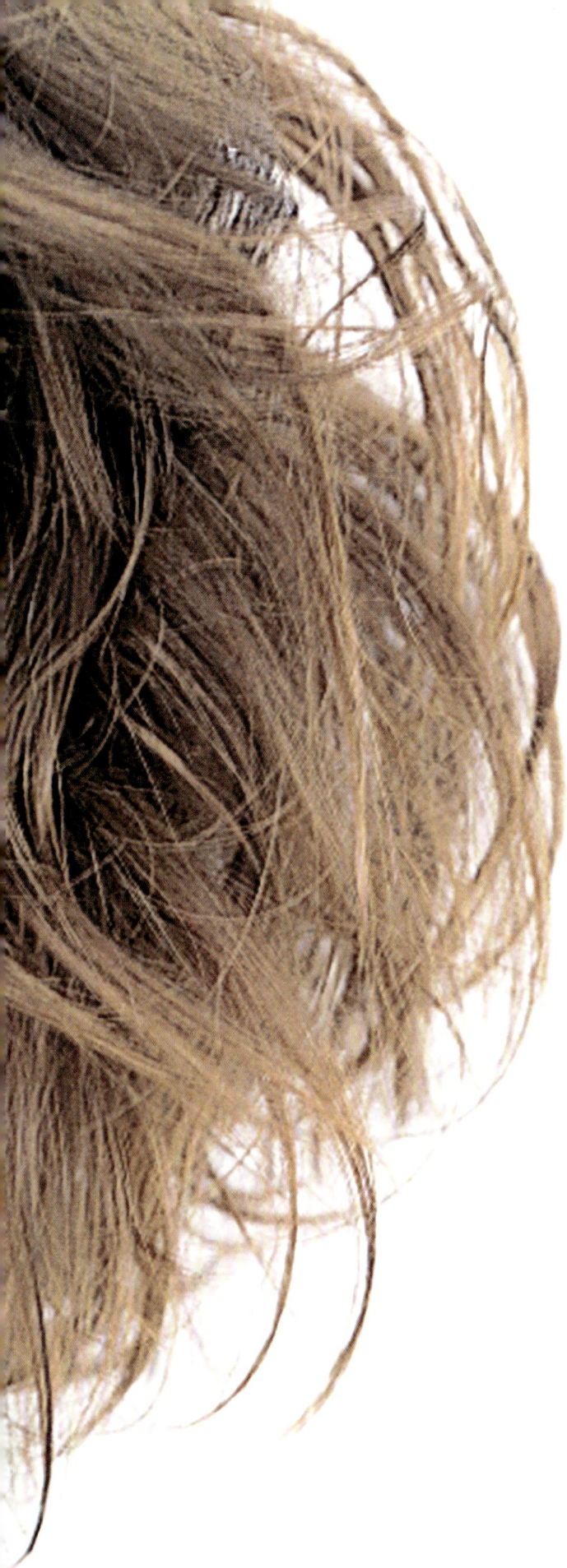

"LINDA LINDA LINDA FOREVER."
– FRANÇOIS NARS

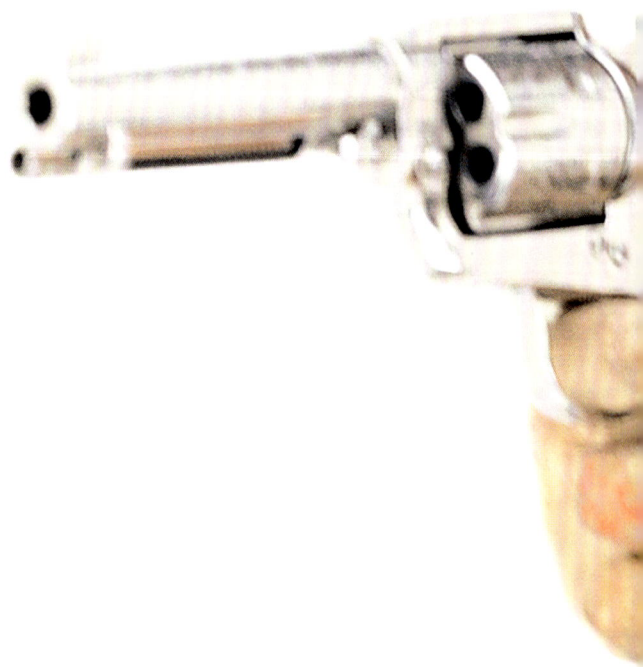

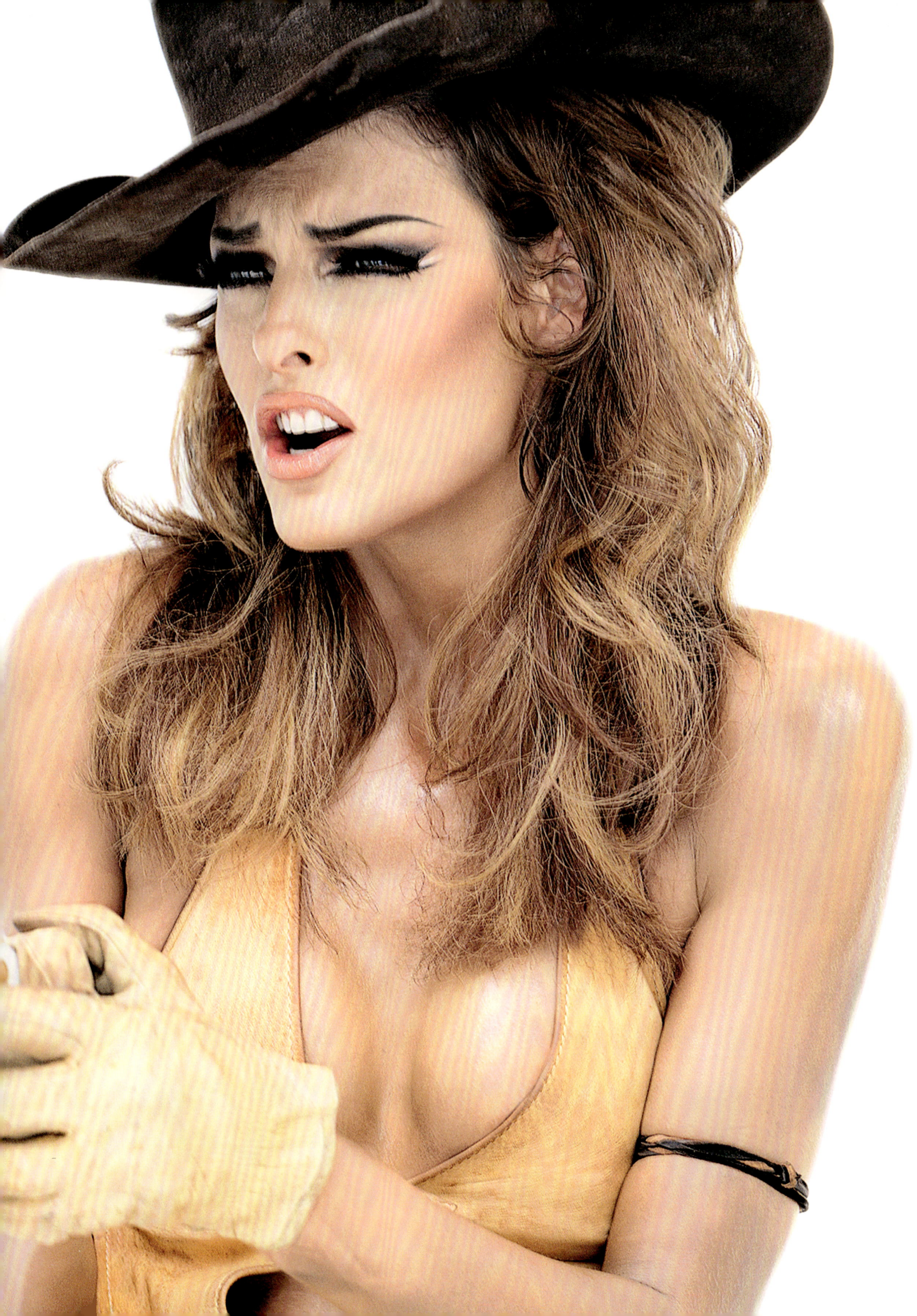

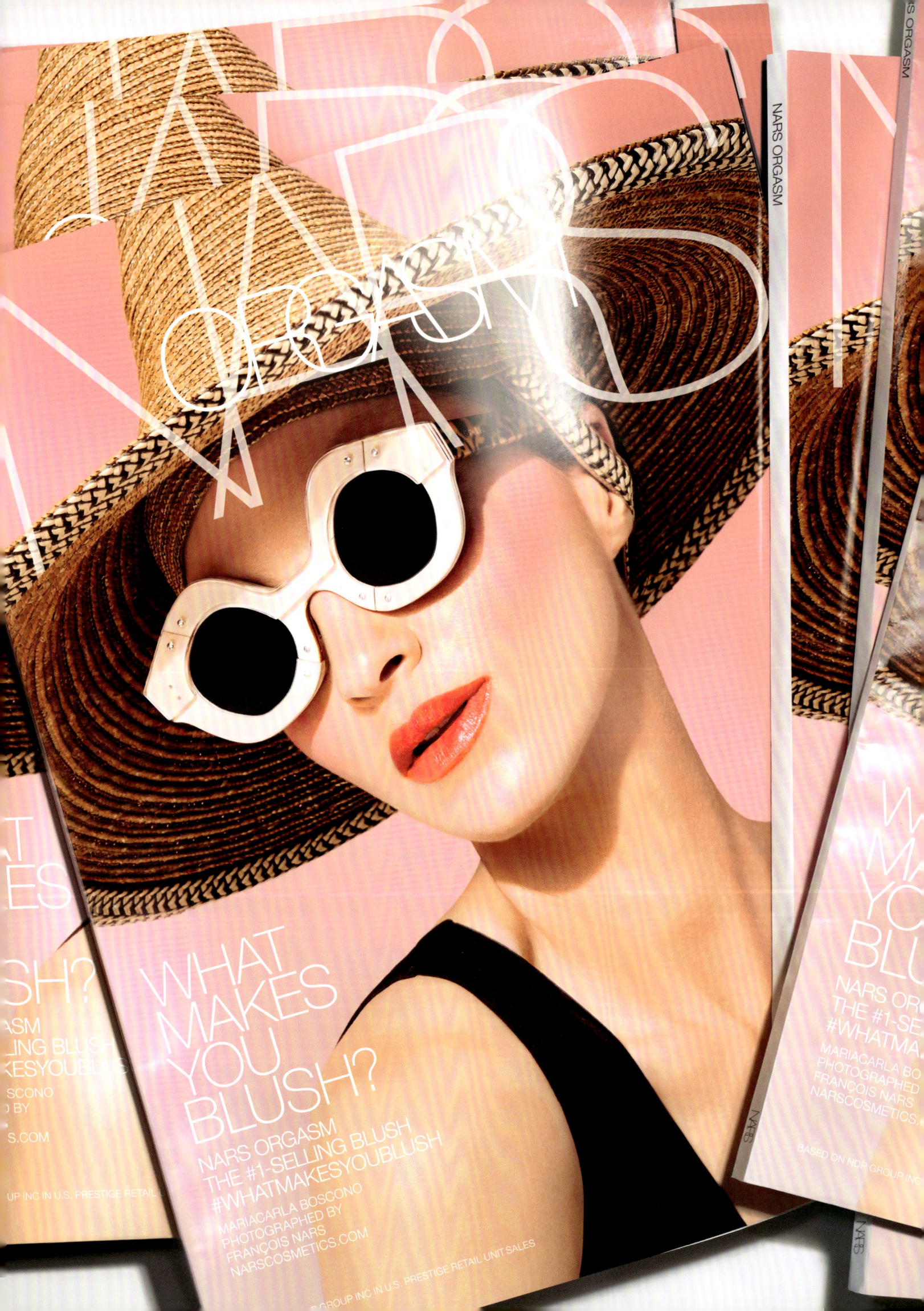

NARS ORGASM

ORGASM

WHAT MAKES YOU BLUSH?

NARS ORGASM
THE #1-SELLING BLUSH
#WHATMAKESYOUBLUSH

MARIACARLA BOSCONO
PHOTOGRAPHED BY
FRANÇOIS NARS
NARSCOSMETICS.COM

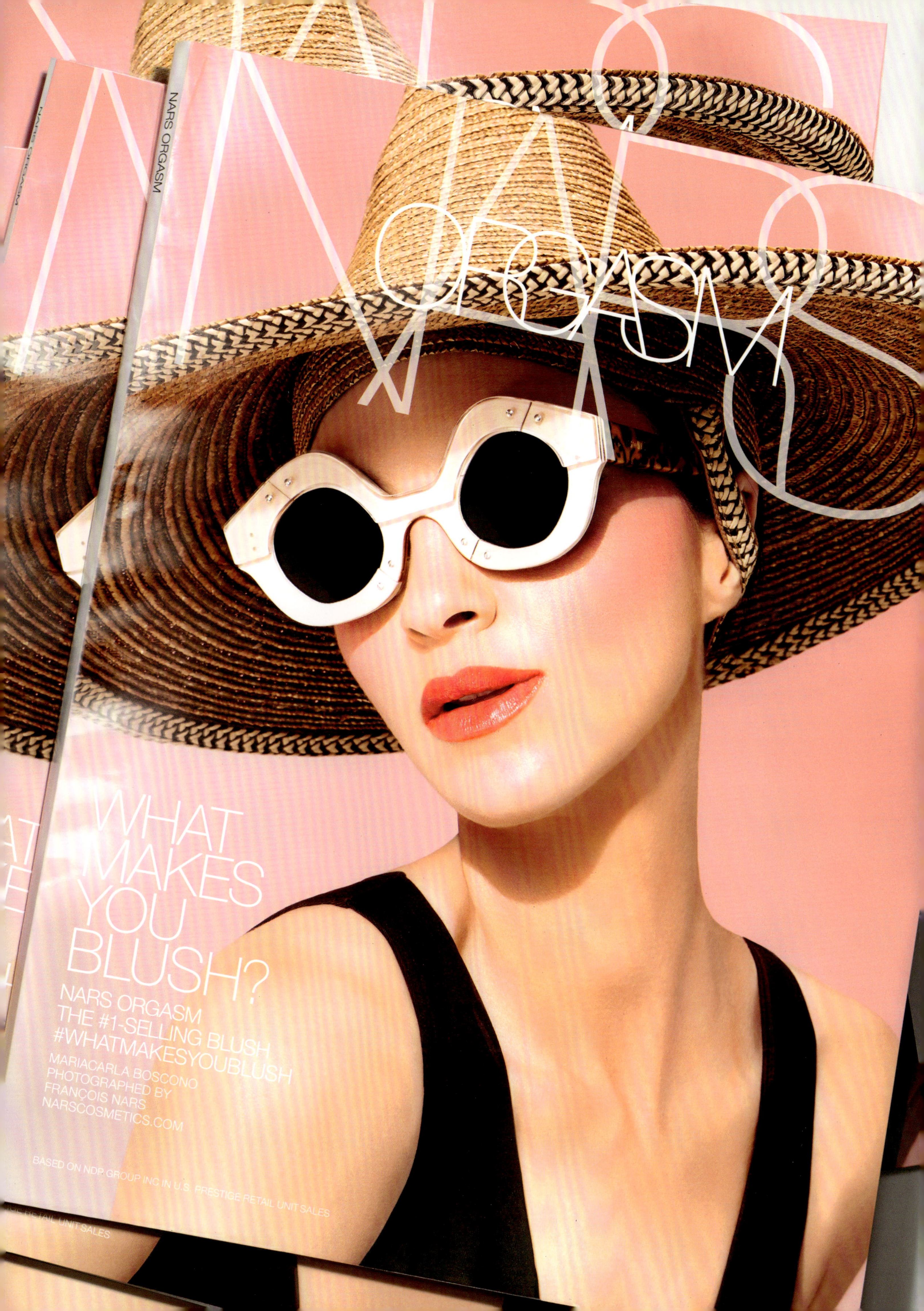

WHAT
MAKES
YOU
BLUSH?

NARS ORGASM
THE #1-SELLING BLUSH
#WHATMAKESYOUBLUSH

MARIACARLA BOSCONO
PHOTOGRAPHED BY
FRANÇOIS NARS
NARSCOSMETICS.COM

BASED ON NDP GROUP INC IN U.S. PRESTIGE RETAIL UNIT SALES

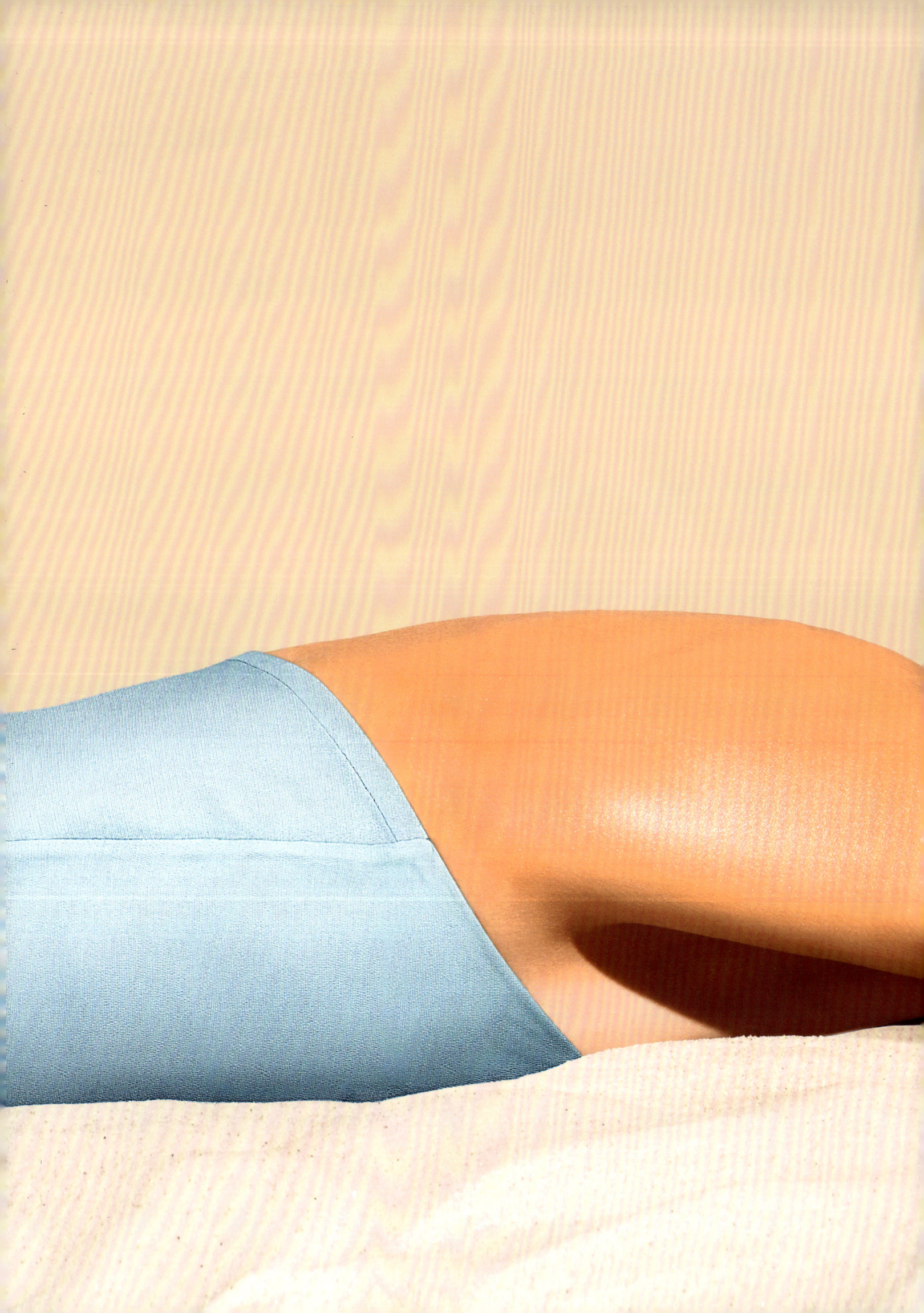

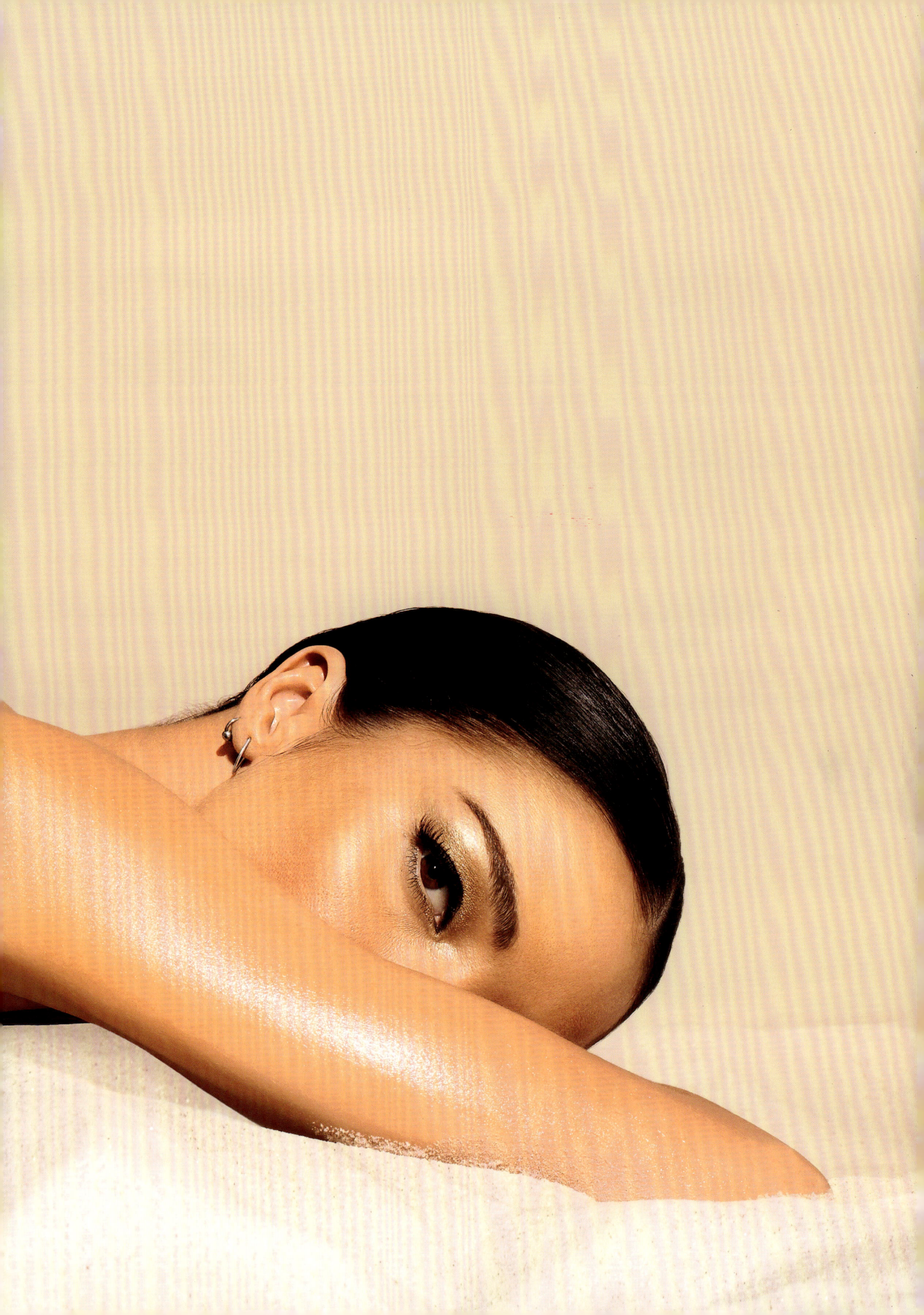

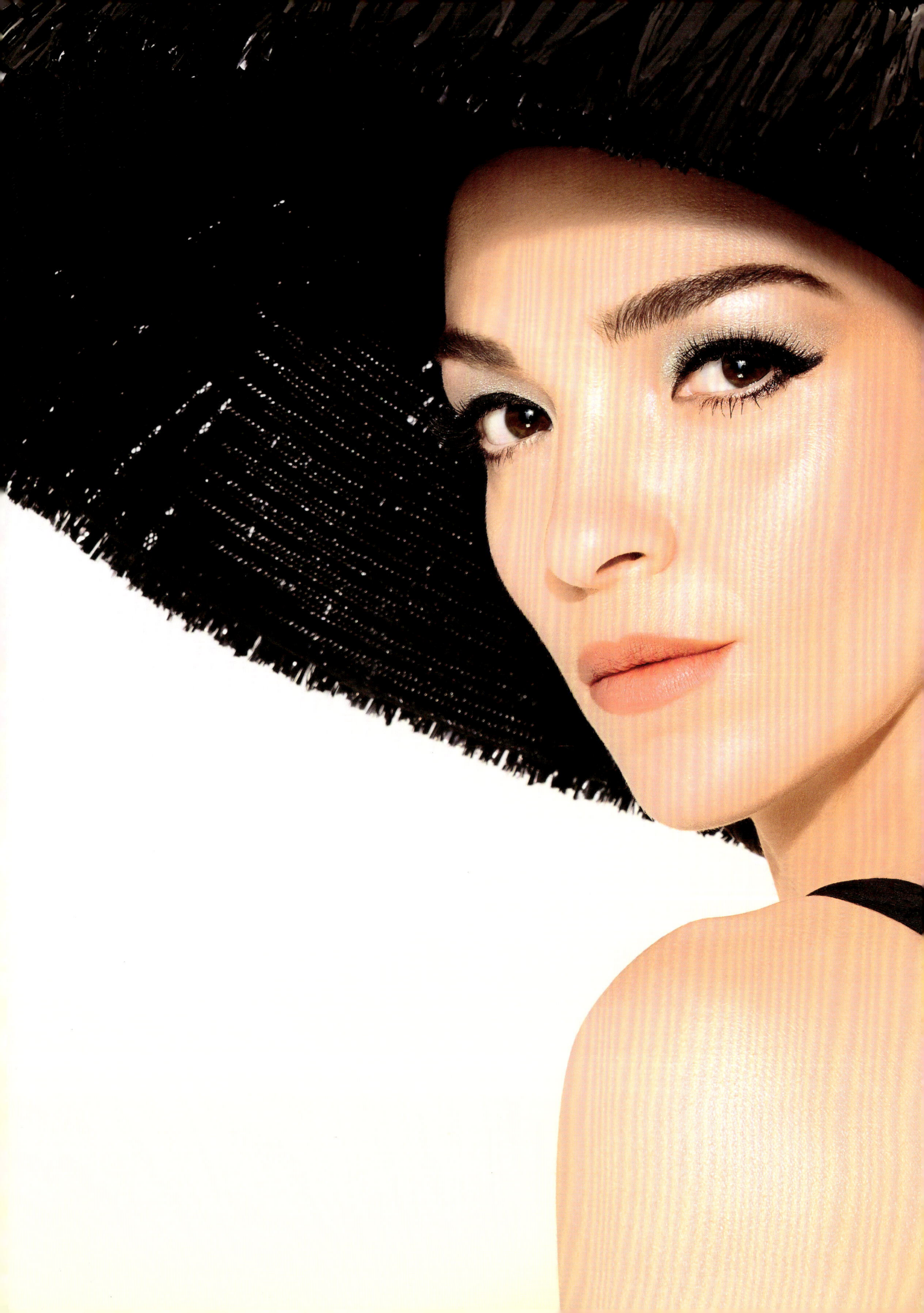

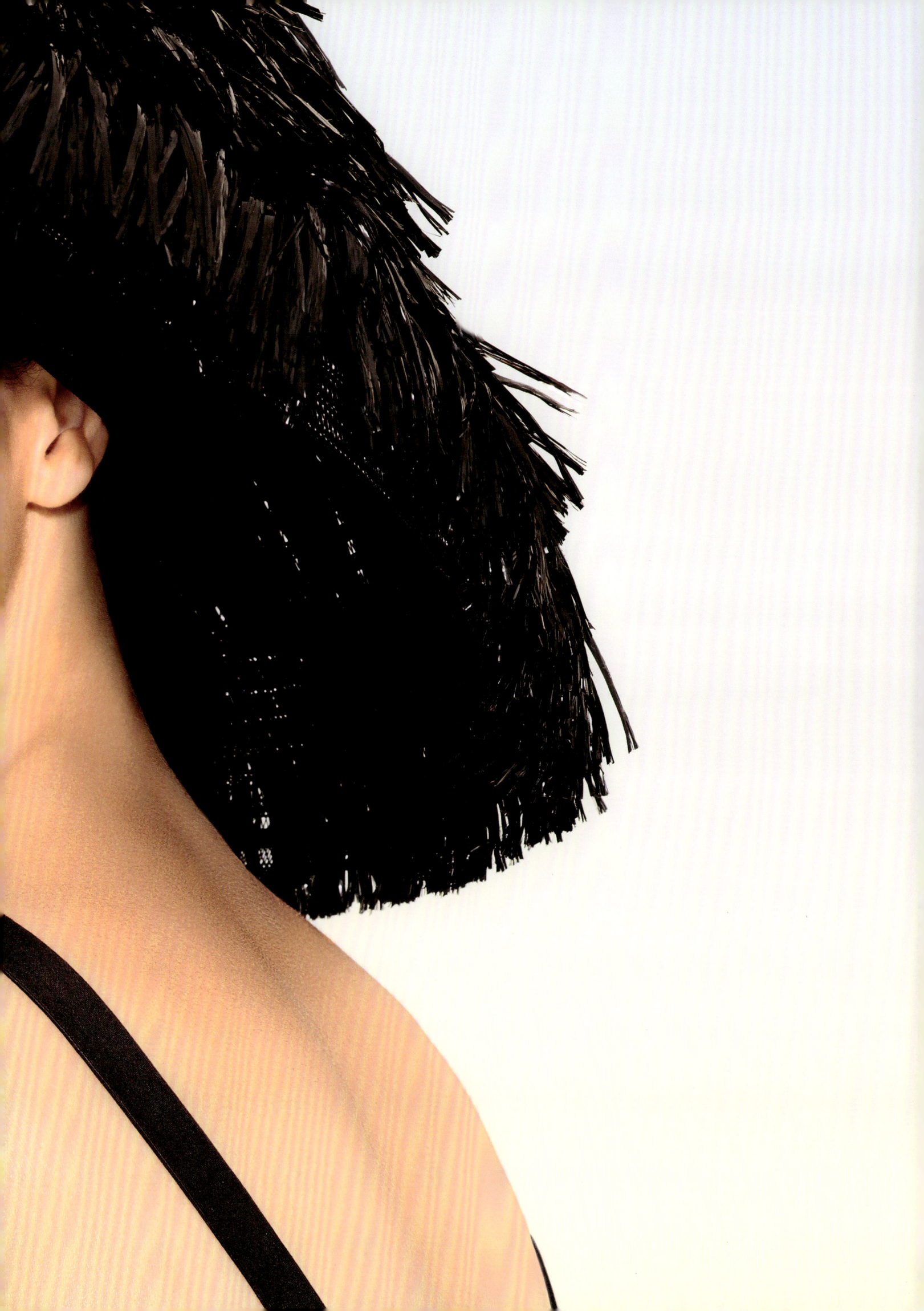

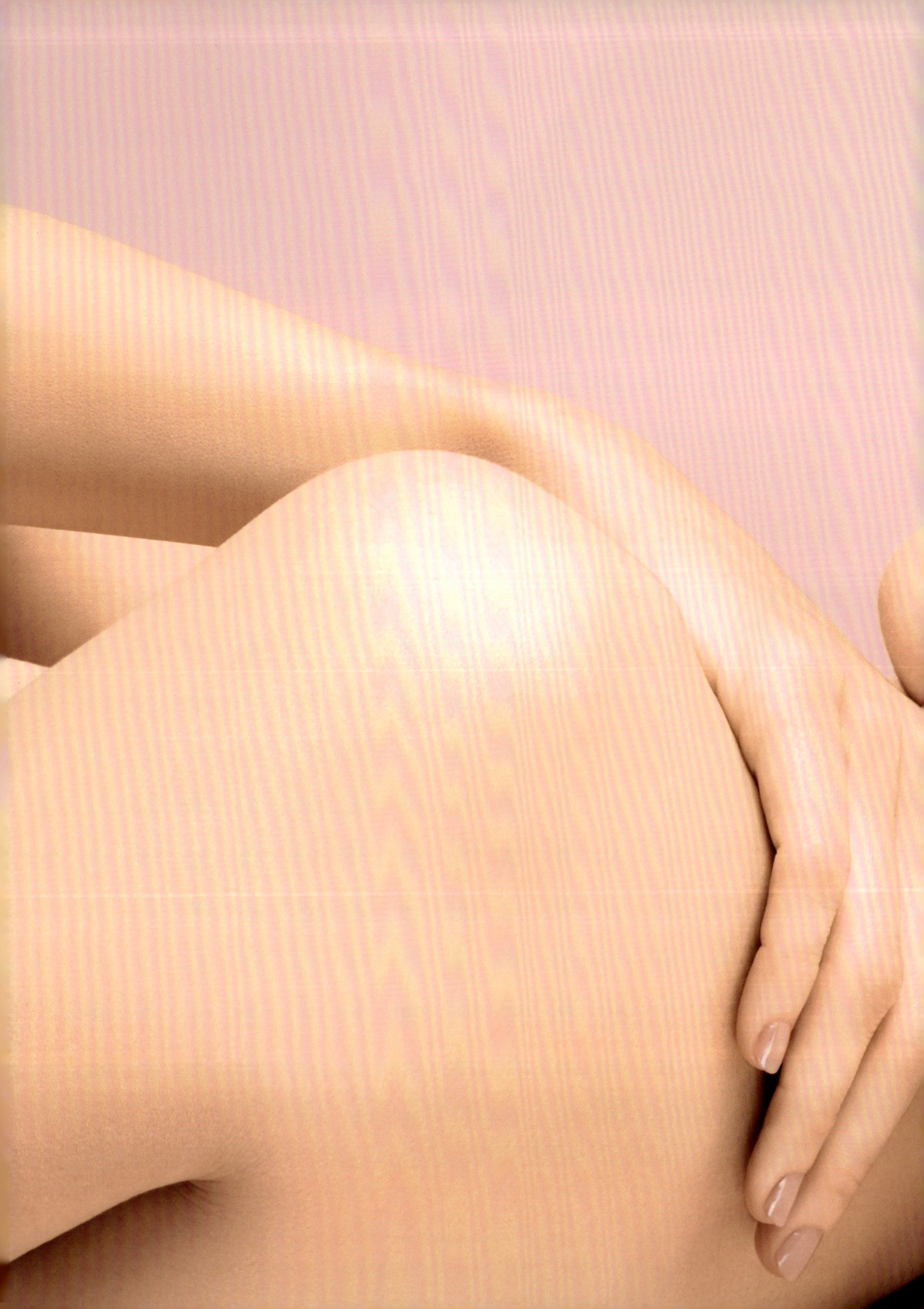

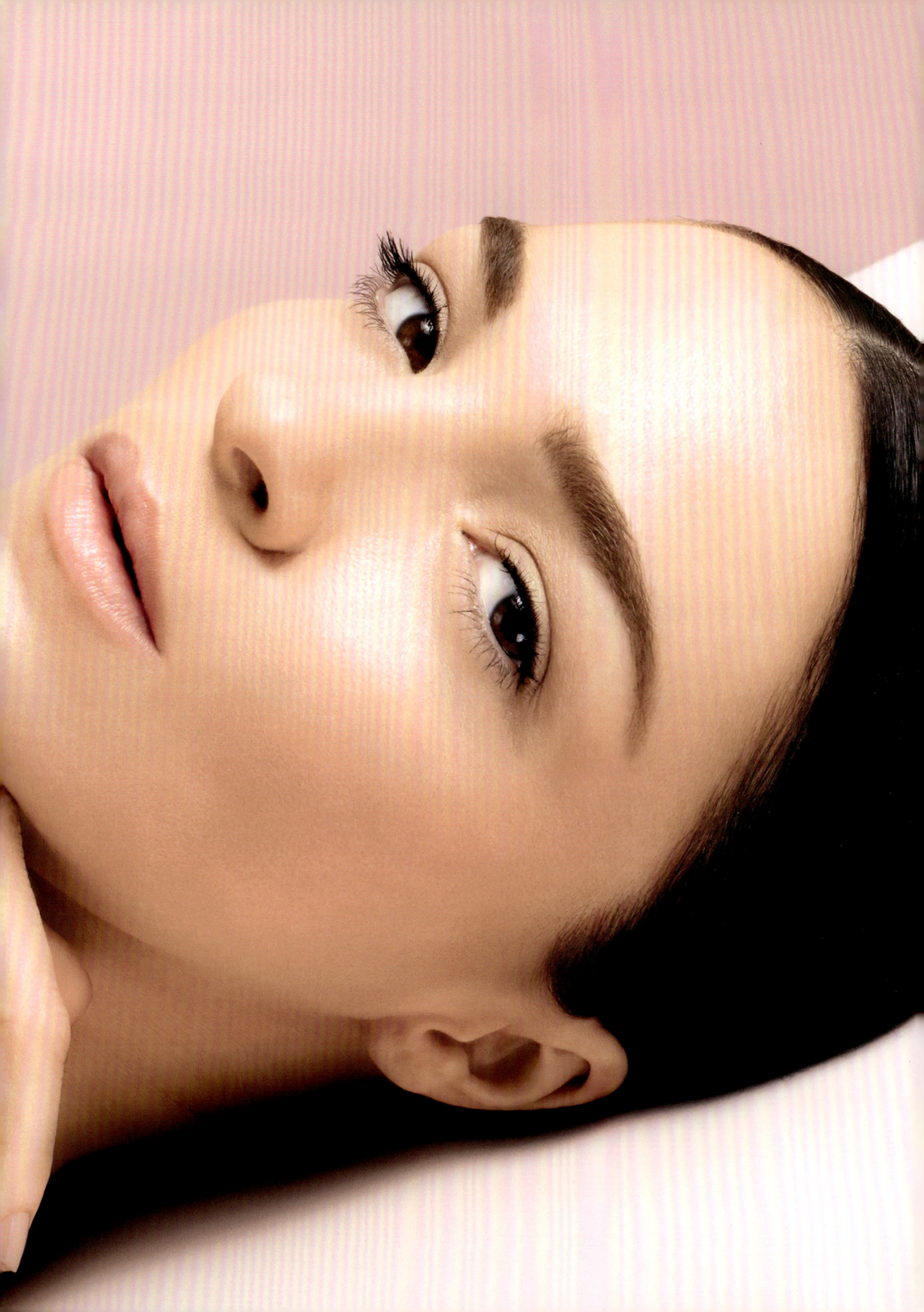

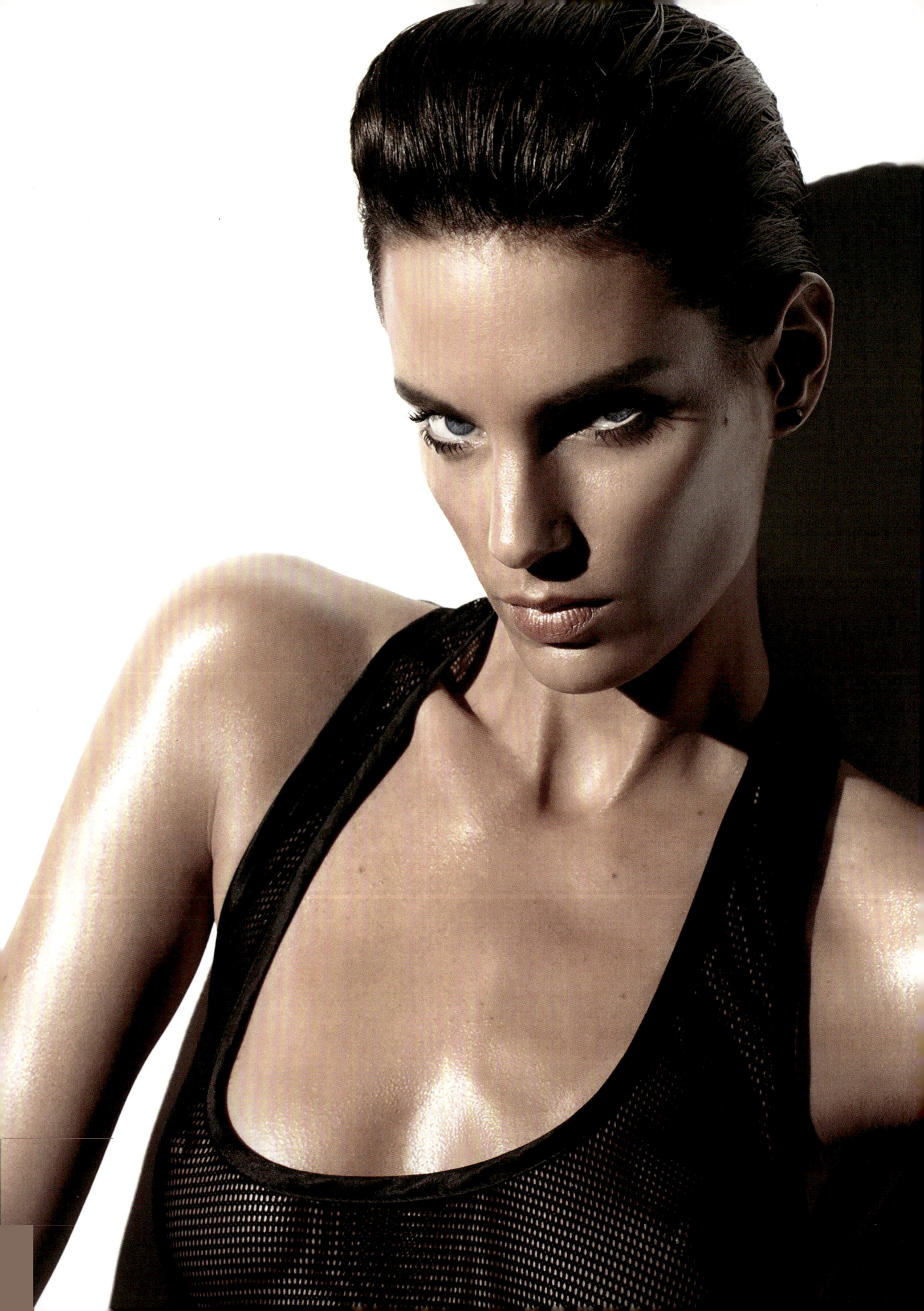

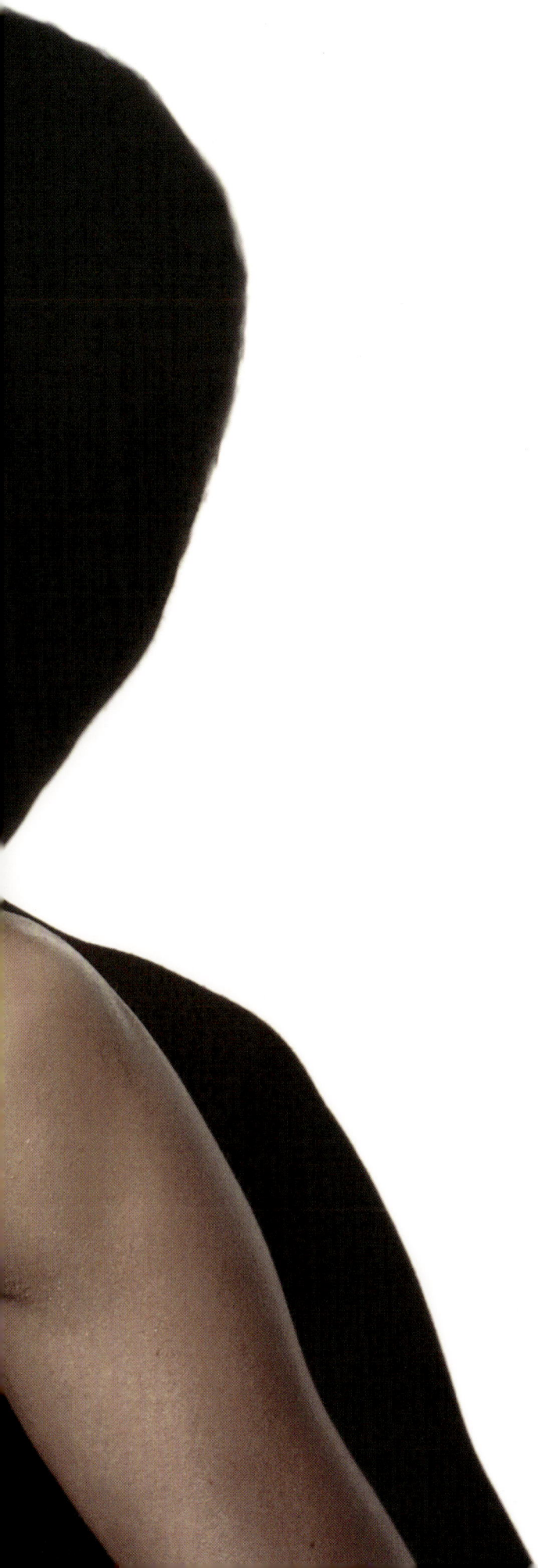

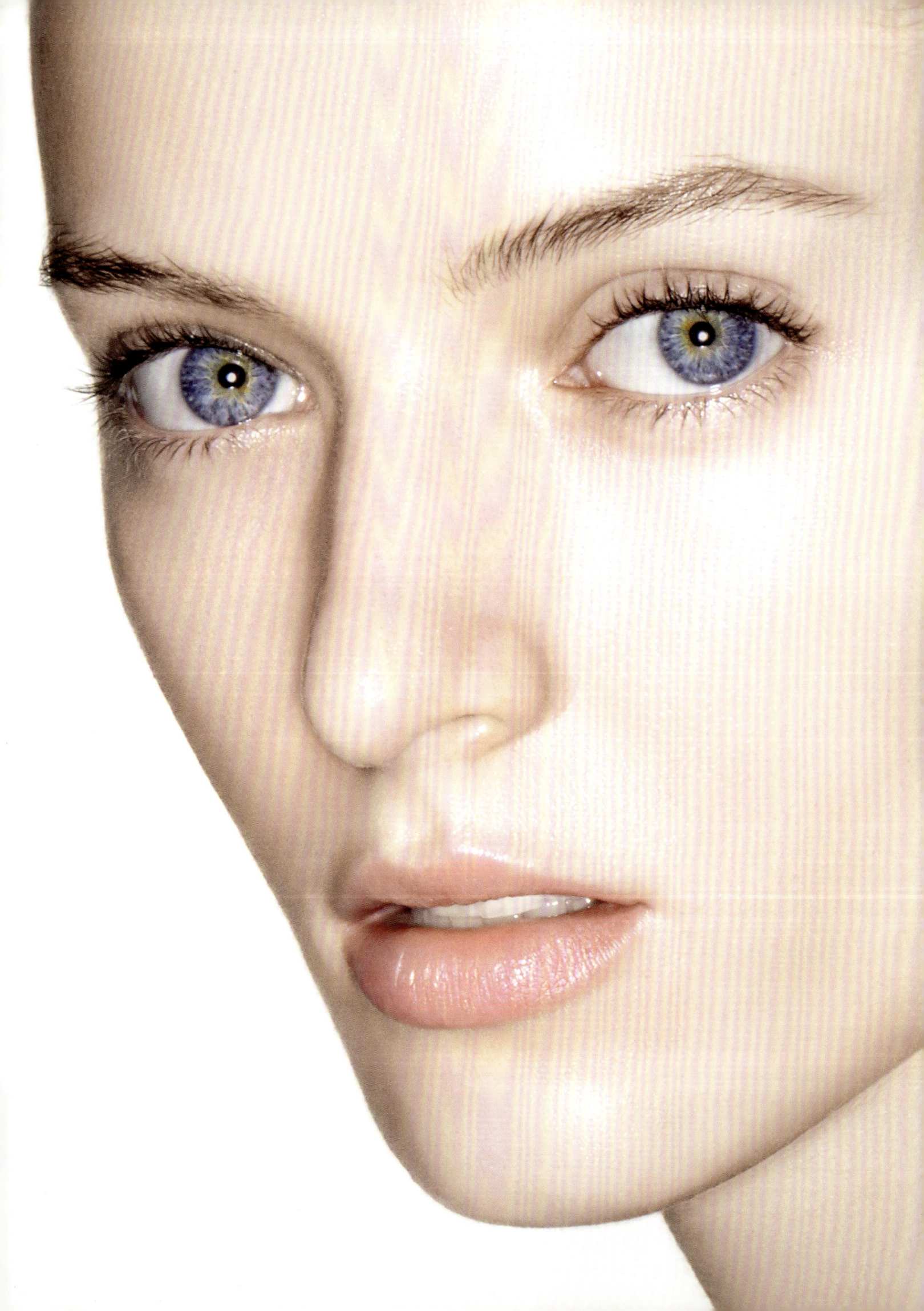

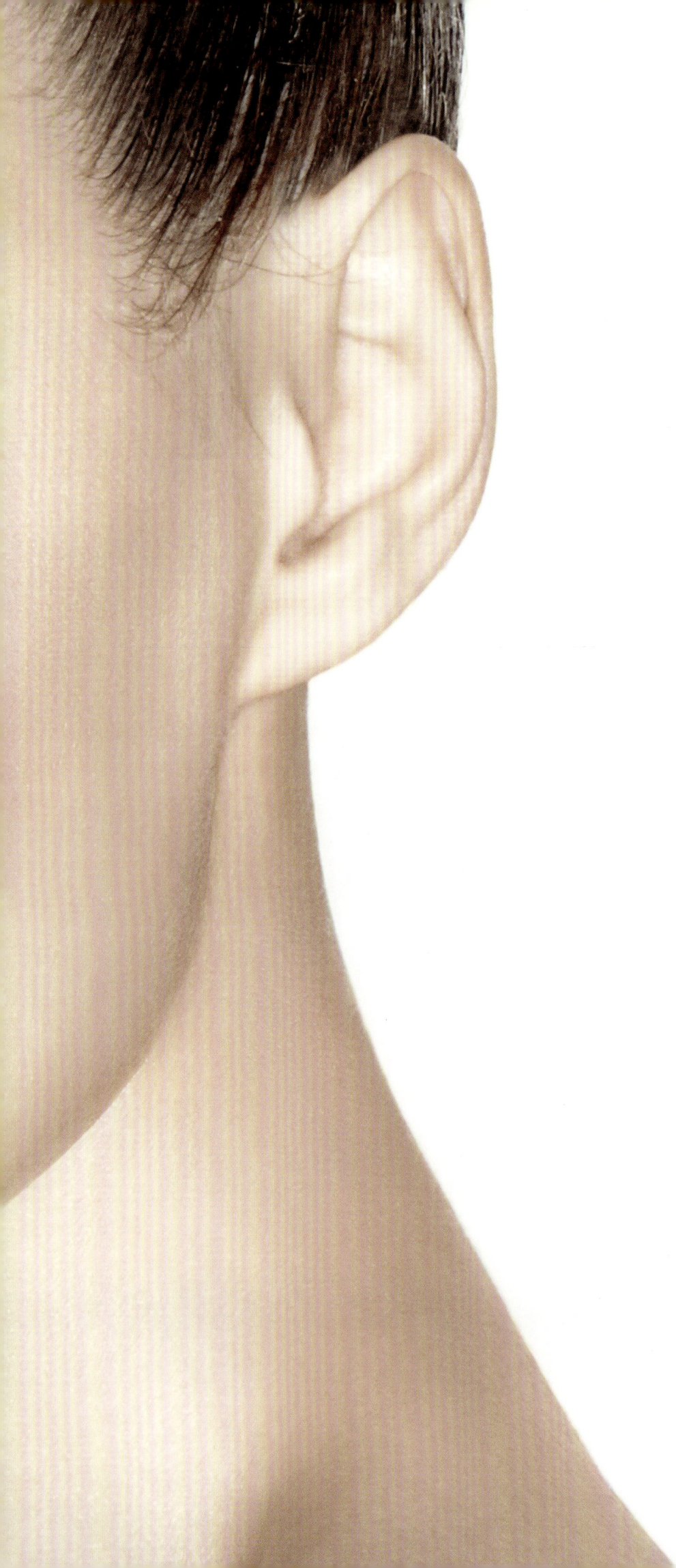

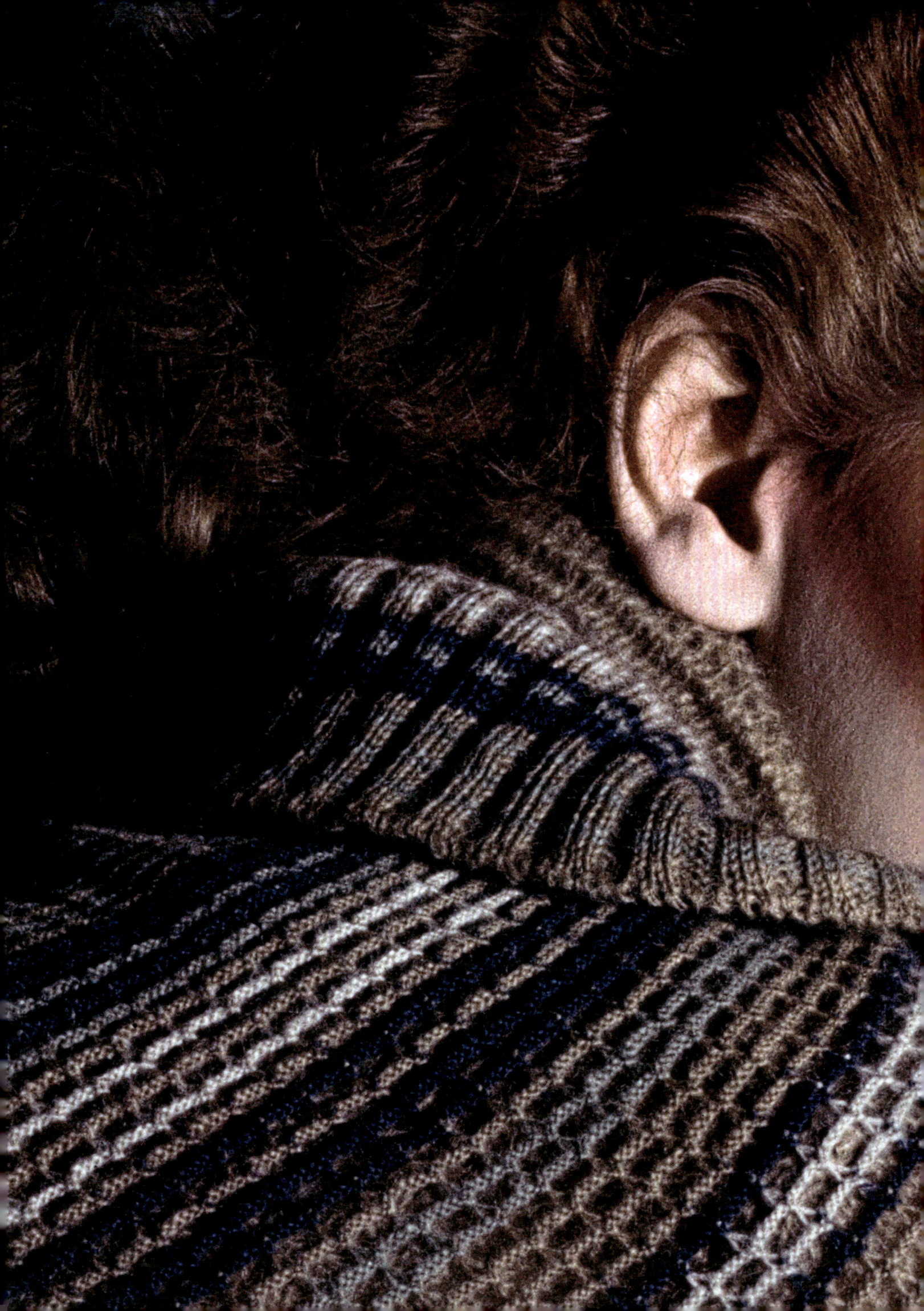

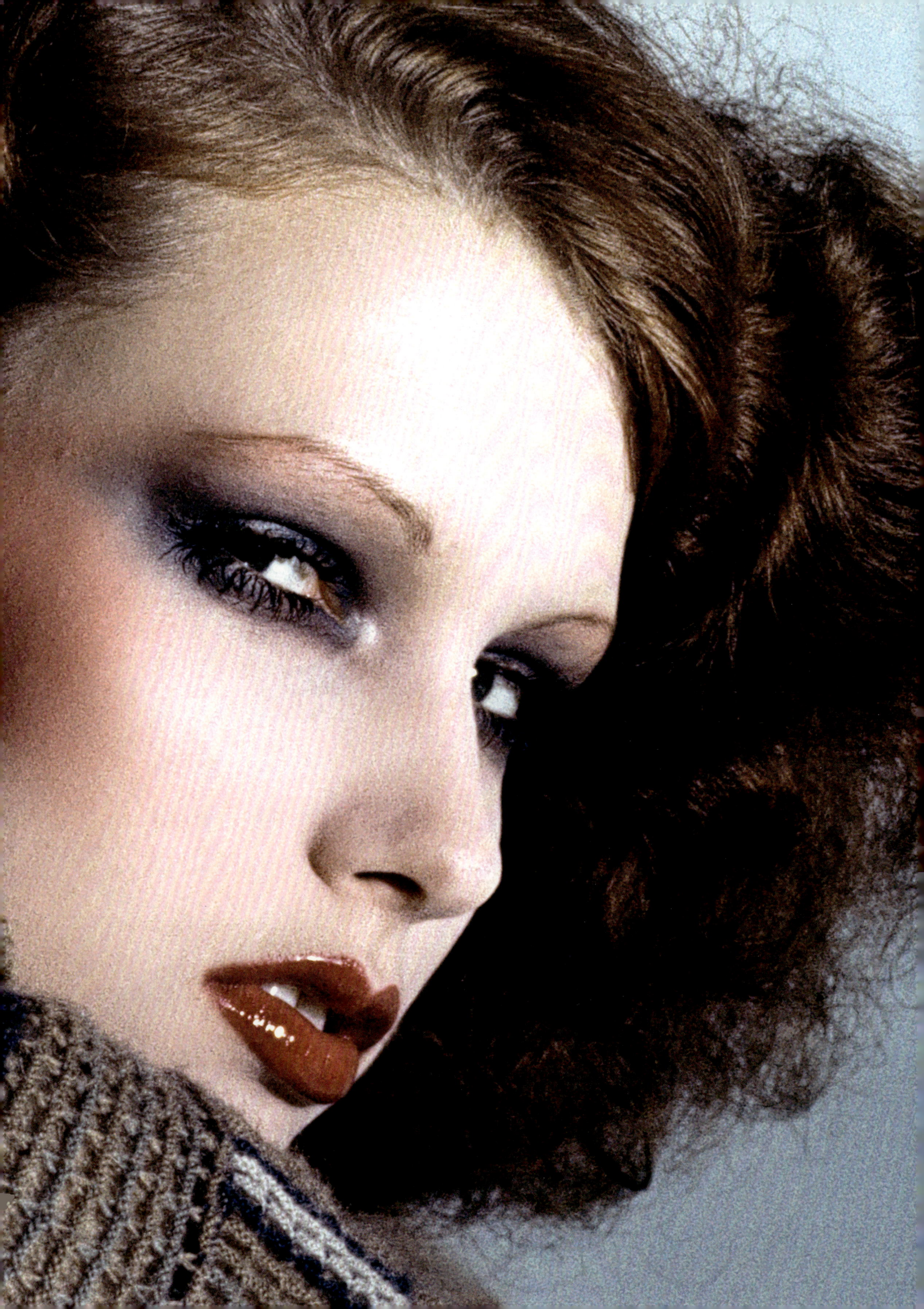

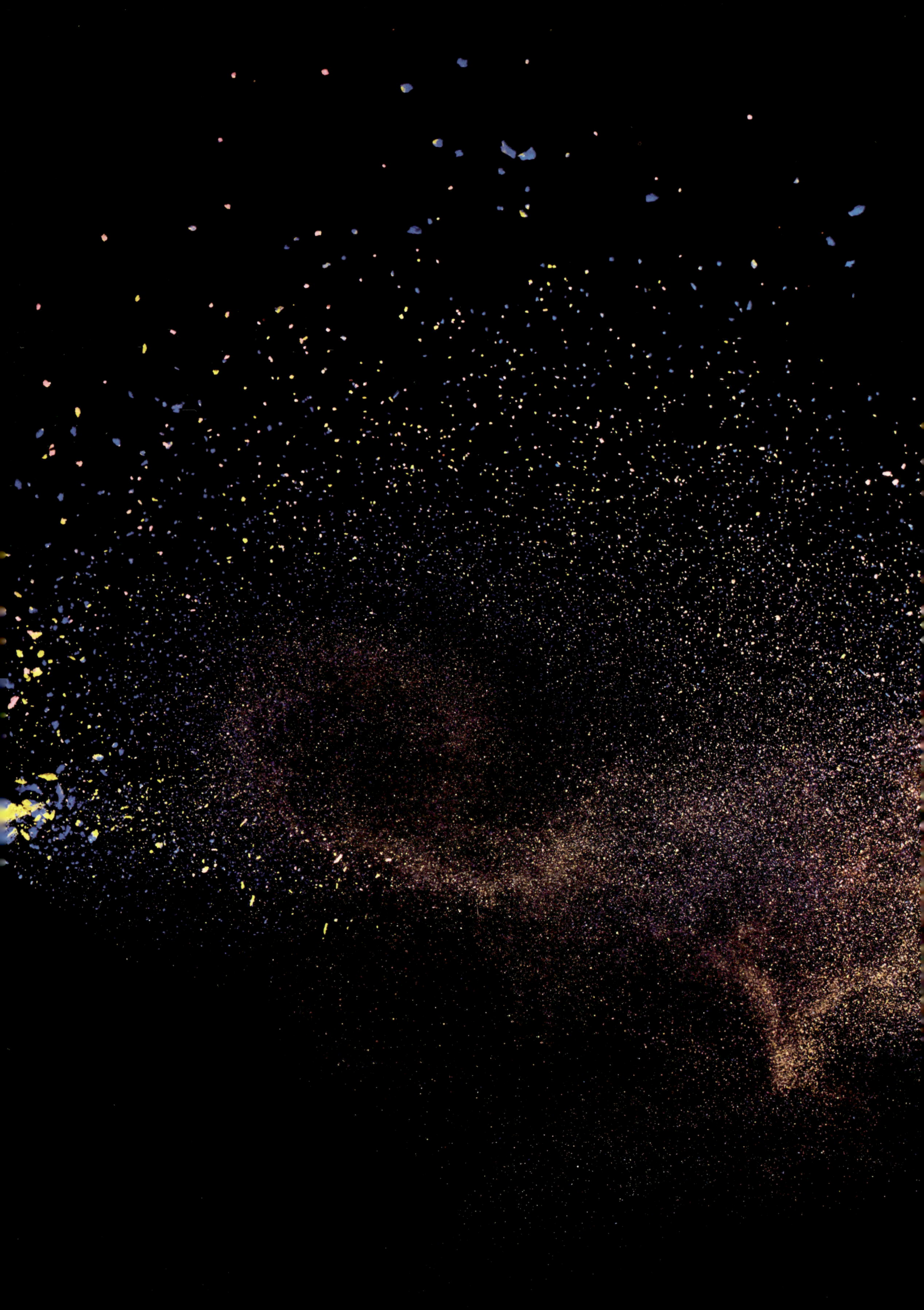

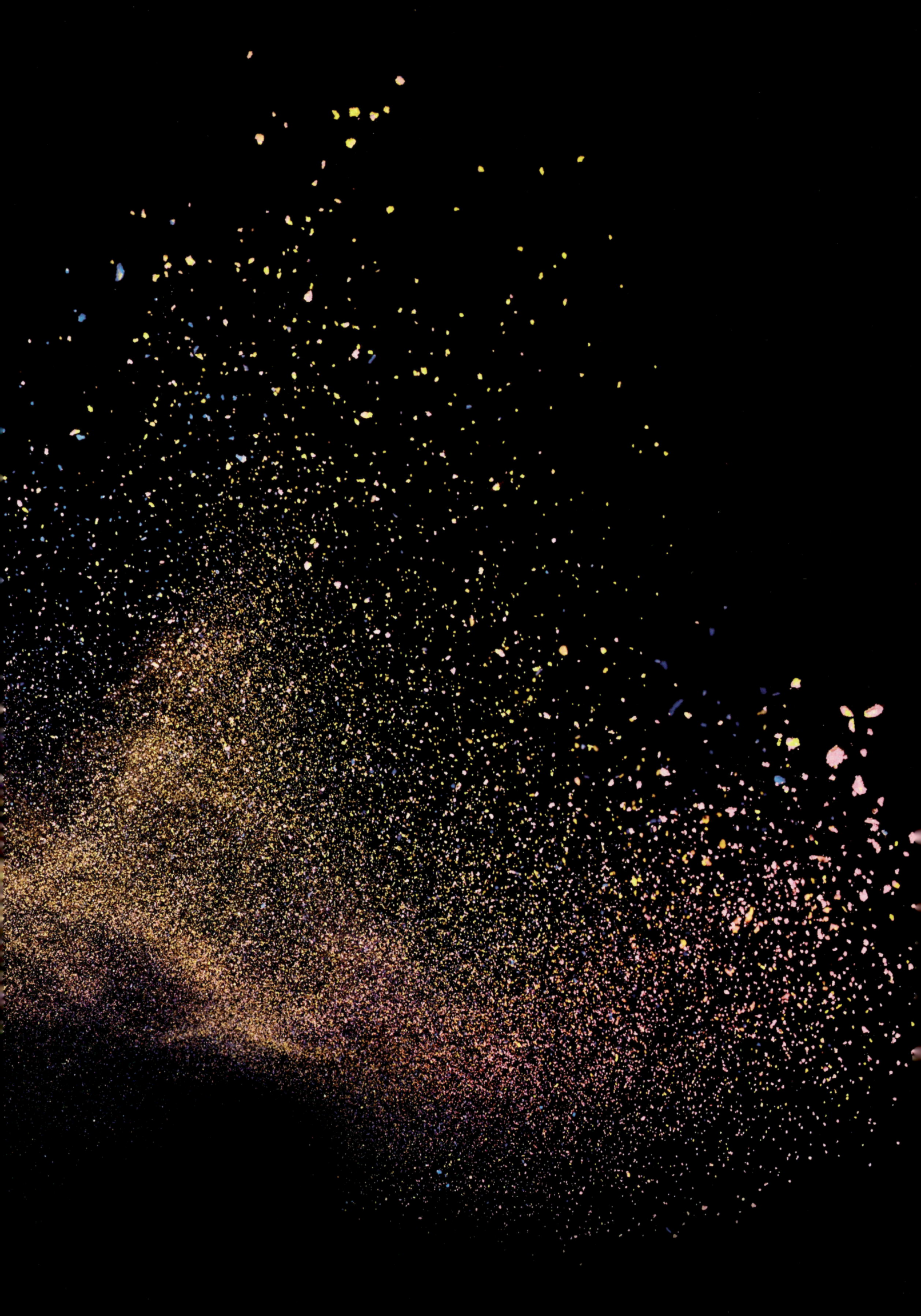

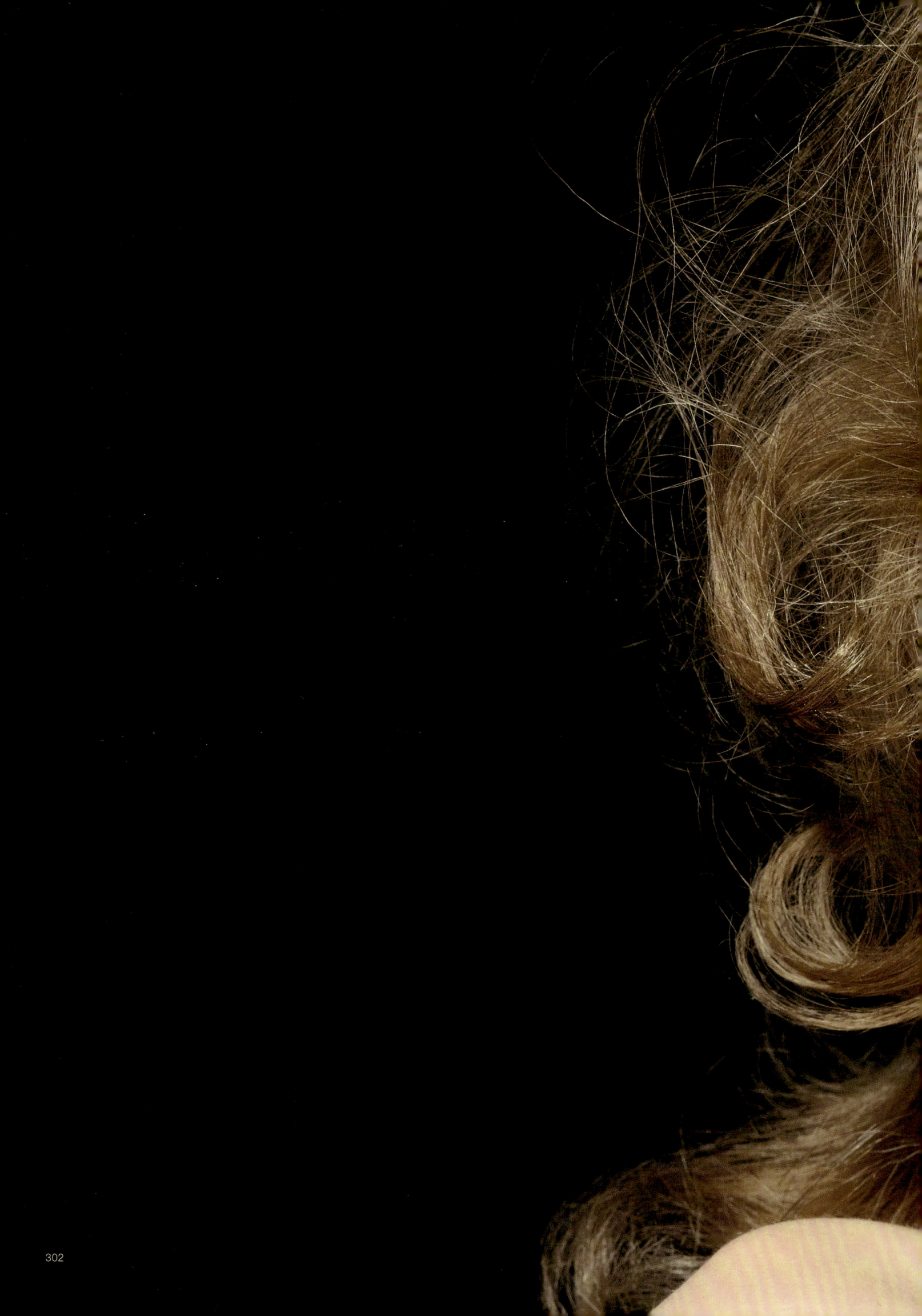

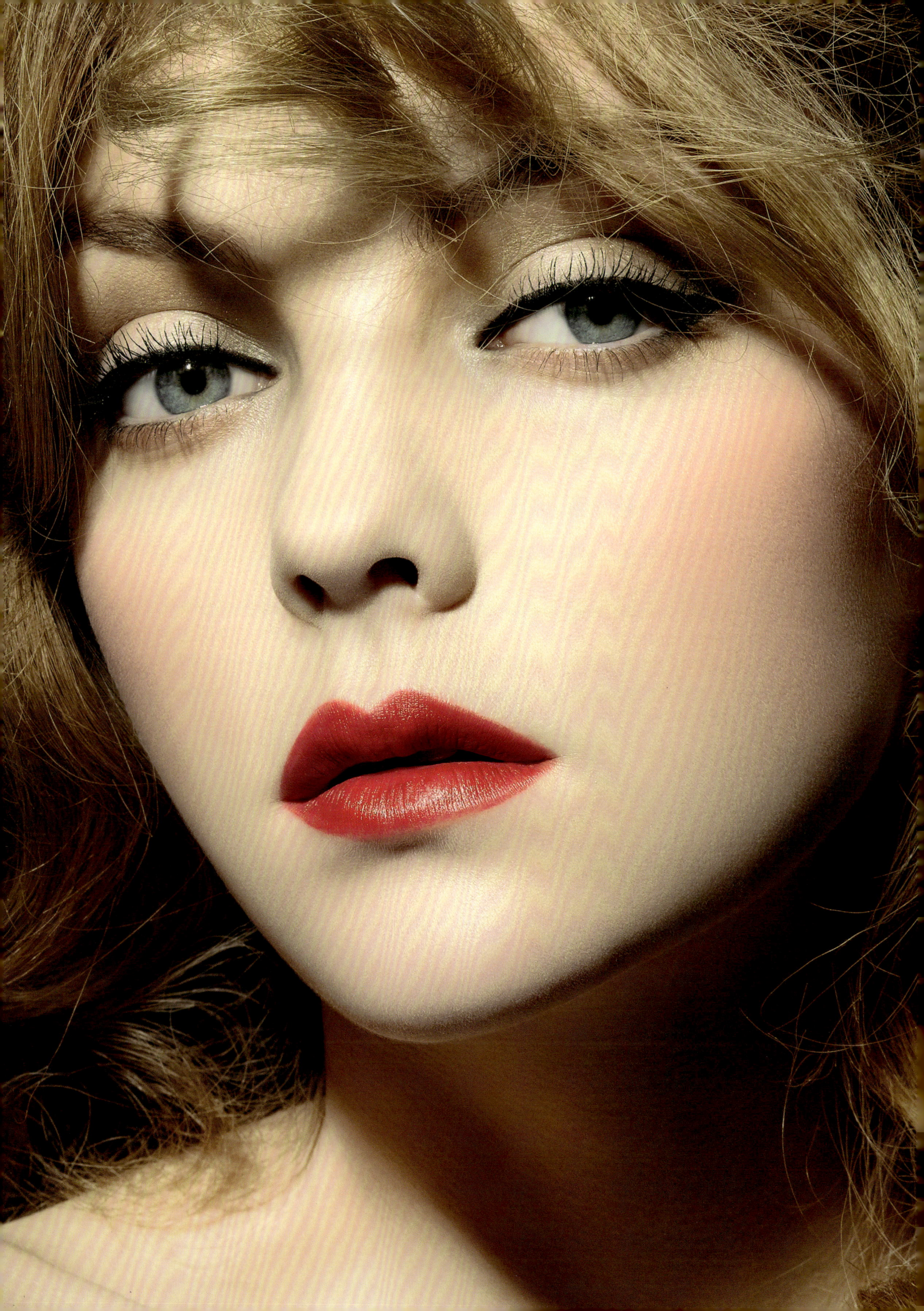

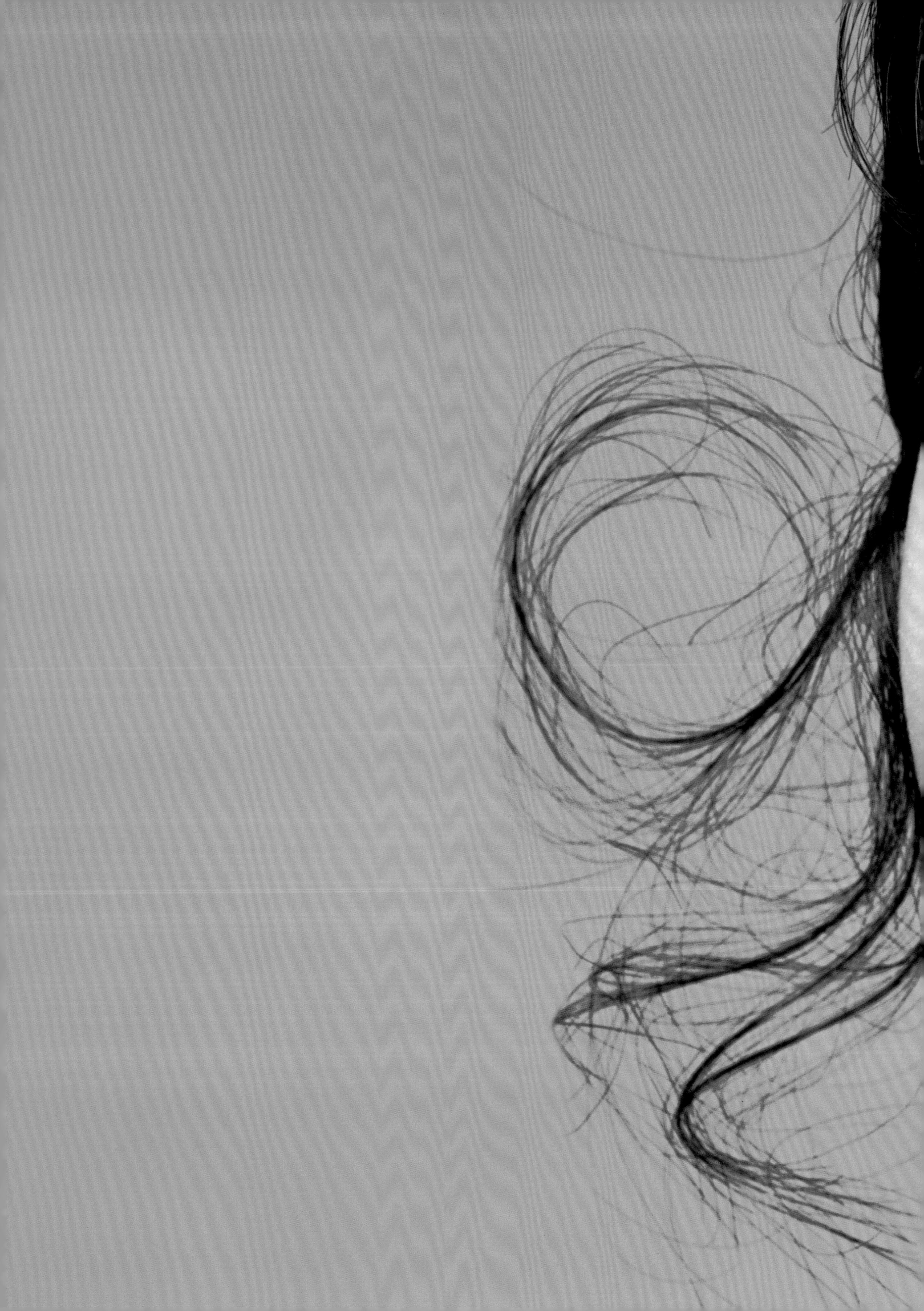

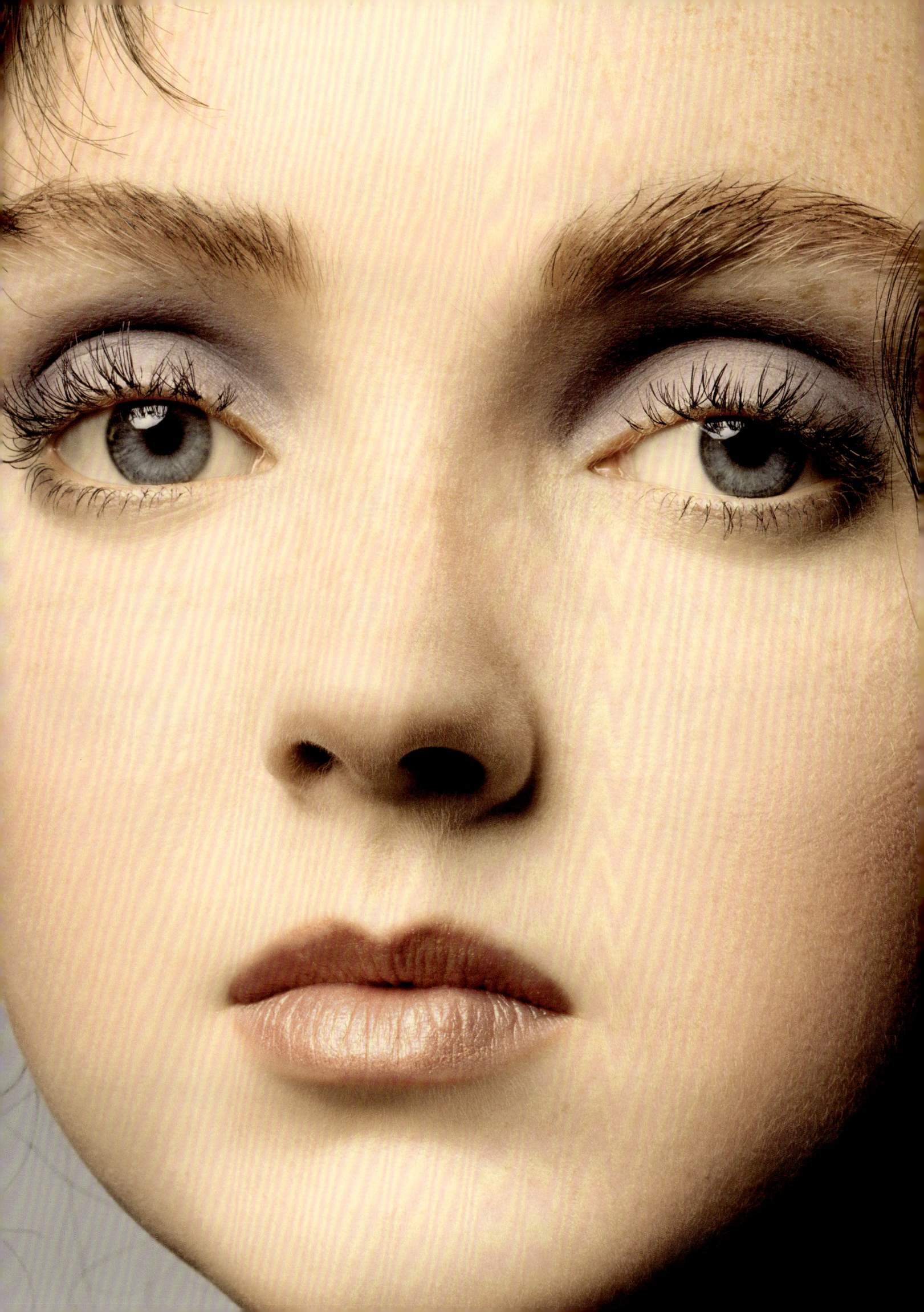

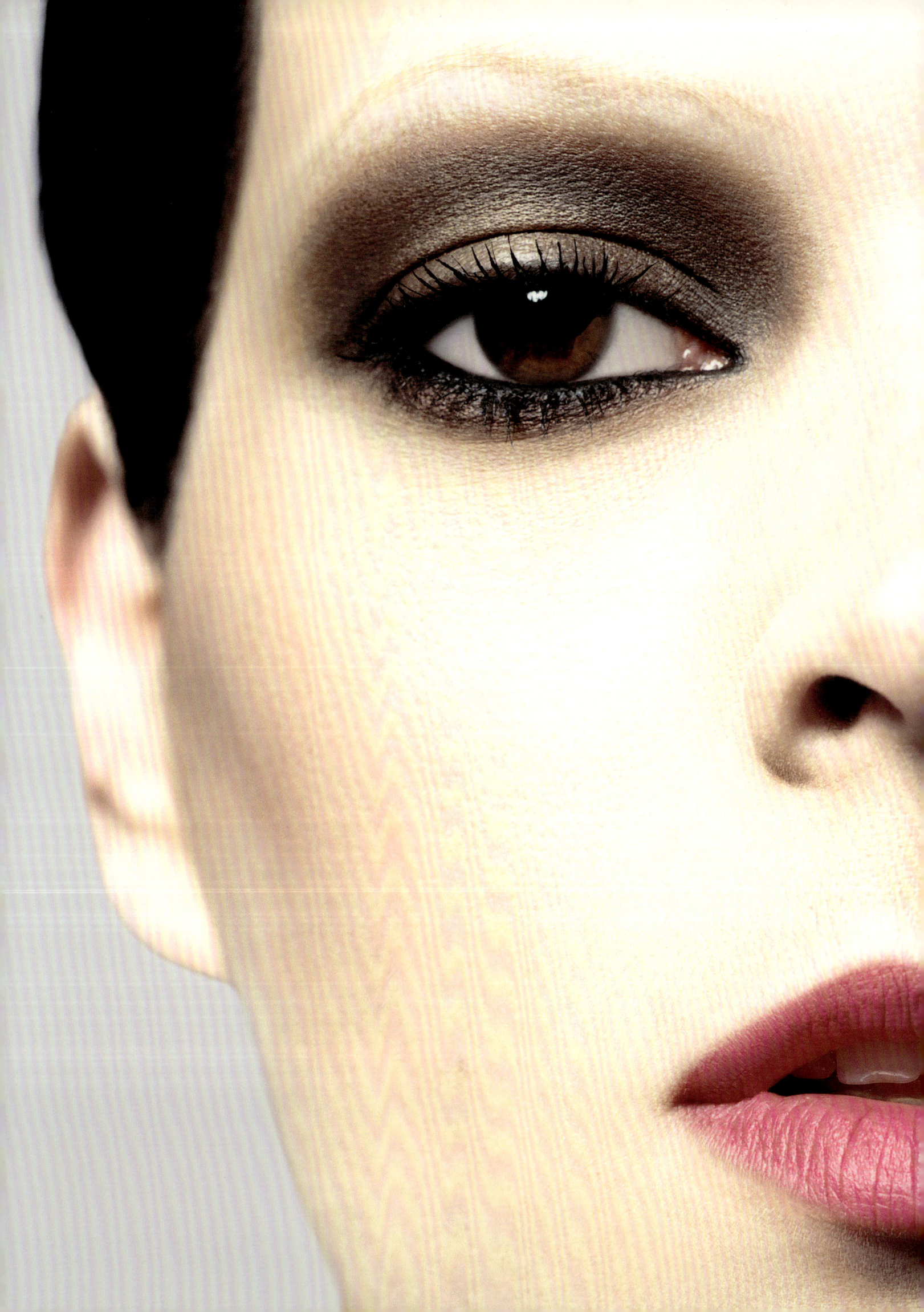

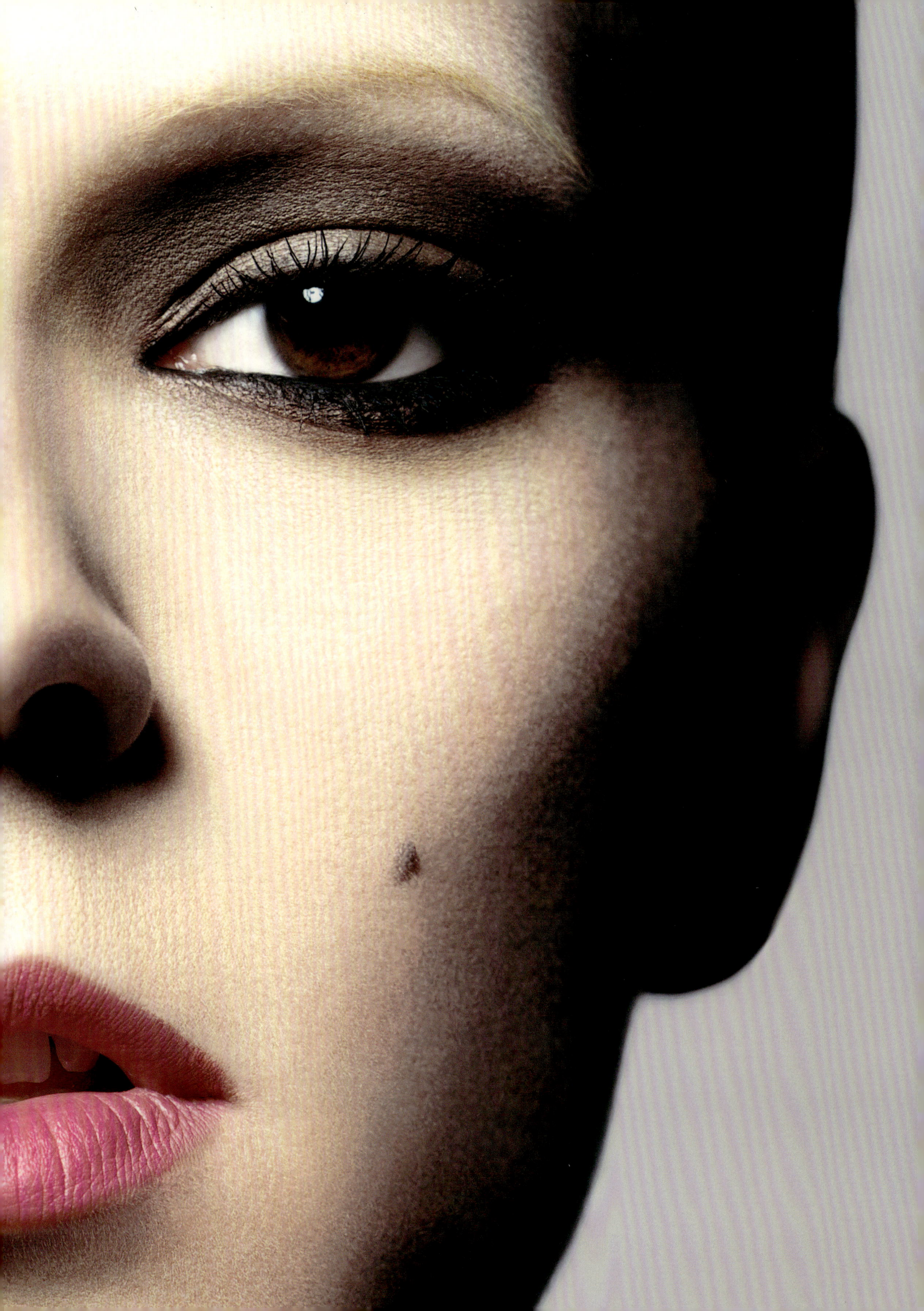

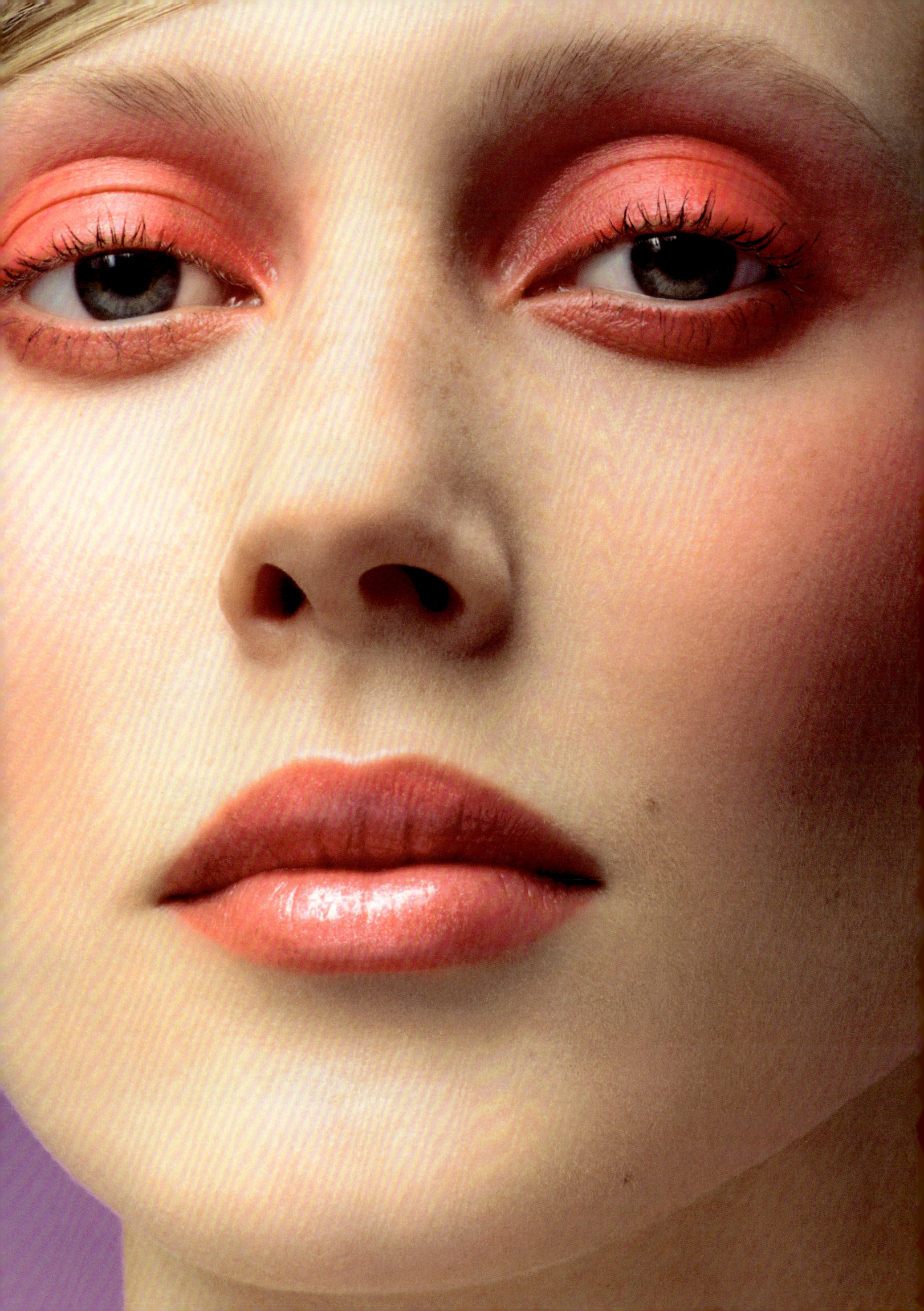

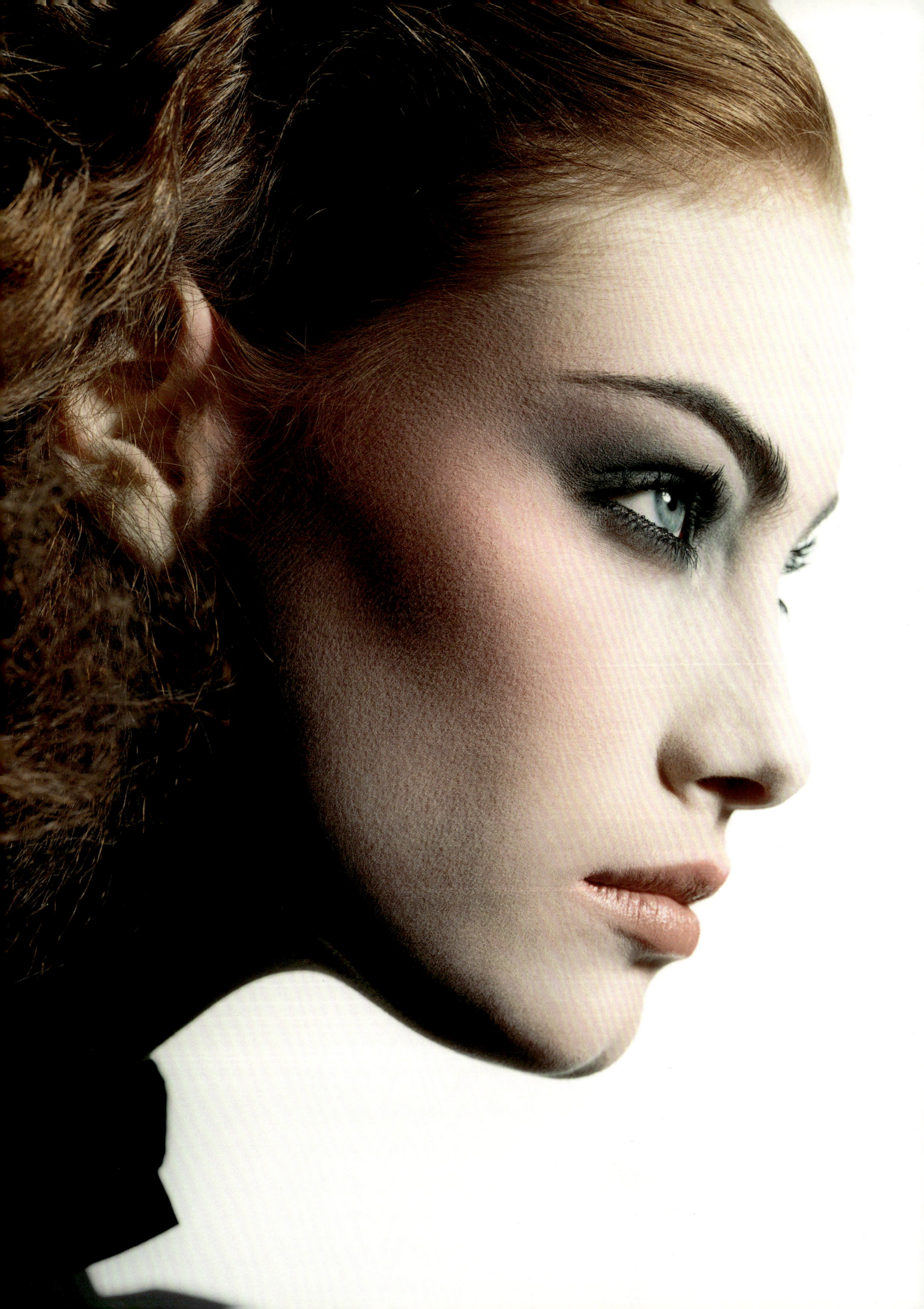

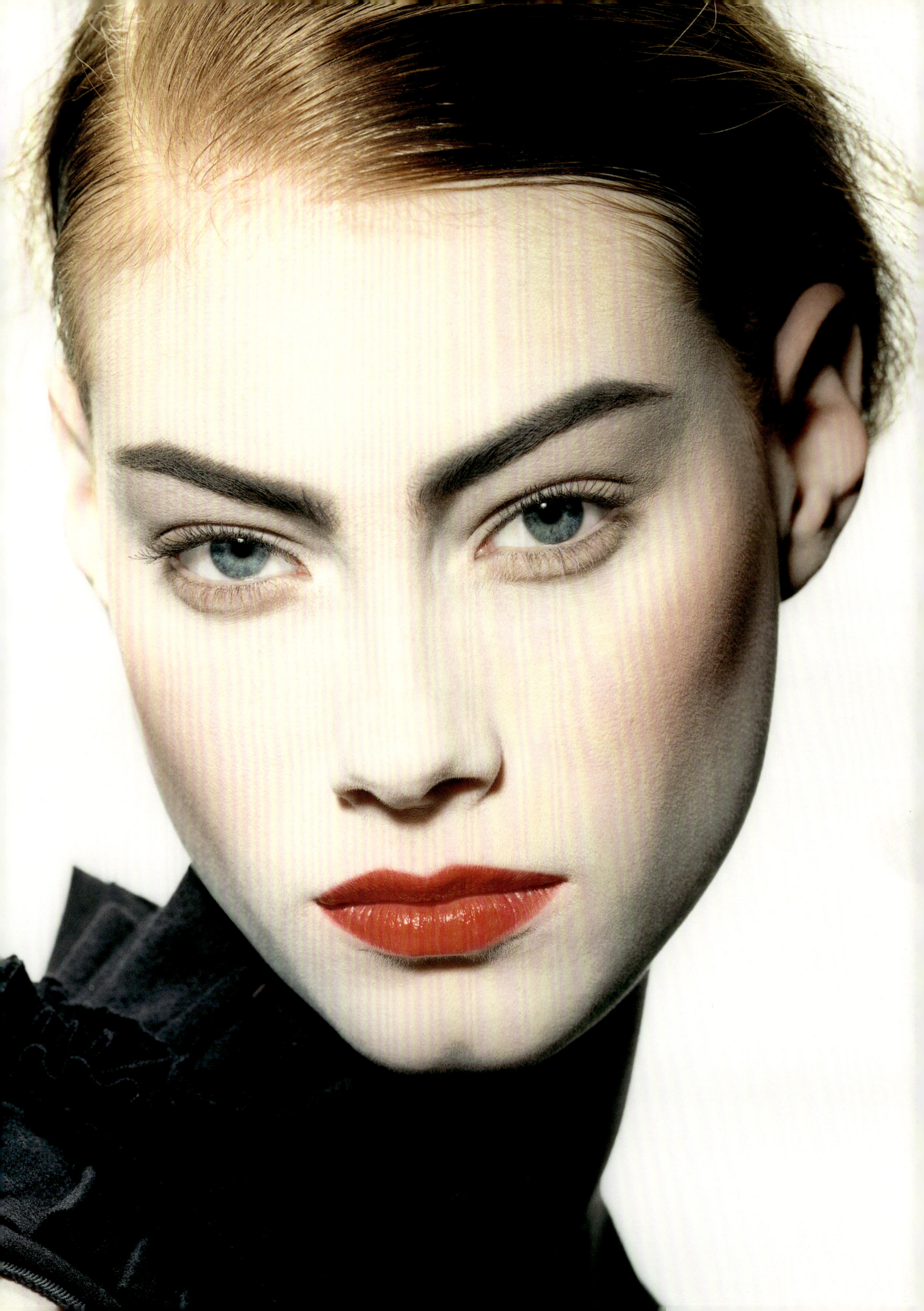

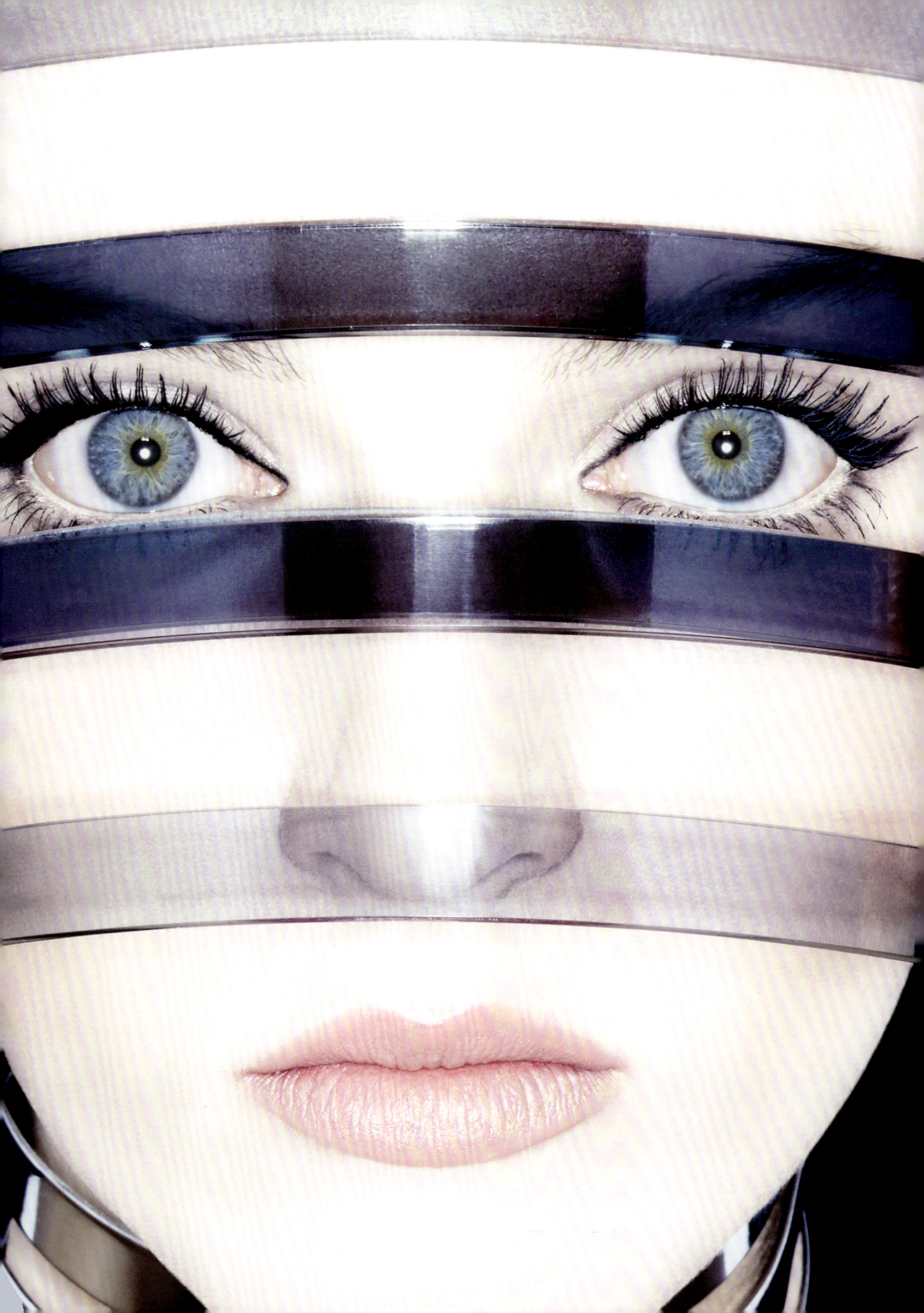

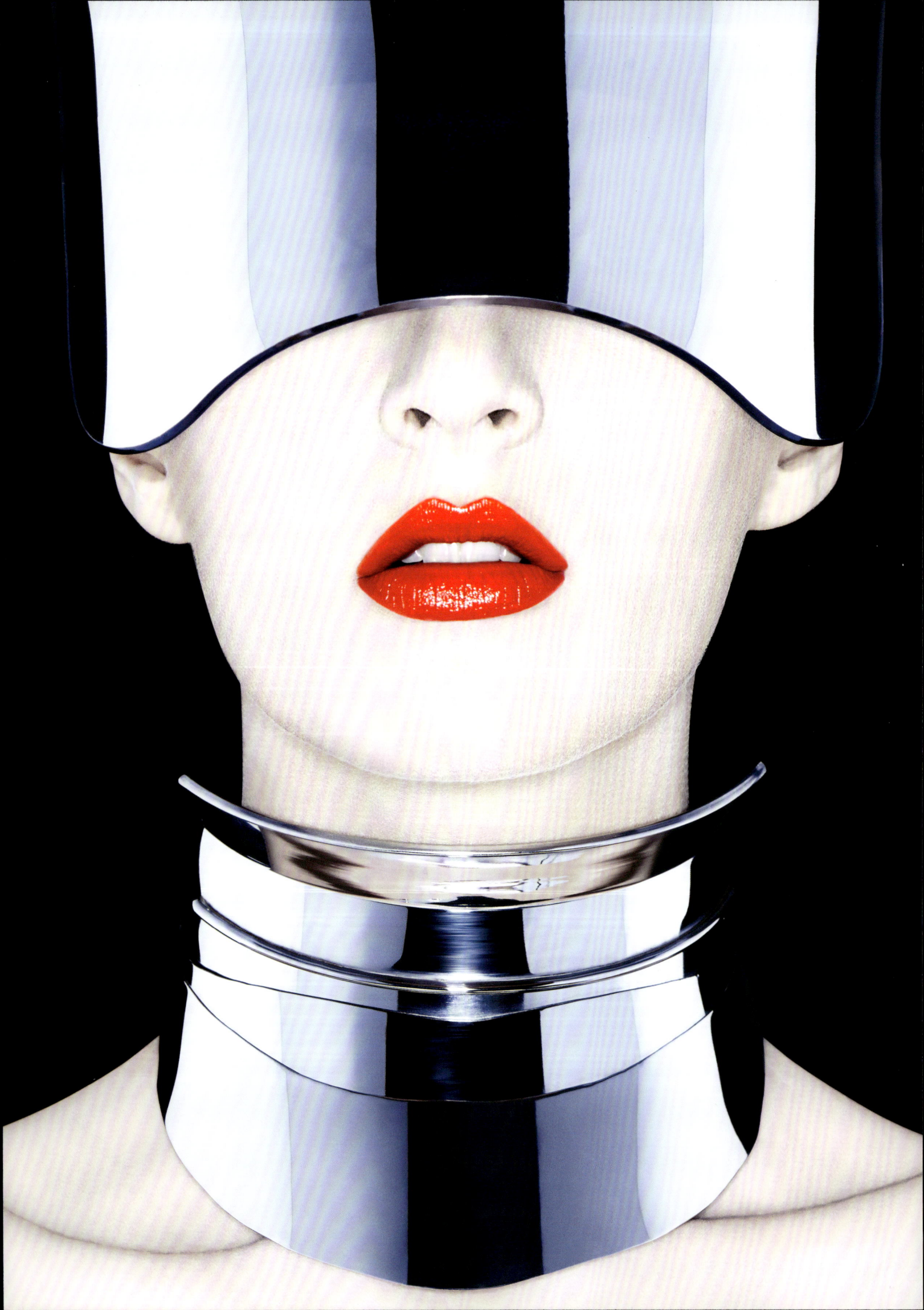

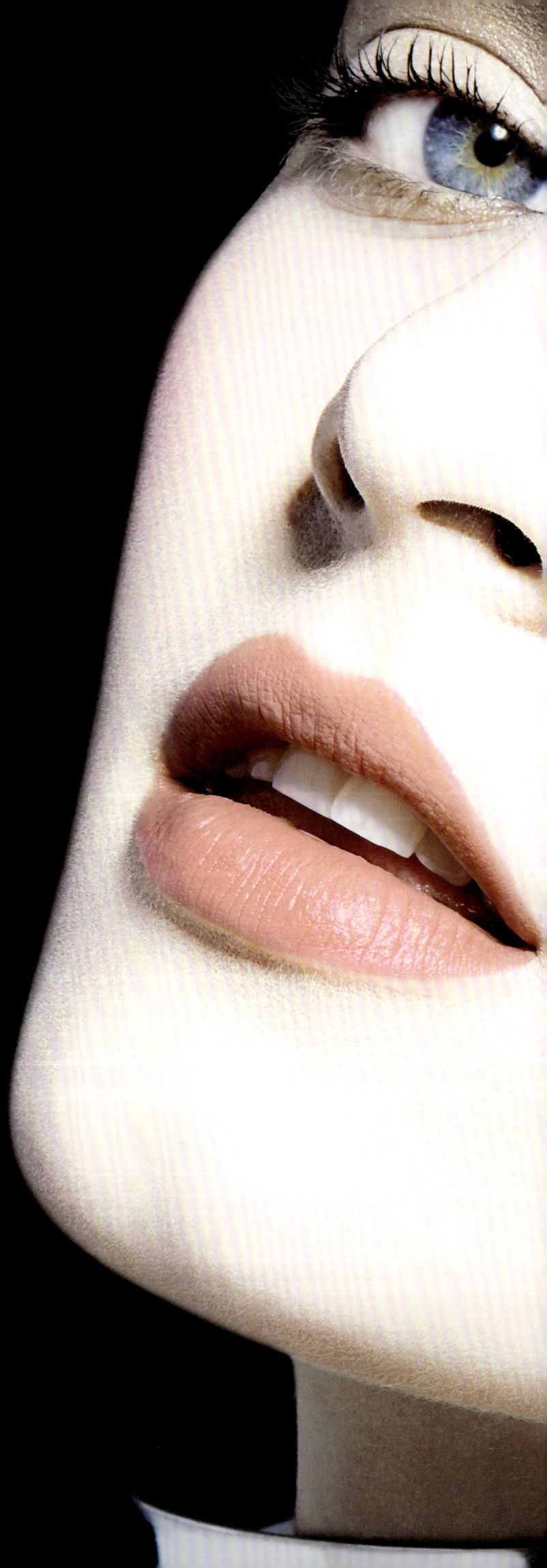

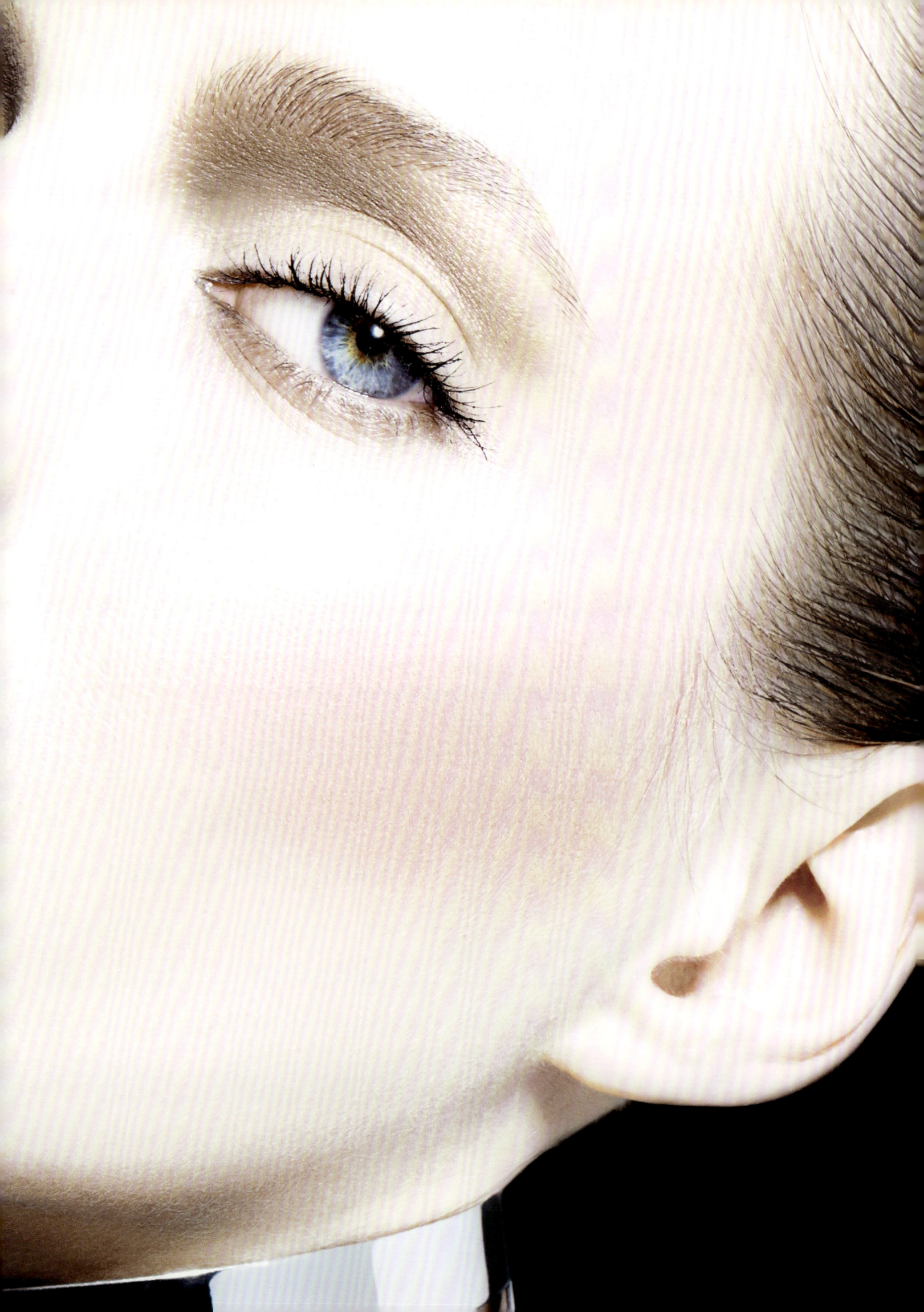

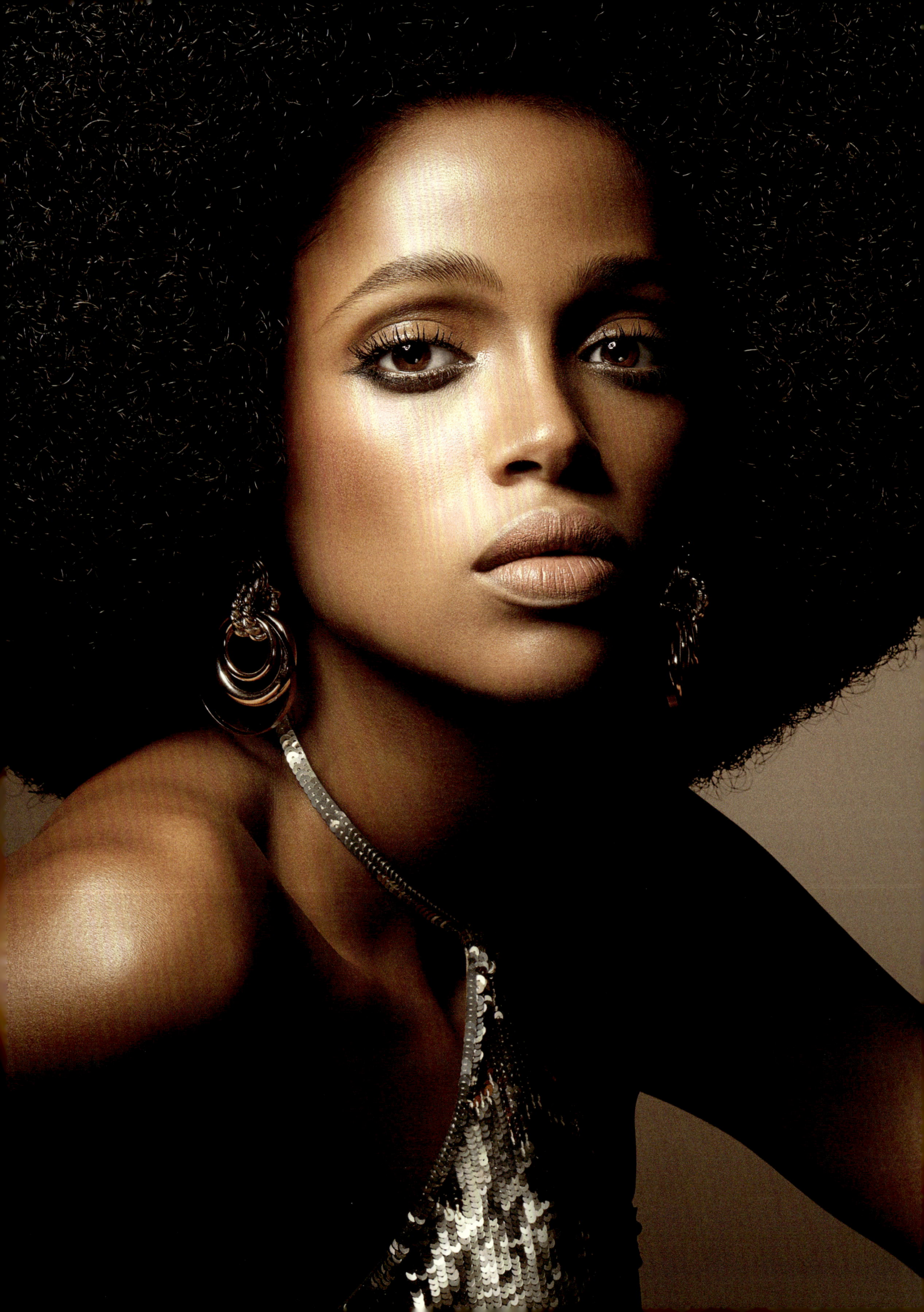

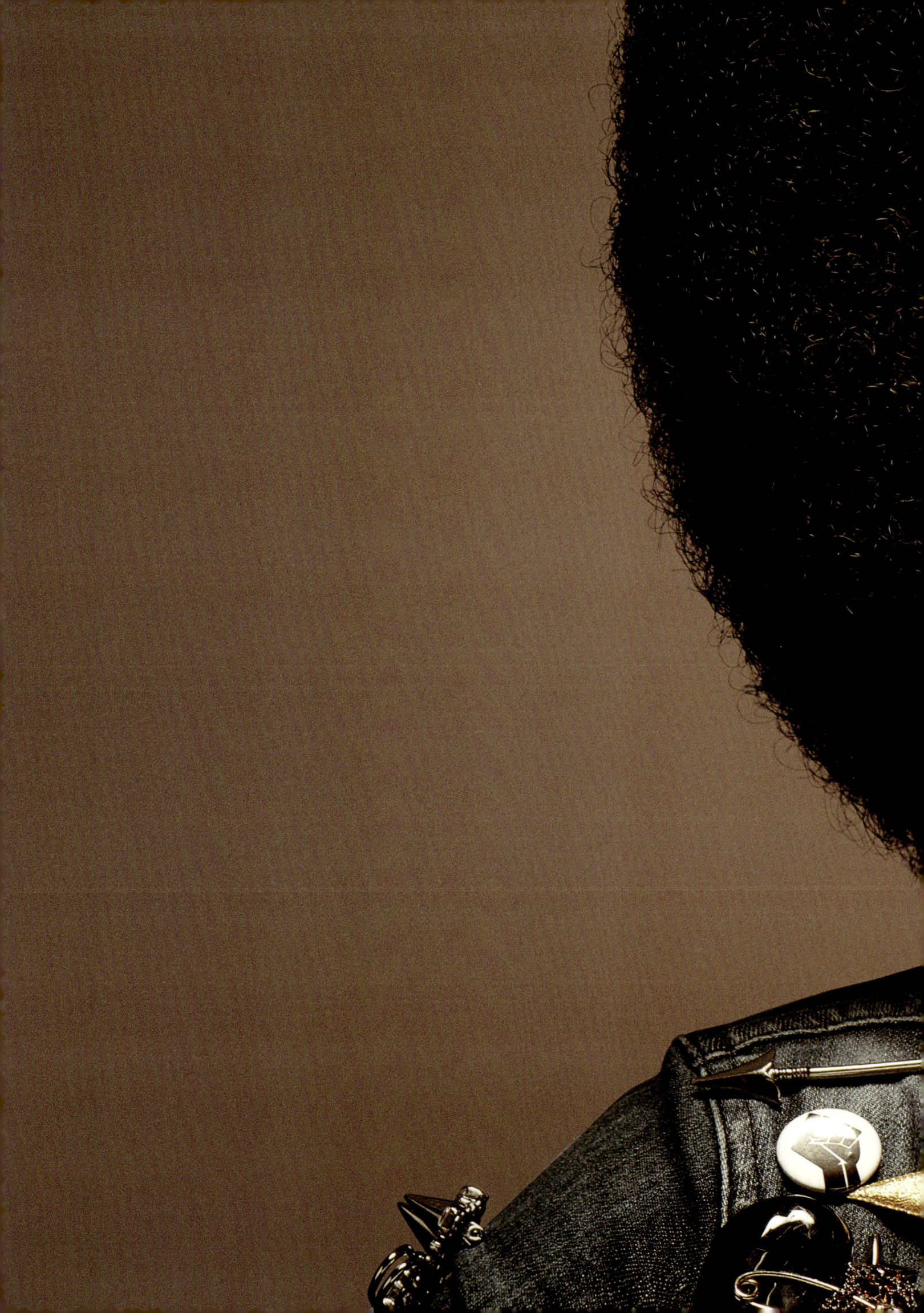

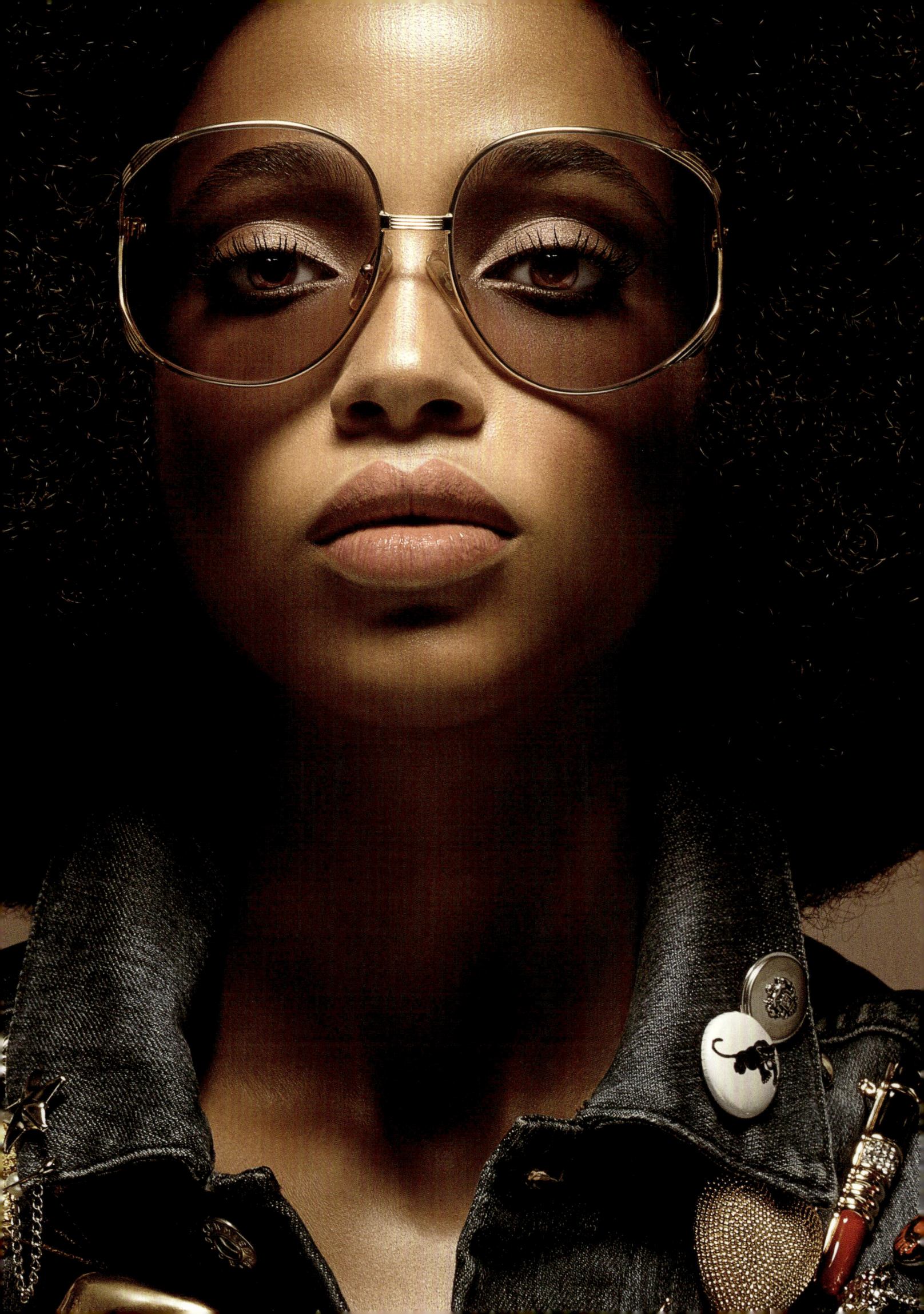

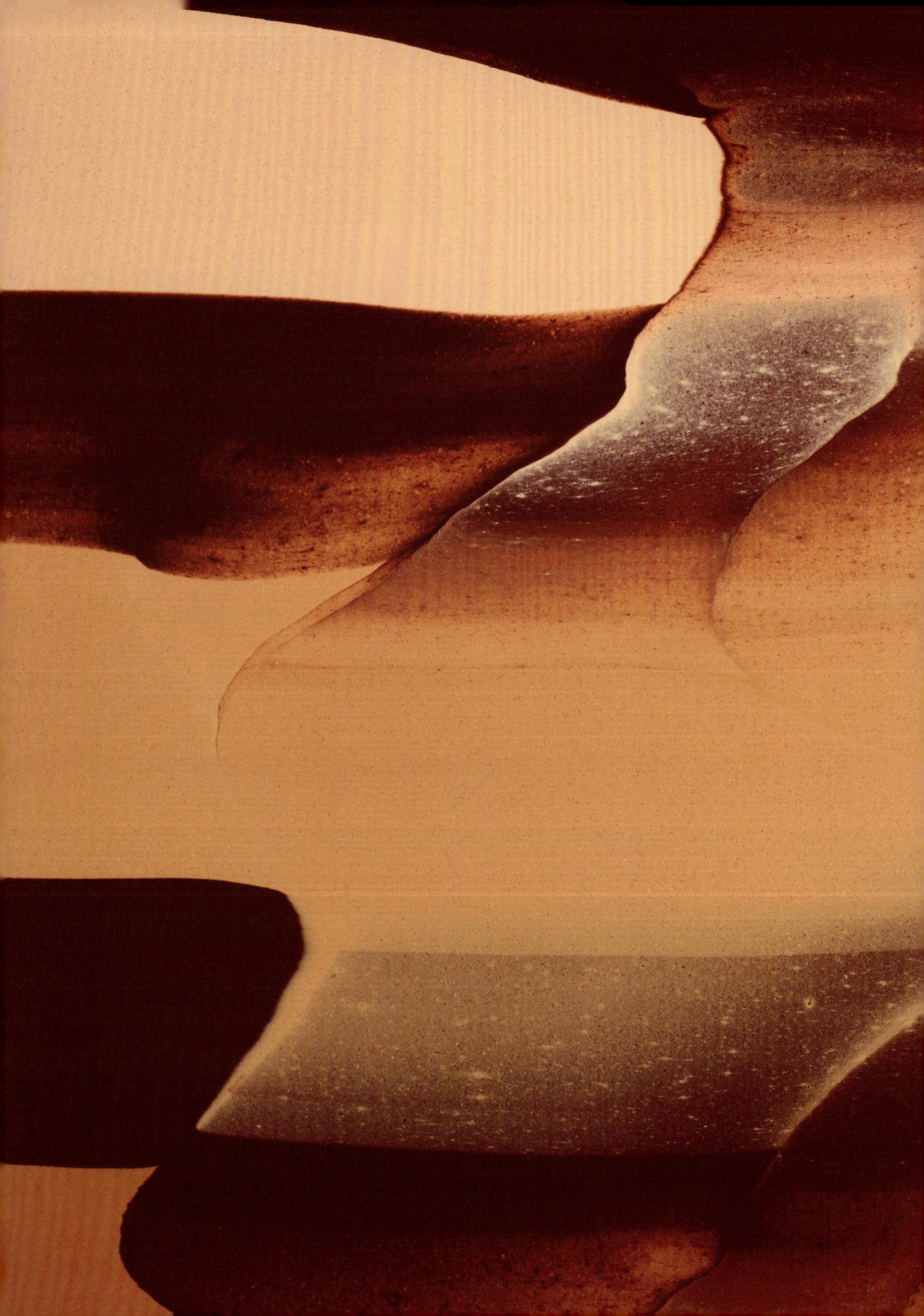

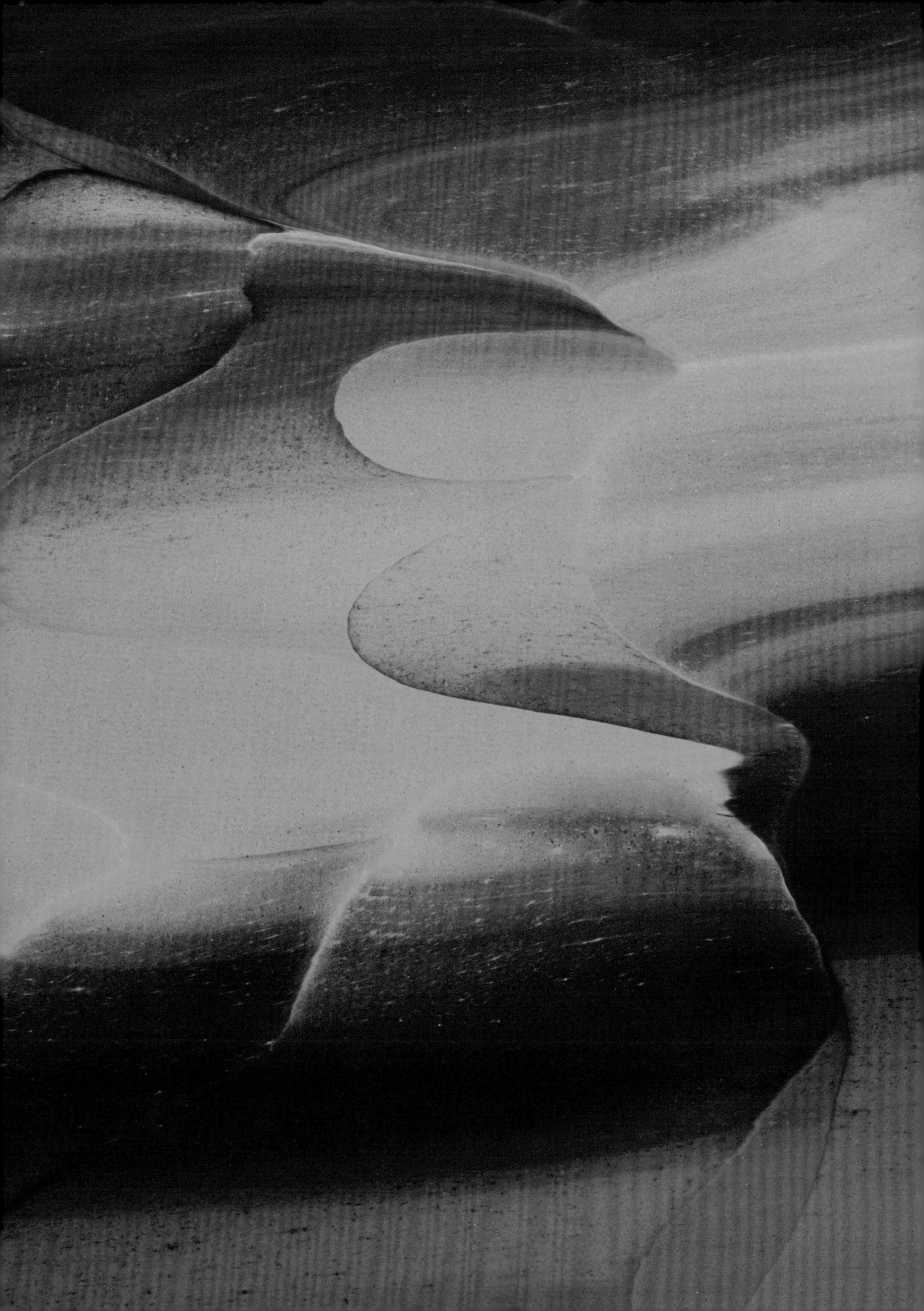

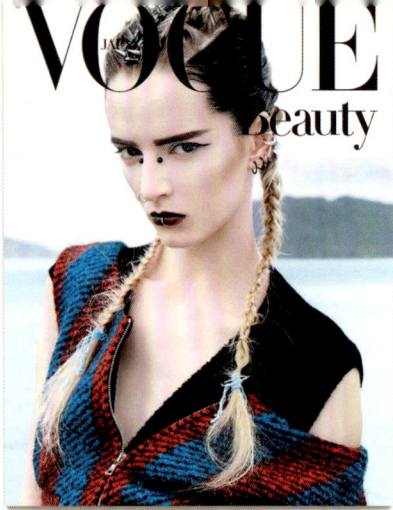

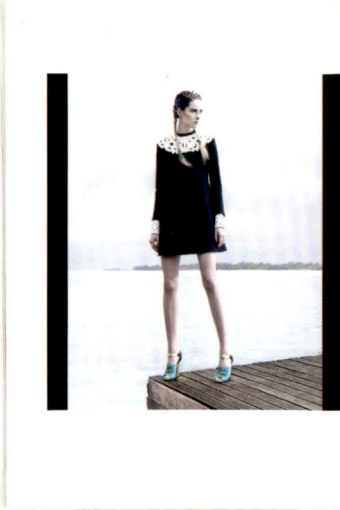

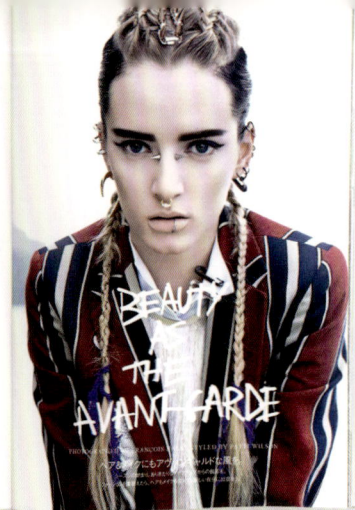

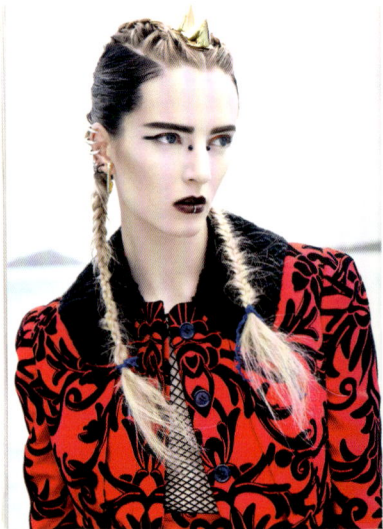

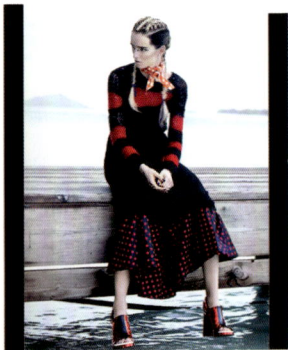

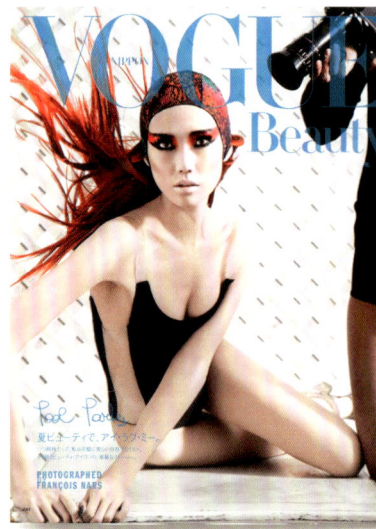

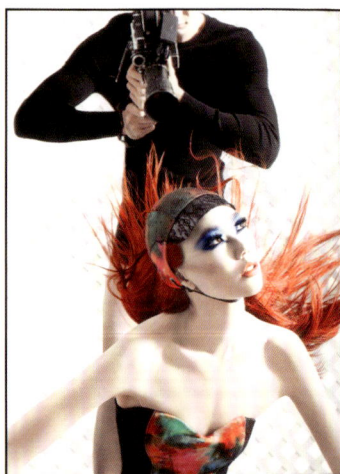

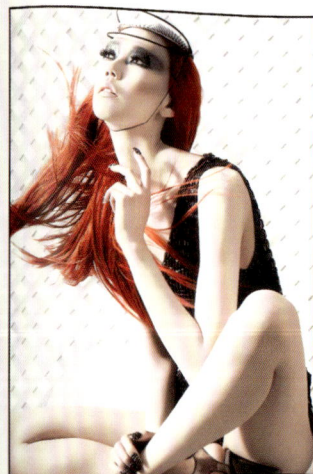

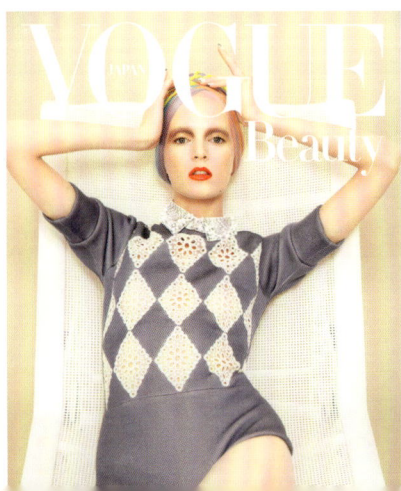

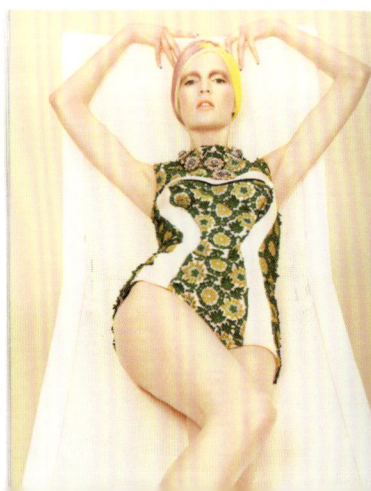

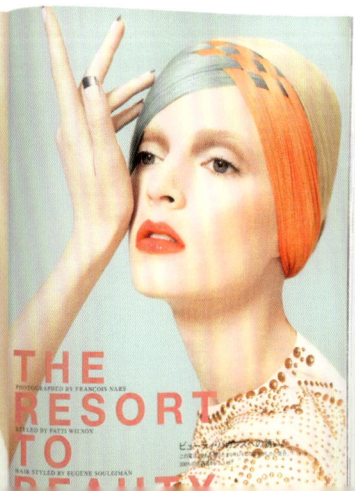

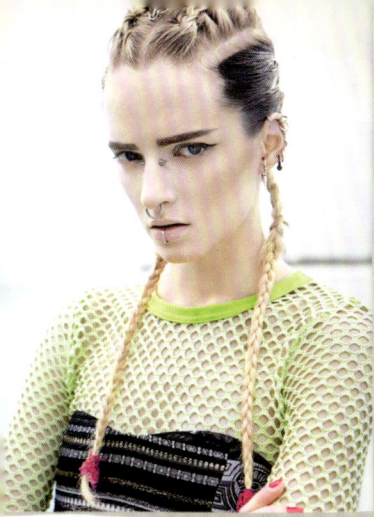

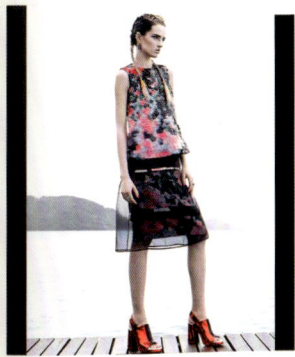

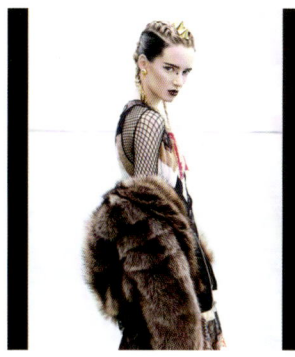

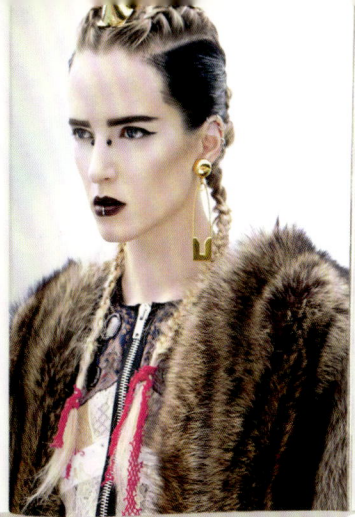

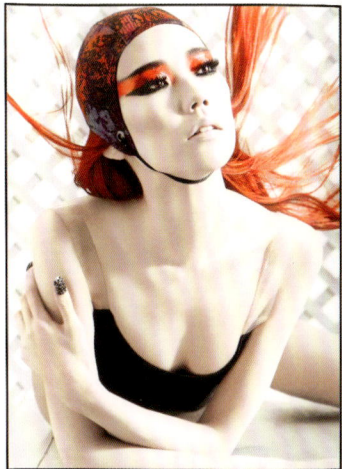

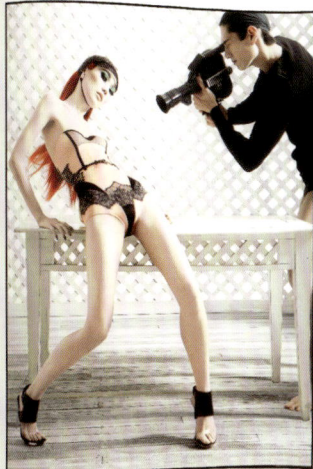

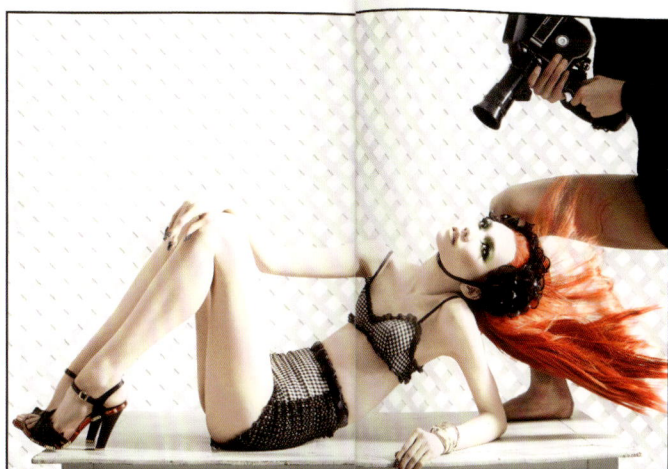

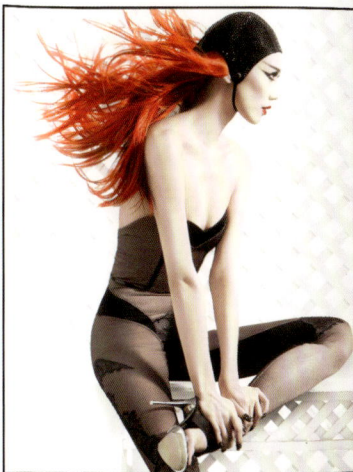

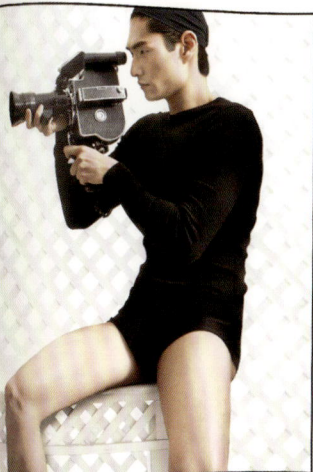

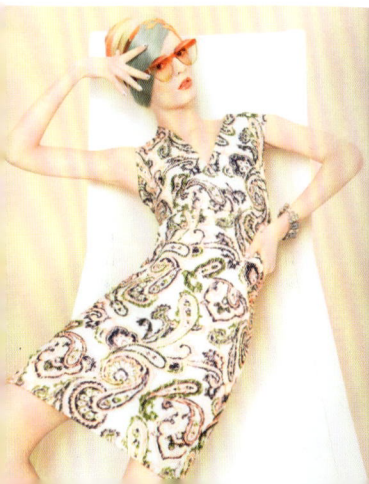

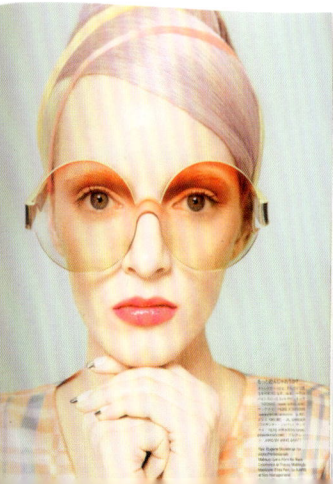

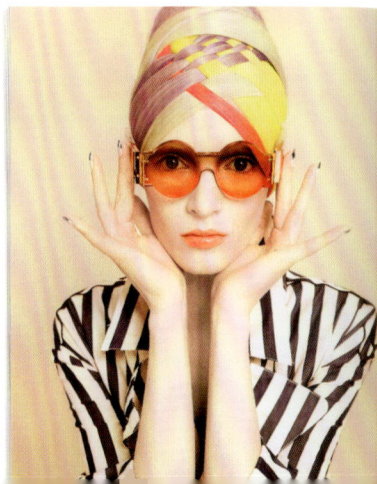

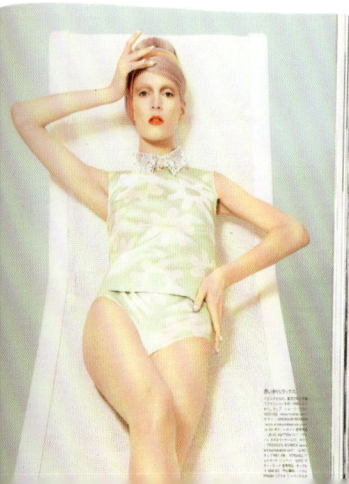

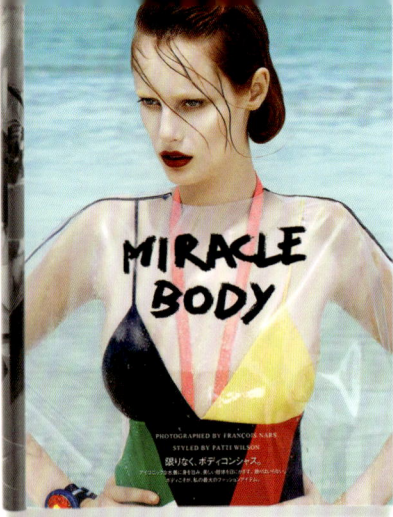

MIRACLE
BODY

PHOTOGRAPHED BY FRANCOIS NARS
STYLED BY PATTI WILSON

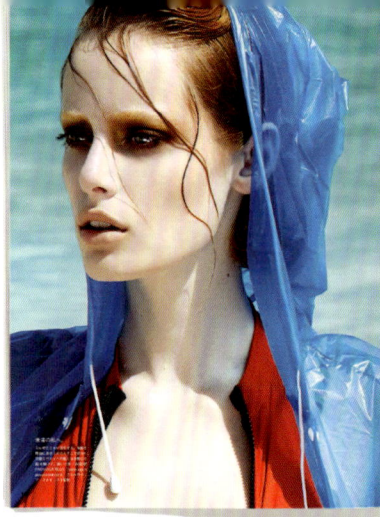

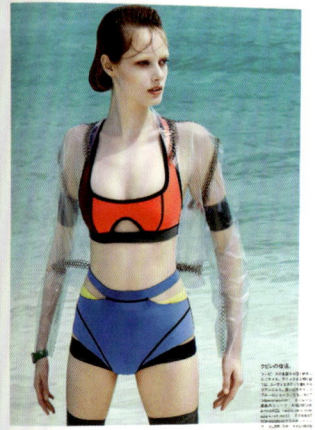

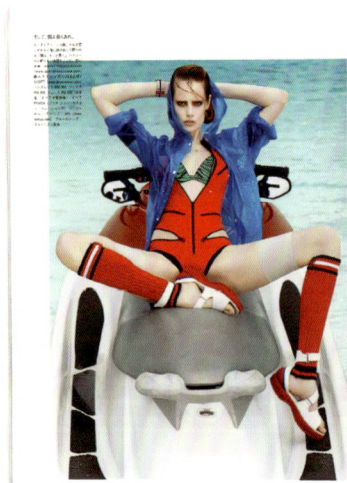

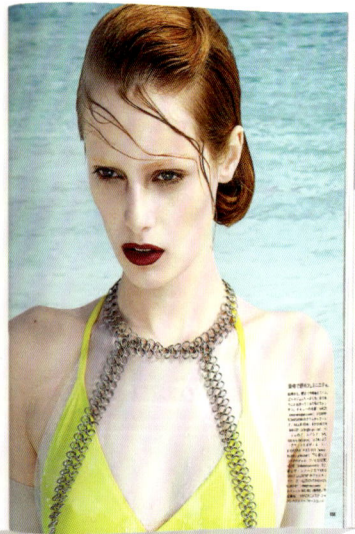

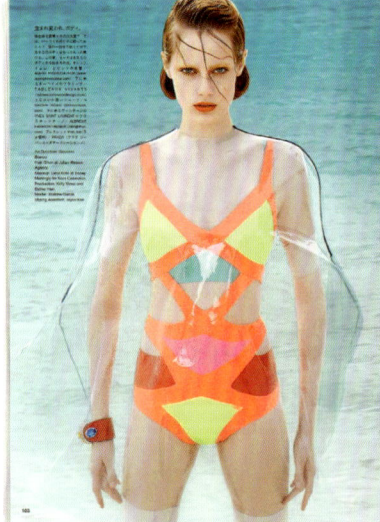

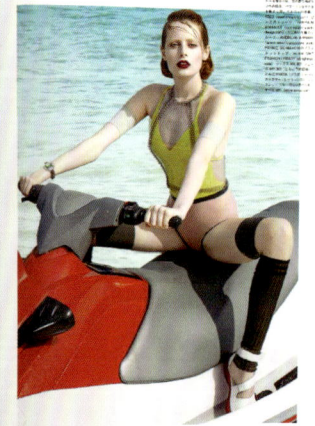

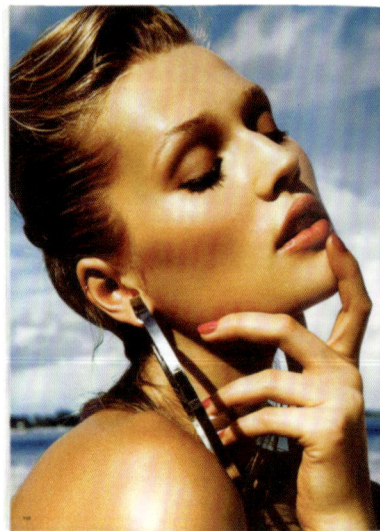

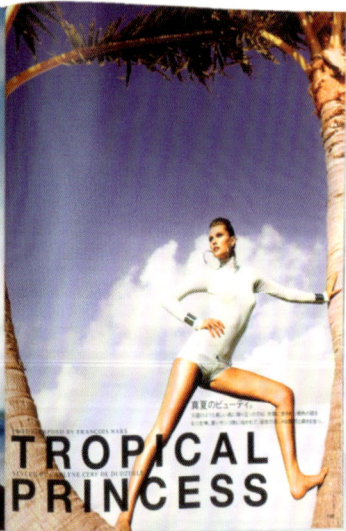

TROPICAL
PRINCESS

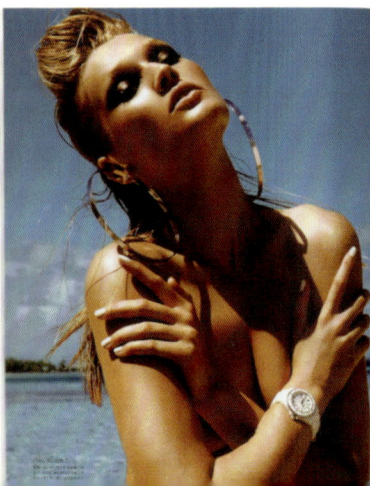

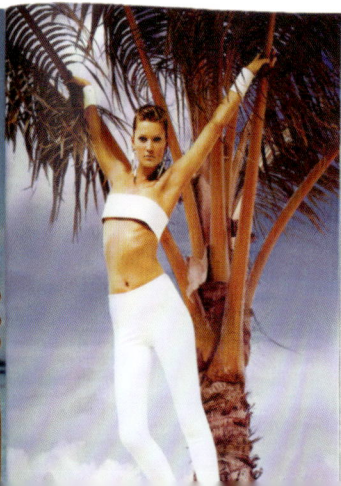

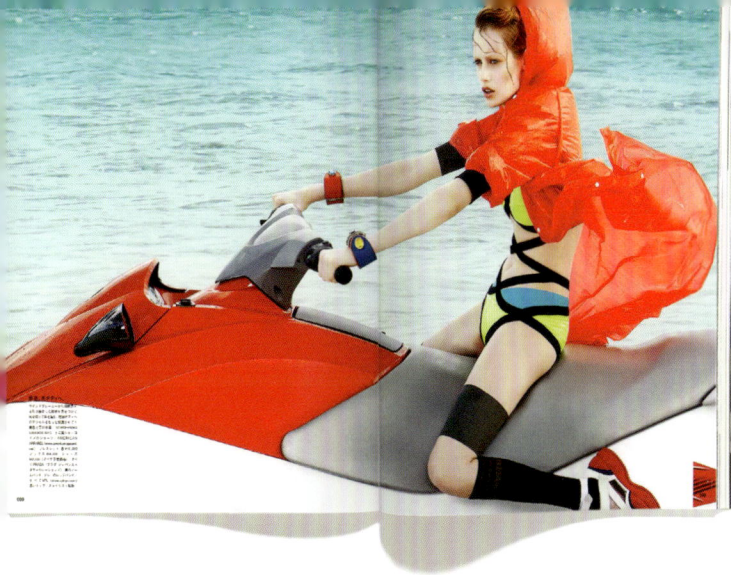

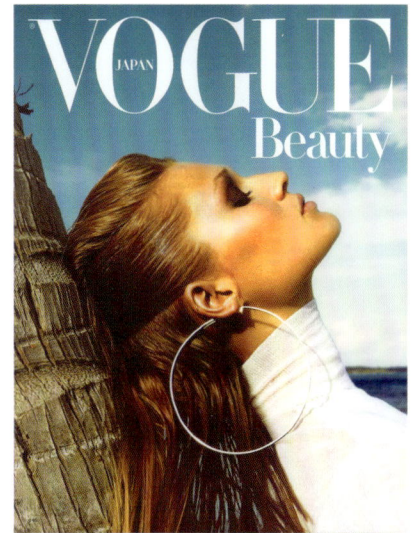

VOGUE JAPAN Beauty

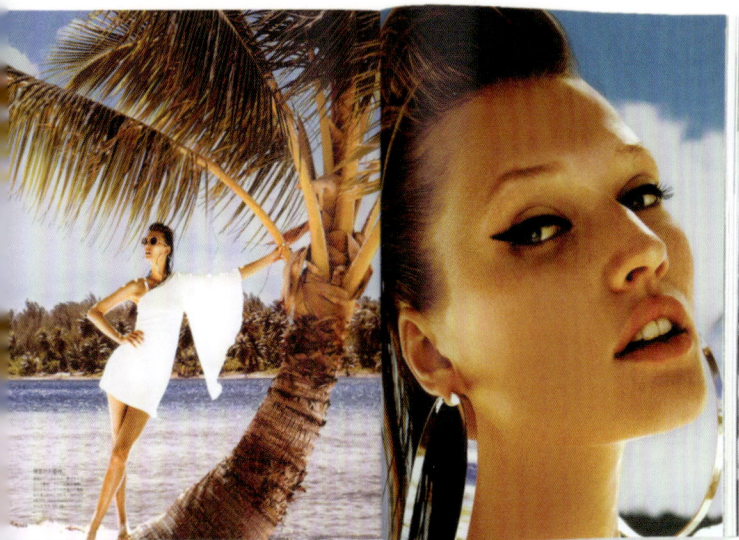

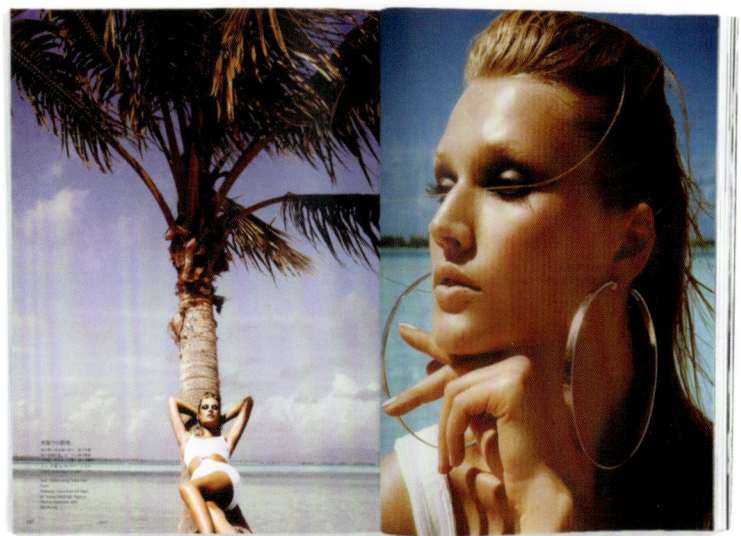

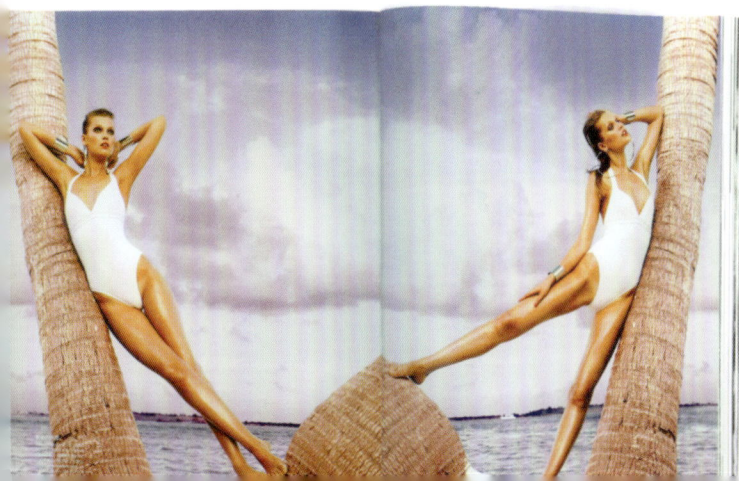

Chloë
Moretz

PHOTO BY
Francois Nars

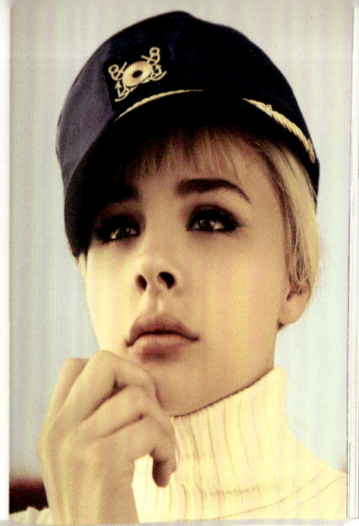

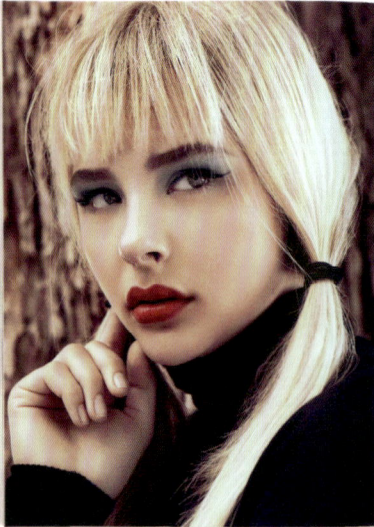

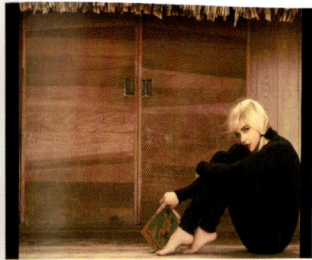

"Red lipstick is to beauty
what the LBD is to fashion.
The difference is that when you
walk into a room wearing a
red lip, people notice you."
—FRANÇOIS NARS

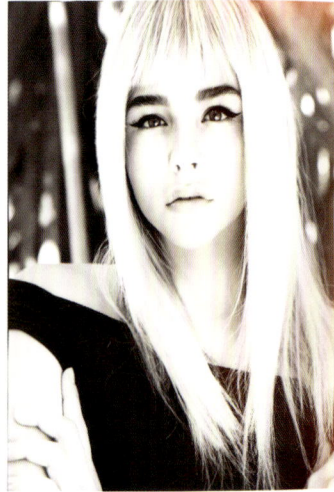

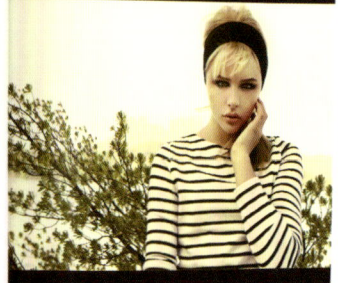

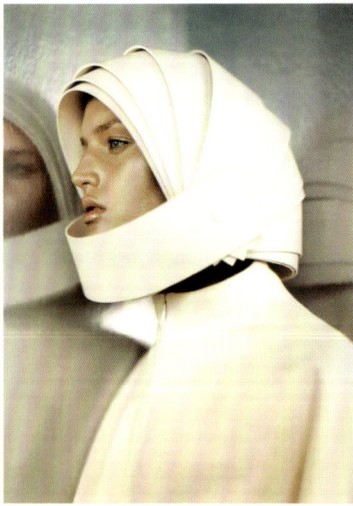

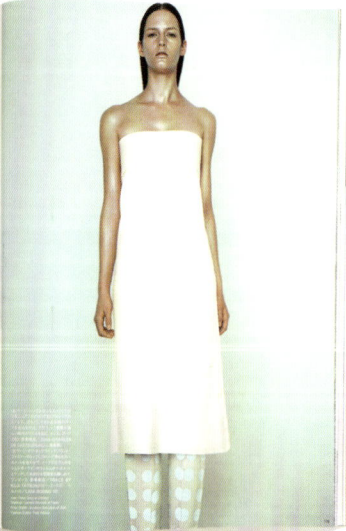

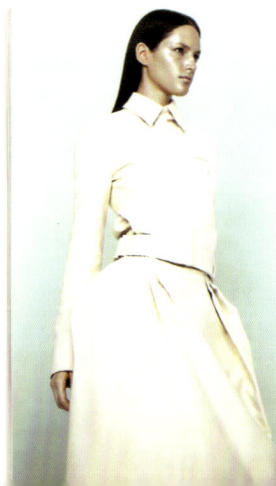

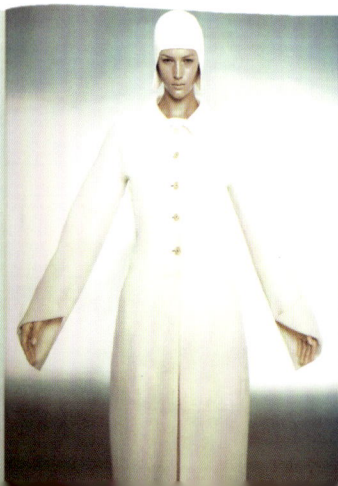

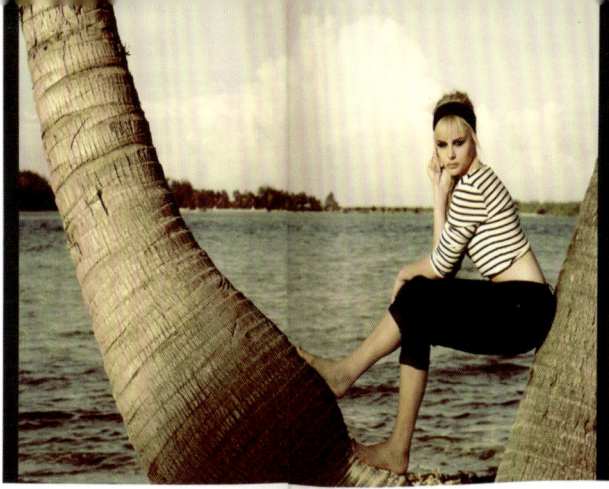

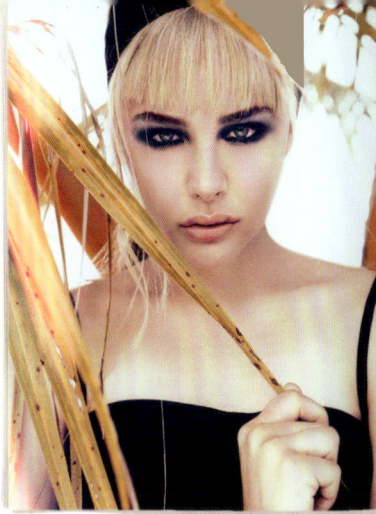

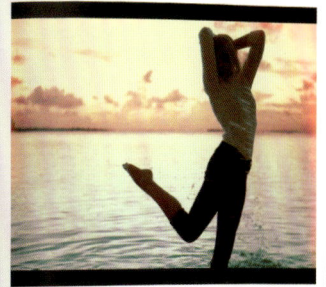

"I've always loved the look of a *smoky eye*—it's fierce! But this one that Mr. Nars gave me couldn't be more perfect. It was like watching an artist paint a beautiful picture."
—CHLOÉ GRACE MORETZ

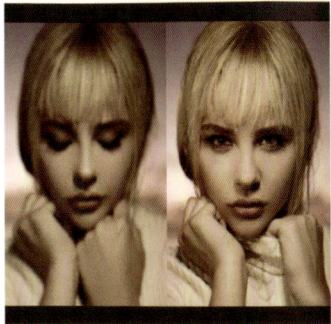

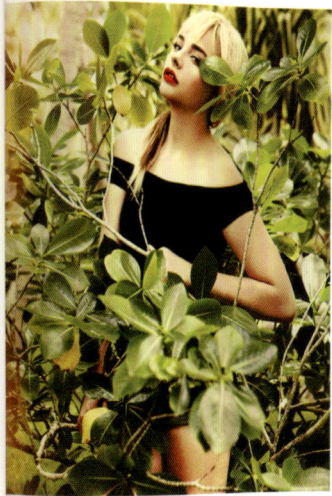

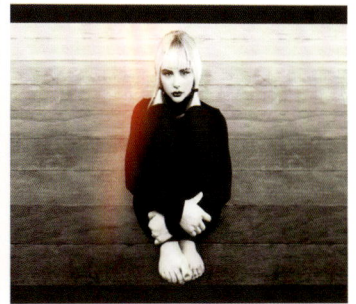

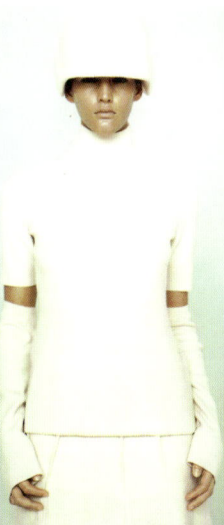

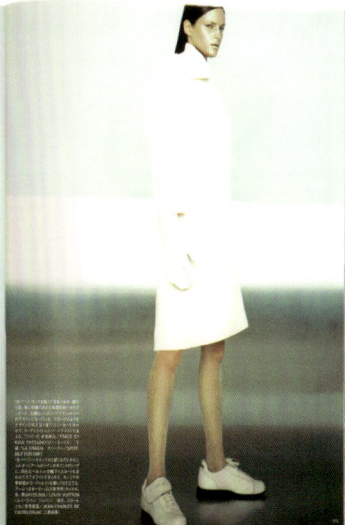

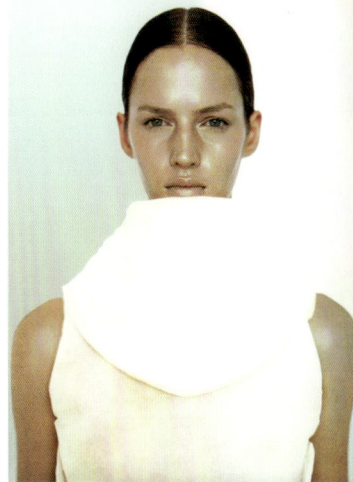

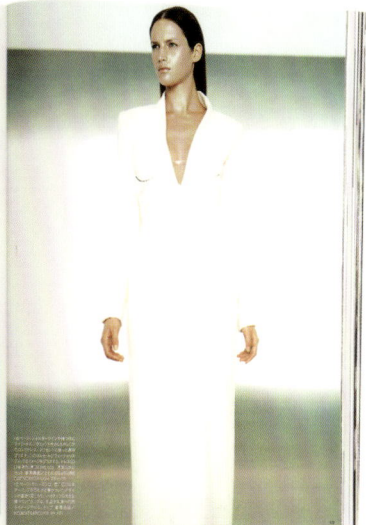

shades of white
未来を予感させる「白」

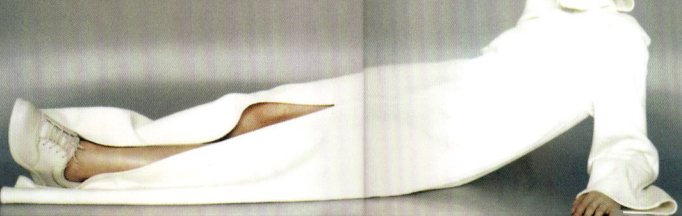

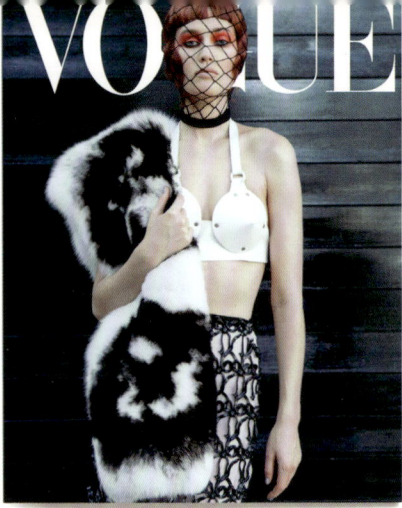

VOGUE

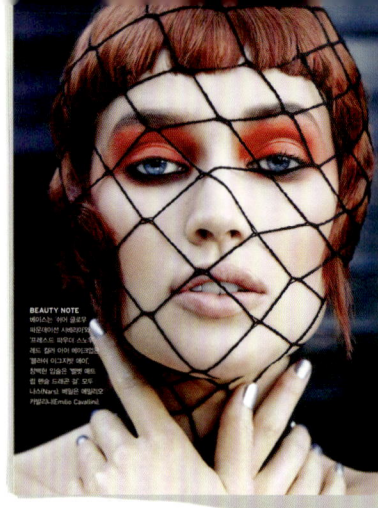

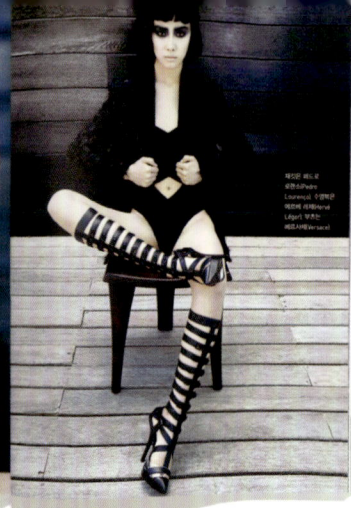

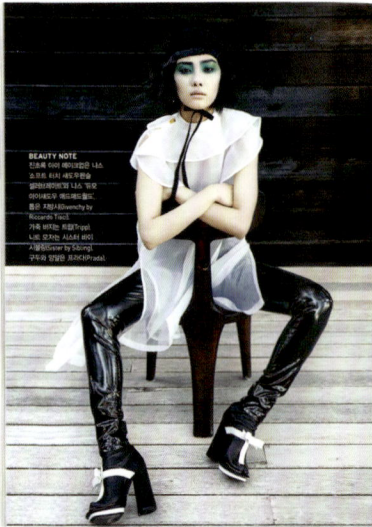

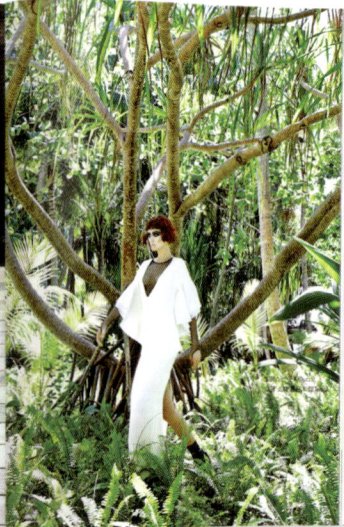

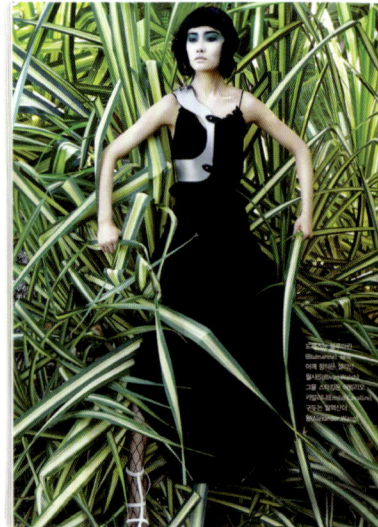

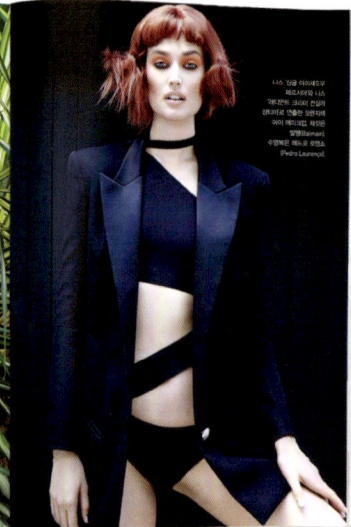

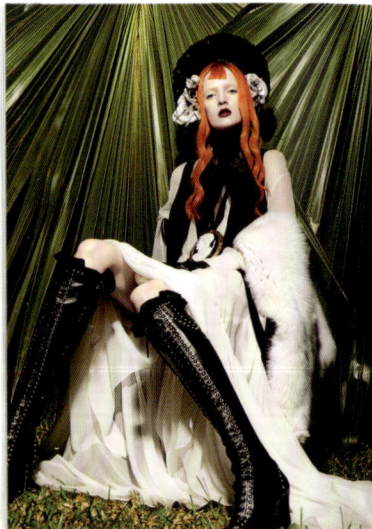

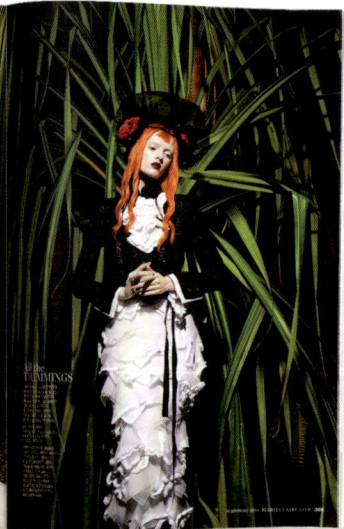

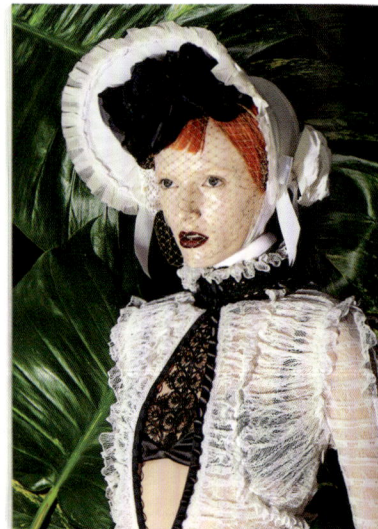

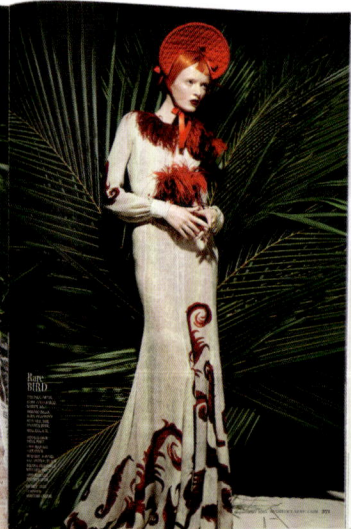

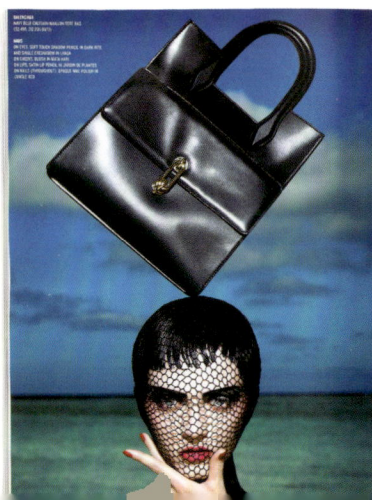

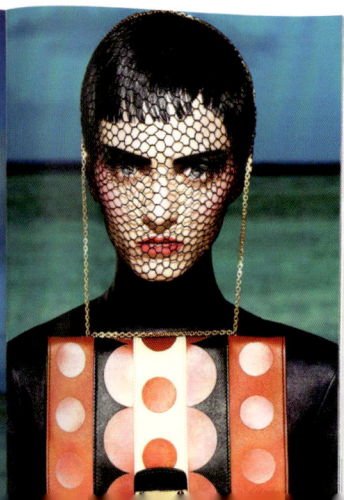

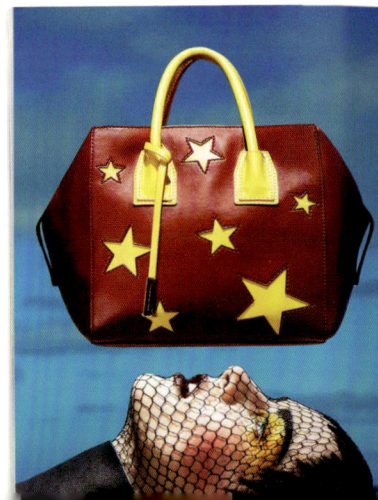

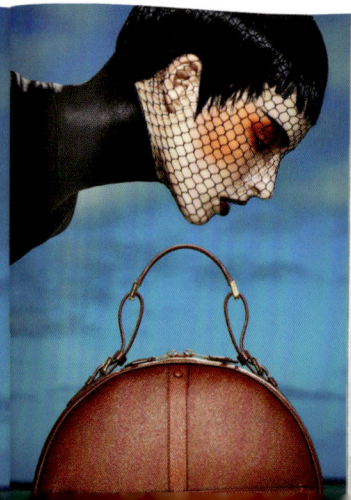

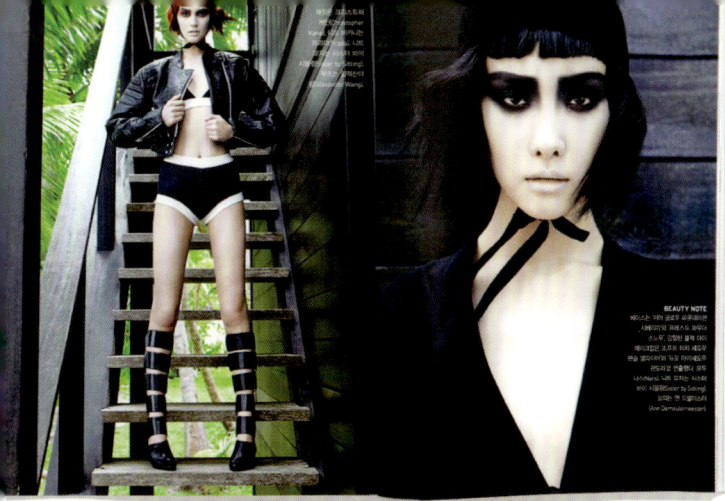

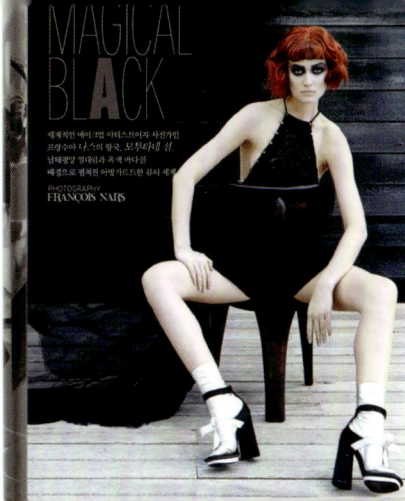

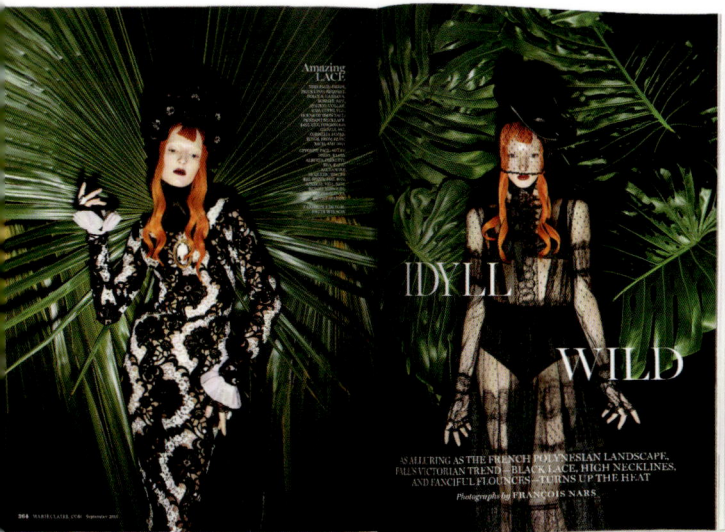

Amazing LACE

IDYLL

WILD

AS ALLURING AS THE FRENCH POLYNESIAN LANDSCAPE,
FALL'S VICTORIAN TREND—BLACK LACE, HIGH NECKLINES,
AND FANCIFUL FLOUNCES—TURNS UP THE HEAT
Photographs by FRANÇOIS NARS

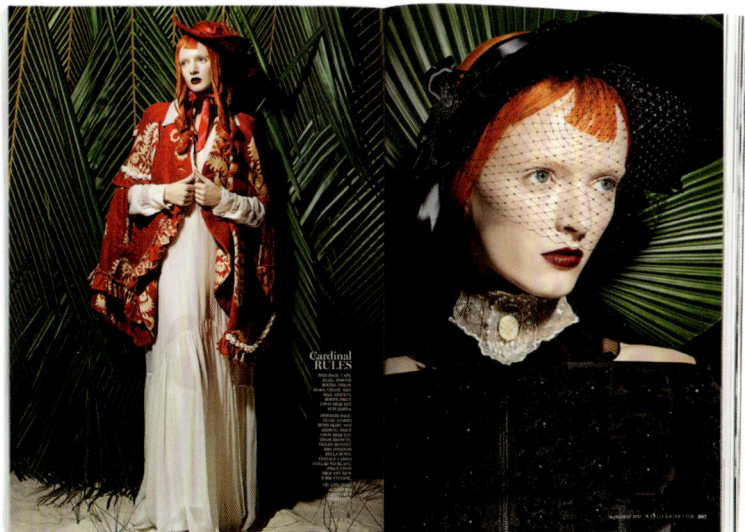

Cardinal RULES

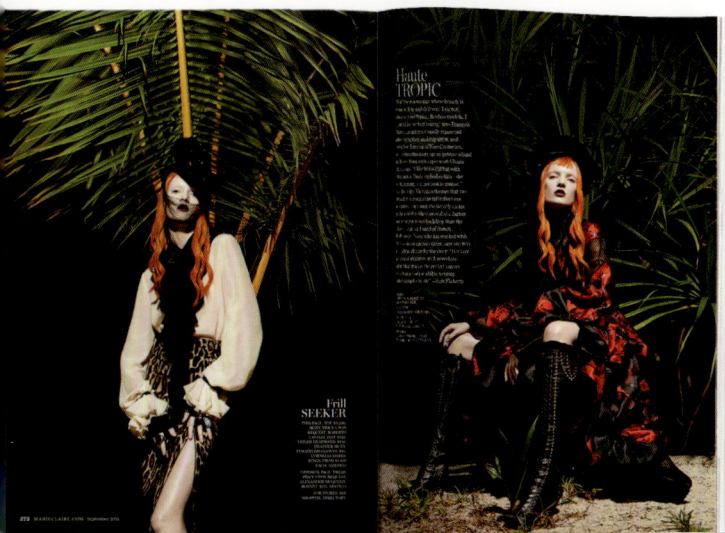

Haute TROPIC

Frill SEEKER

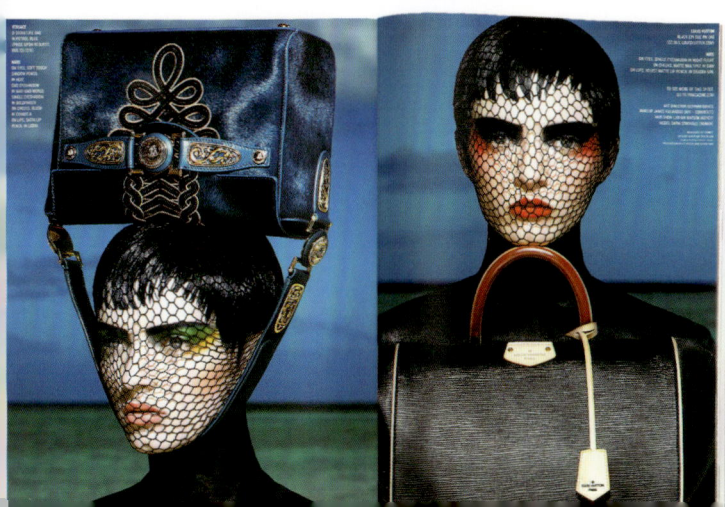

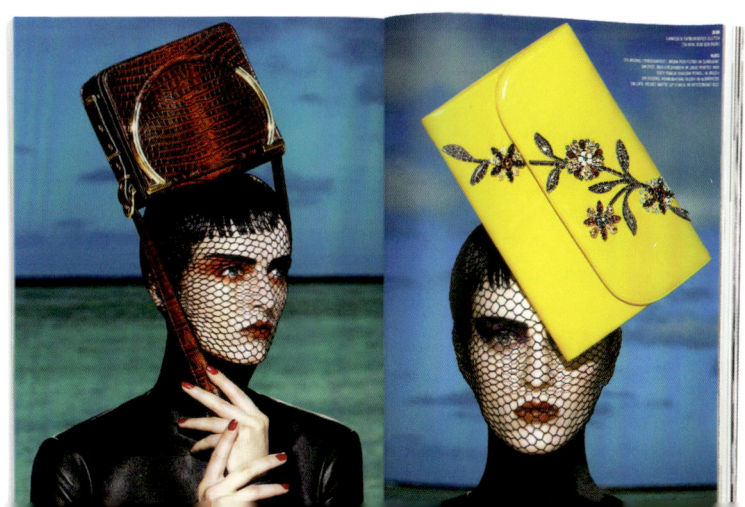

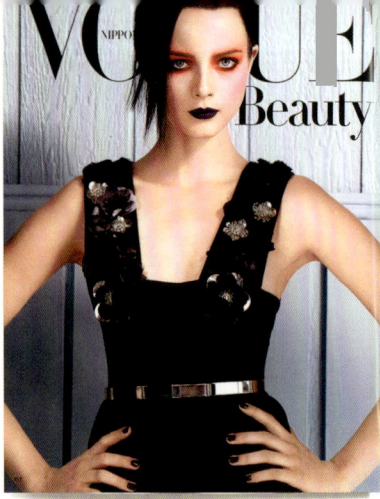

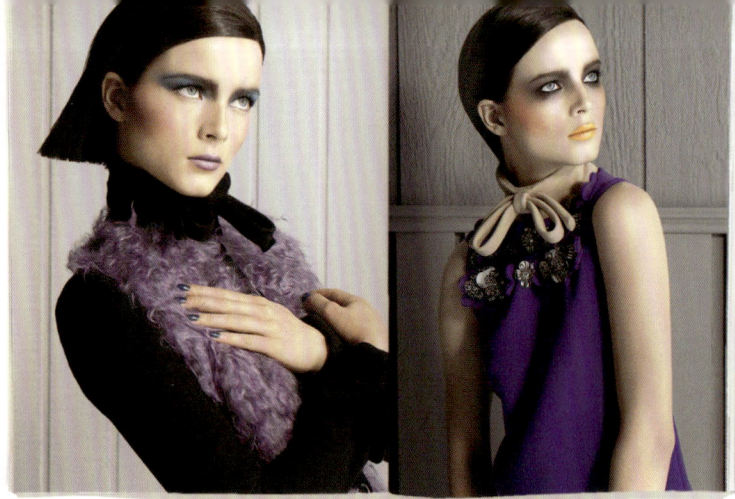

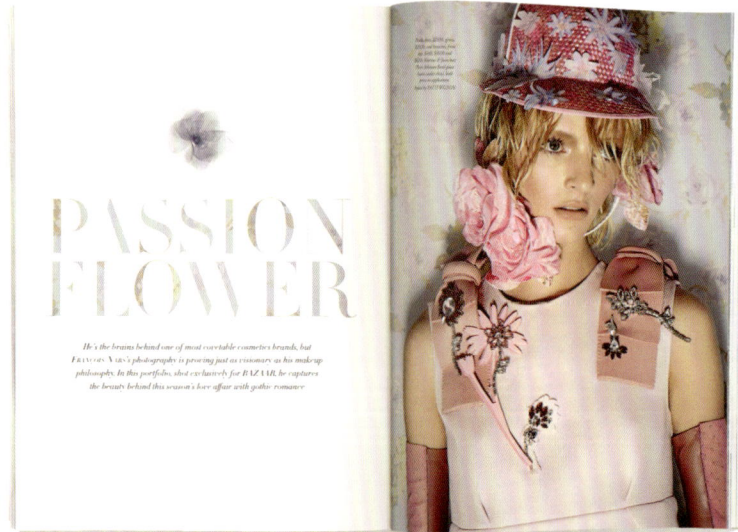

PASSION FLOWER

He's the brains behind one of most covetable cosmetics brands, but François Nars's photography is proving just as covetous as his makeup philosophy. In this portfolio, shot exclusively for BAZAAR, he captures the beauty behind this season's love affair with gothic romance

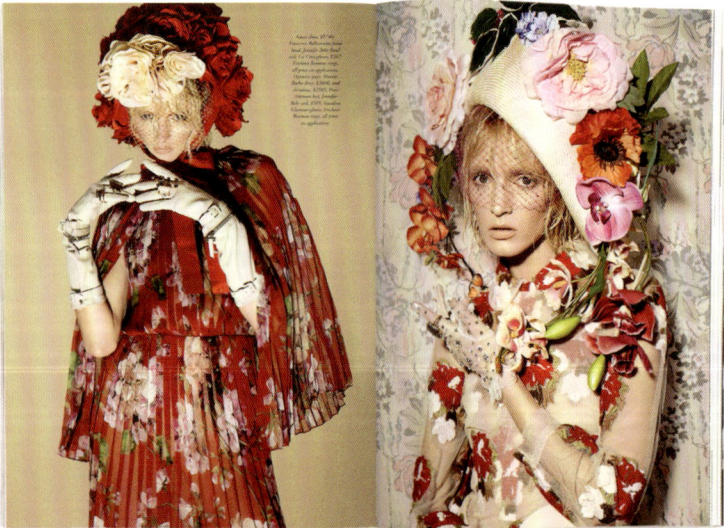

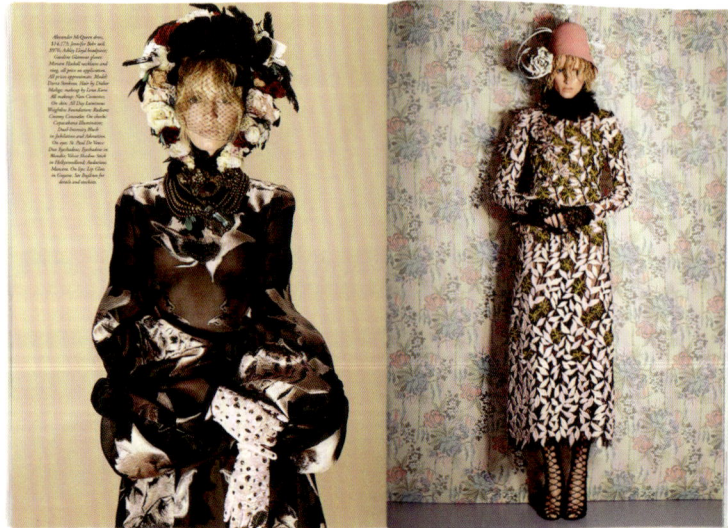

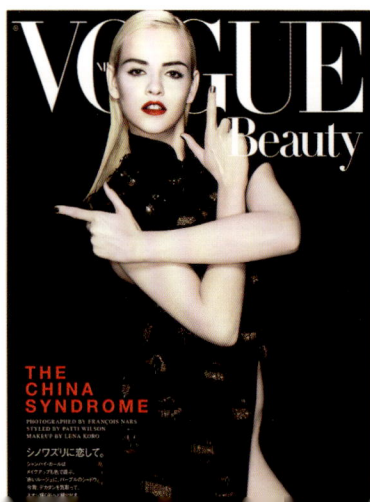

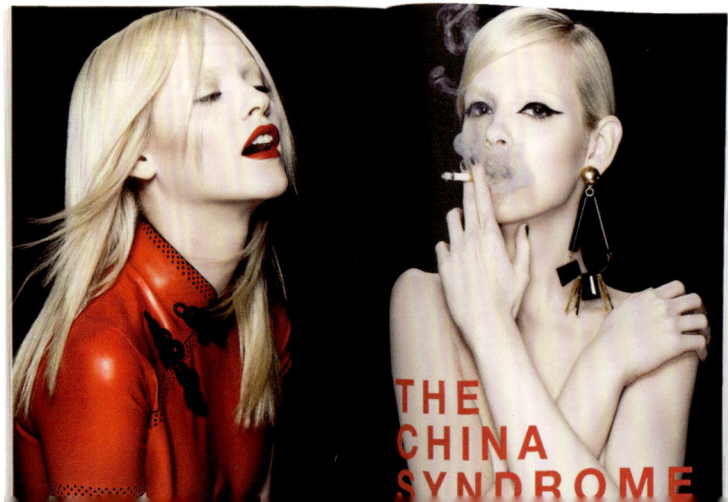

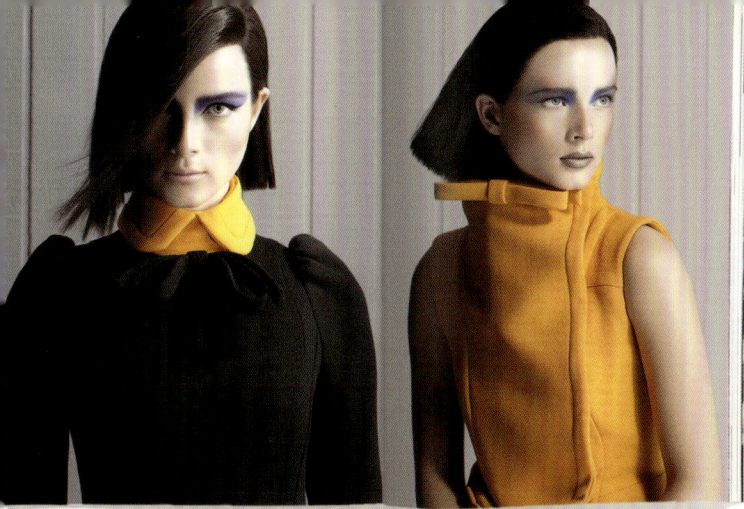

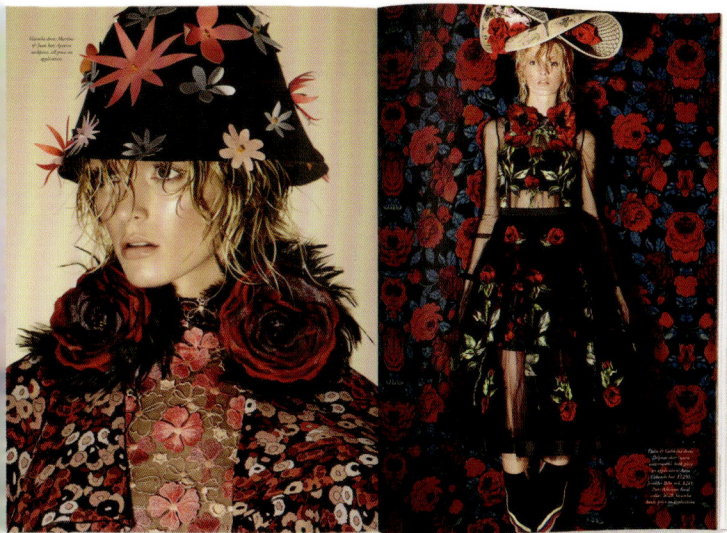

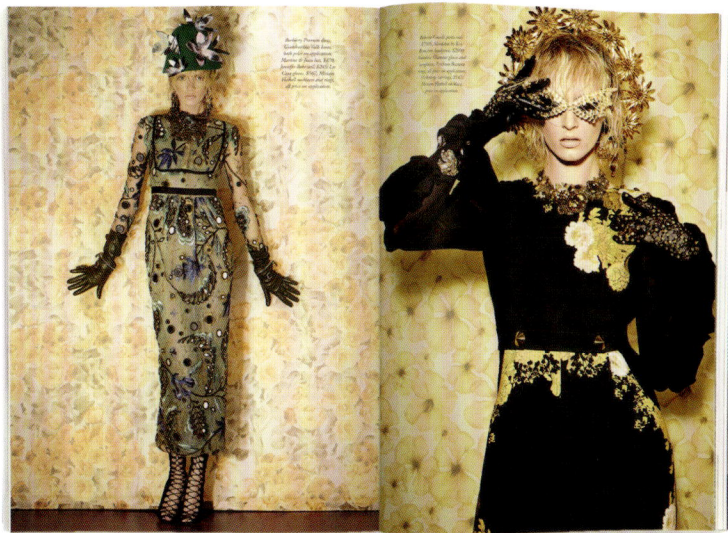

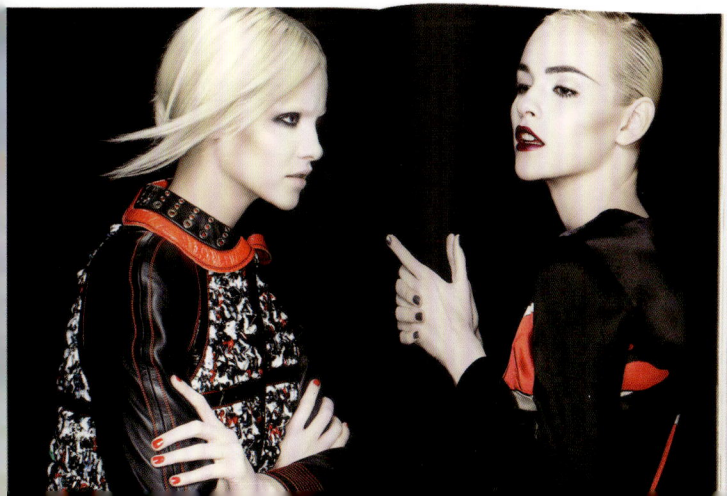

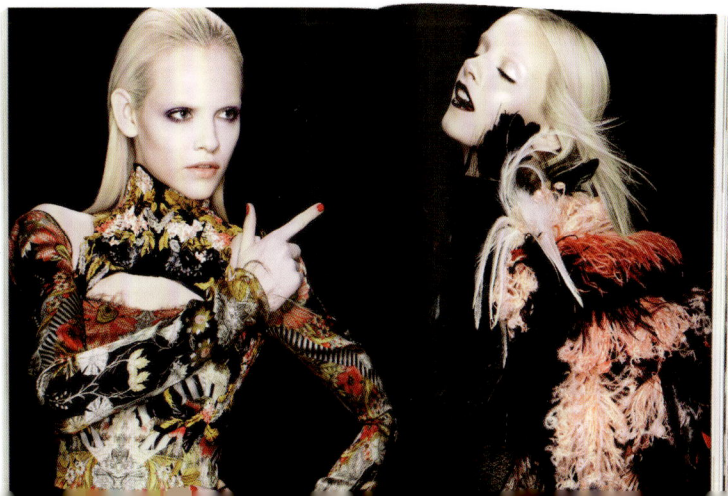

VOGUE

GISELE
100%
DOMINADO

TIM-TIM
Do look ao drinque,
um guia completo
para brilhar
no fim de ano

FRANÇOIS NARS

GISELE

A ÜBERMODEL CONVERSA COM GIOVANNI BIANCO SOBRE OS BASTIDORES
DO LIVRO QUE CELEBRA SEUS 20 ANOS DE CARREIRA

GIOVANNI BIANCO

DÉBAUCHE
DE *PIGMENTS*

Carte blanche à *François Nars* qui,
pour *célébrer* les 15 ans de sa
marque, farde et *photographie* les
trois nouveaux visages de la *mode*.
Trois tops en pleine ascension, trois
femmes en libre *exhibition*, trois
maquillages à forte *impression*...

Par FRÉDÉRIQUE VERLEY.
Photographe et maquillage FRANÇOIS NARS.
Réalisation CARINE ROITFELD.

ANNA SELEZNEVA

TAO OKAMOTO

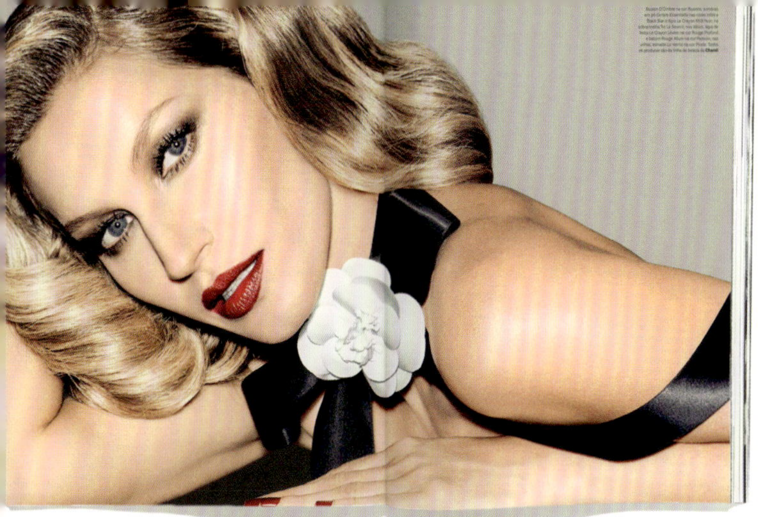

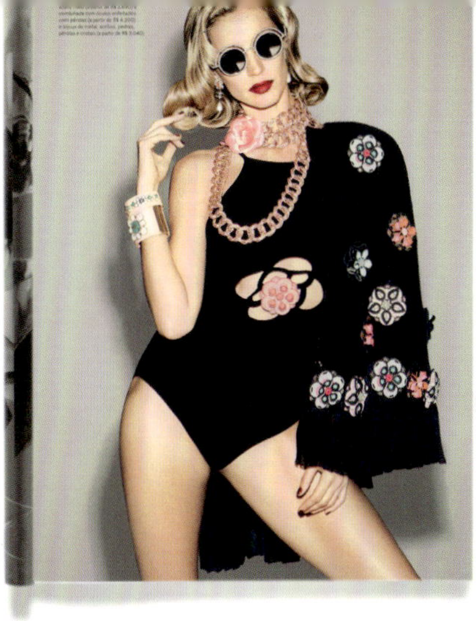

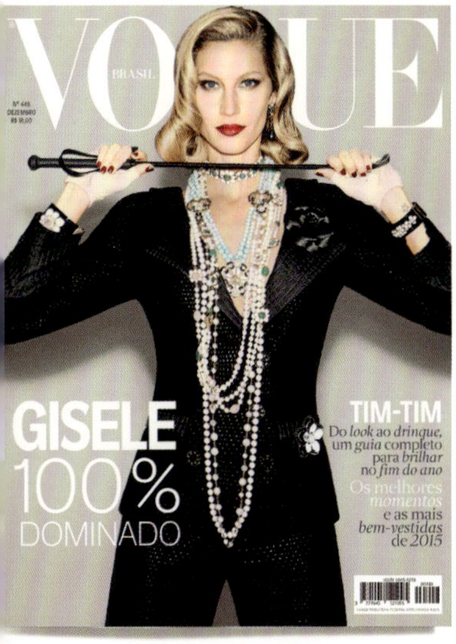

VOGUE

**GISELE
100%
DOMINADO**

TIM-TIM
Do *look* ao *drinque*,
um *guia* completo
para *brilhar*
no fim do ano
Os melhores
momentos
e as mais
bem-vestidas
de 2015

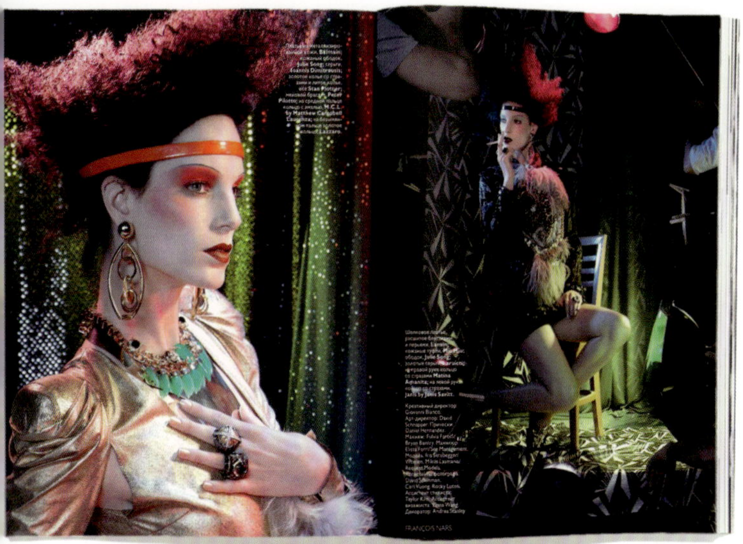

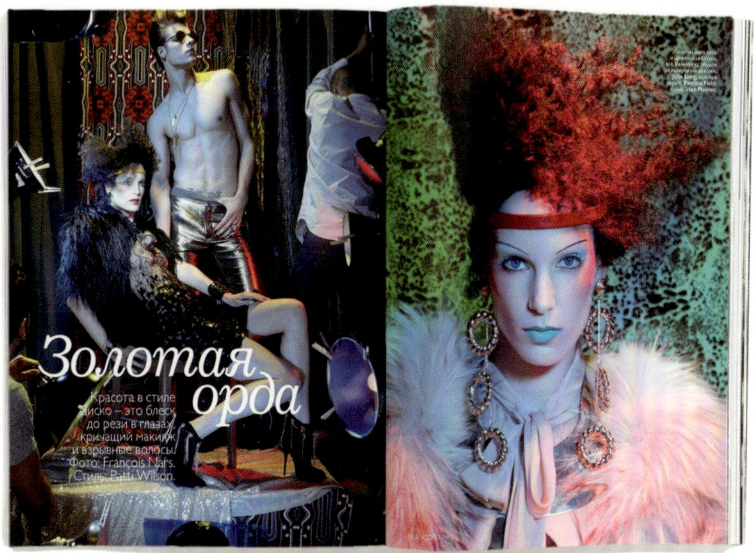

Золотая
орда

Красота в стиле
диско — это блеск
до рези в глазах,
кричащий макияж
и взрывные волосы.
Фото: Francois Nars.
Стиль: Patti Wilson

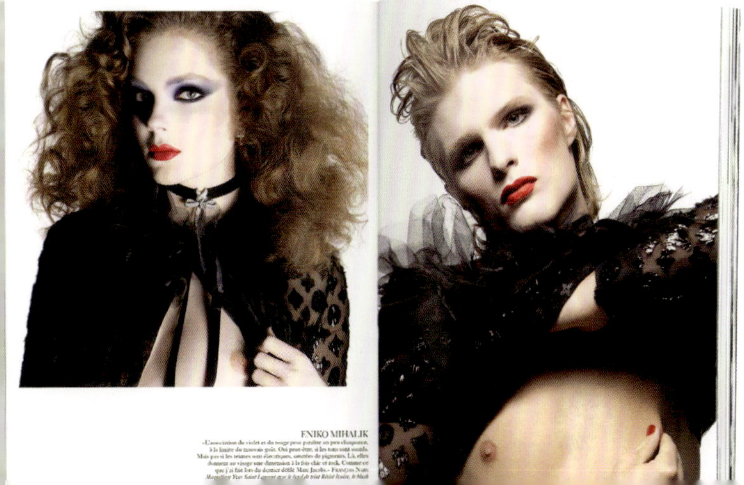

FRANCOIS NARS

ENIKO MIHALIK

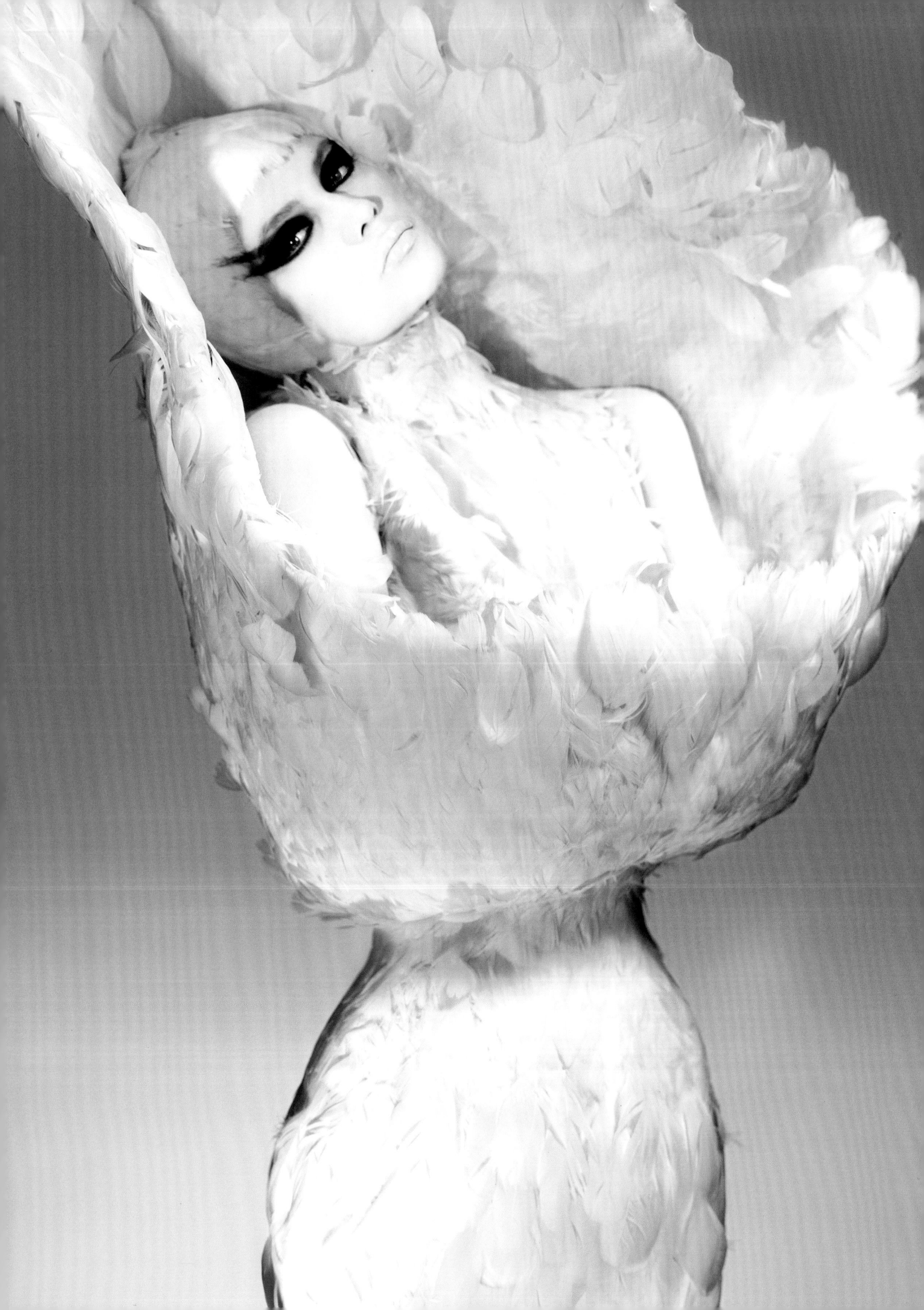

NEW
ORDER

FRANÇOIS NARS WANTS YOU TO FALL IN LOVE WITH YOUR MAKEUP. DEEPLY, MADLY, WILDLY. IT SHOULD TRANSPORT YOU, BREAK OPEN A NEW WORLD FROM THE PALM OF YOUR HAND. HIS PROFOUND CONNECTION TO PRODUCT STARTS WITH PIGMENT PURITY AND TRANSLUCENCY—KEY FOR MAINTAINING THE INTEGRITY OF COLOR. "IN THE NATURAL PURSUIT OF BEAUTY, WOMEN CHANGE CONSTANTLY—GREAT PRODUCTS GUIDE THIS PROCESS," SAYS FRANÇOIS. "IT'S ALL ABOUT FINDING DIFFERENT WAYS TO EXPRESS INDIVIDUAL BEAUTY AND PERSONALITY."

IN REALIZING HIS OWN VISION, FRANÇOIS BEGAN CHALLENGING BOTH CONVENTIONAL BEAUTY AND THE COSMETICS USED TO CONSTRUCT IT. HE FOUND THE HEAVY FEEL AND LIMITED PALETTES OF THE 90s INSUFFICIENT FOR CREATING HIS SIGNATURE MODERN, RADIANT LOOKS. IF IT DIDN'T EXIST, HE WOULD SIMPLY HAVE TO INVENT IT. DESIGNED TO MEET HIS OWN ARTISTRY NEEDS AND EXACTING STANDARDS, FRANÇOIS LAUNCHED A LINEUP OF TWELVE LIPSTICKS AT BARNEYS NEW YORK IN NOVEMBER 1994. FUSING UNPRECEDENTED PIGMENTATION WITH LUXURIOUS TEXTURE, EACH LIPSTICK BULLET—DRESSED IN AN ICONIC SOFT-TOUCH CASE DESIGNED BY CREATIVE DIRECTOR FABIEN BARON—DEFINED A NEW FORMULA FOR SUCCESS. OVER TWO DECADES OF REVOLUTIONARY BEAUTY LATER, NARS HAS GROWN TO BECOME A CULT-CLASSIC BRAND WITH A FULL-RANGE COLLECTION OFFERED IN STORES AND NAMESAKE BOUTIQUES AROUND THE GLOBE.

FRANÇOIS'S CREATIVE FORCE REMAINS AT THE CORE OF NARS'S ESSENCE, INSPIRING CREATIVITY, SELF EXPRESSION, AND BOLD ARTISTRY. FROM PROVOCATIVE SHADE NAMES LIKE ORGASM TO HIS BOUNDARY-PUSHING, NO-RULES APPROACH TO BEAUTY, HE EMBRACES THE AUDACIOUS AT EVERY TURN—CONTINUING TO BRING HIGH-FASHION, HIGH-STYLE, AND FORWARD-THINKING TO BEAUTY.

"I FIRST MET FRANÇOIS IN THE EARLY 90s AT A BARNEYS SHOOT. I WAS STAGGERED BY HIS COMBO OF AUDACITY AND SKILL. FOR EXAMPLE, HE COVERED LINDA EVANGELISTA'S EYEBROWS WITH CONCEALER AND THEN PAINTED FAKE ONES HALFWAY UP HER FOREHEAD. IT SOUNDS INSANE, BUT IN THE PHOTOGRAPHS, IT LOOKS MAGNIFIQUE!"
– SIMON DOONAN, CREATIVE AMBASSADOR, BARNEYS NEW YORK

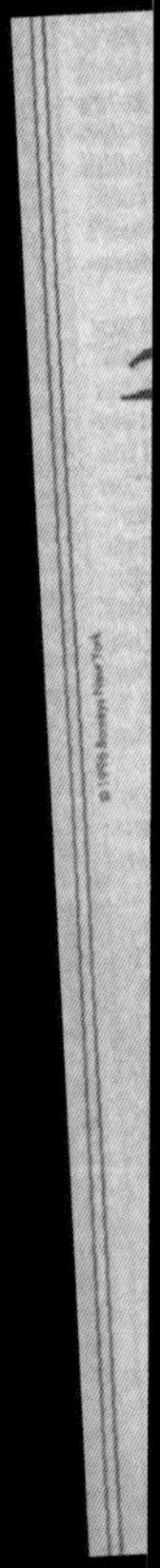

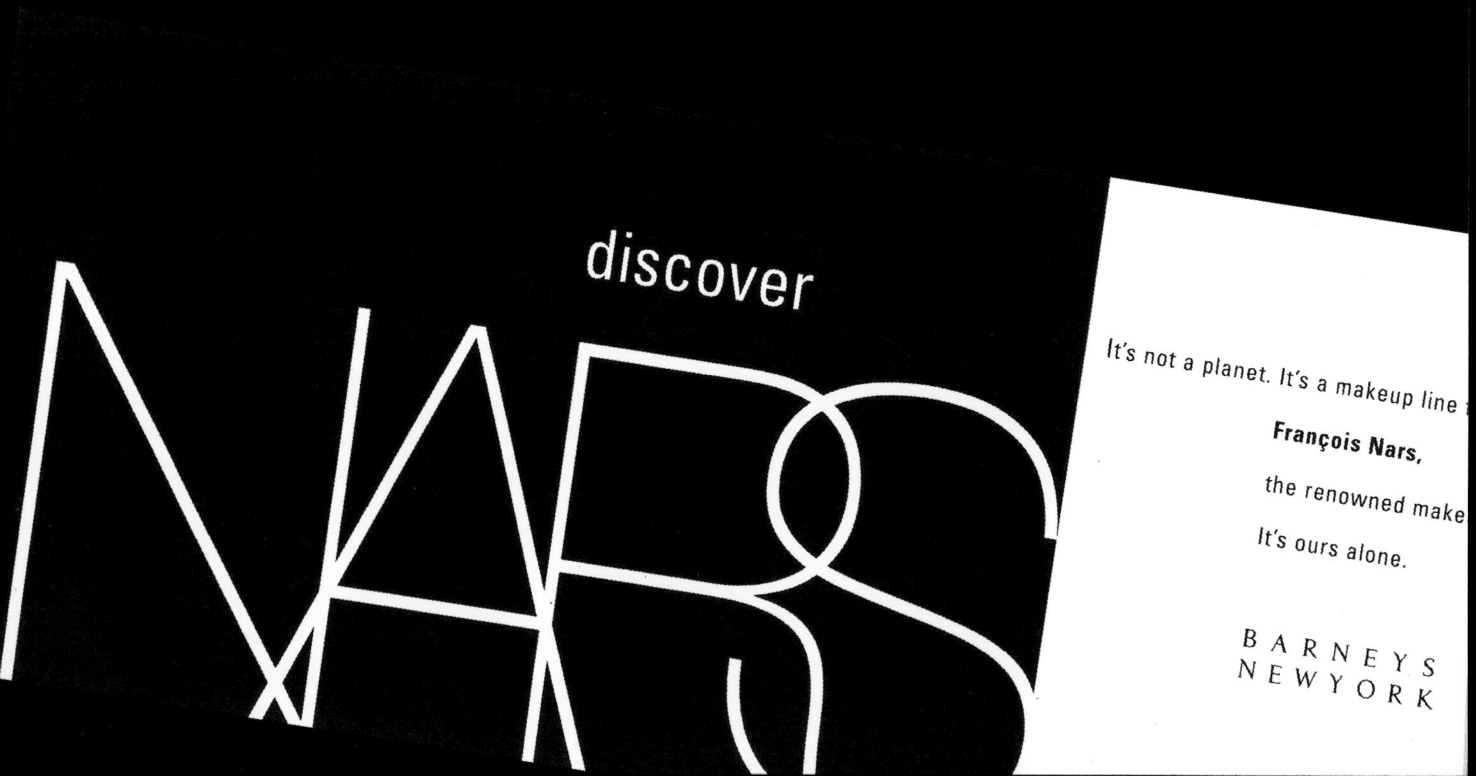

discover

NARS

It's not a planet. It's a makeup line

François Nars,

the renowned make

It's ours alone.

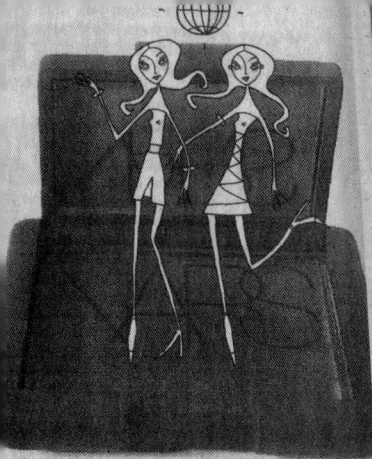

NARS NIGHT LIFE

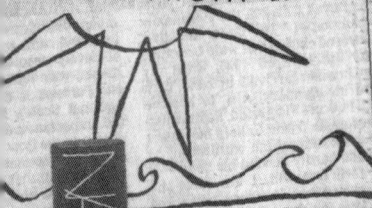

Naturally Nars.

New from Nars, **The Multiple**, lends a natural summ___
___w all year long. Color sweeps from eyes to lips to sho___
___le in four shades inspired by Malibu, Waikiki, South ___
___ Copa Cabana, $32 each. At all of our stores.

A R N E Y

___mme's Here. Think Sheer!

___ew from Nars - clear **nail polishes** with a hint of color.
___roducing three sheer nail glosses in **Funny Girl pink**,
___s **Stop orange** and **Ultra Violet purple**, $15 each.

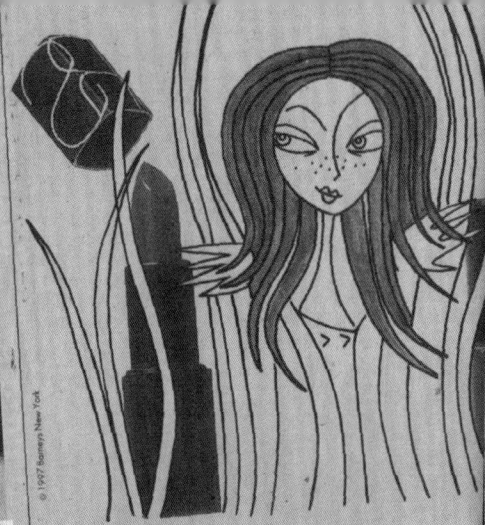

IT'S A JUNGLE OUT TH___

New from **Nars**. Jungle Red nail color $15 ___
$19. Get back to sexy with the ___

Bond with the **Nars** team of make-up ___
Avenue store Oct. 29th, 30th & 3___

A tip for
Hip lips

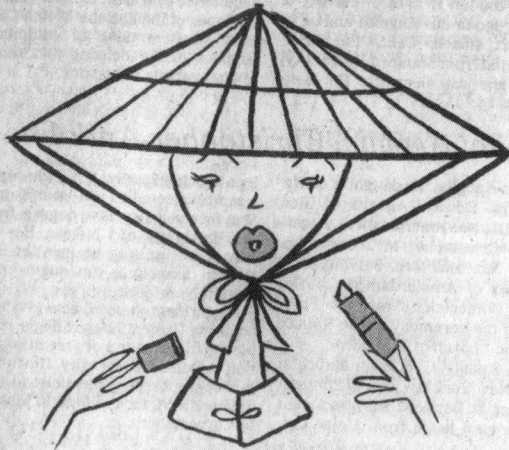

Master makeup artist **François Nars** has created his own lipsticks in
twelve intriguing and immediate colors. They're ours alone. $19 each

B A R N E Y S
N E W Y O R K

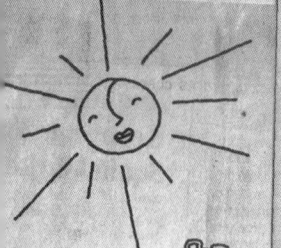

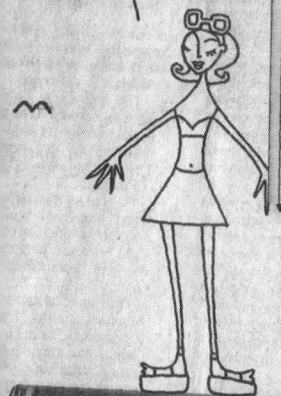

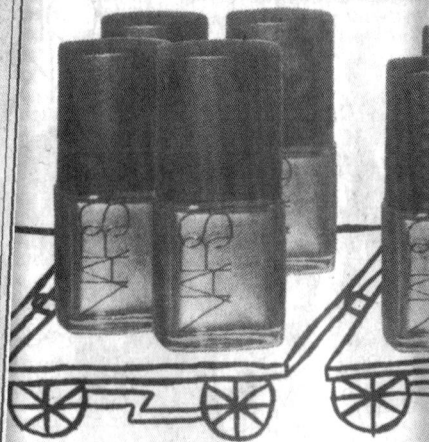

MADISON AVENUE AND SIXTY-FIRST STREET   212 826 8900
SEVENTH AVENUE AND SEVENTEENTH STREET   212 929 9000

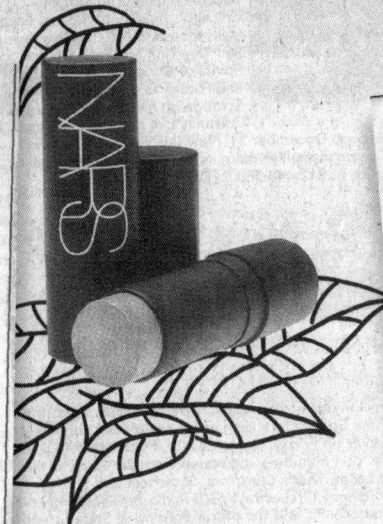

RS Nail Packs To Go

Necessary Nars

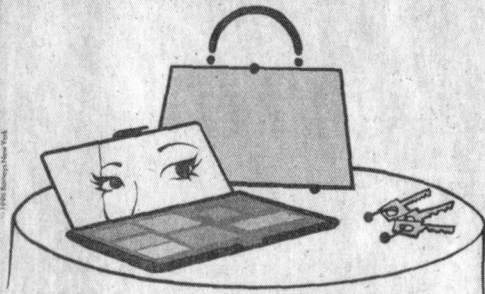

NARS by François Nars makes it easy. Everything you need in
one sleek portable compact. Four perfectly designed color palettes offering
3 eyeshadows, 2 blushes, 3 lip colors and a great mirror, $75.
One of life's wonderful necessities, and it's ours alone.

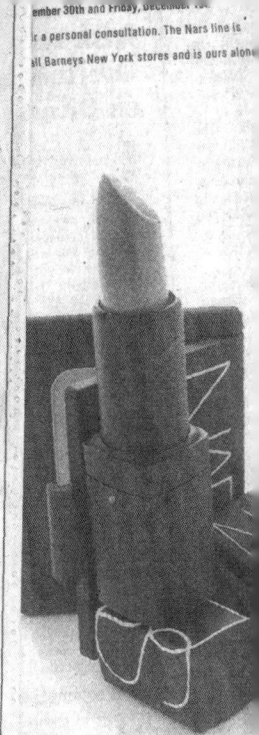

Fall for Nars

___ew from Nars, **The Multiple**, gives you that natural glow.
___ps from eyes to lips to cheeks and shoulders. Available in four shades
___ed by beaches around the world $32 each. At all of our stores.

A R N E Y S
N E W Y O R K

Nars of the stars

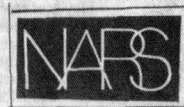

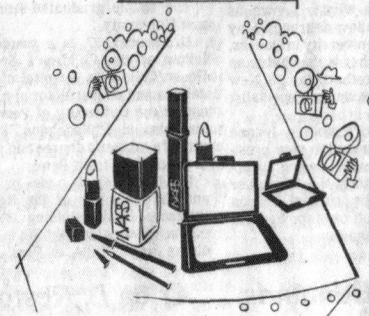

NARS

Nars - it isn't just for lips anymore. Now you'll find the entire line
of cosmetics by renowned makeup artist, François Nars, at all of our
Eye shadow, eyeliner, eyebrow pencils, mascara, lipstick, lipline
foundation, pressed powder, concealer. And it's ours alone.

B A R N E Y
N E W Y O R

___ember 30th and Friday, December 1___
___r a personal consultation. The Nars line is
___ll Barneys New York stores and is ours alone.

BONJOUR
FRANÇOIS!

Meet François Nars
and his international make-up team
Thursday, Oct. 15; 12pm - 3pm —
they will be conducting personal
consultations using the **NARS** make up line;
including Colette Lipstick, $19 and
Tallulah for Nails, $15.

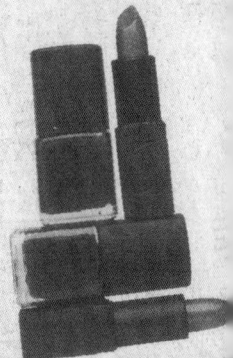

B A R N E Y
N E W Y O R K

25 East Oak Street, Chicago 312.587.1

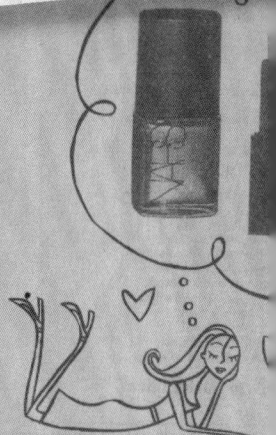

THINK PINK

Belle de Jour is a groovy sub___
available in both lipstick $19 a___
François Nars uses this classic col___
statement for spring 1997. Le___

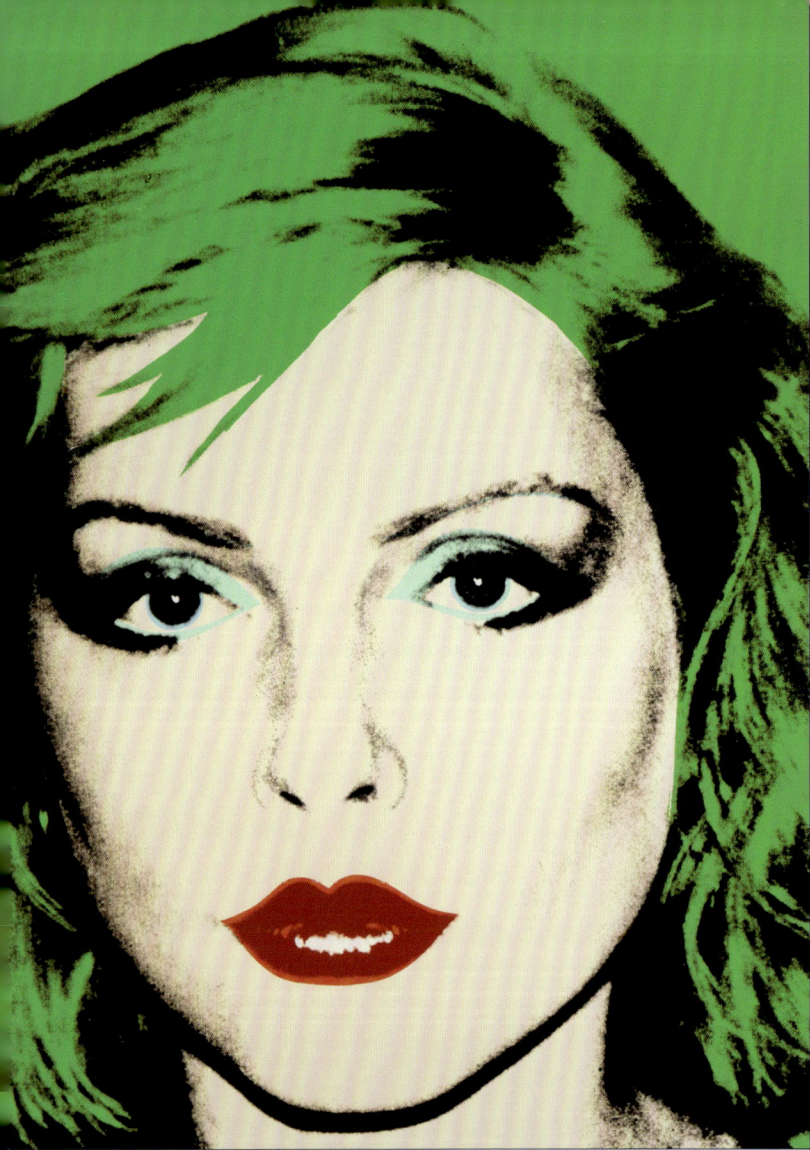

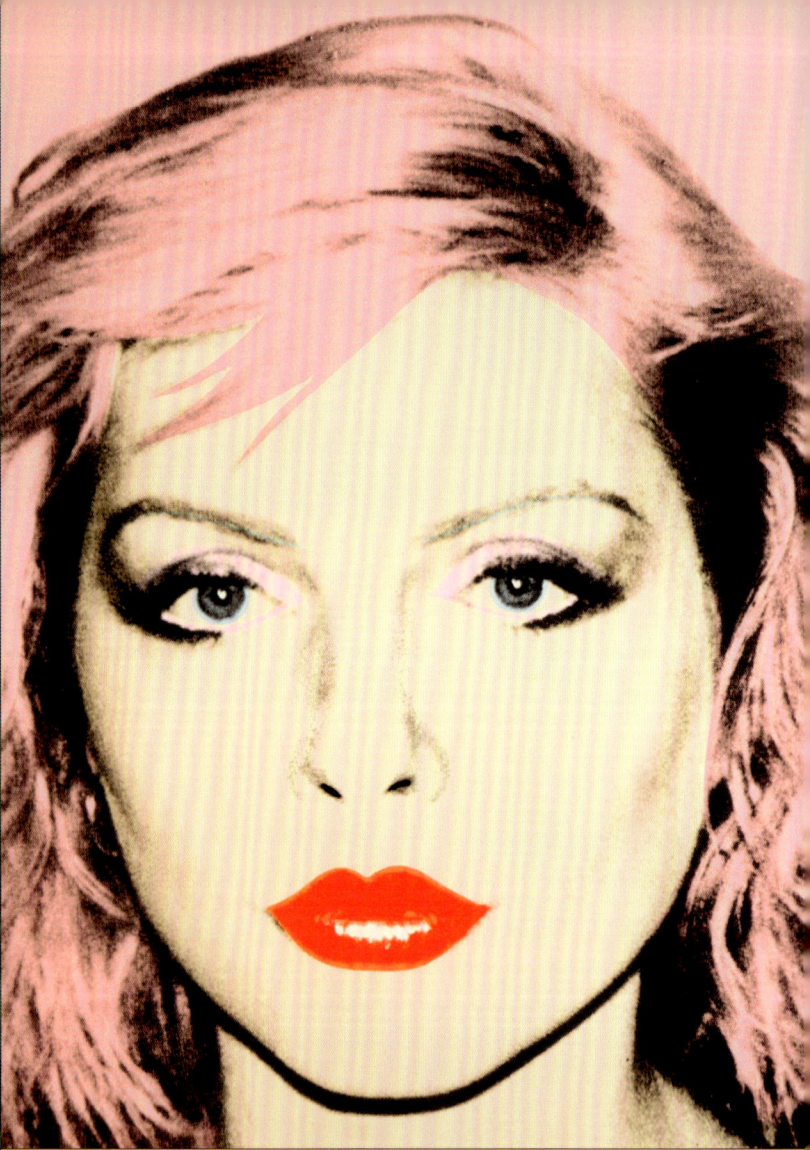

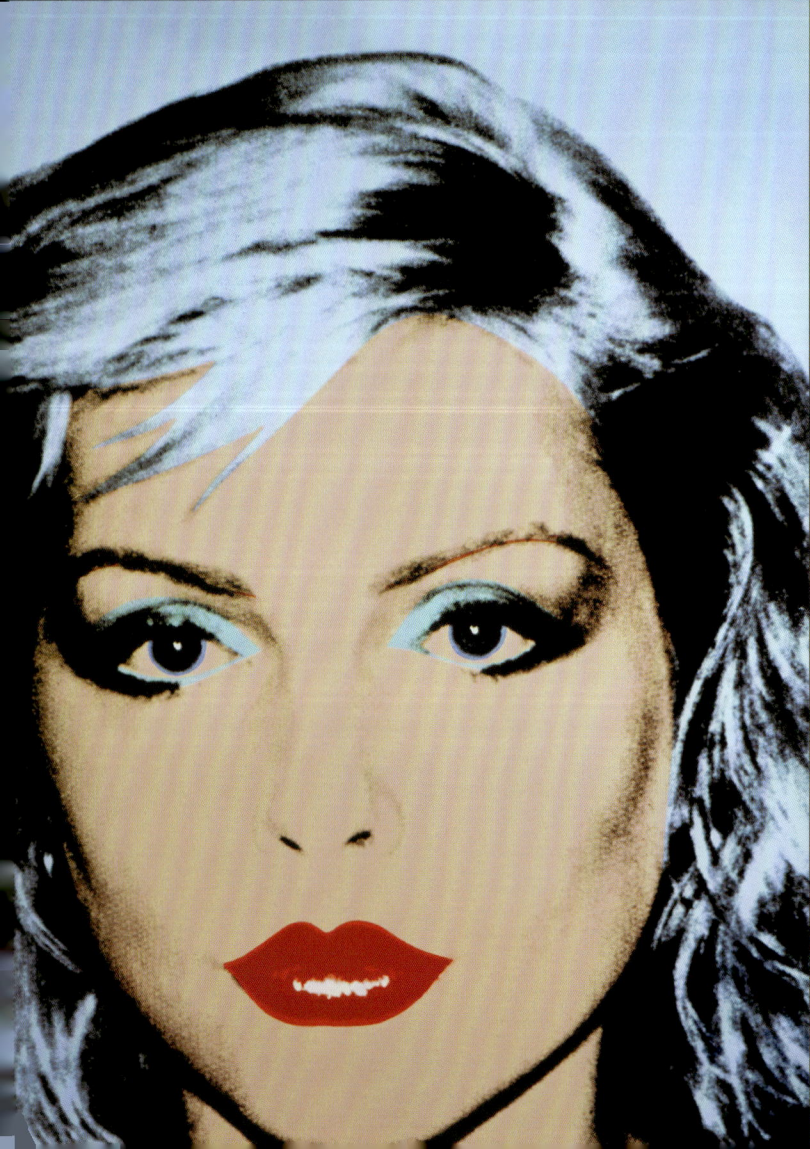

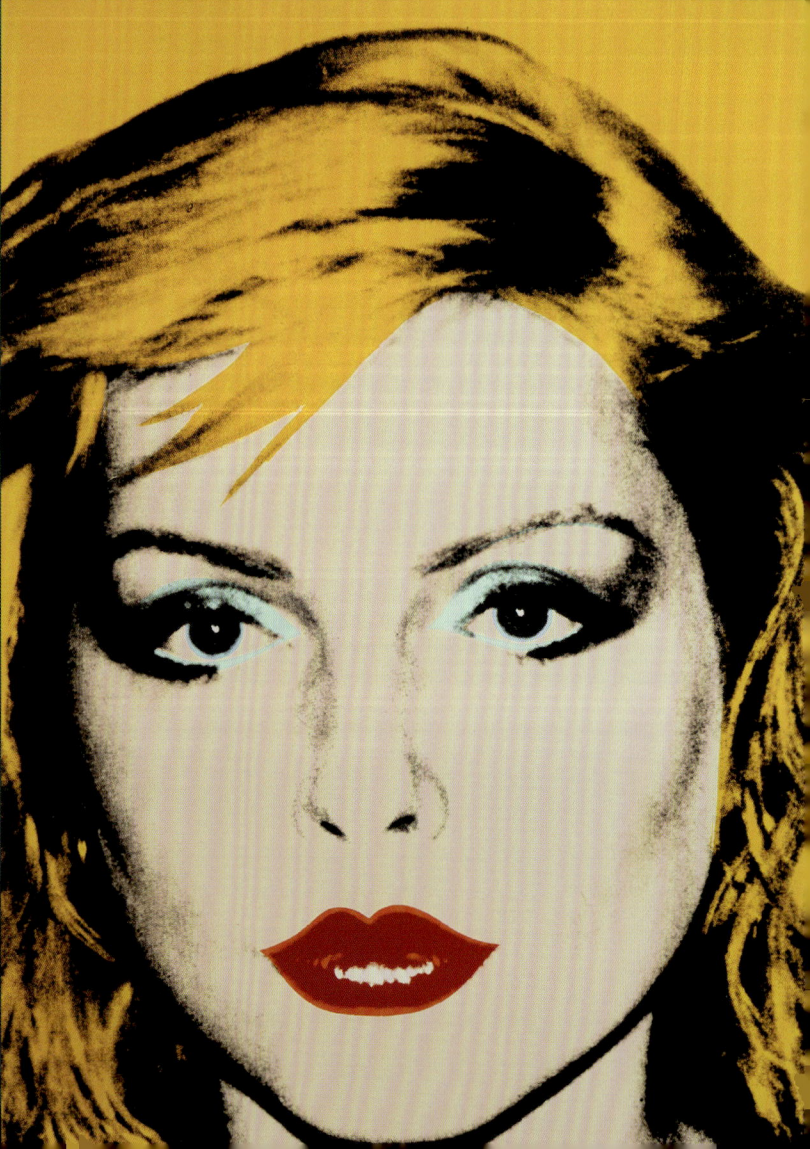

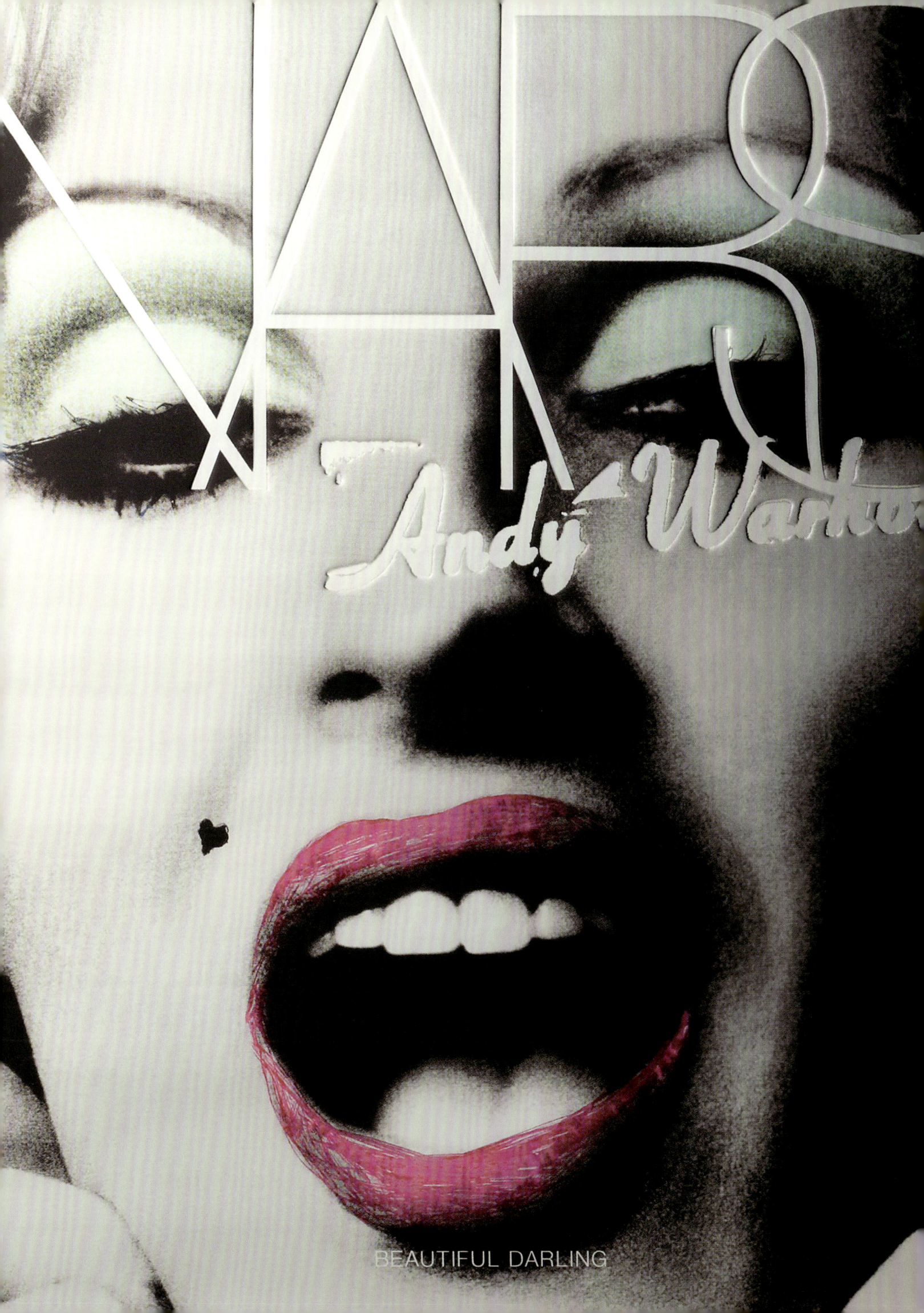

STARS

Andy Warhol

BEAUTIFUL DARLING

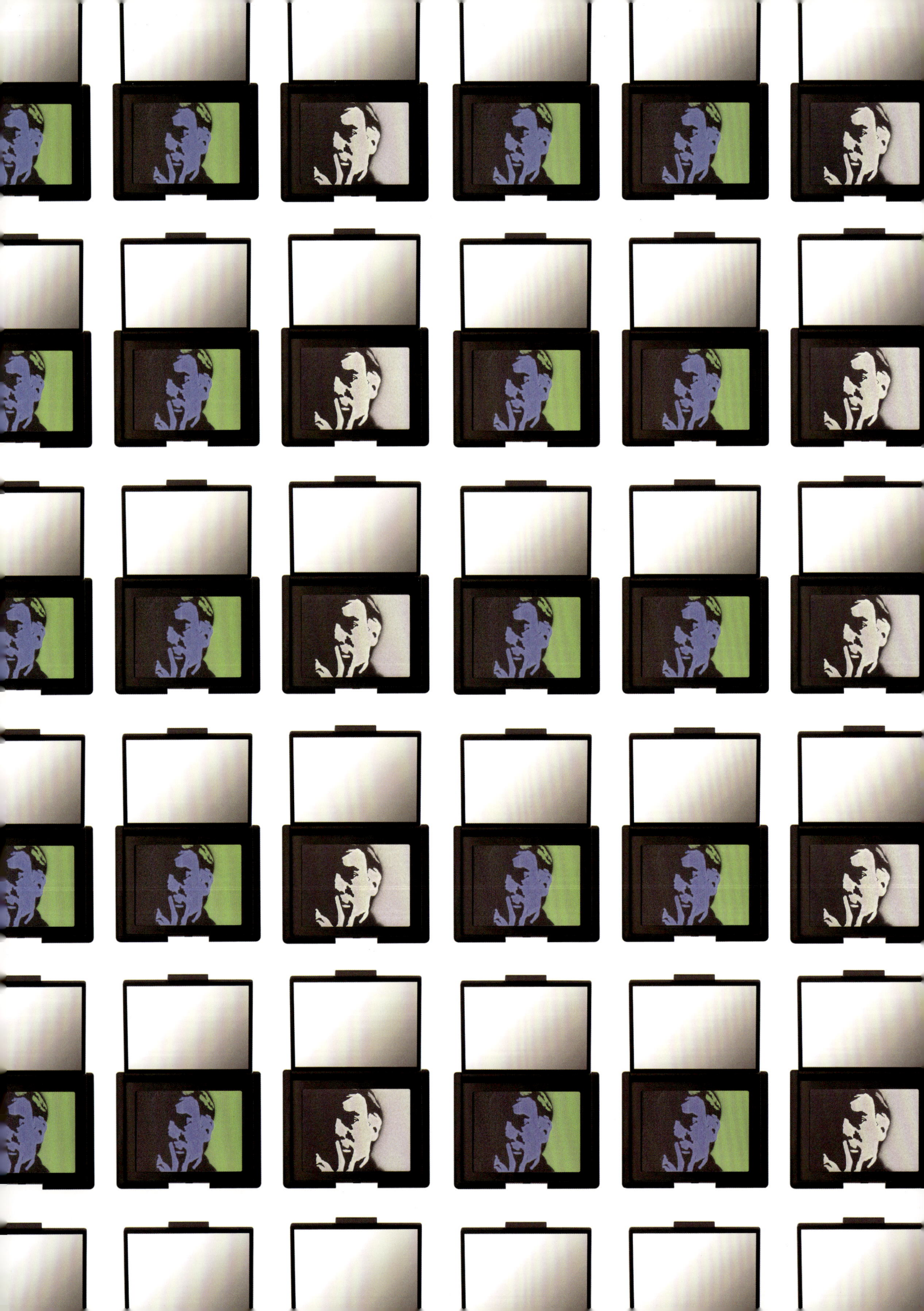

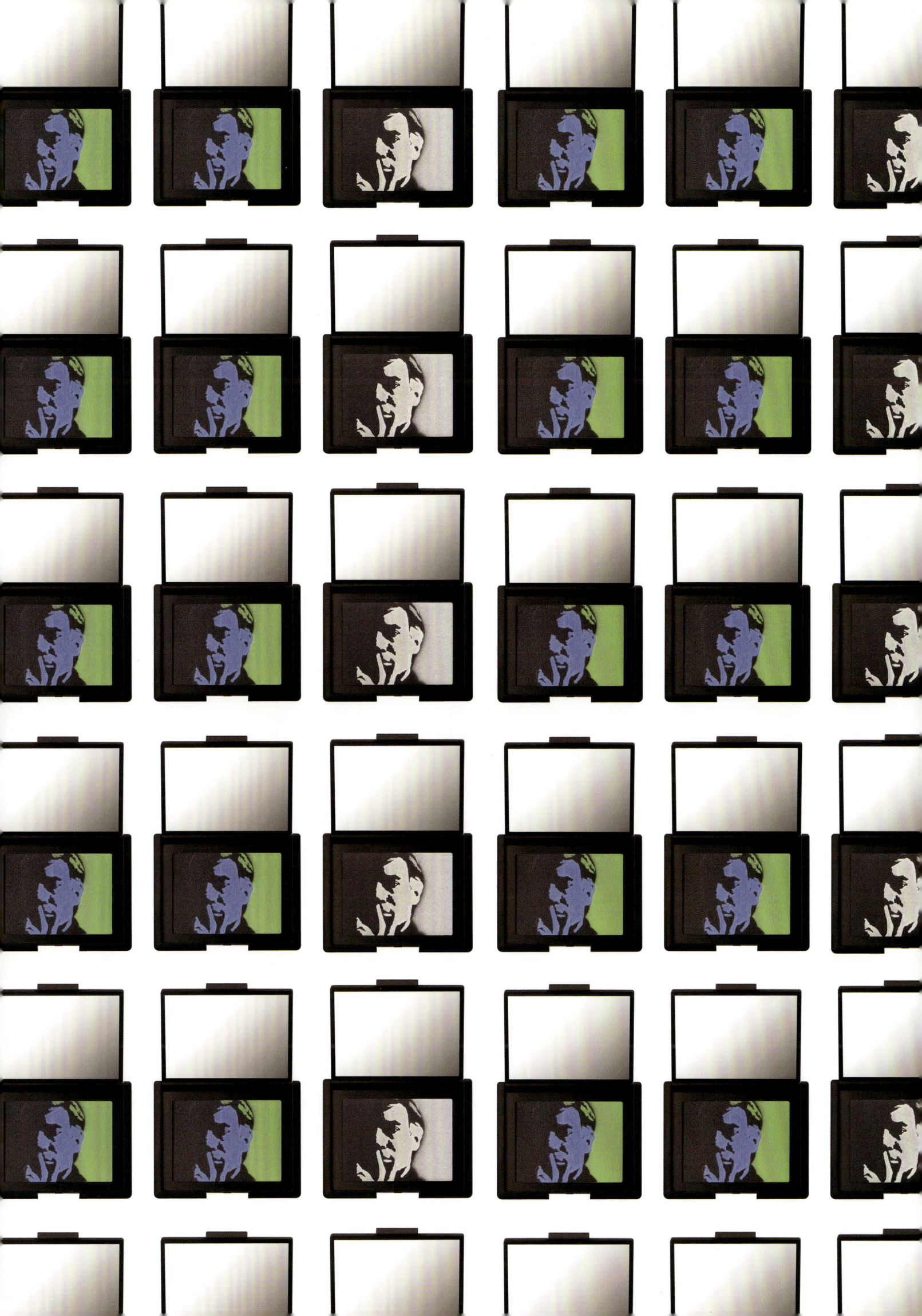

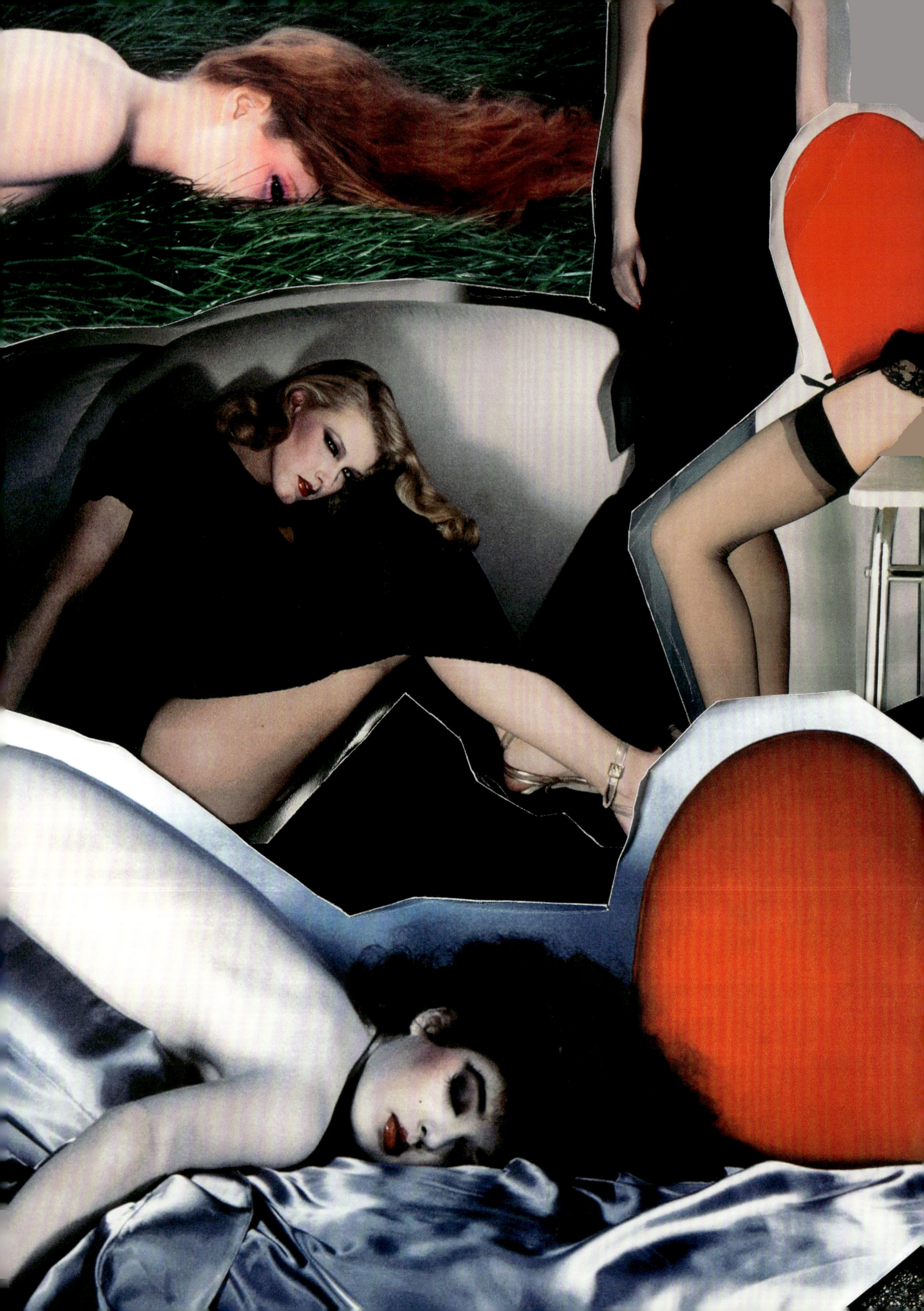

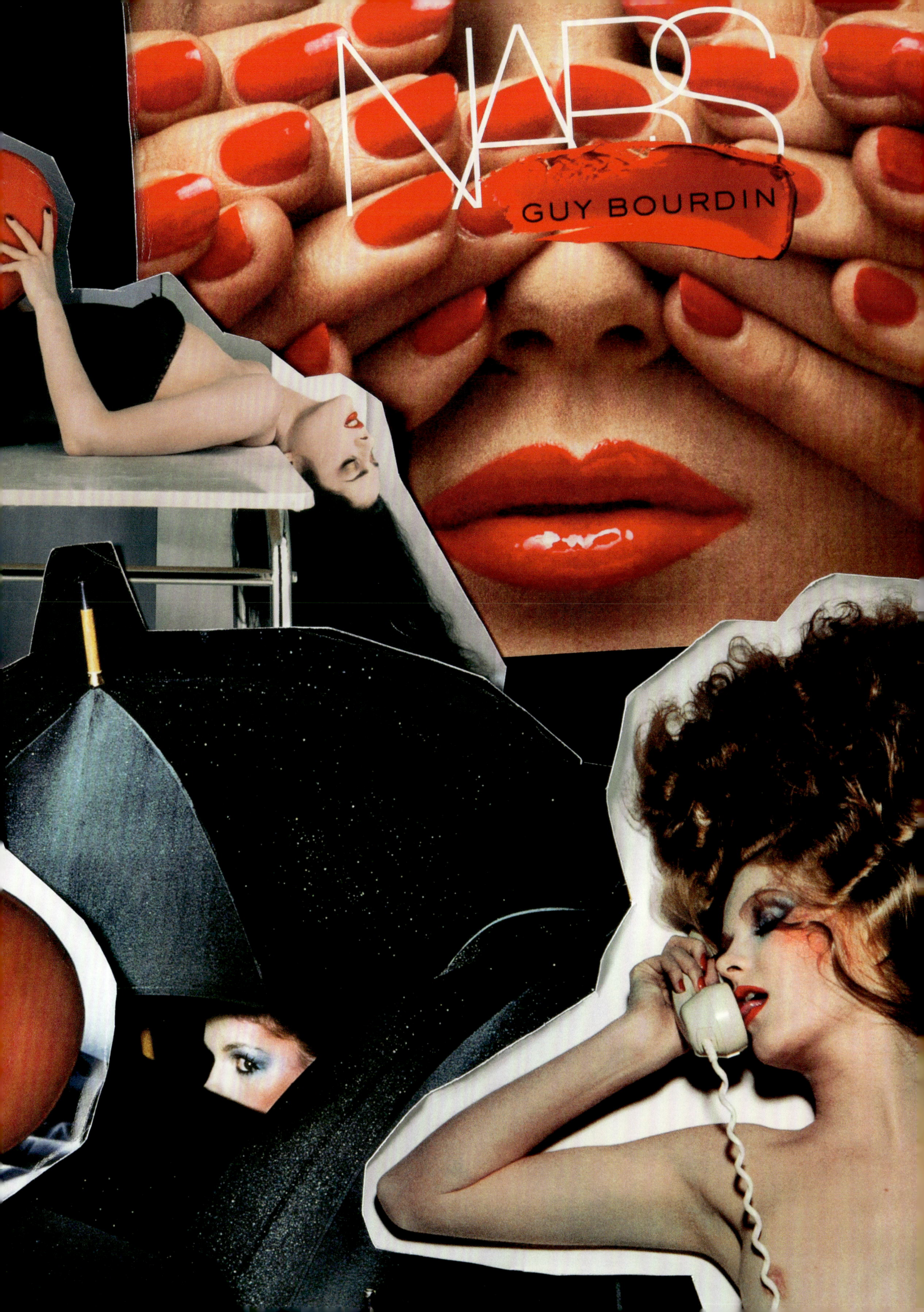

NARS

GUY BOURDIN

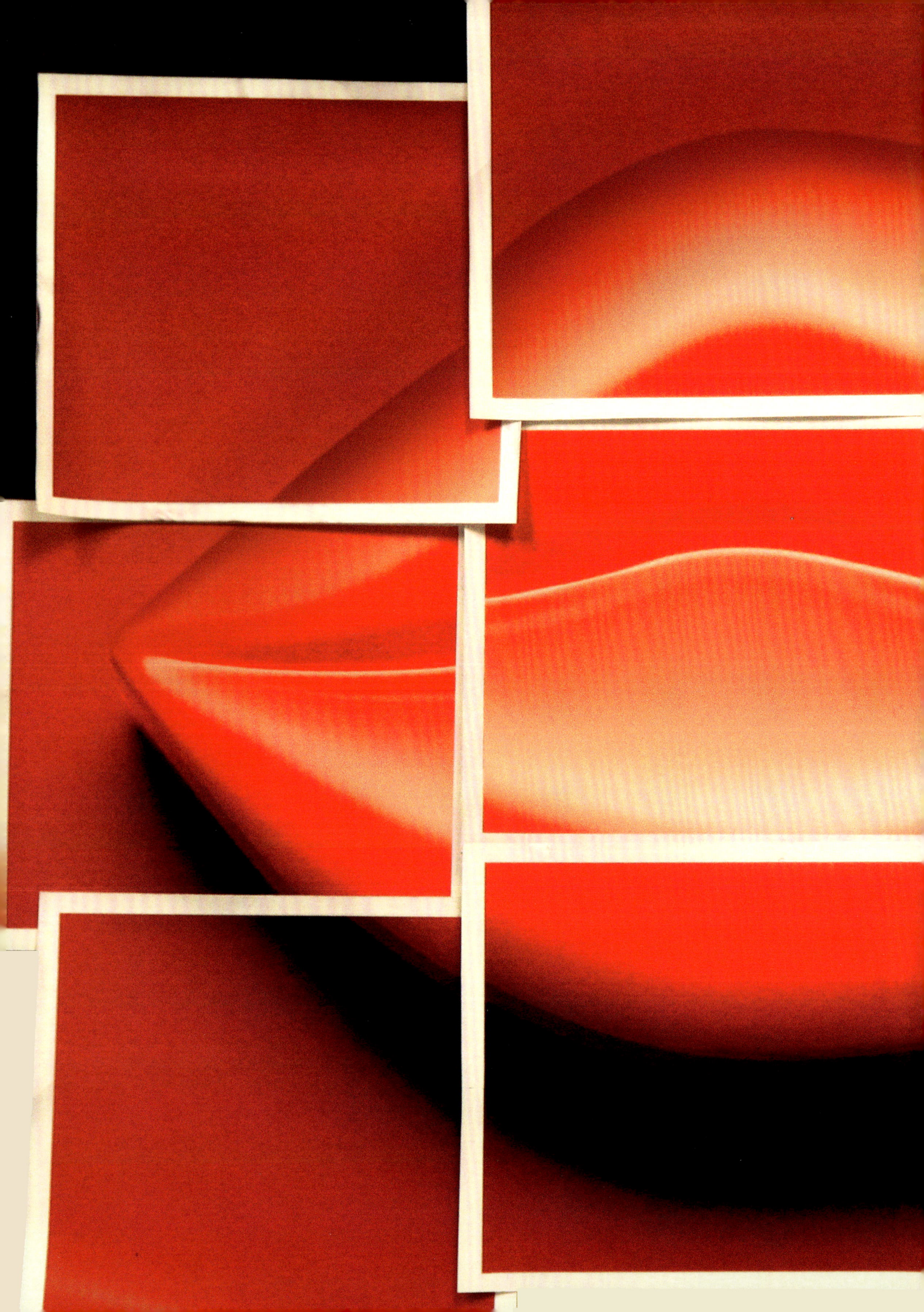

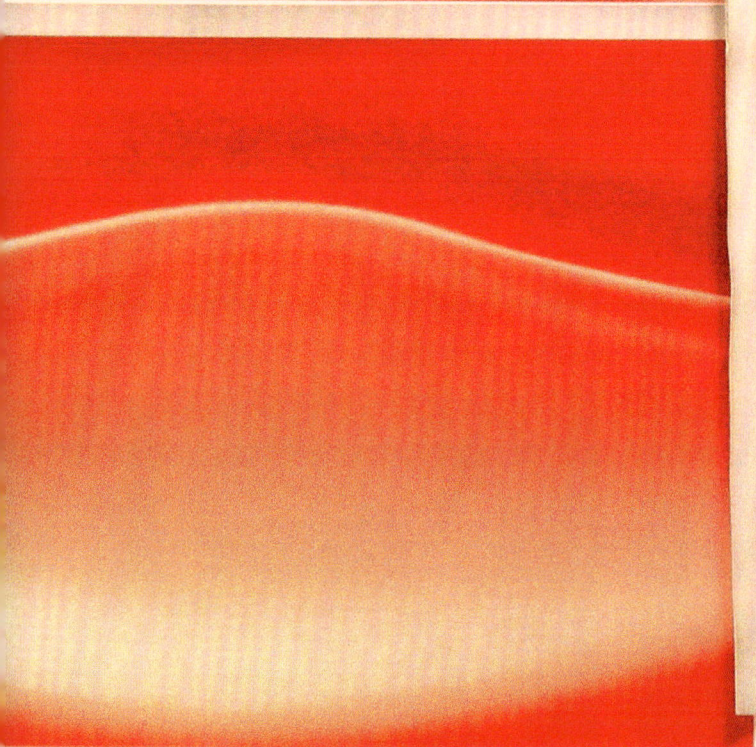

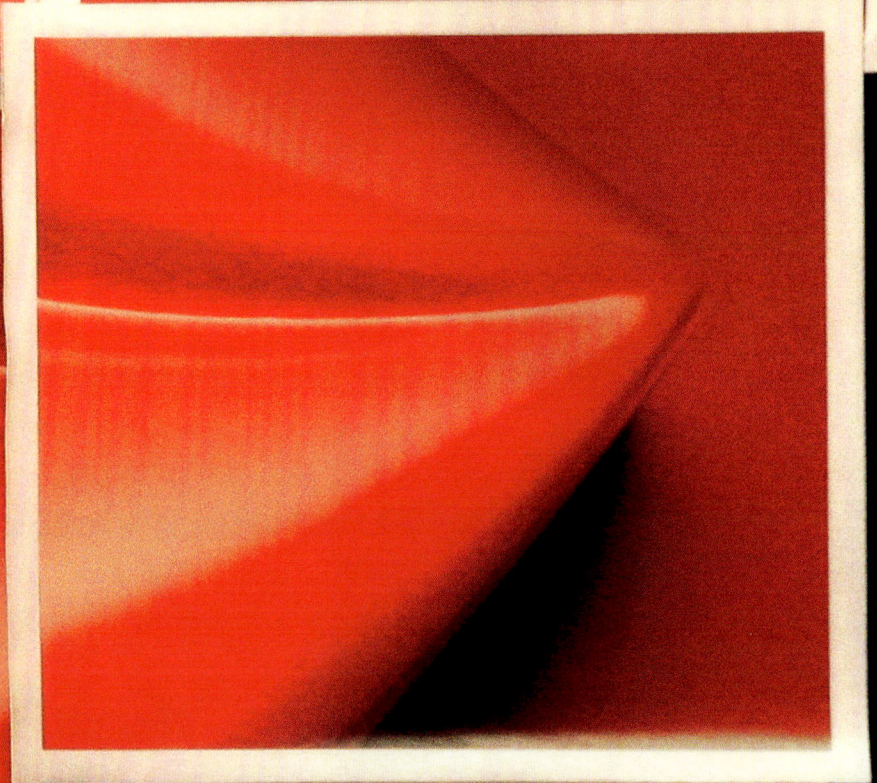

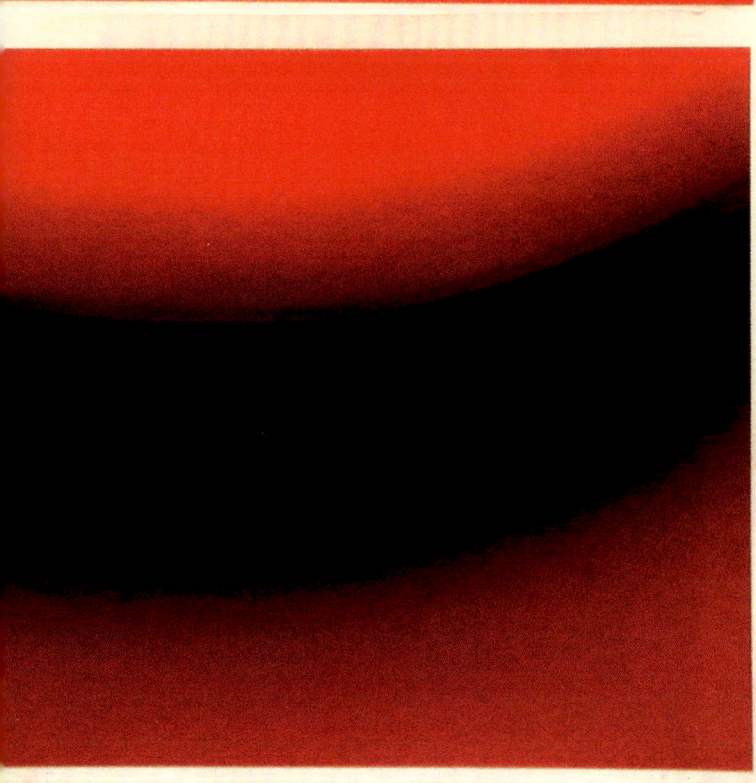

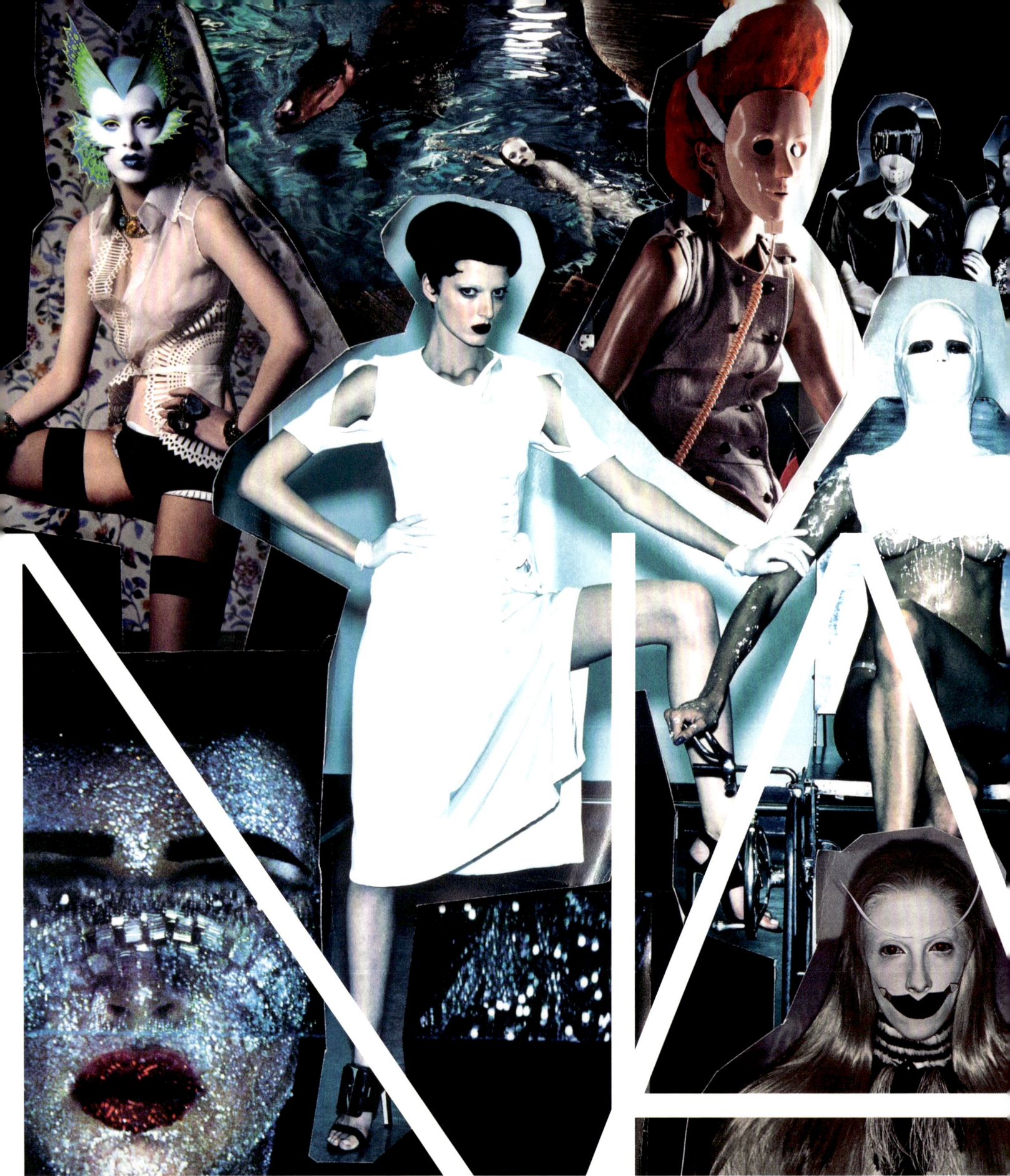

STEVEN

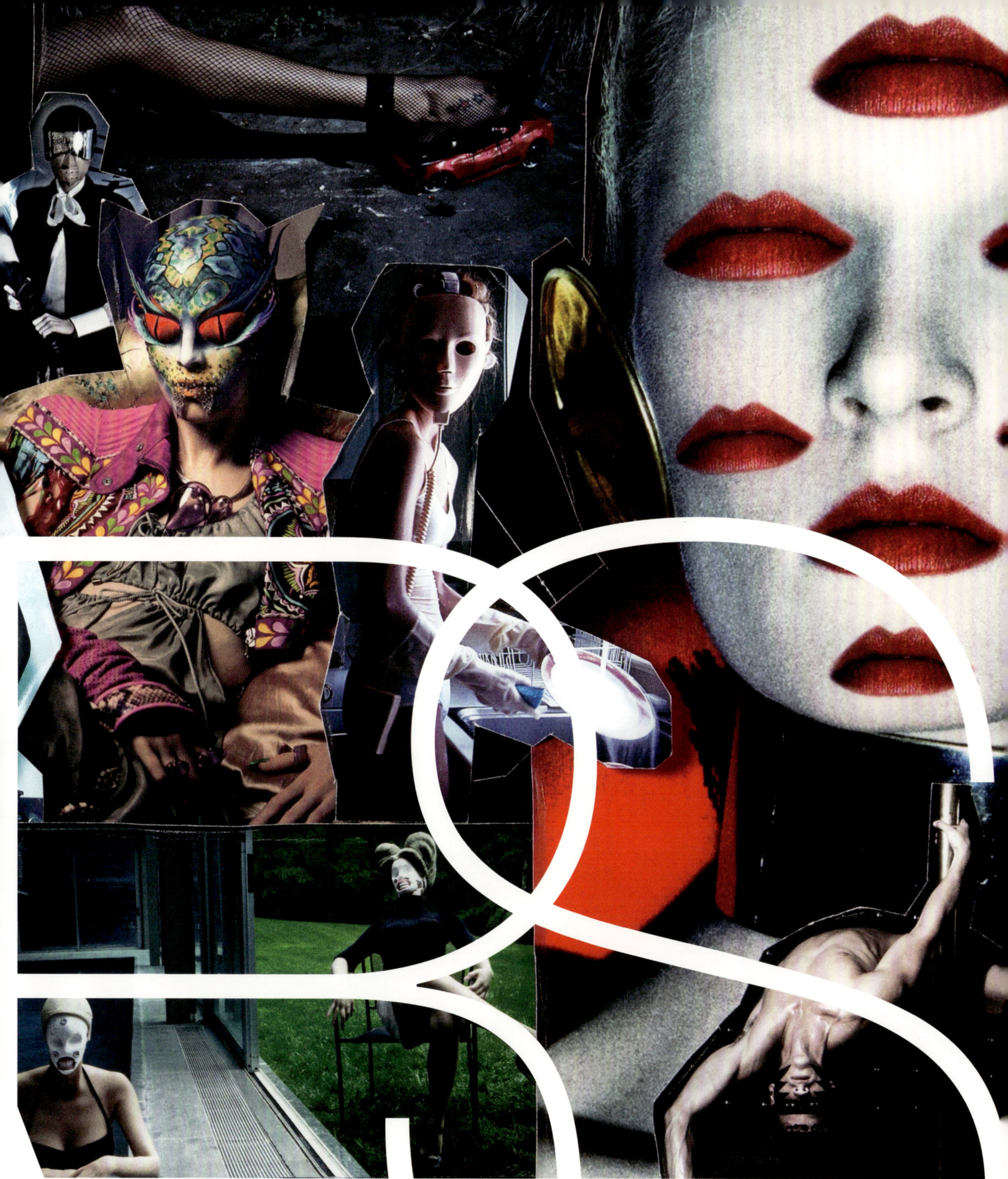

KLEIN

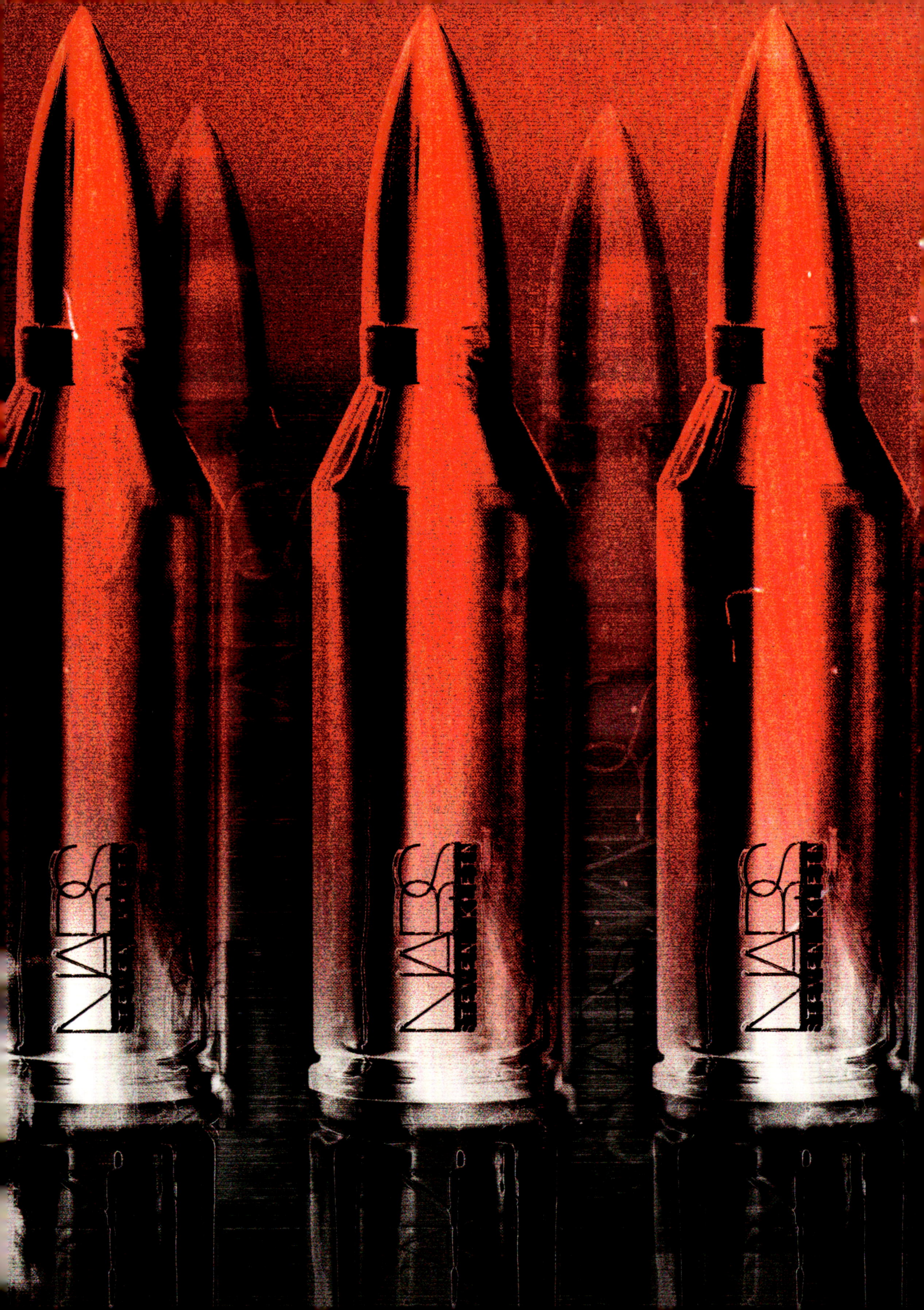

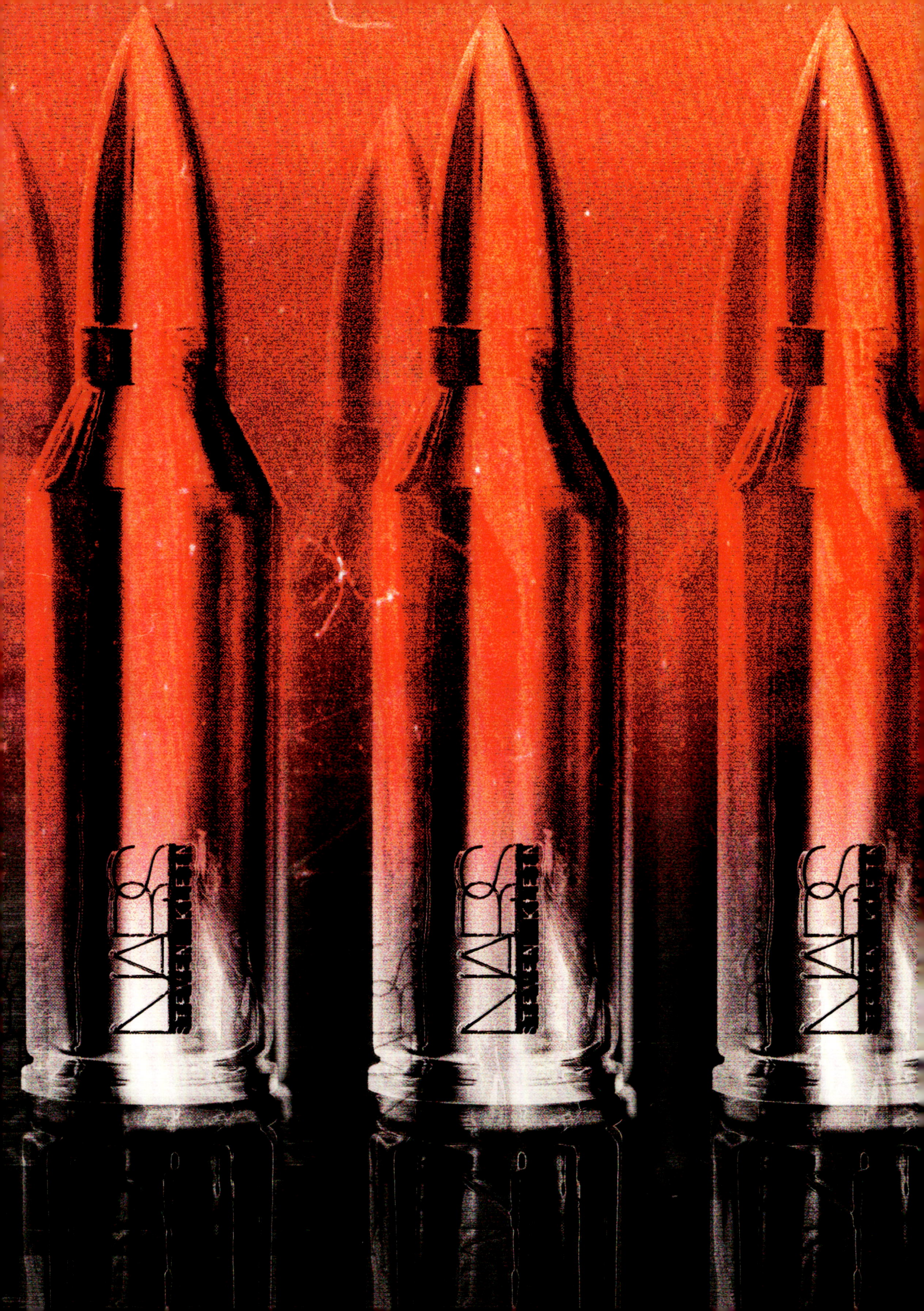

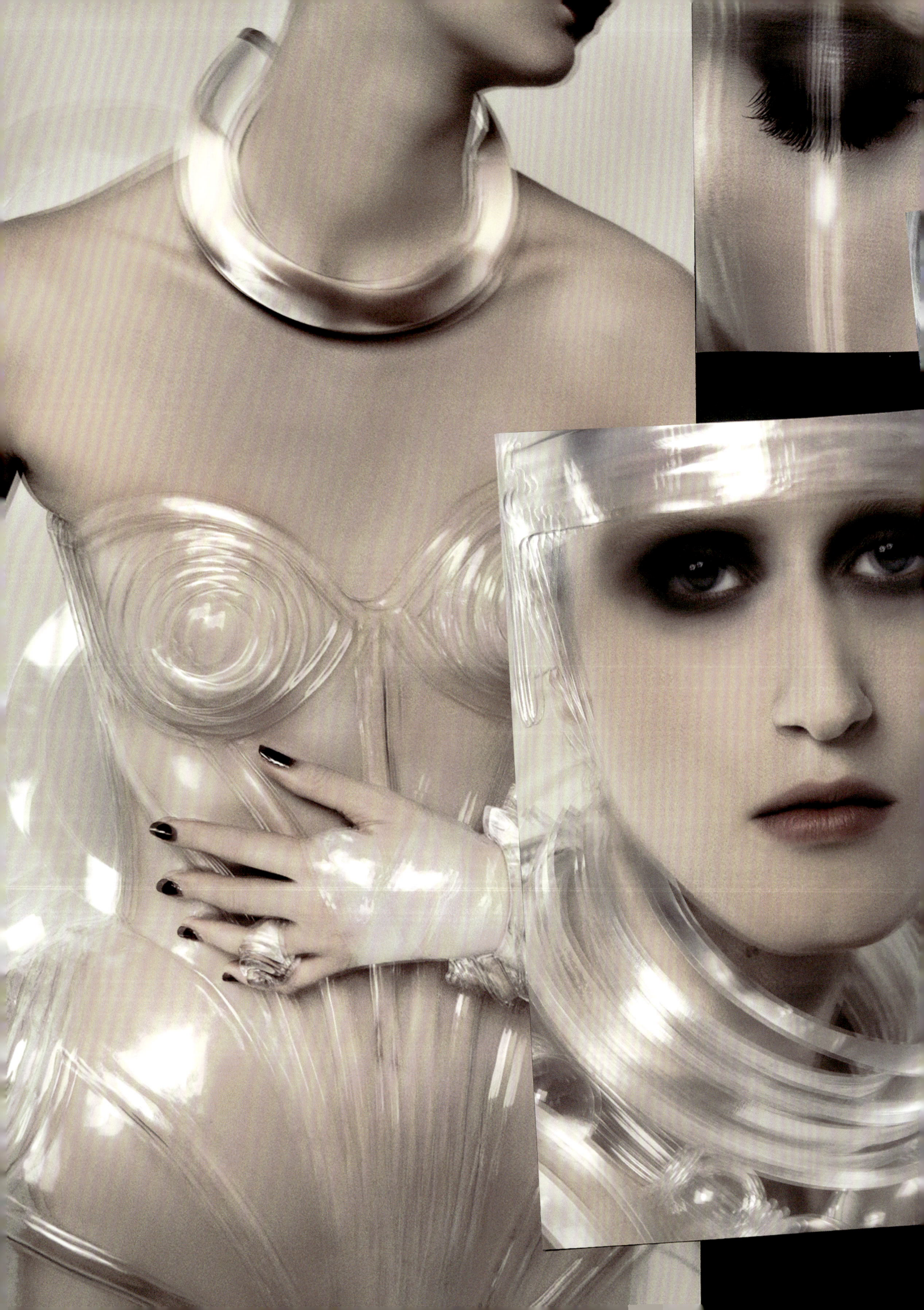

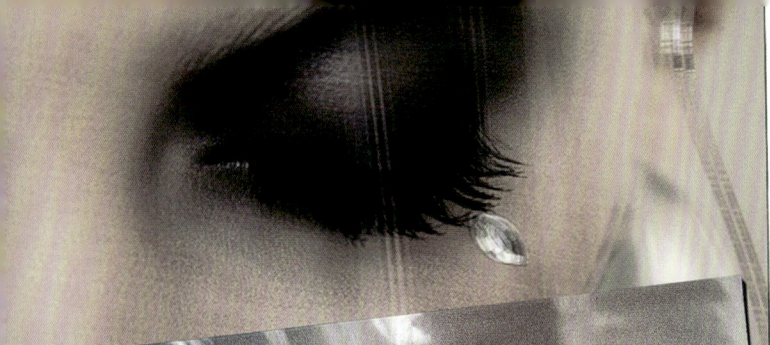

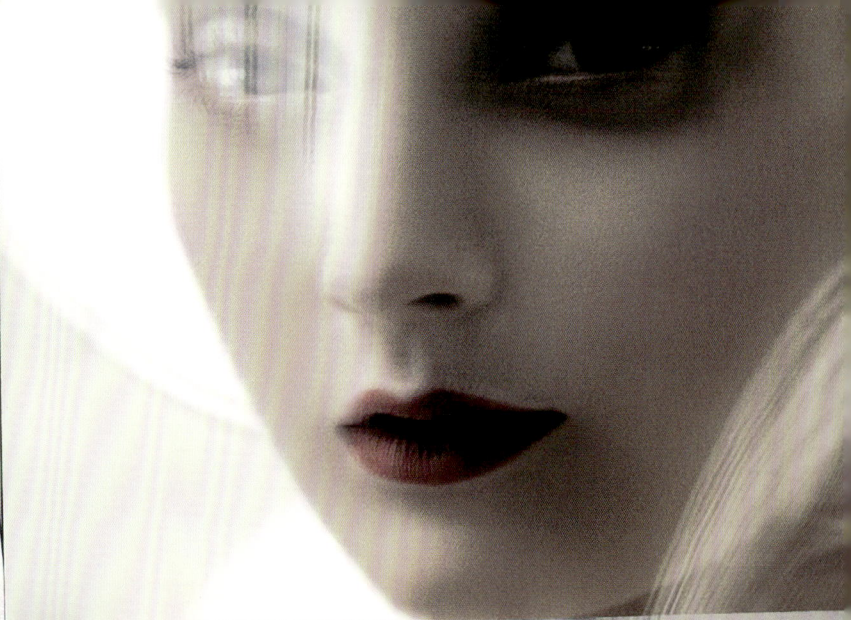

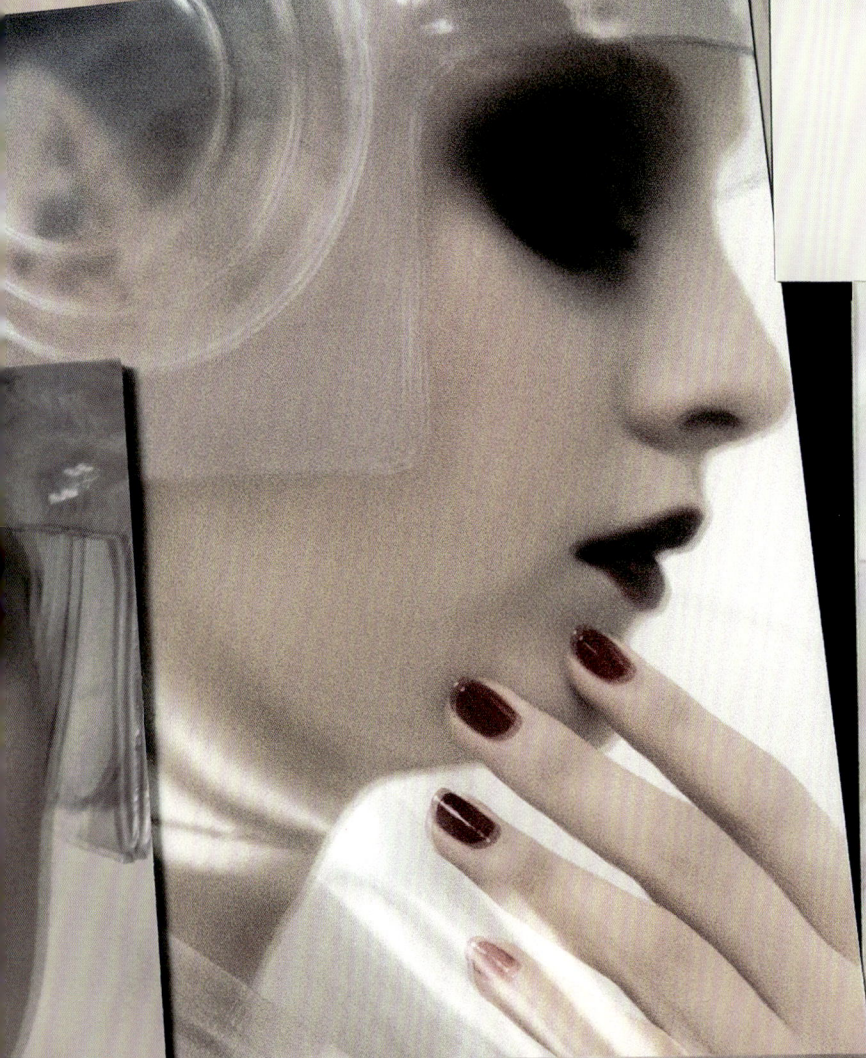

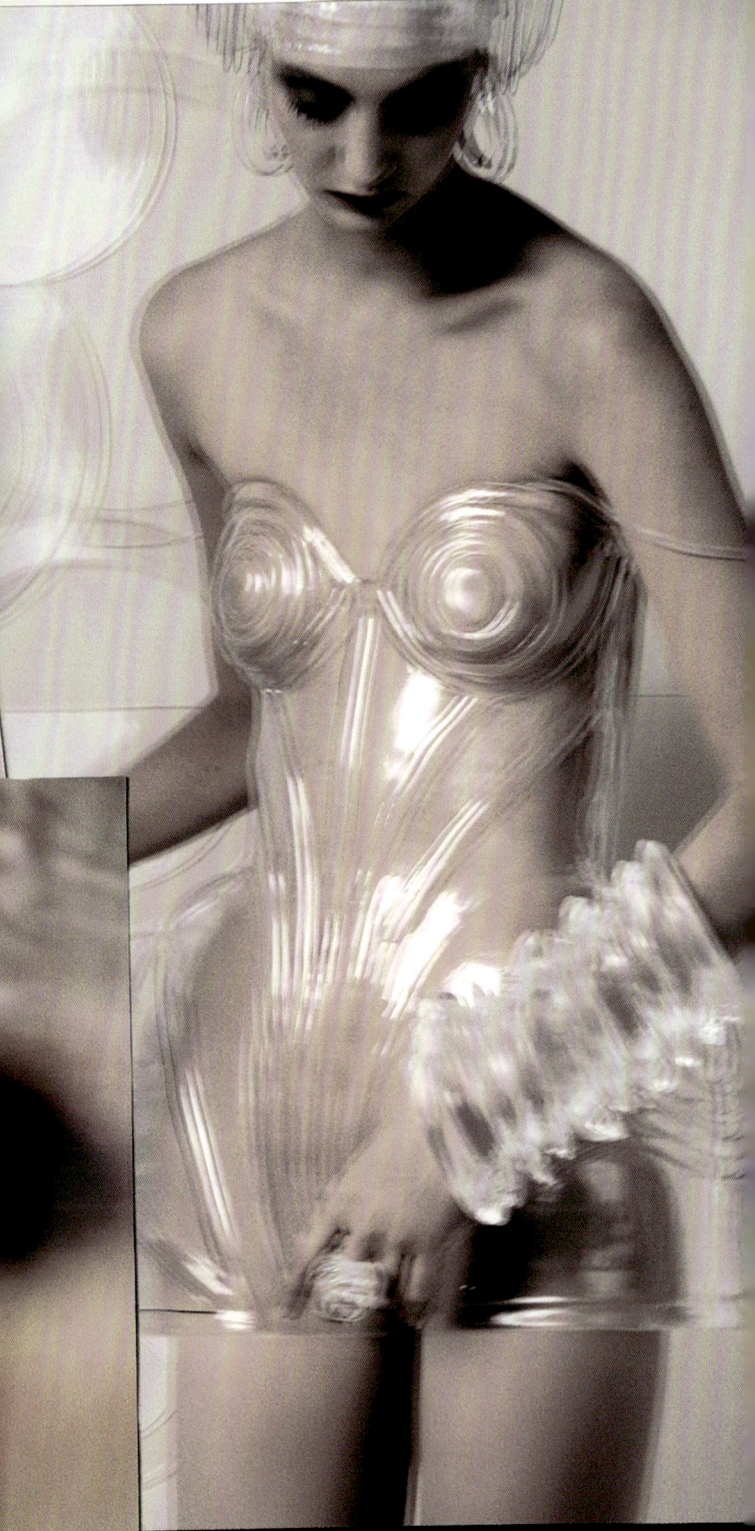

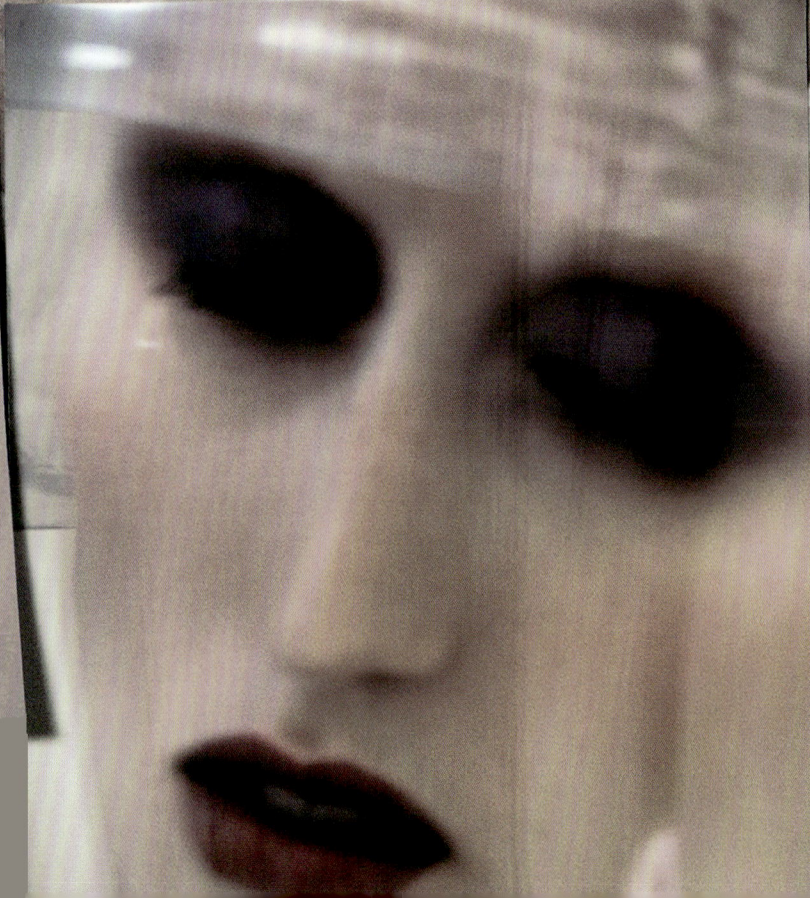

NARS

SARAH
MOON

MOON
HALL

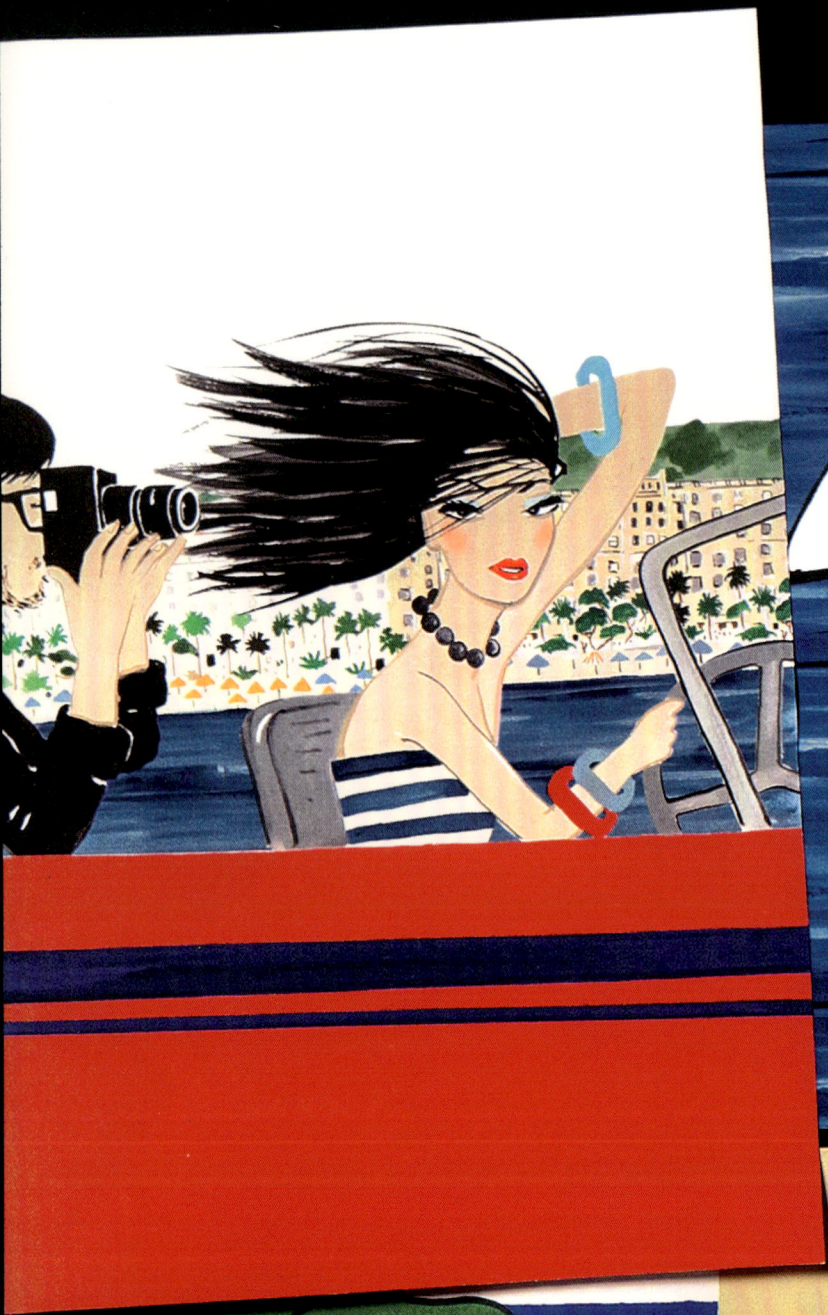

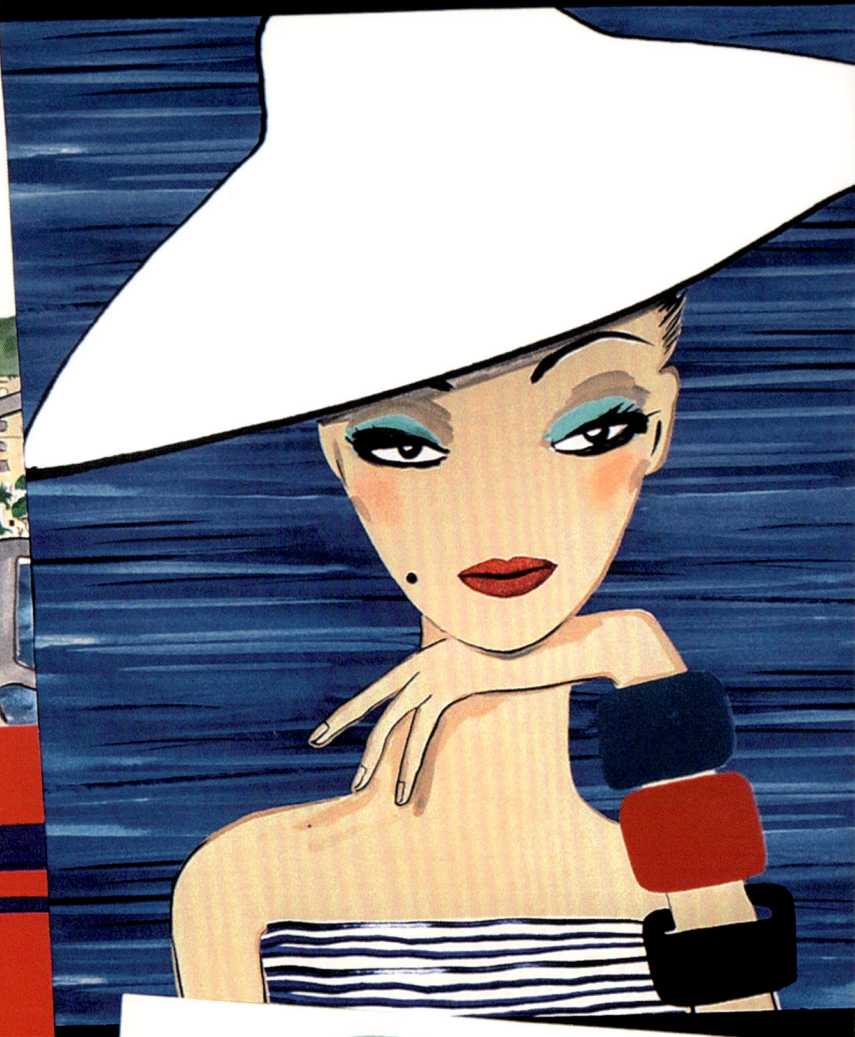

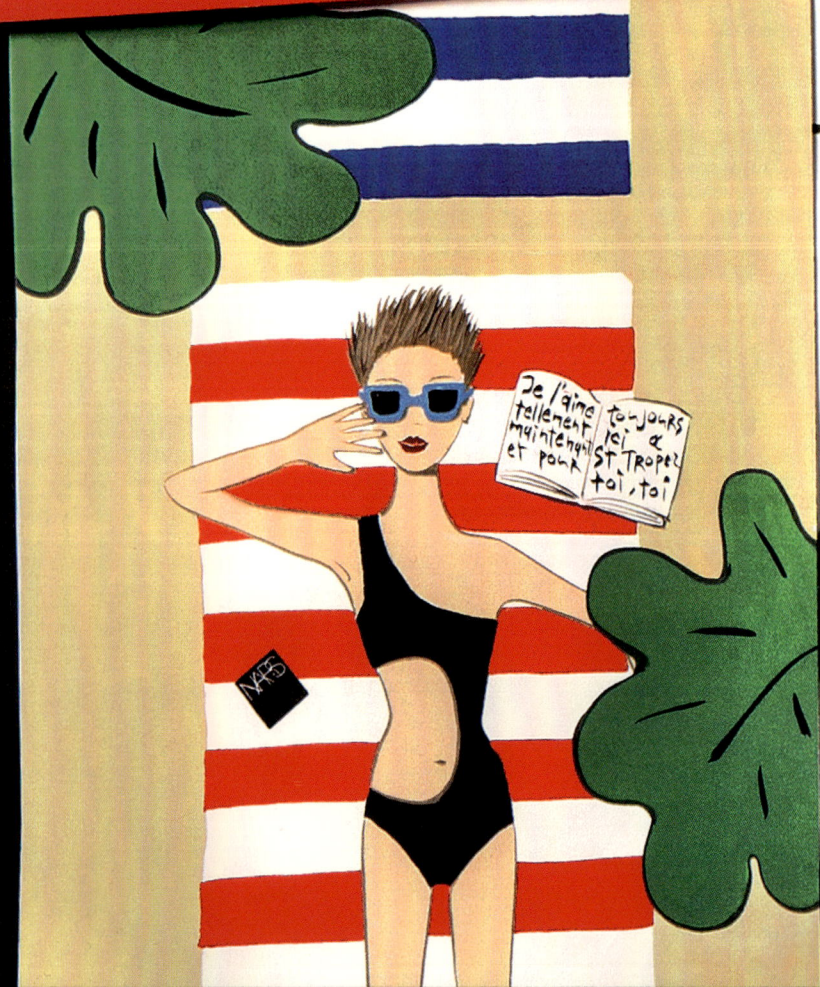

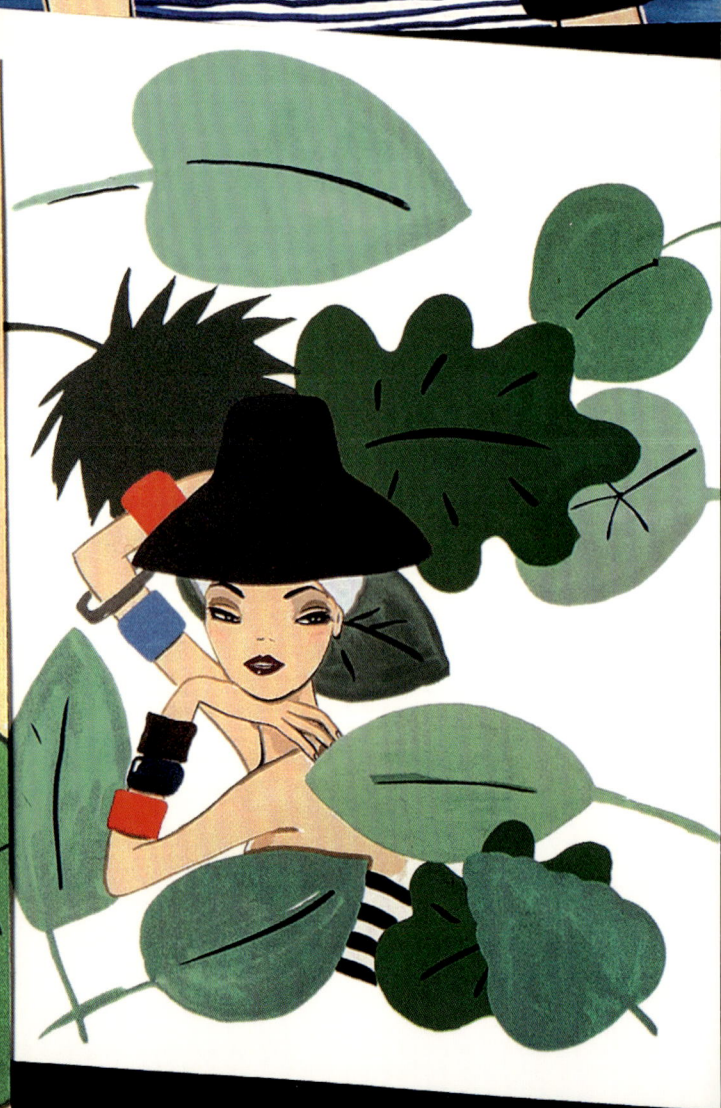

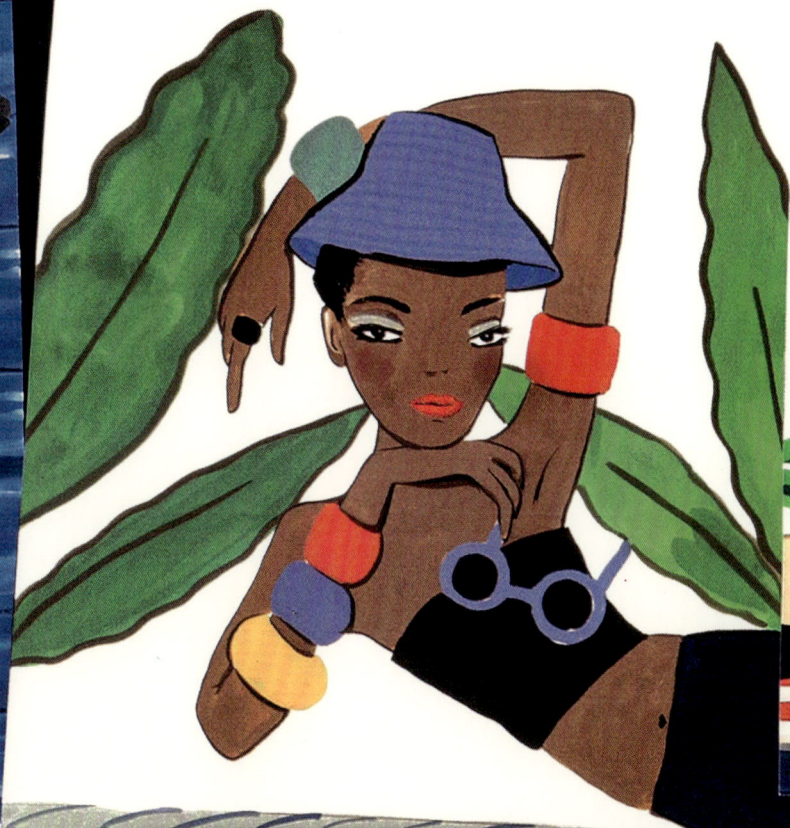

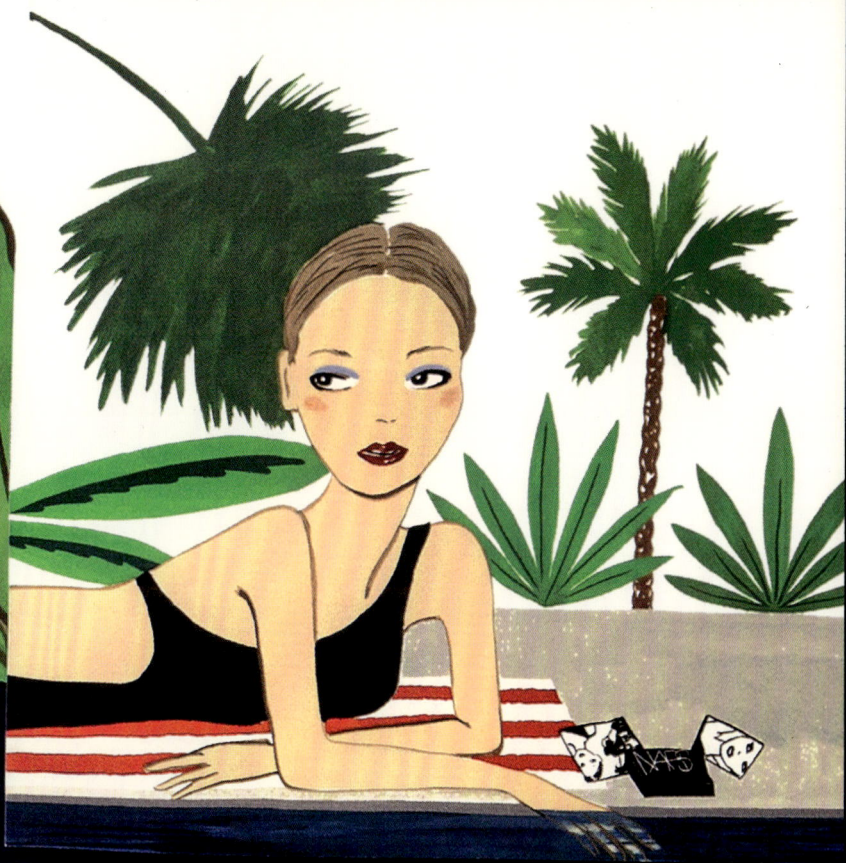

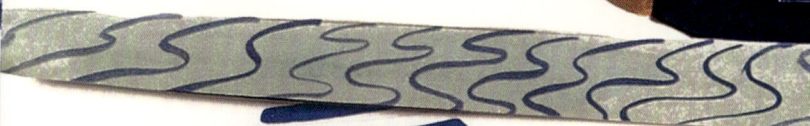

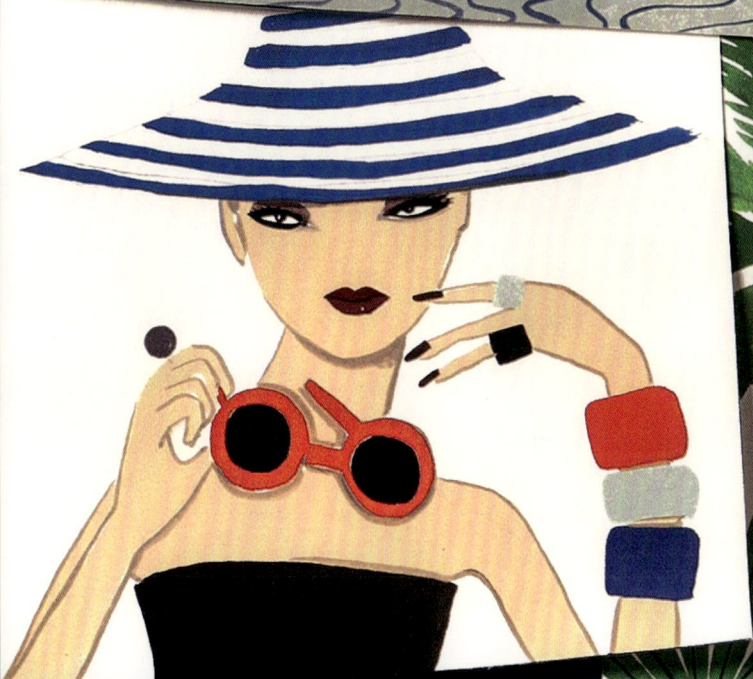

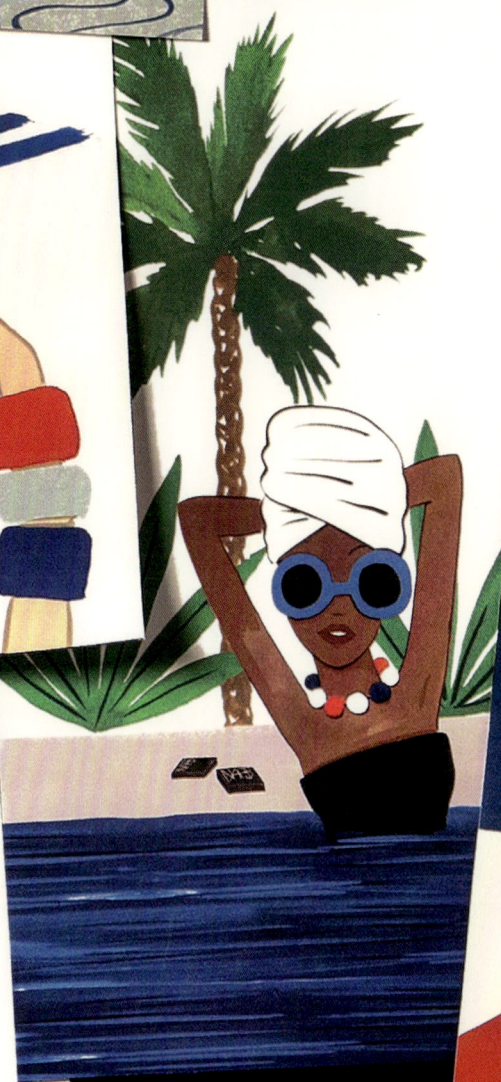

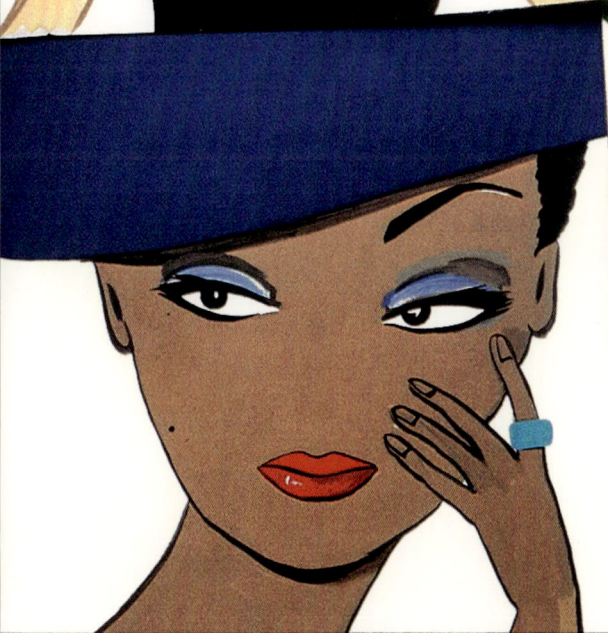

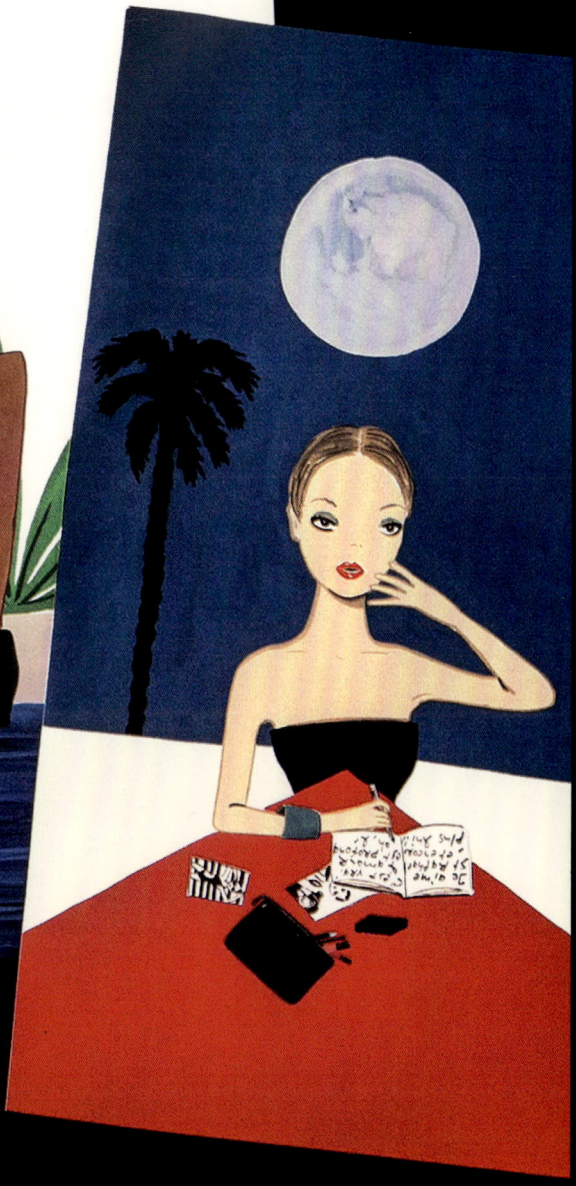

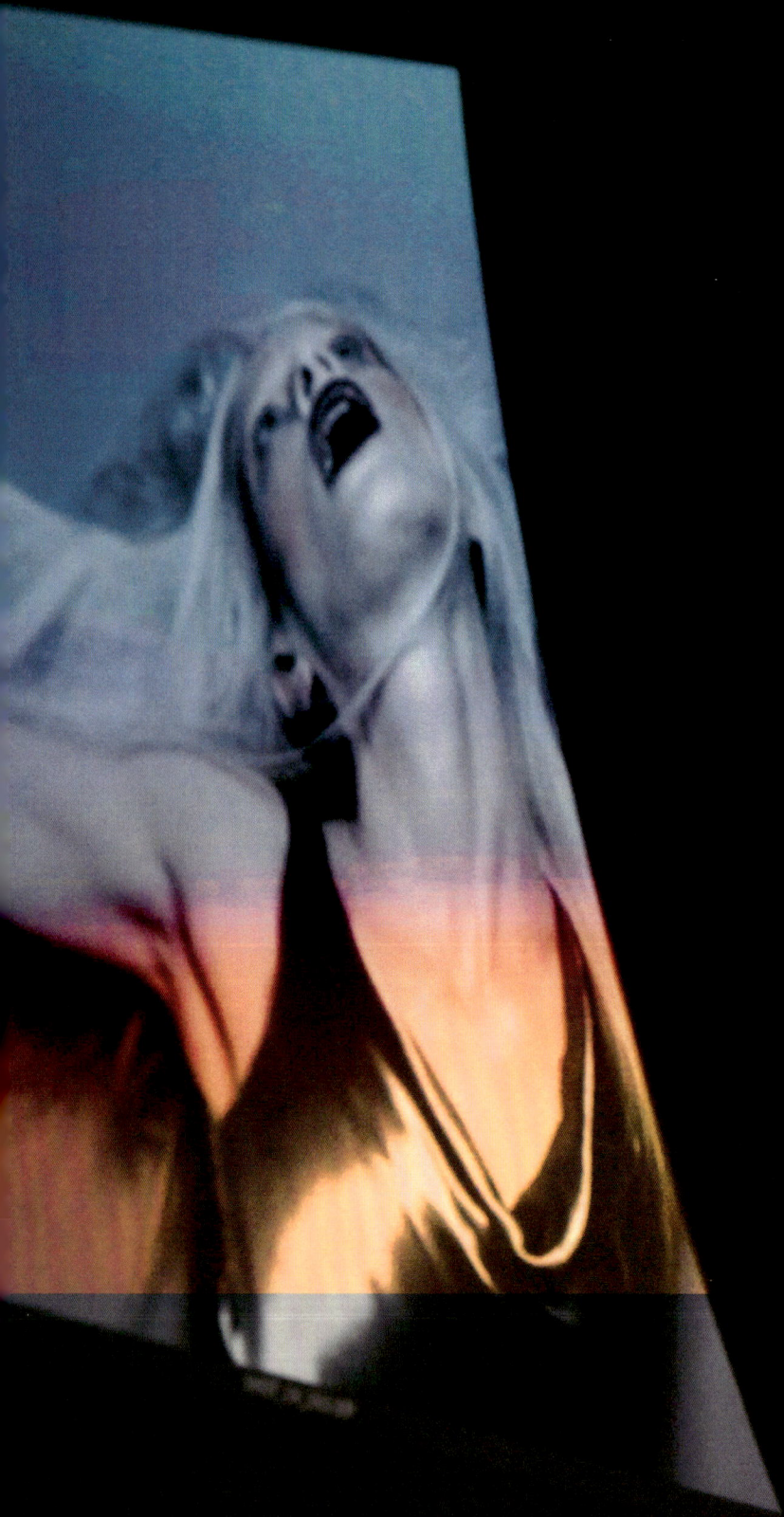

"I ADORE SHOOTING CAMPAIGNS FOR NARS, IT'S SO MUCH FUN TO CREATE AN IMAGE FOR THE BRAND AND FIND A FACE TO REPRESENT WHAT I AM LOOKING FOR – A BEAUTIFUL GIRL WITH STRENGTH AND CHARISMA."
– FRANÇOIS NARS

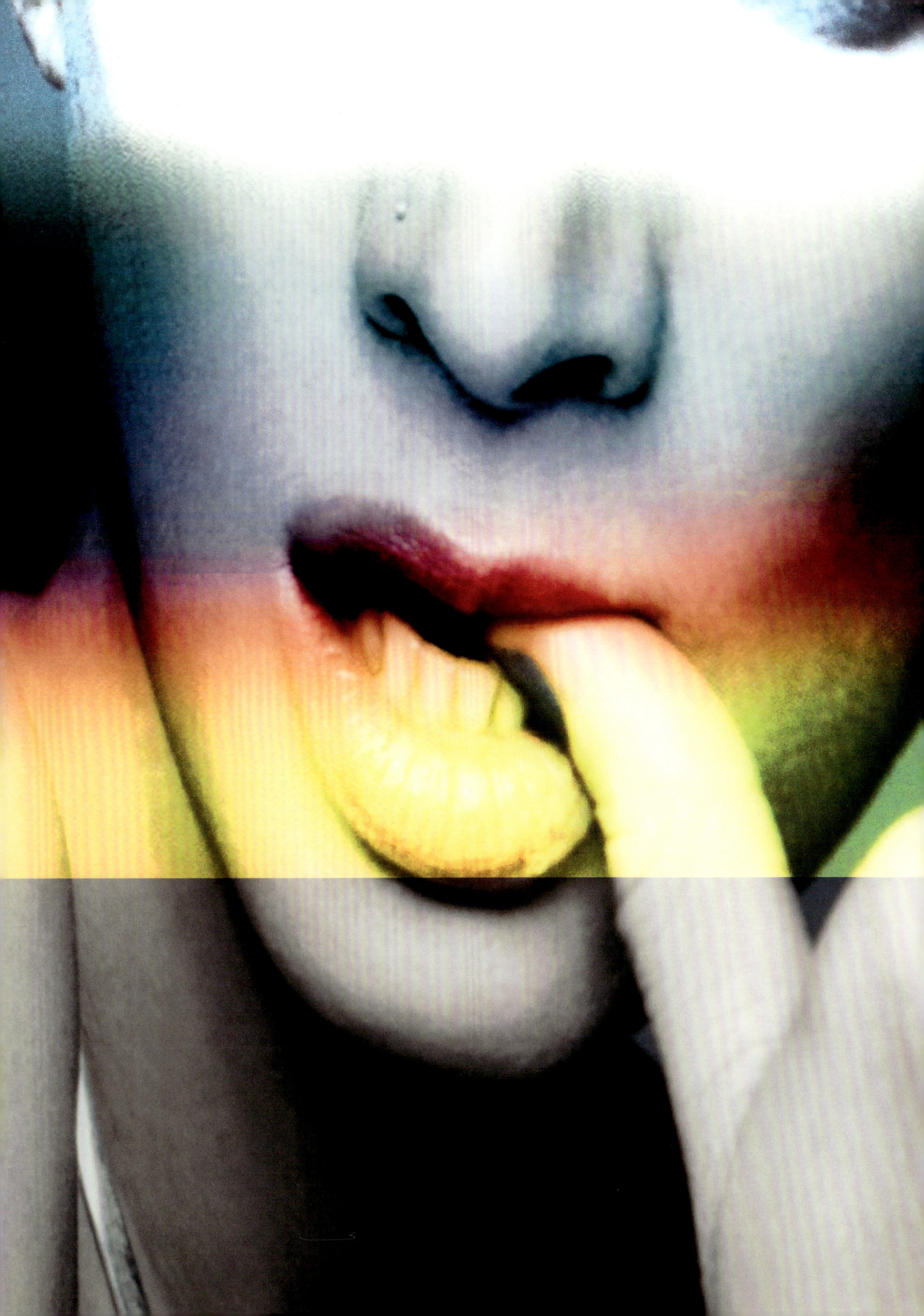

"FRANÇOIS NARS IS THE
MOST INFLUENCIAL ICON
IN BEAUTY TODAY. HE
HAS TAUGHT ME SOME
OF THE MOST IMPORTANT
LESSONS IN MY CAREER.
BE AUTHENTIC. BE THE
BEST. BE PASSIONATE
AND LOVE WHAT YOU DO.
TAKE RISKS. PUSH THE
BOUNDARIES. NEVER
SETTLE. HIS VALUES
ARE DEEPLY EMBEDDED
IN THE CULTURE AND
LEADERSHIP AT NARS.
I AM HONORED TO HAVE
HIM AS A MENTOR."
– BARBARA CALCAGNI,
PRESIDENT OF NARS
COSMETICS SINCE 2015

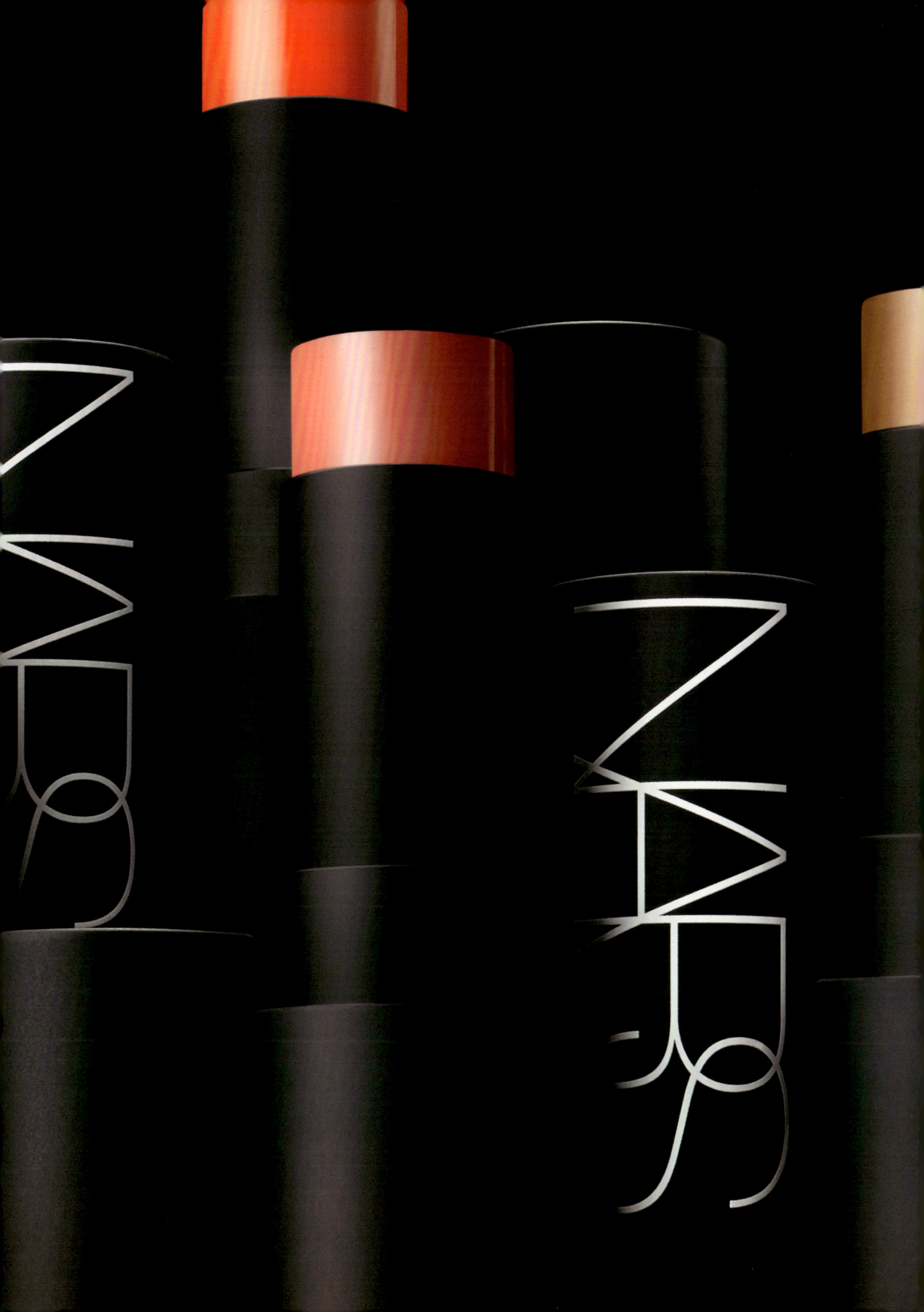

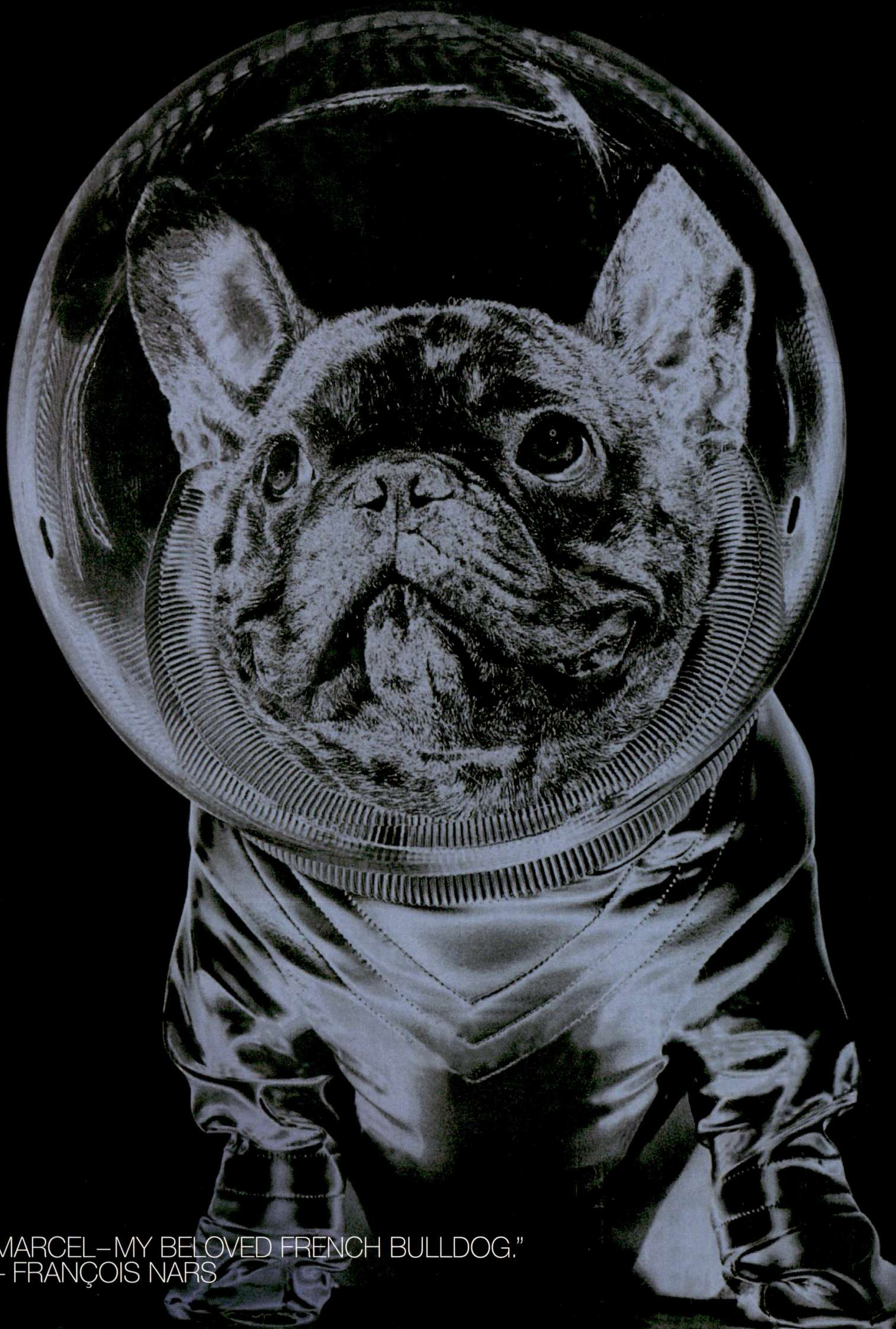

"MARCEL—MY BELOVED FRENCH BULLDOG."
– FRANÇOIS NARS

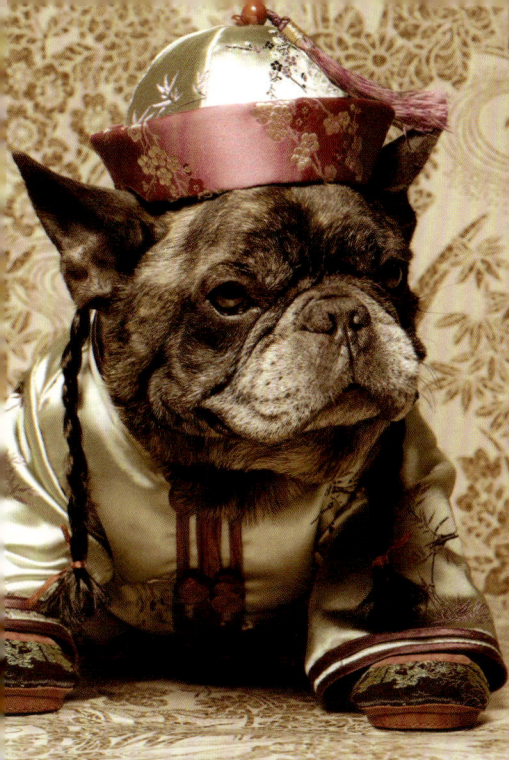

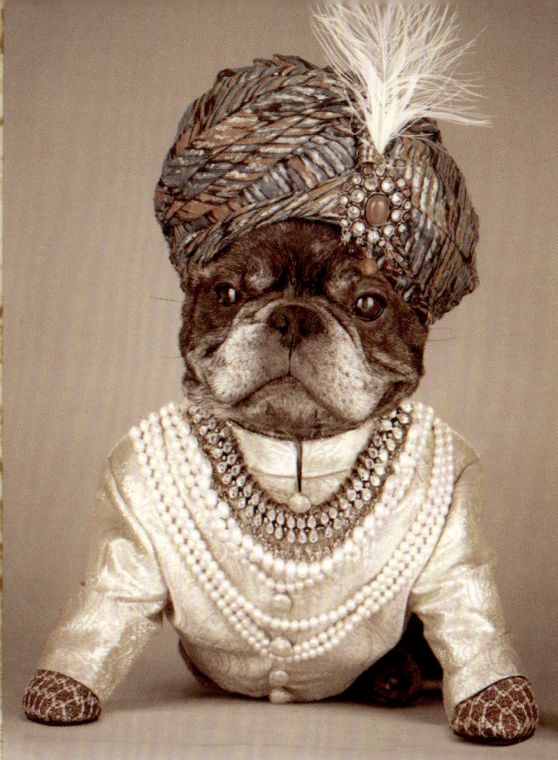

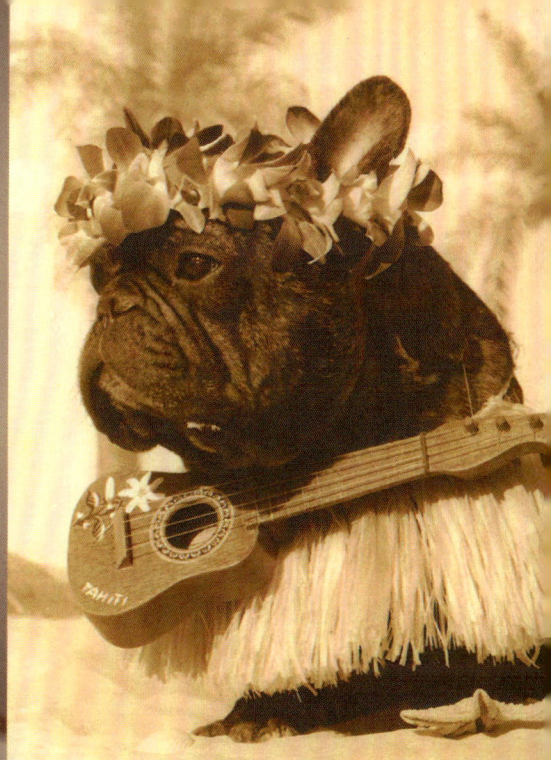

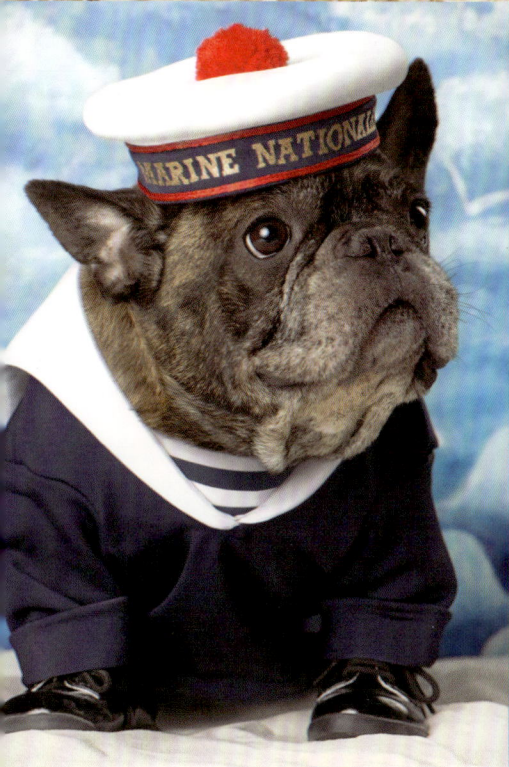

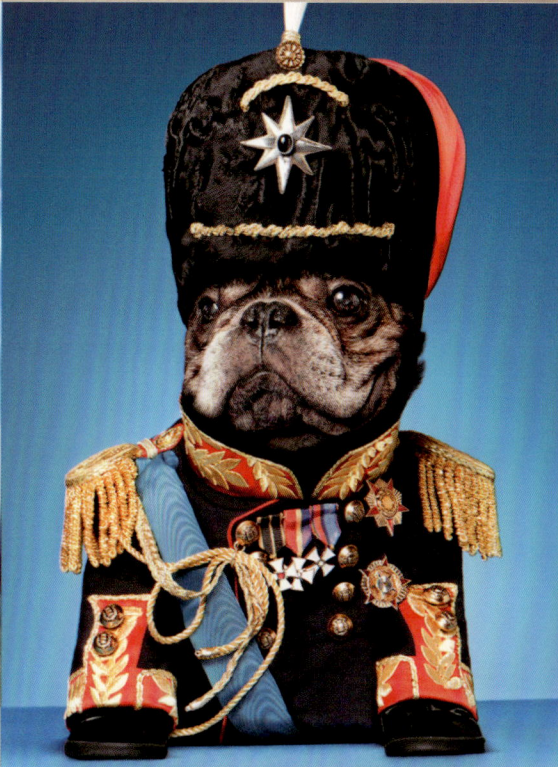

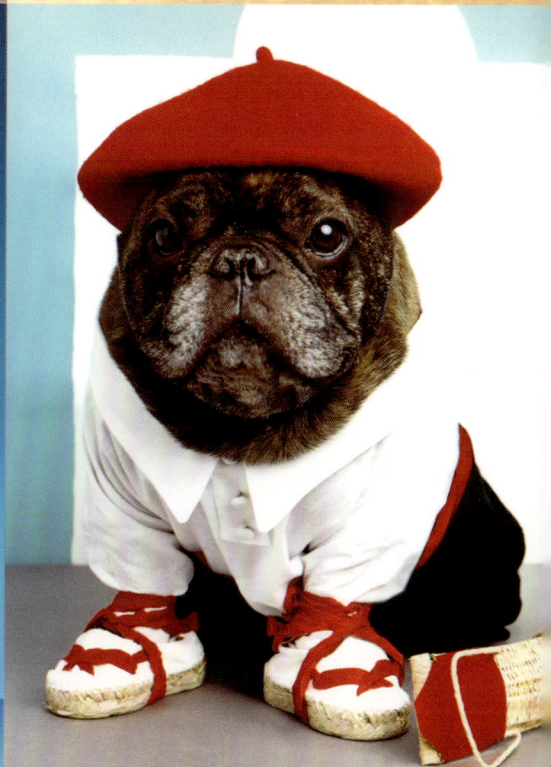

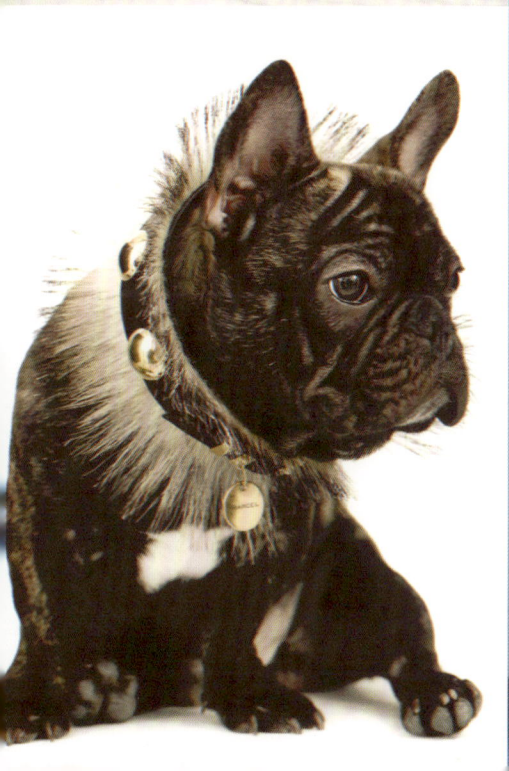

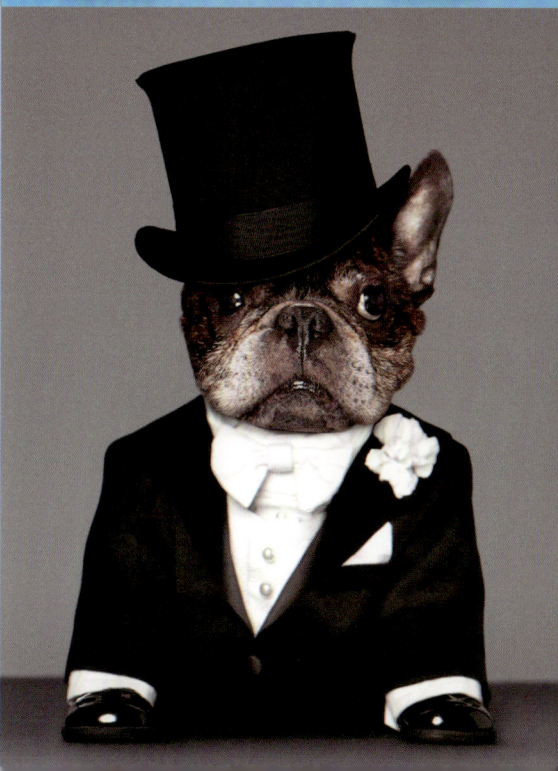

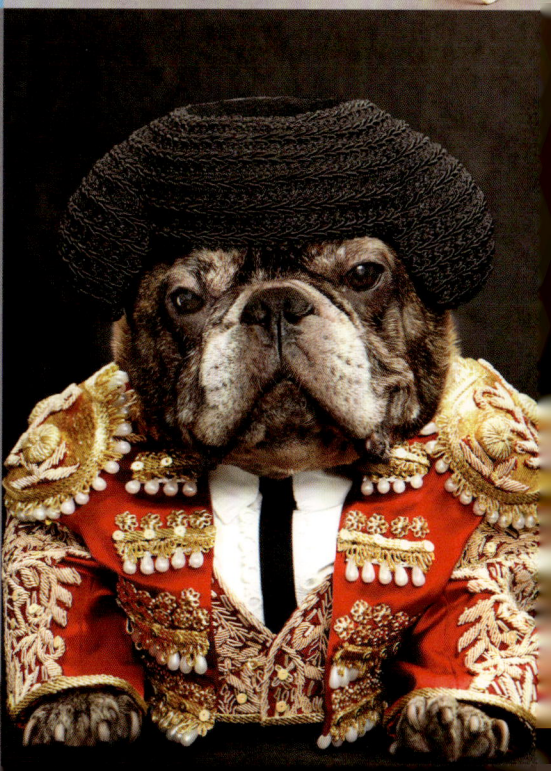

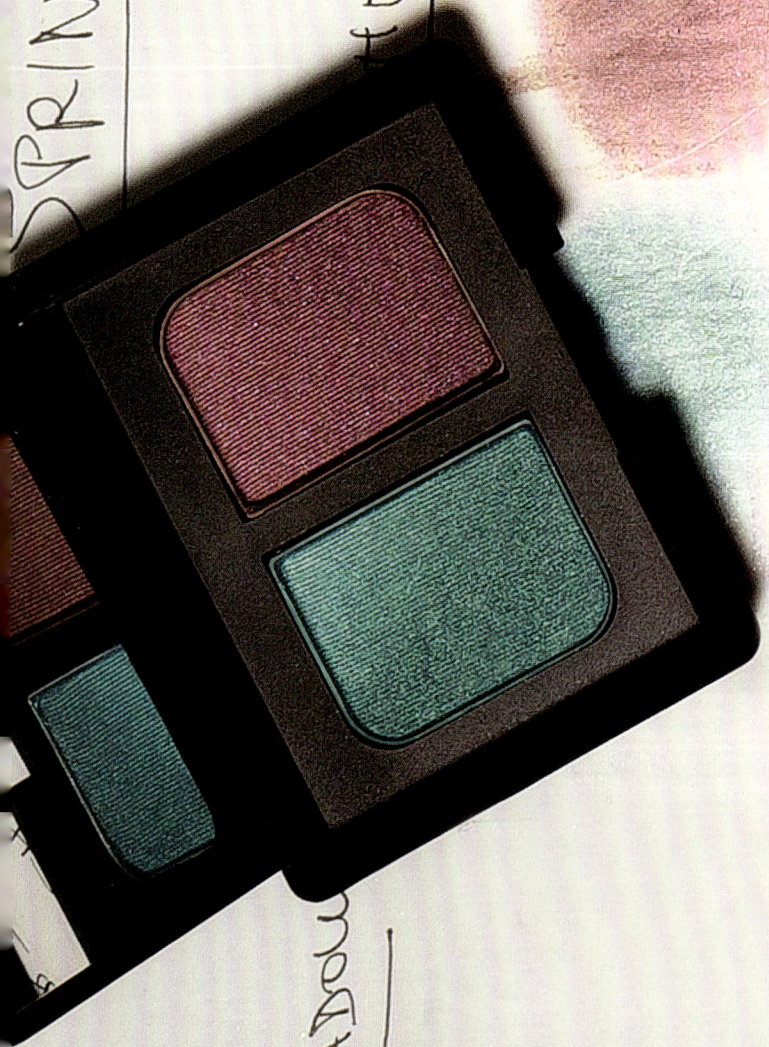
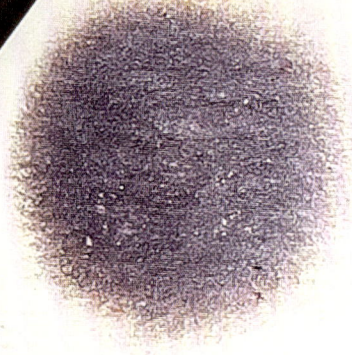
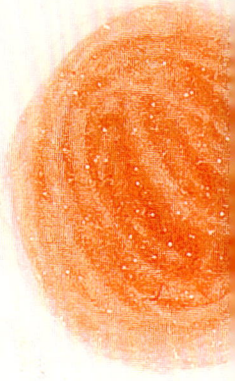

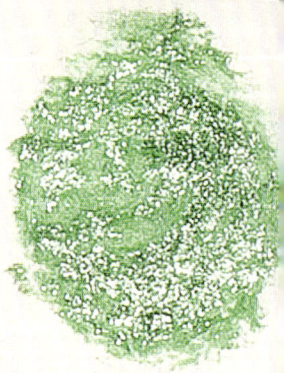
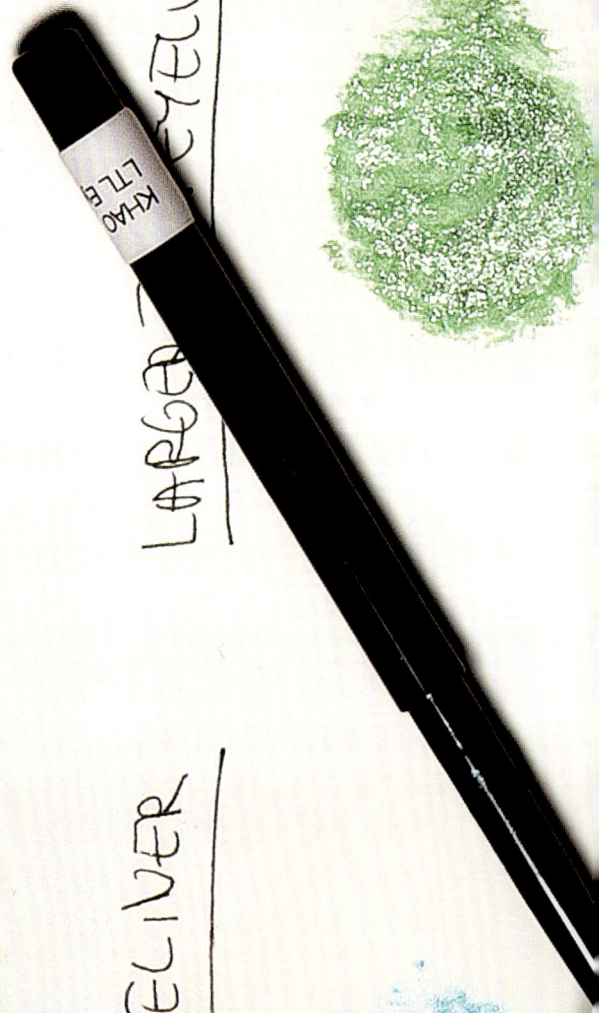
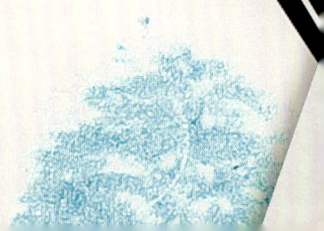

SPRING 2014

DUO

EYESHADOW

"ISKANDAR"

SATIN LIP PENCIL

"CHINA SEAS"

LARGE EYELINER

"KHAO LTE E"

EYESHADOW

"SNOW"

EYELINER

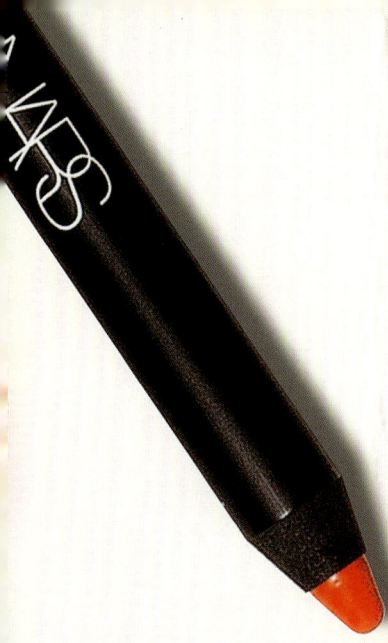

NARS

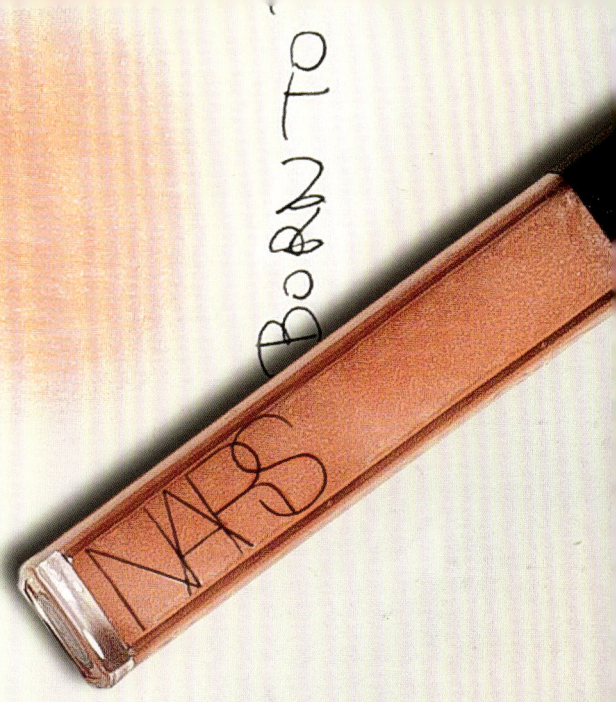

BORN TO

NARS

COAST "

SOL
(MADRI SQUARE "
POLI

PU
LTL

" I DON'T HAVE RULES !
JUST HAVE FUN ! .
YOU CAN'T GO WRONG WITH
MAKE UP . AND IF YOU DO .
WASH IT OFF AND TRY SOMETHING
ELSE . LIFE IS SHORT AND YOU
SHOULD ENJOY IT !! "
— FRANÇOIS NARS

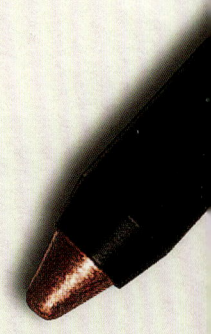

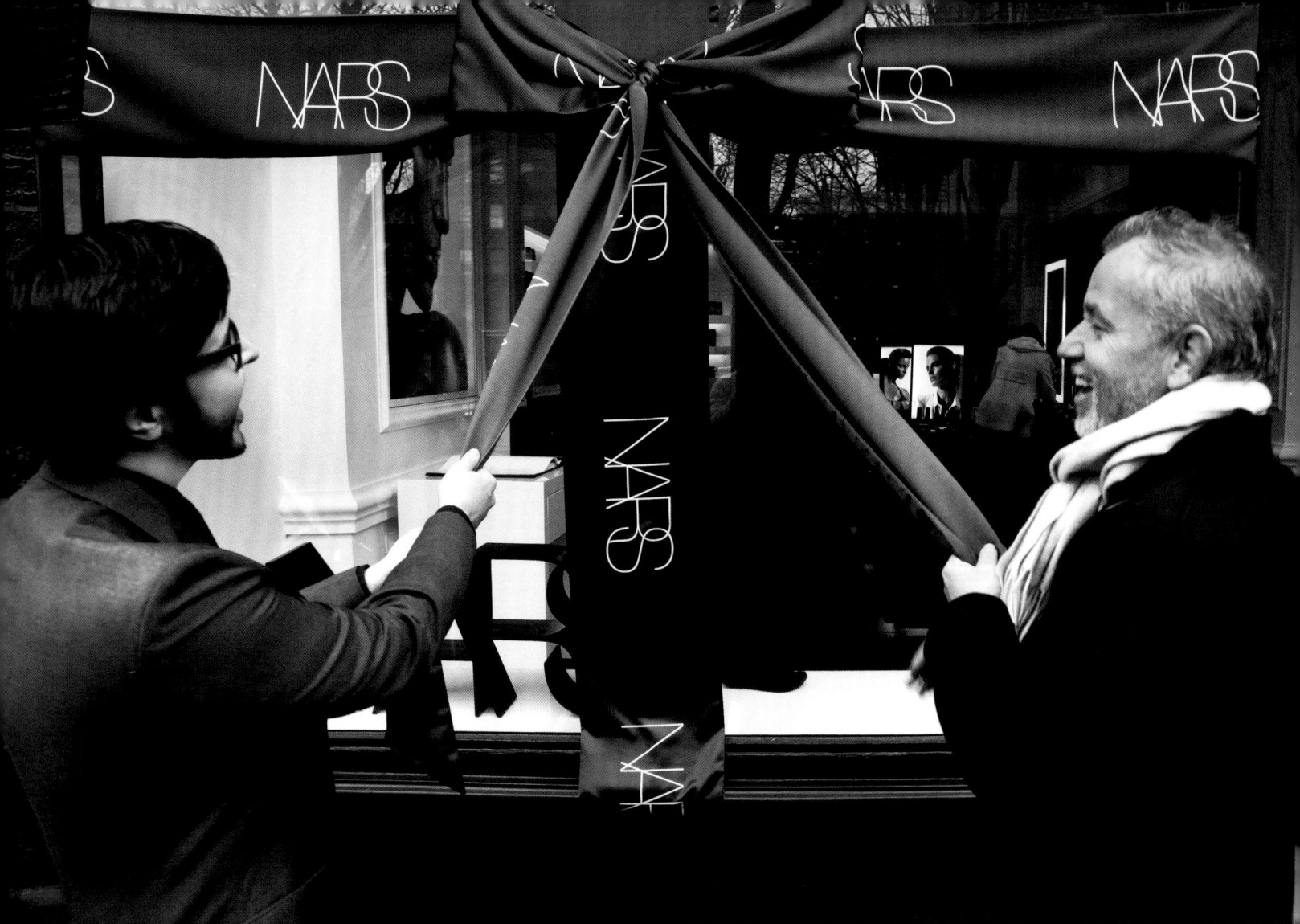

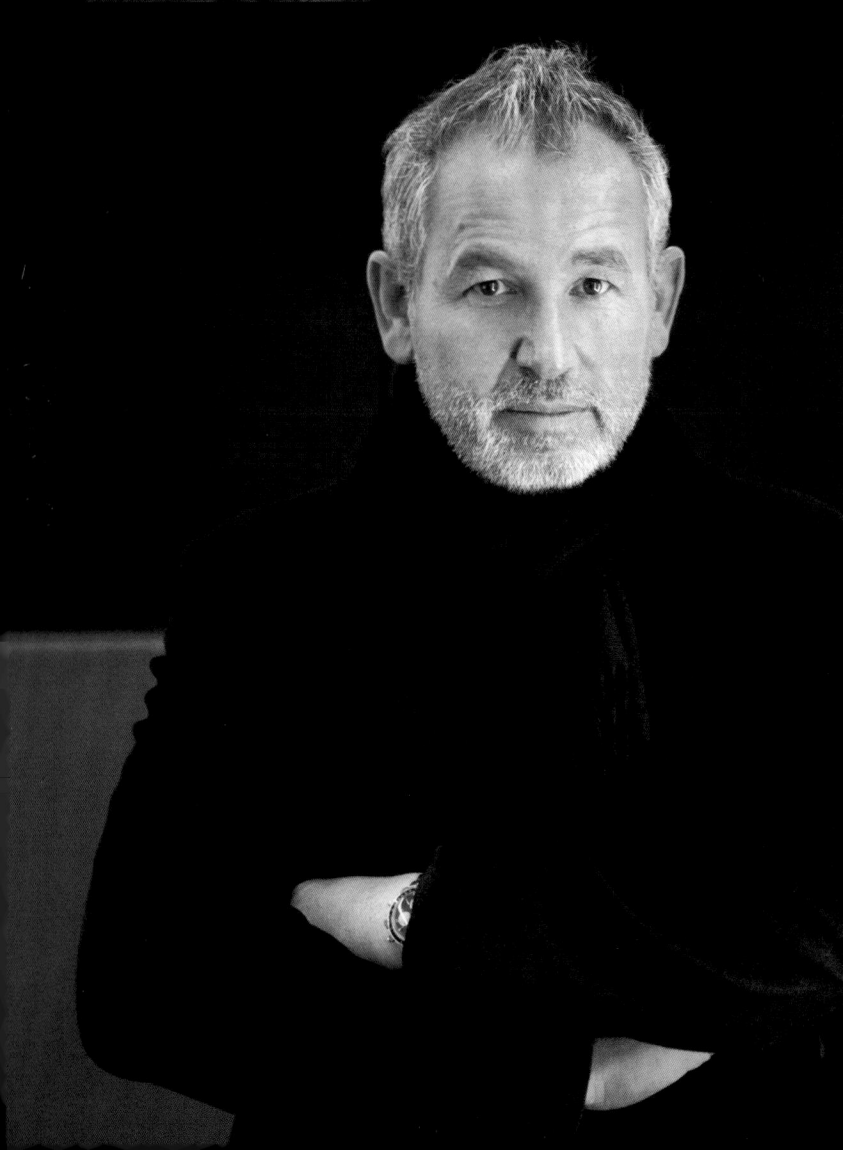

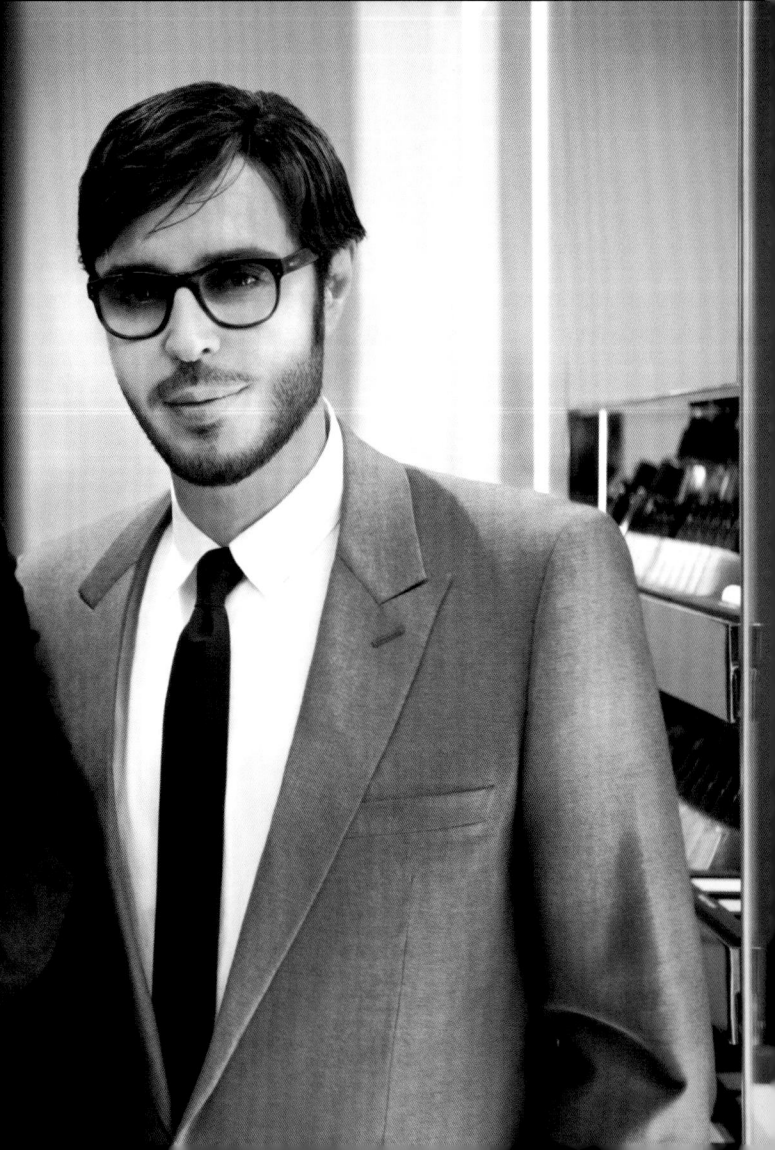

"FABIEN AND I, A CREATIVE PARTNERSHIP OF TWENTY YEARS AND A FRIENDSHIP OF MANY MORE. THERE IS ONLY ONE FABIEN. HE IS JUST AMAZING."
– FRANÇOIS NARS

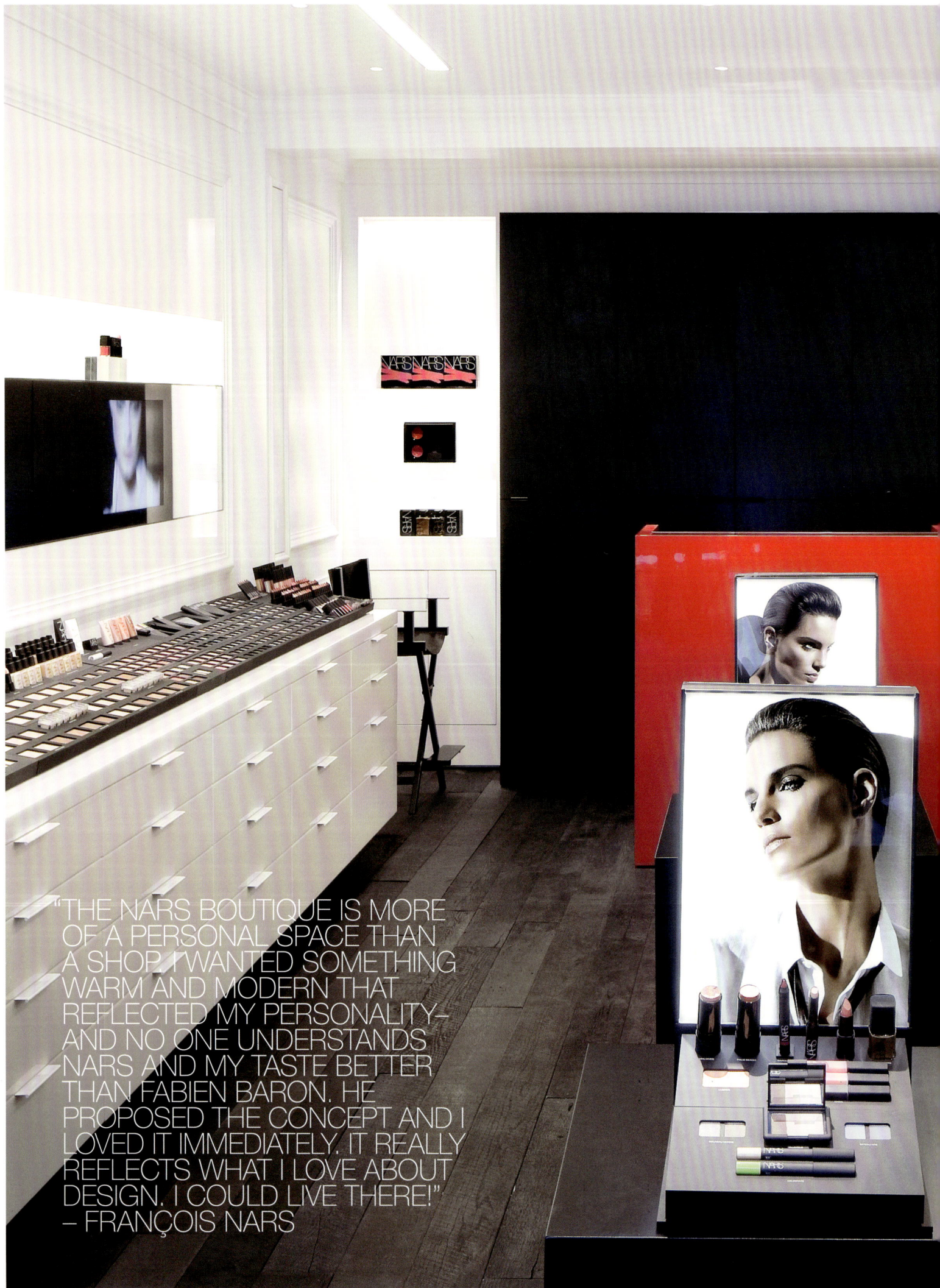

"THE NARS BOUTIQUE IS MORE OF A PERSONAL SPACE THAN A SHOP. I WANTED SOMETHING WARM AND MODERN THAT REFLECTED MY PERSONALITY— AND NO ONE UNDERSTANDS NARS AND MY TASTE BETTER THAN FABIEN BARON. HE PROPOSED THE CONCEPT AND I LOVED IT IMMEDIATELY. IT REALLY REFLECTS WHAT I LOVE ABOUT DESIGN. I COULD LIVE THERE!"
– FRANÇOIS NARS

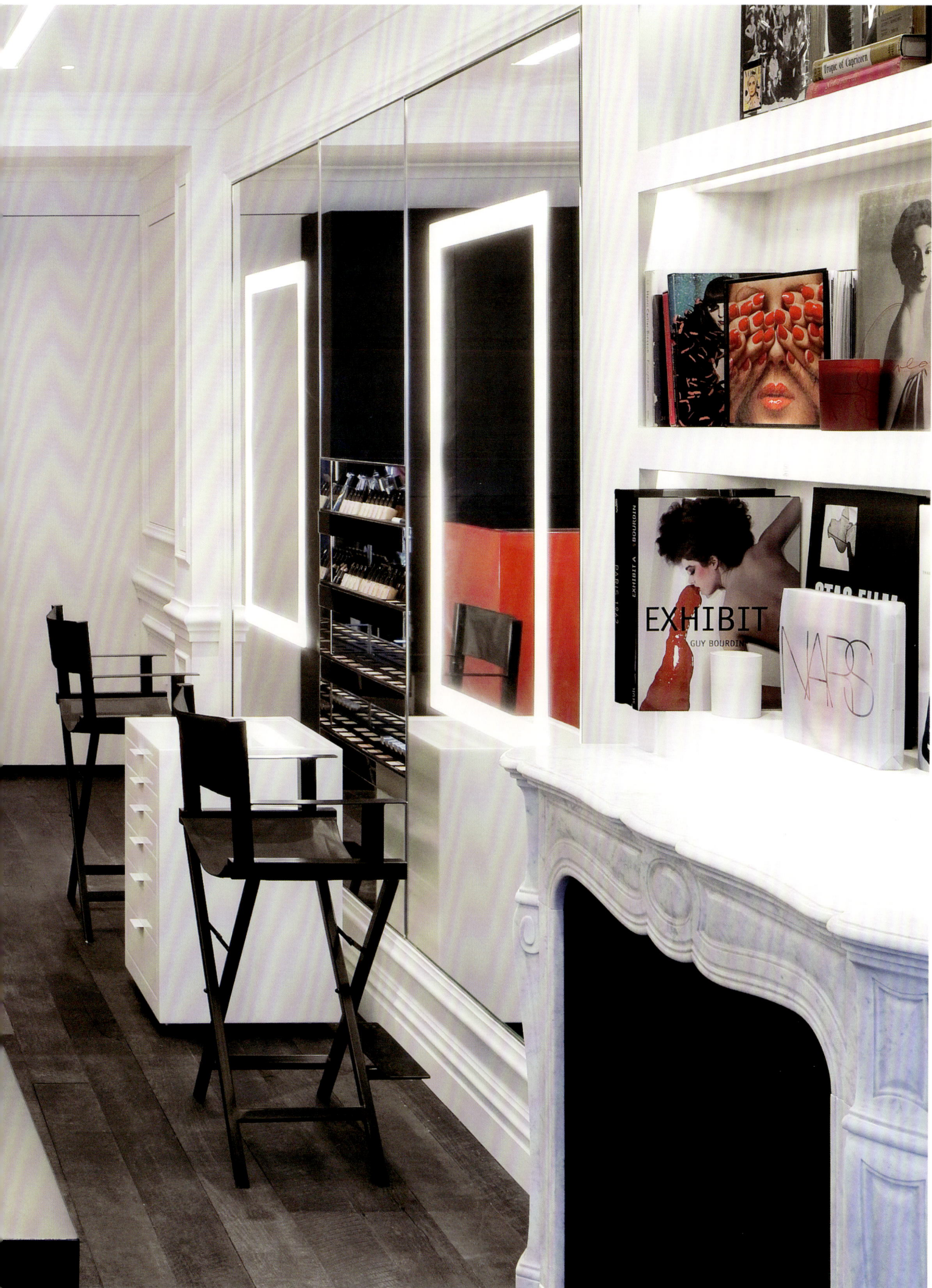

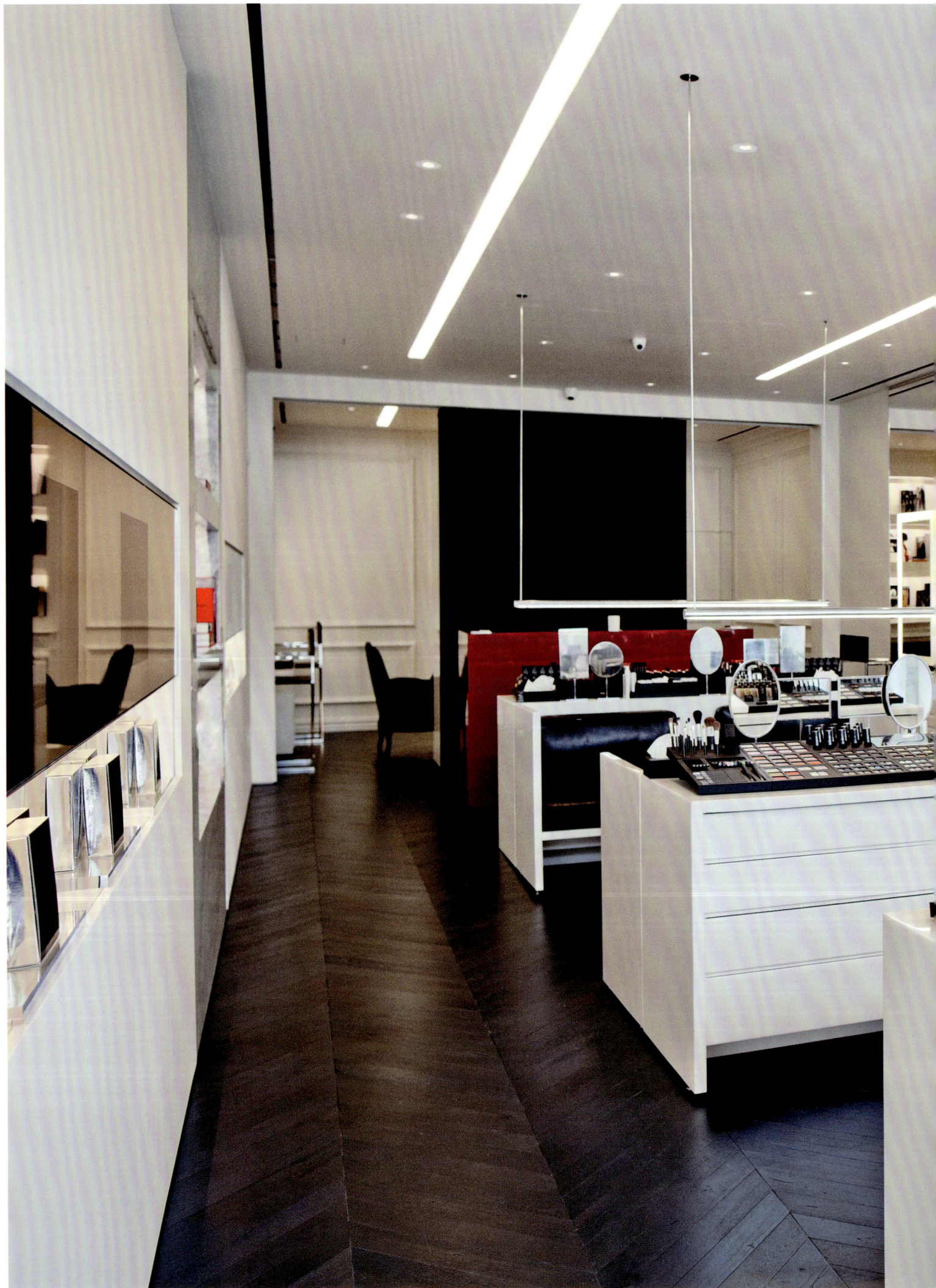

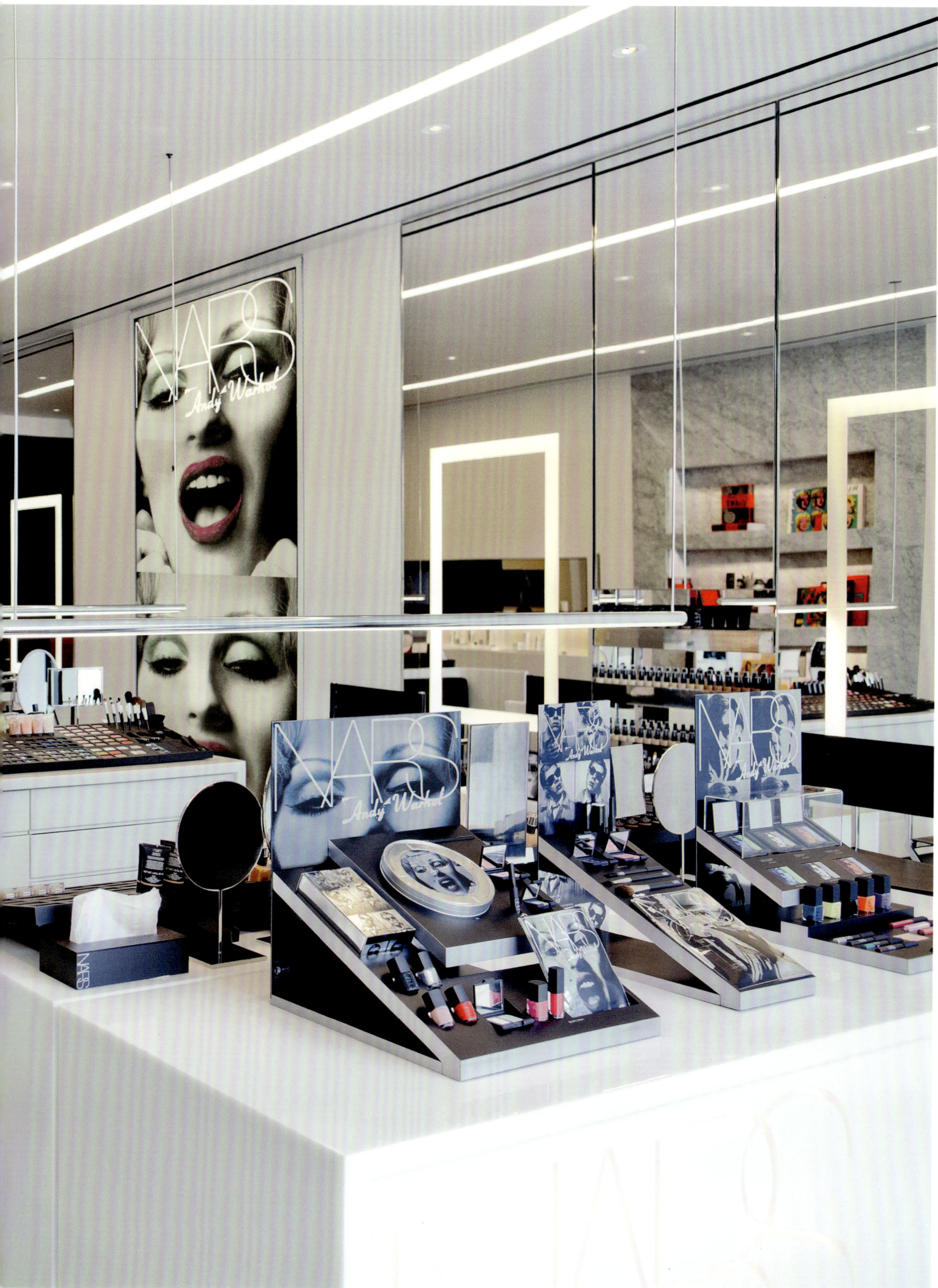

"IN ALL MY YEARS WORKING WITH FRANÇOIS NARS, I HAVE COME TO BELIEVE THAT HE IS TO MAKEUP WHAT YVES SAINT LAURENT IS TO FASHION: A VISIONARY, A RULE BREAKER, A GAME CHANGER. I FEEL IMMENSELY PRIVILEGED TO BE WORKING WITH HIM."
— LOUIS DESAZARS, CEO OF NARS COSMETICS FROM 2008 TO 2015

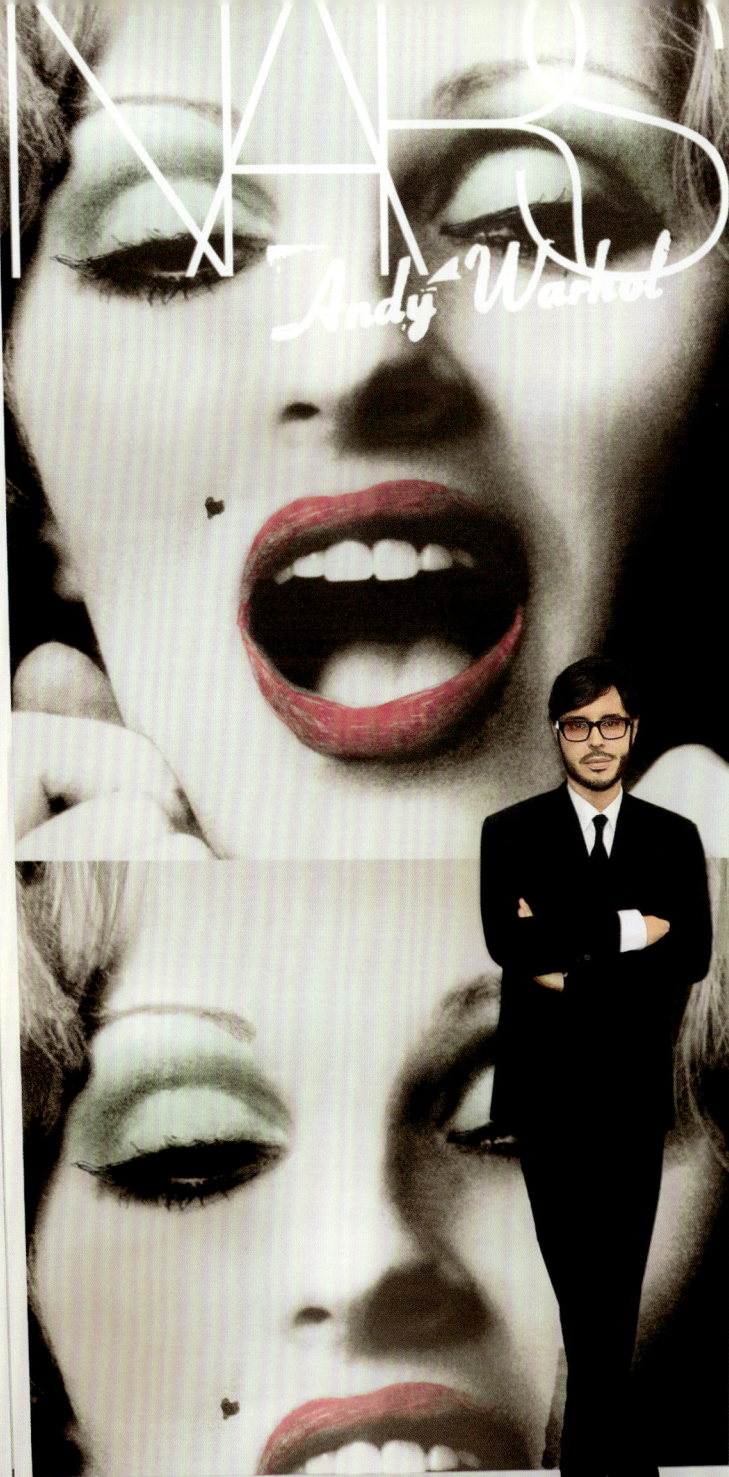

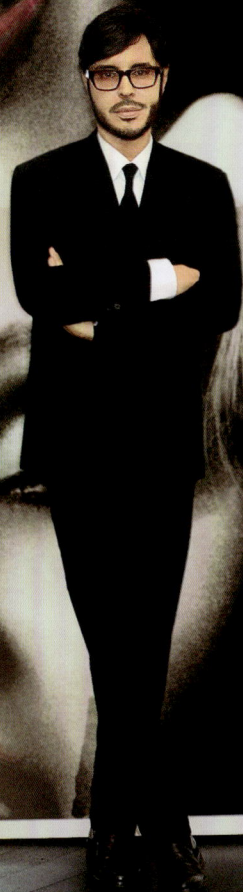

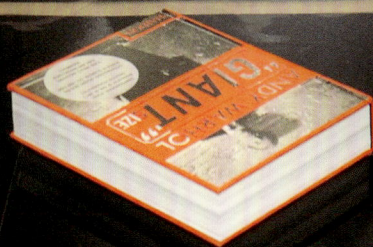

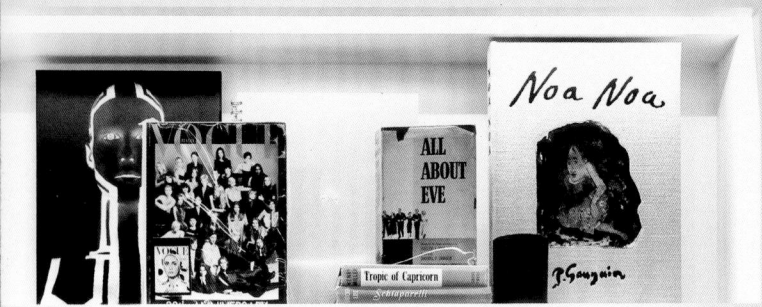

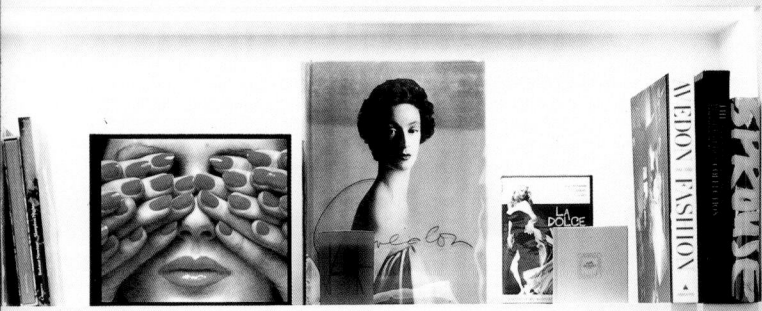

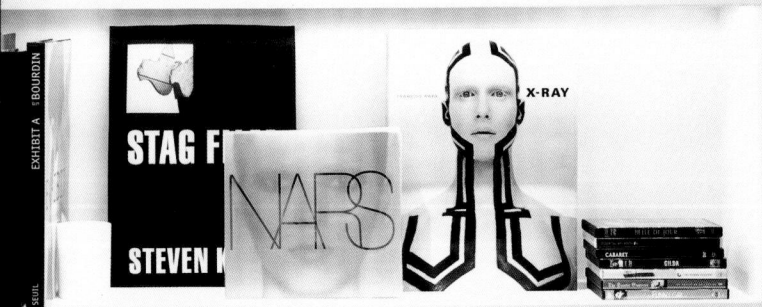

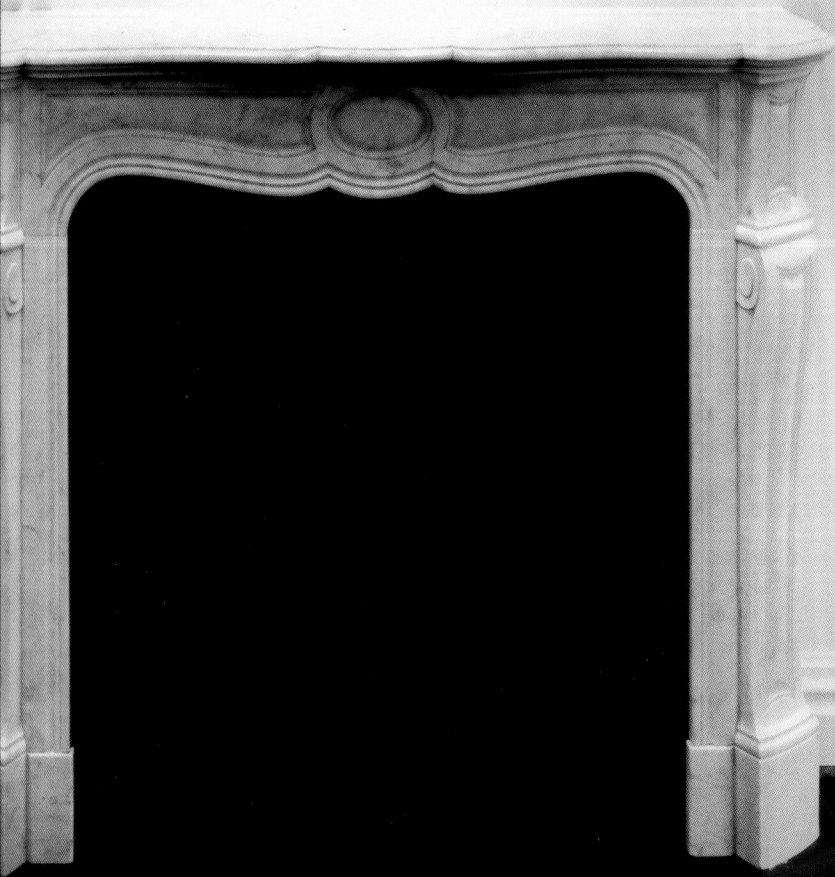

"THE BOUTIQUES ARE
FULL OF INSPIRATION
FROM PERSONAL ICONS
AND PLACES I'VE VISITED
OR DREAM OF VISITING.
I TRAVEL THROUGH
BOOKS, MOVIES, AND
MUSIC. IMAGINATION
IS VERY POWERFUL."
– FRANÇOIS NARS

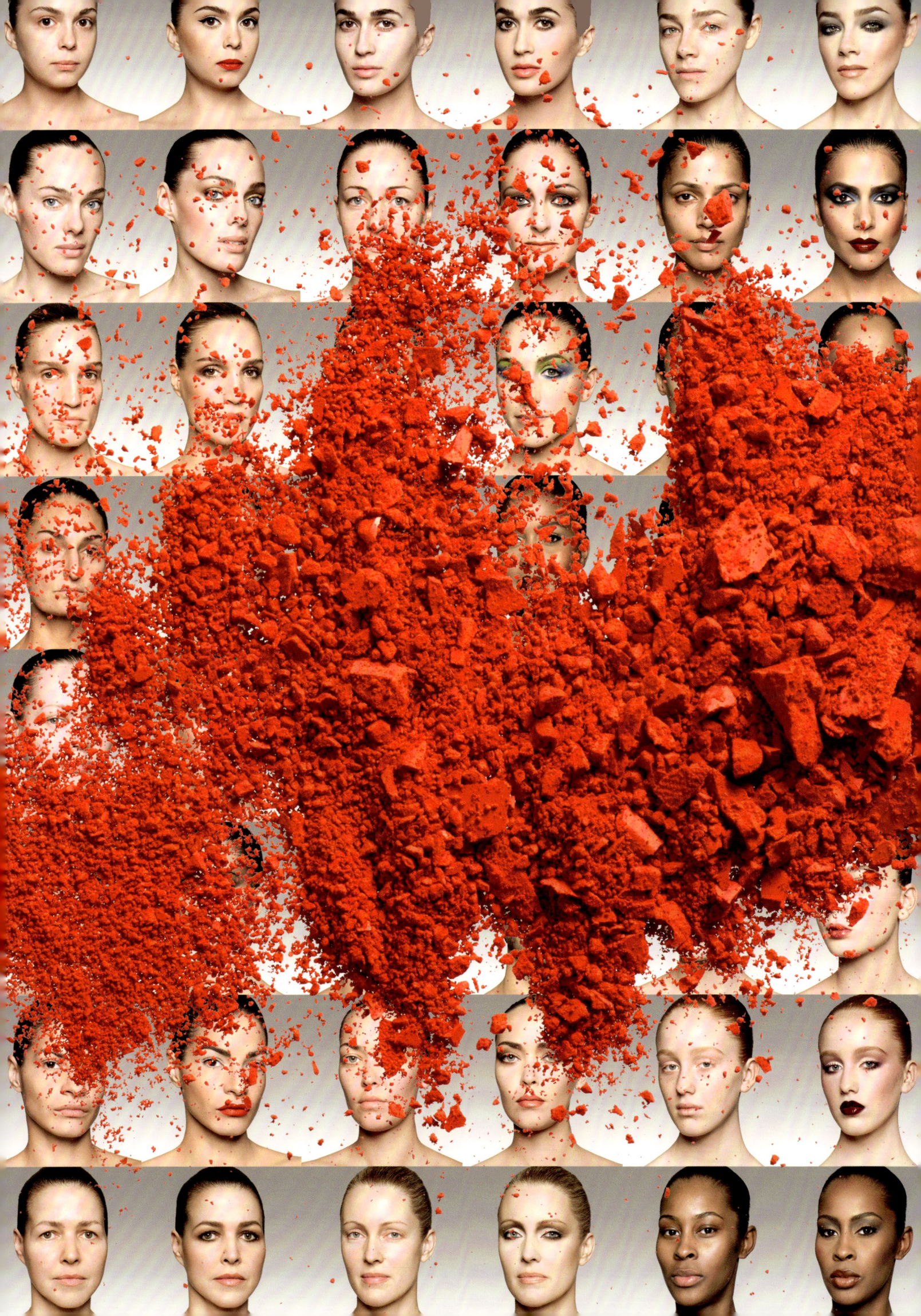

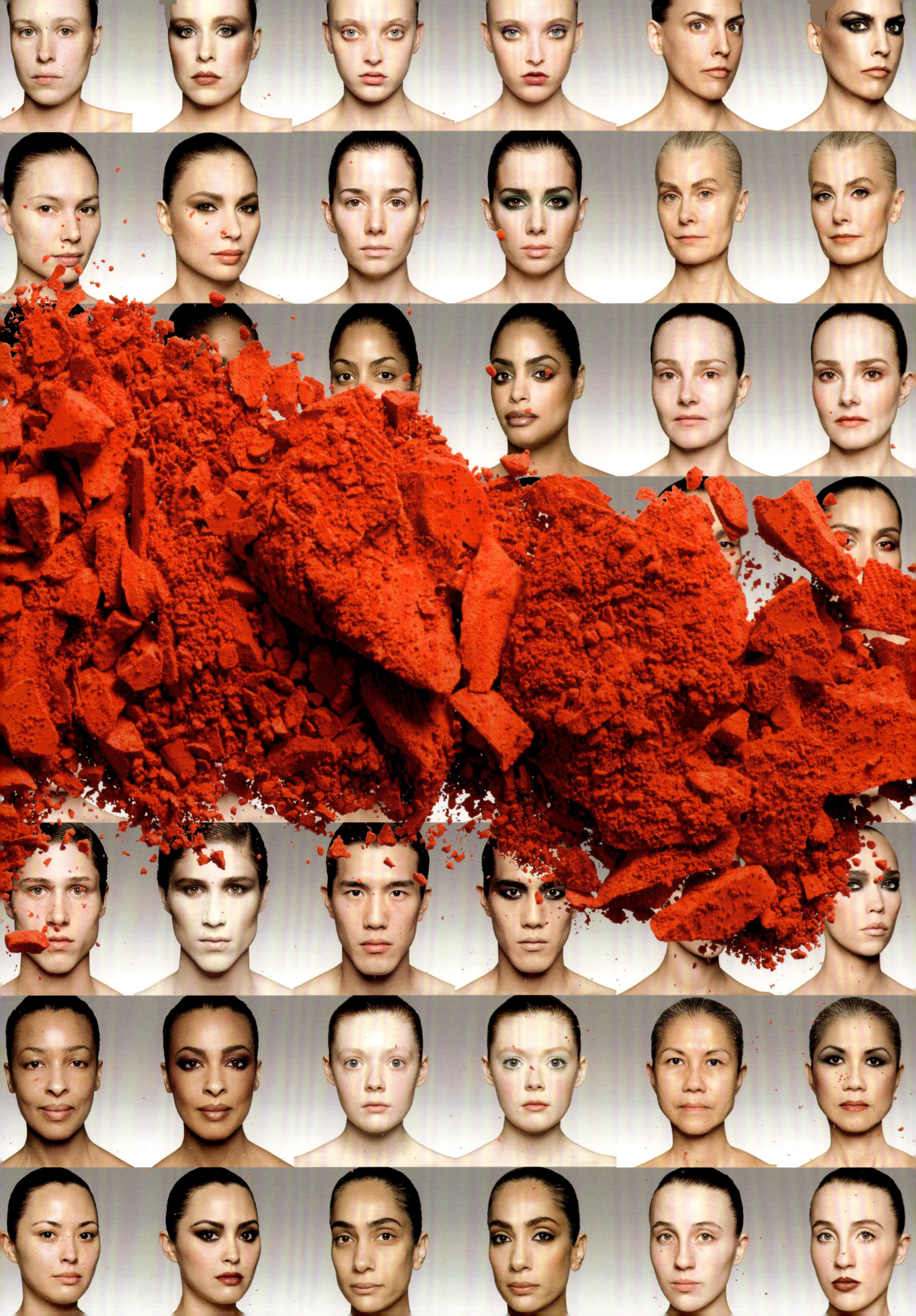

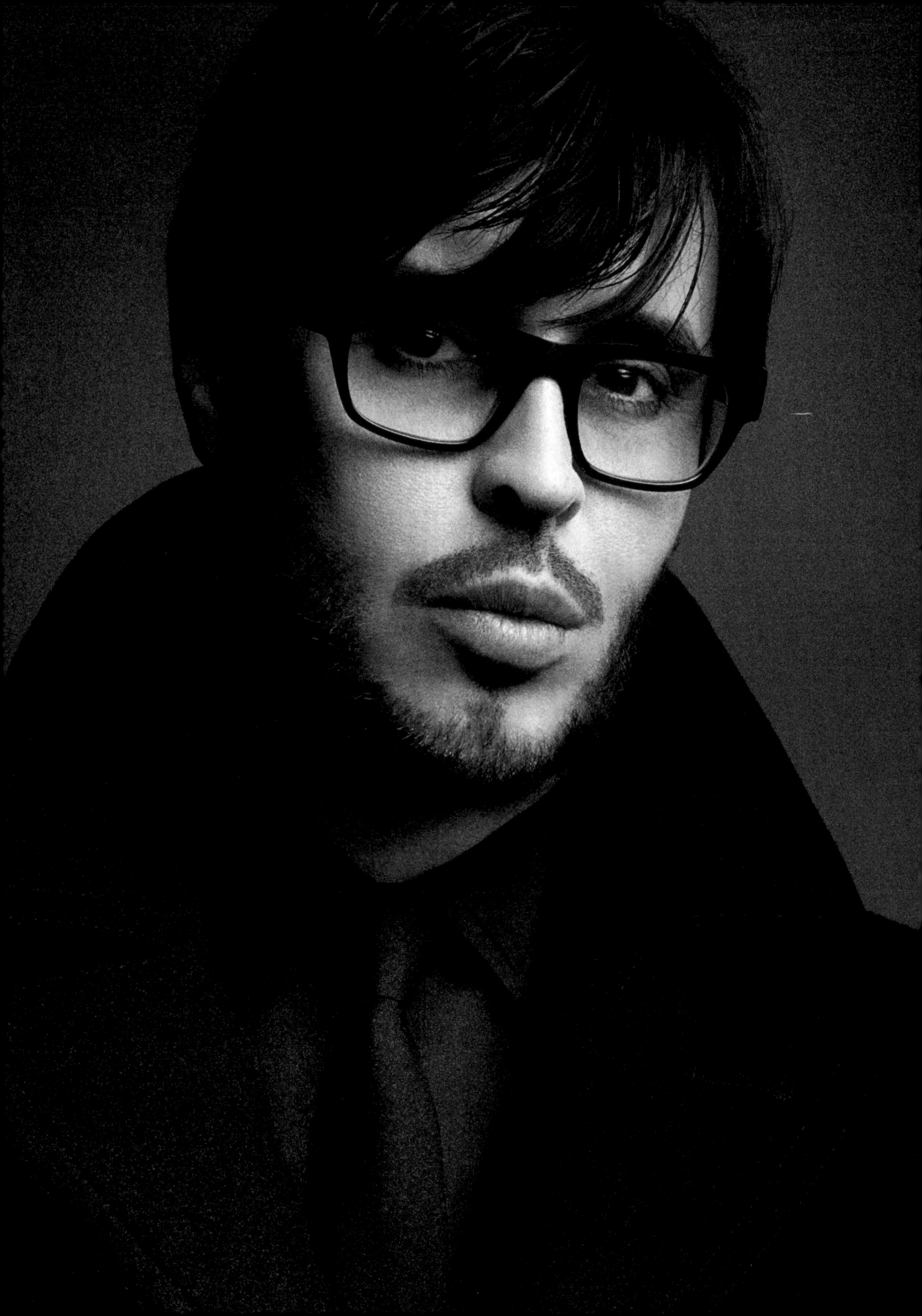

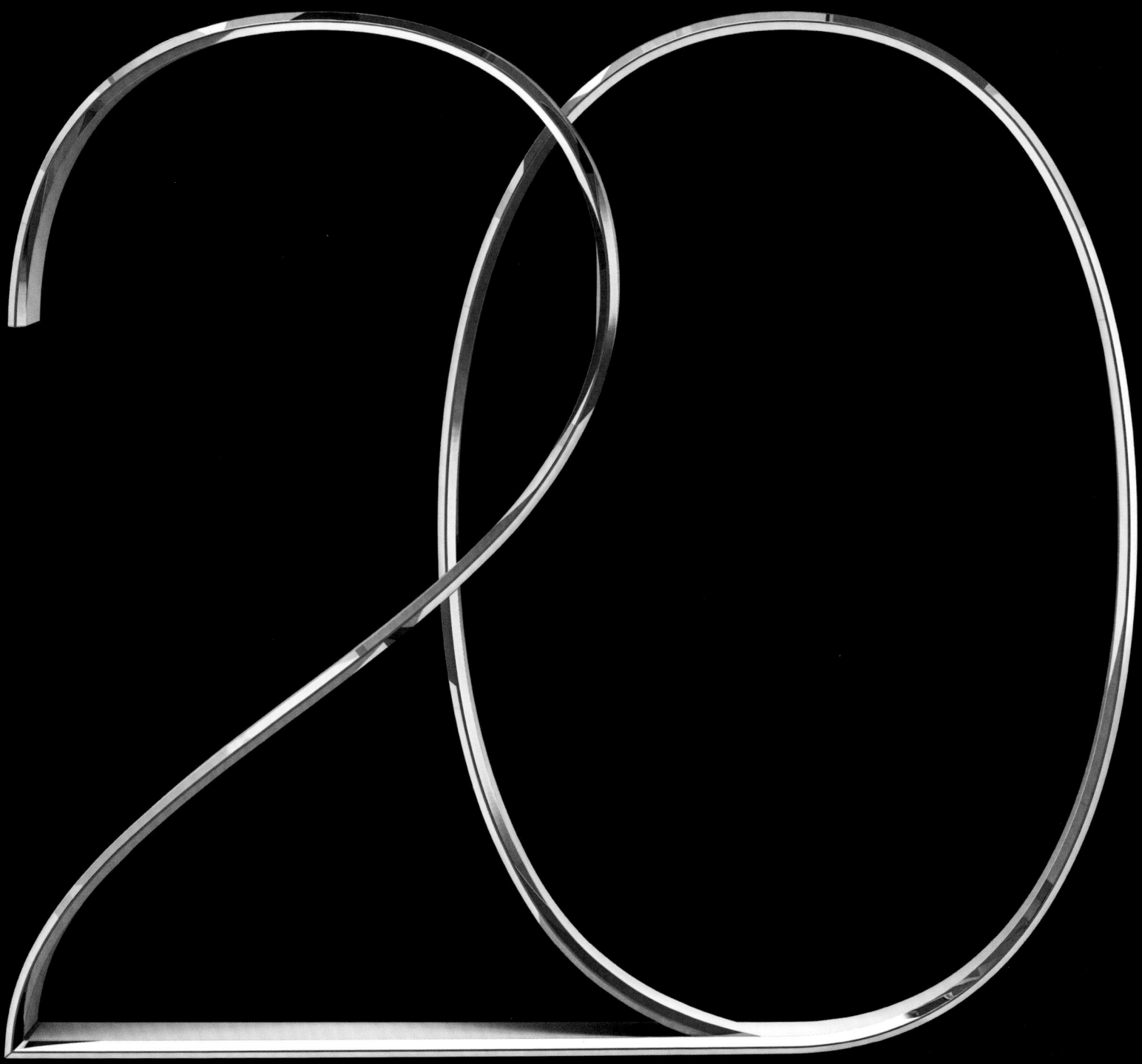

ISLAND FEVER

"MAKEUP ARTISTS ARE ALMOST LIKE PAINTERS. WE NEED TO BE INSPIRED BY OUR SURROUNDINGS, AND HERE, NATURE IS SO EXTRAVAGANT. IT KEEPS ME CREATIVE, FRESH, NEW, AND MODERN." — FRANÇOIS NARS

MORE THAN A PRIVATE WORLD—A DREAM COME TRUE. MOTU TANÉ, ONE OF 118 ISLANDS STREWN ACROSS THE CERULEAN EXPANSE OF FRENCH POLYNESIA, IS FRANÇOIS'S PERSONAL PARADISE AND A PLACE TO CALL HOME. KNOWN AS THE "ISLAND OF UNIVERSAL LOVE," ITS LUSH LANDSCAPE SCULPTED BY ARCHITECT PASCAL CRIBIER SERVES AS AN INTIMATE GETAWAY FOR FRIENDS AND FAMILY, AS WELL AS FRANÇOIS'S PART-TIME RESIDENCE. ITS VERDANT MOUNTAINS, POWDERY BEACHES, EMERALD LAGOONS, PEOPLE, AND CULTURE SERVE AS HIS LIMITLESS SOURCE OF INSPIRATION.

PREVIOUSLY INHABITED BY FRENCH EXPLORER AND WRITER PAUL-ÉMILE VICTOR, FRANÇOIS ACQUIRED MOTU TANÉ IN THE EARLY 2000s, FULFILLING A LIFELONG ASPIRATION OF LIVING ON AN ISLAND IN THE SOUTH PACIFIC. MUCH LIKE FRANÇOIS'S CREATIVE FORCE, THE ISLAND THRIVES IN A WORLD OF FERTILE IMAGINATION—REMOTE, SINGULAR, A WORLD UNTO ITSELF.

THATCHED ROOF BUNGALOWS WITH INTERIORS BY FAMED FRENCH DESIGNER CHRISTIAN LIAIGRE BALANCE THE WONDER OF LUXURY WITH THE WILD UNKNOWN. HERE, FRANÇOIS IS REJUVENATED BY ITS TOTAL ESCAPE. HE REVELS IN AN UNINTERRUPTED CONNECTION TO THE ELEMENTS, ENGAGING ALL FIVE SENSES IN THE PRIMAL THRILL OF THE ISLAND'S UNIMAGINABLE DYNAMIC—ALL RICHLY CAPTURED IN HIS 2013 PHOTOGRAPHY COLLECTION, *FAERY LANDS*, A MESMERIZING ODE TO FRENCH POLYNESIA.

"WHAT IS BEAUTY TO ME? A DESERTED BEACH," HE SAYS.

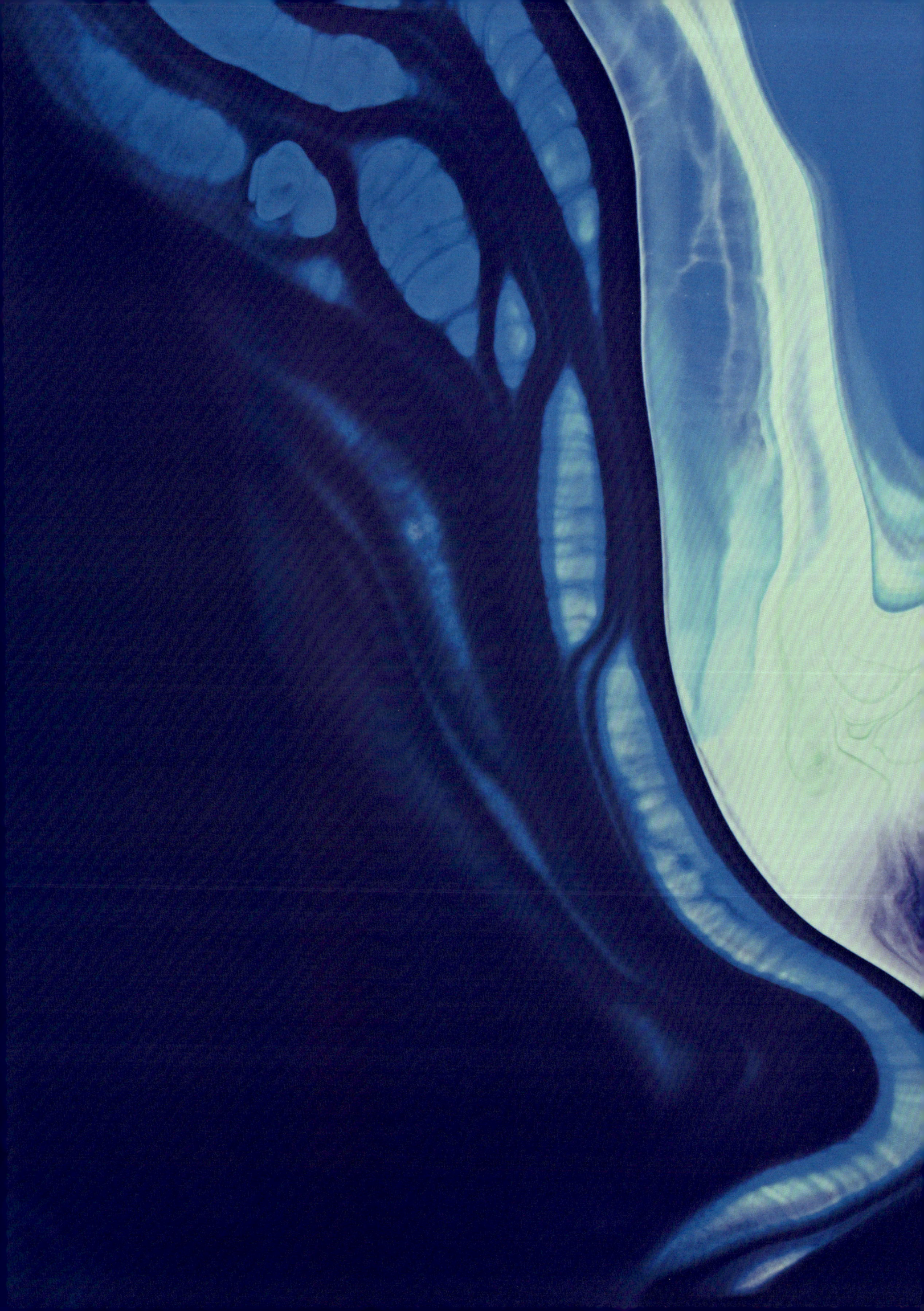

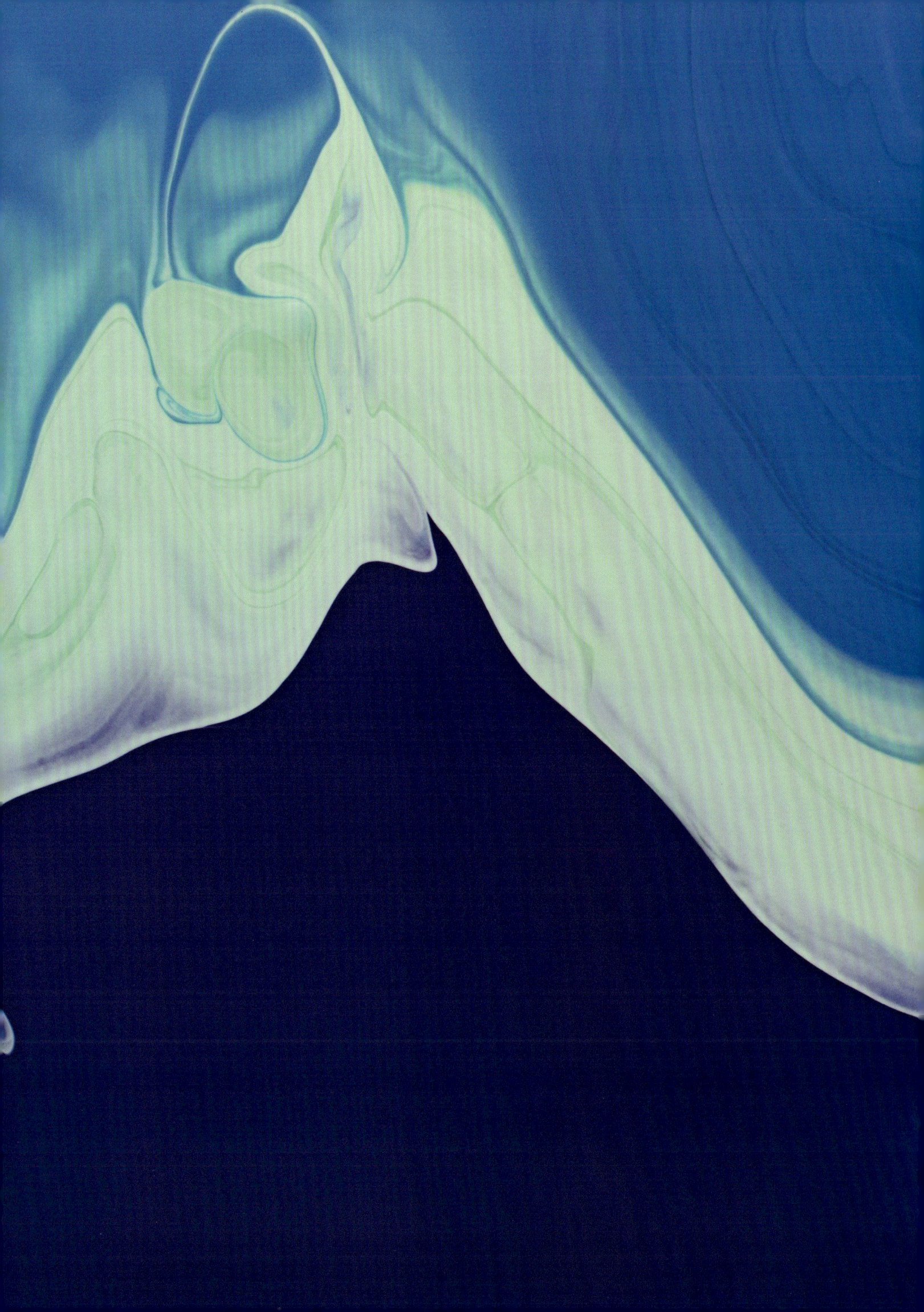

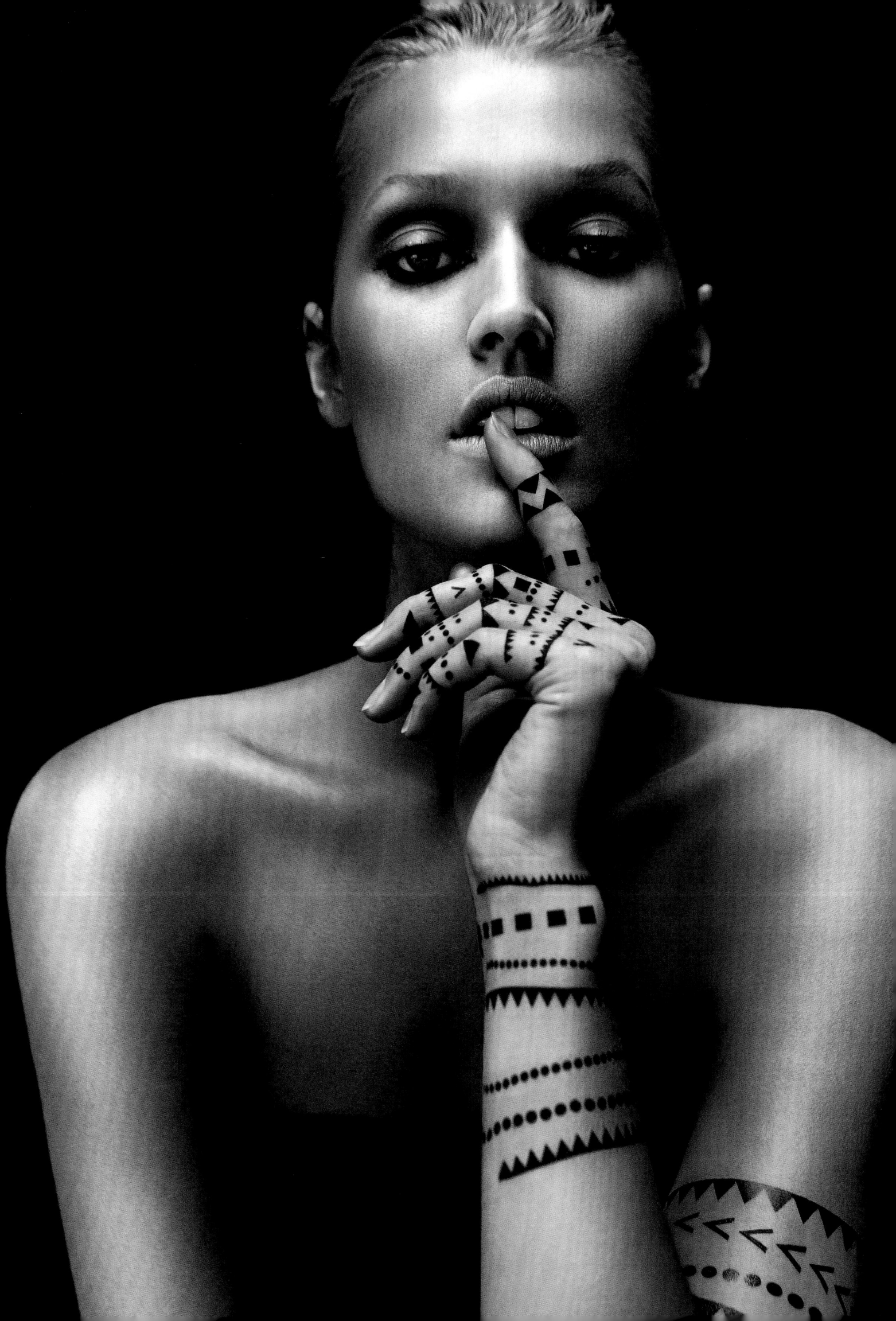

"MOTU TANÉ IN BORA BORA IS PERHAPS MY FAVORITE PLACE ON EARTH. I WOULD SPEND THE REST OF MY LIFE THERE IF I COULD."
– FRANÇOIS NARS

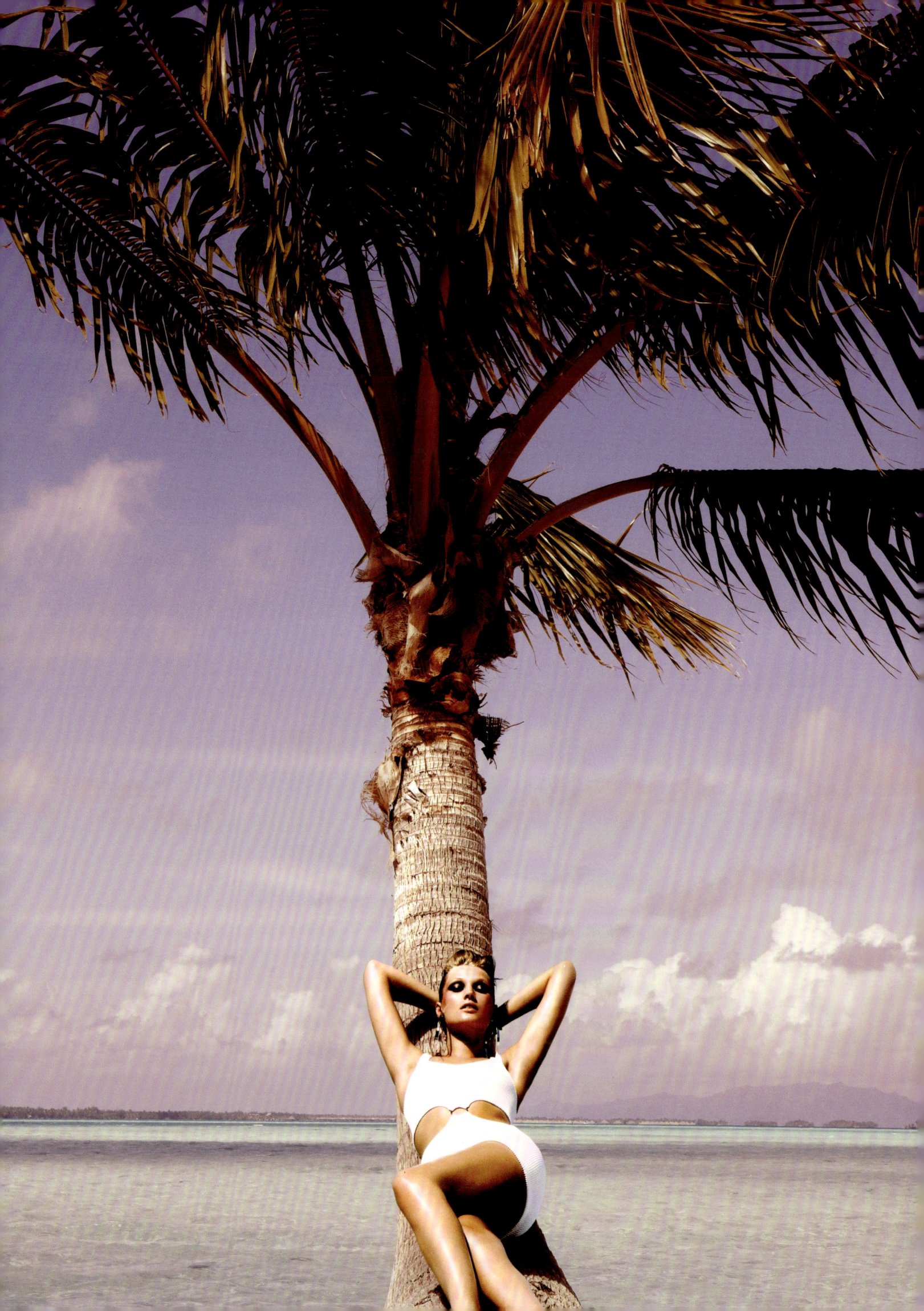

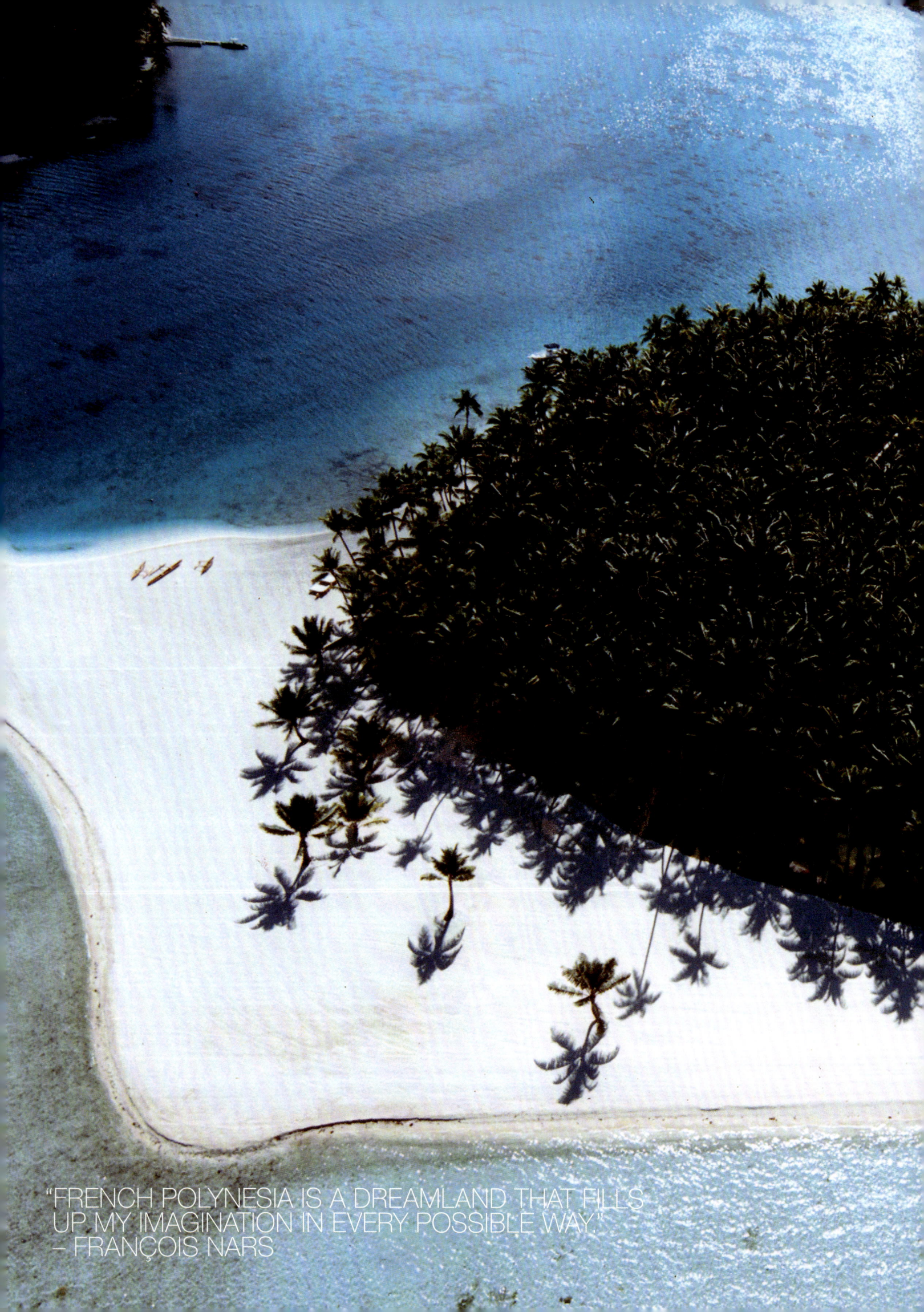

"FRENCH POLYNESIA IS A DREAMLAND THAT FILLS
UP MY IMAGINATION IN EVERY POSSIBLE WAY."
– FRANÇOIS NARS

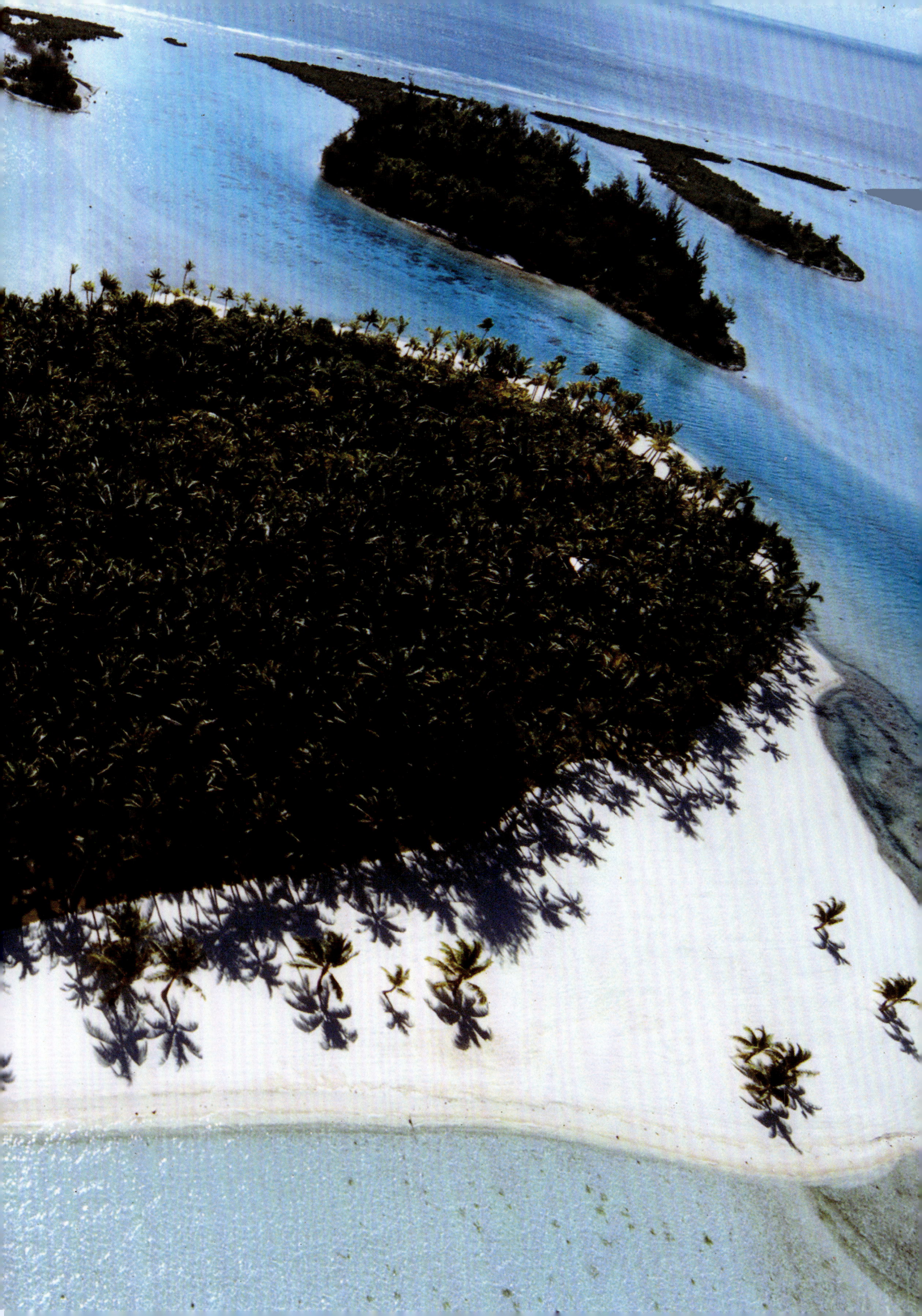

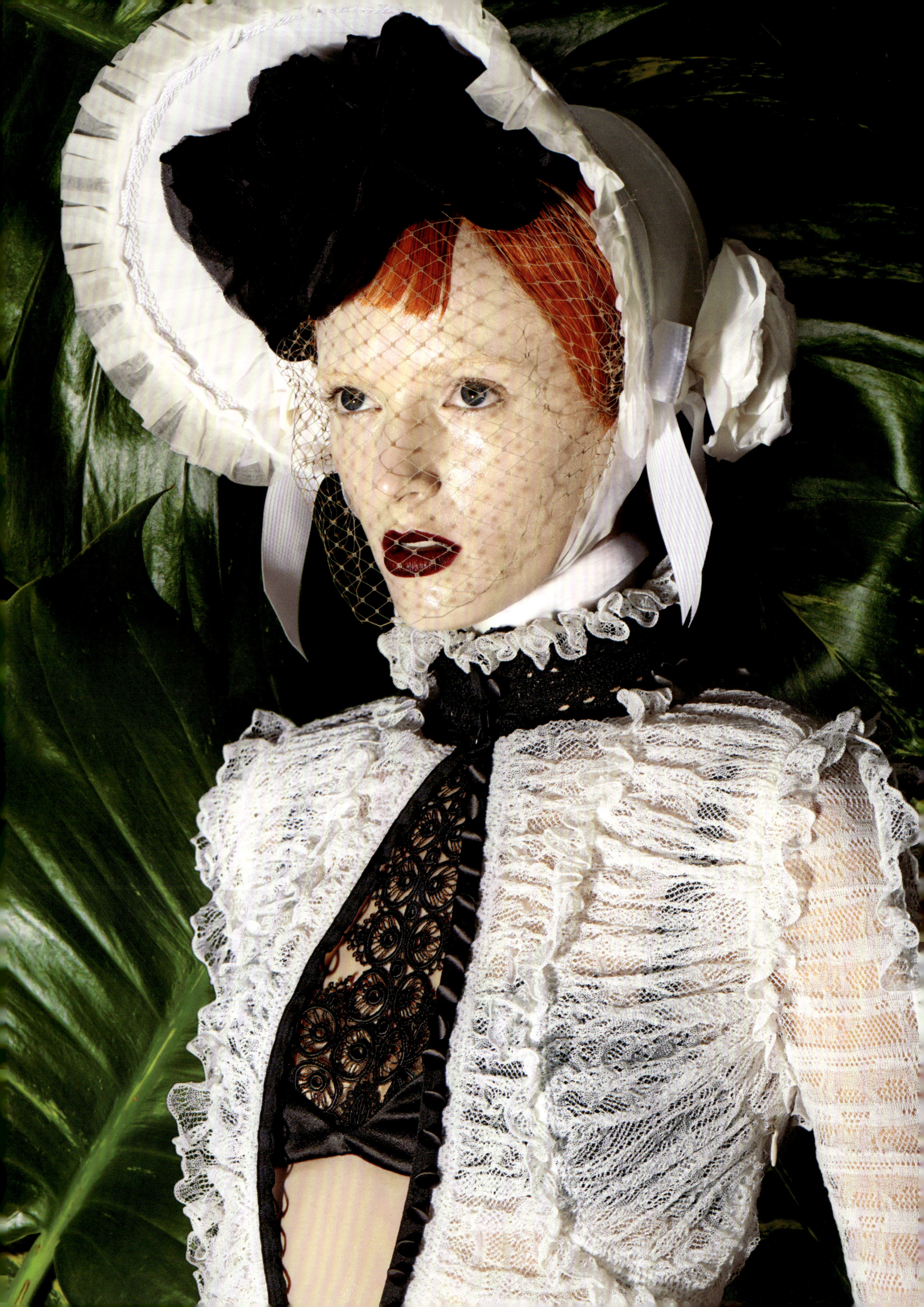

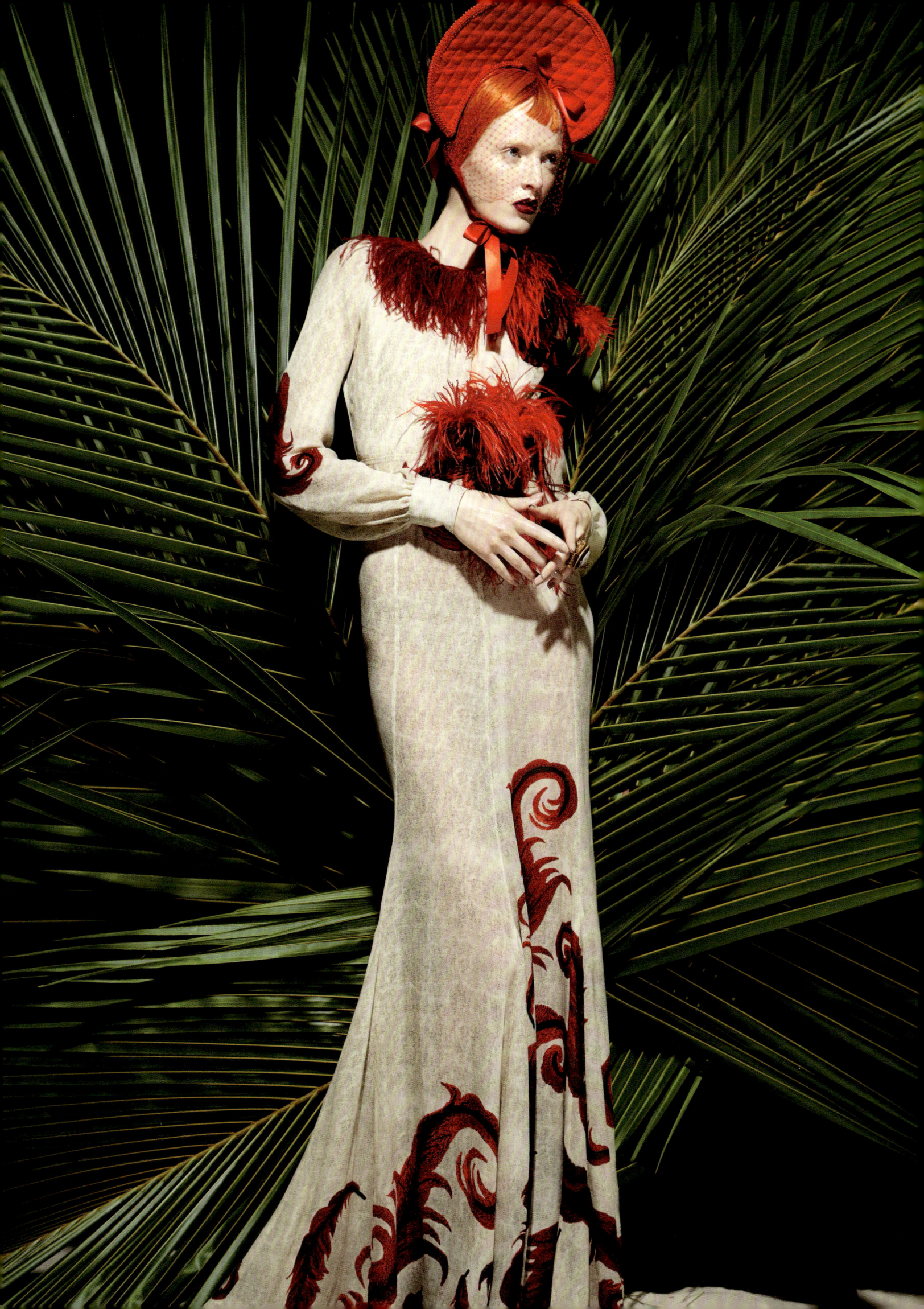

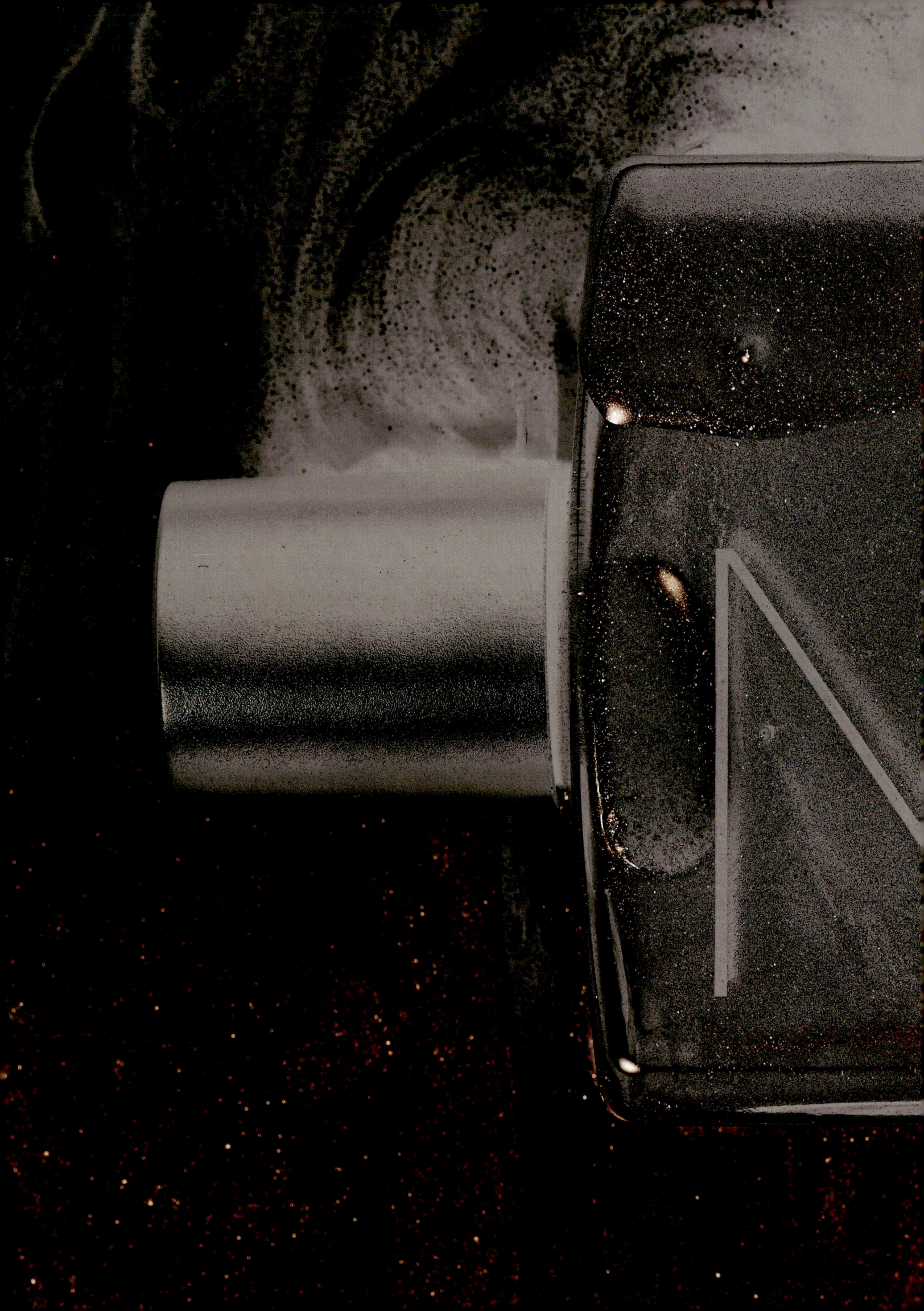

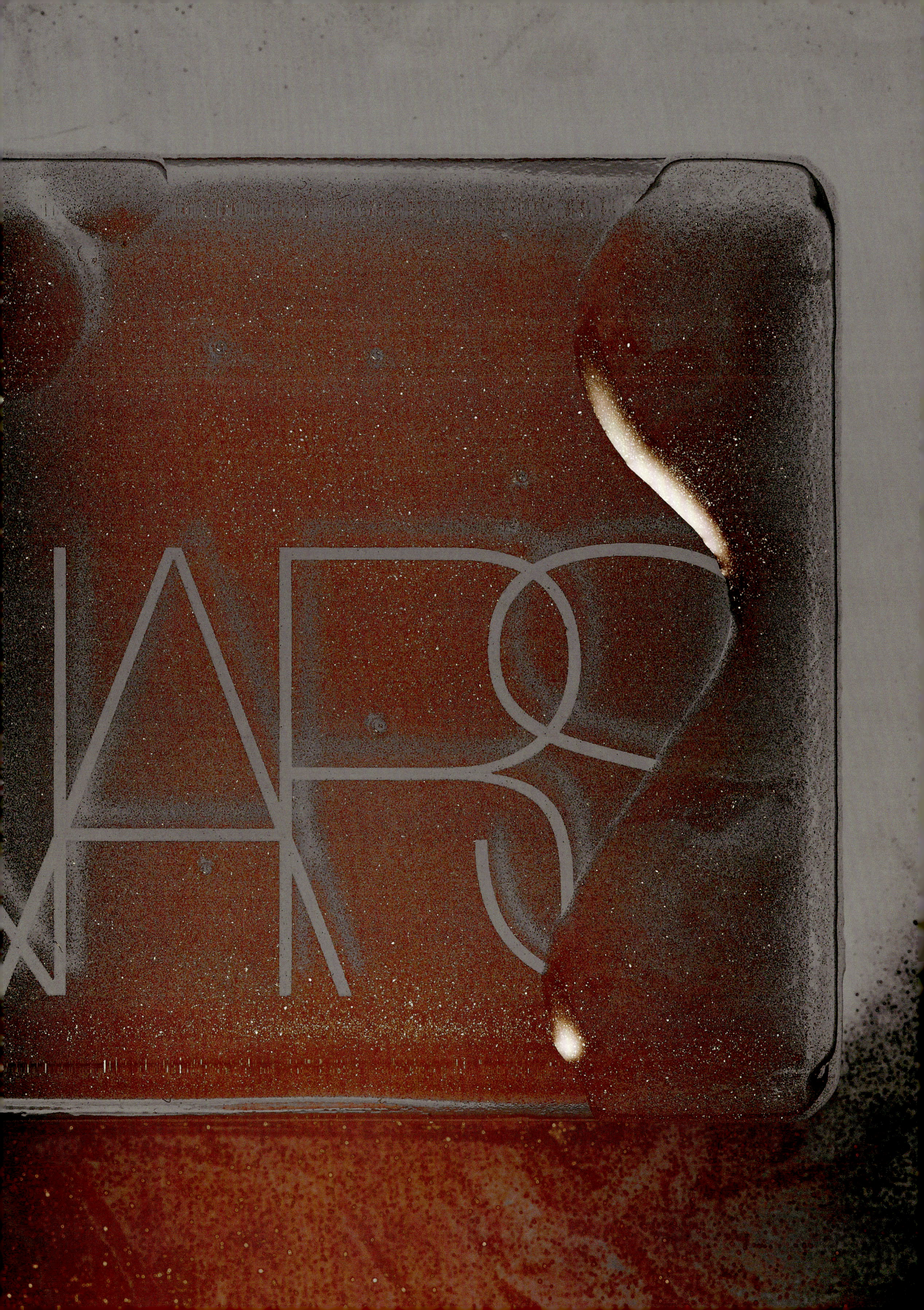

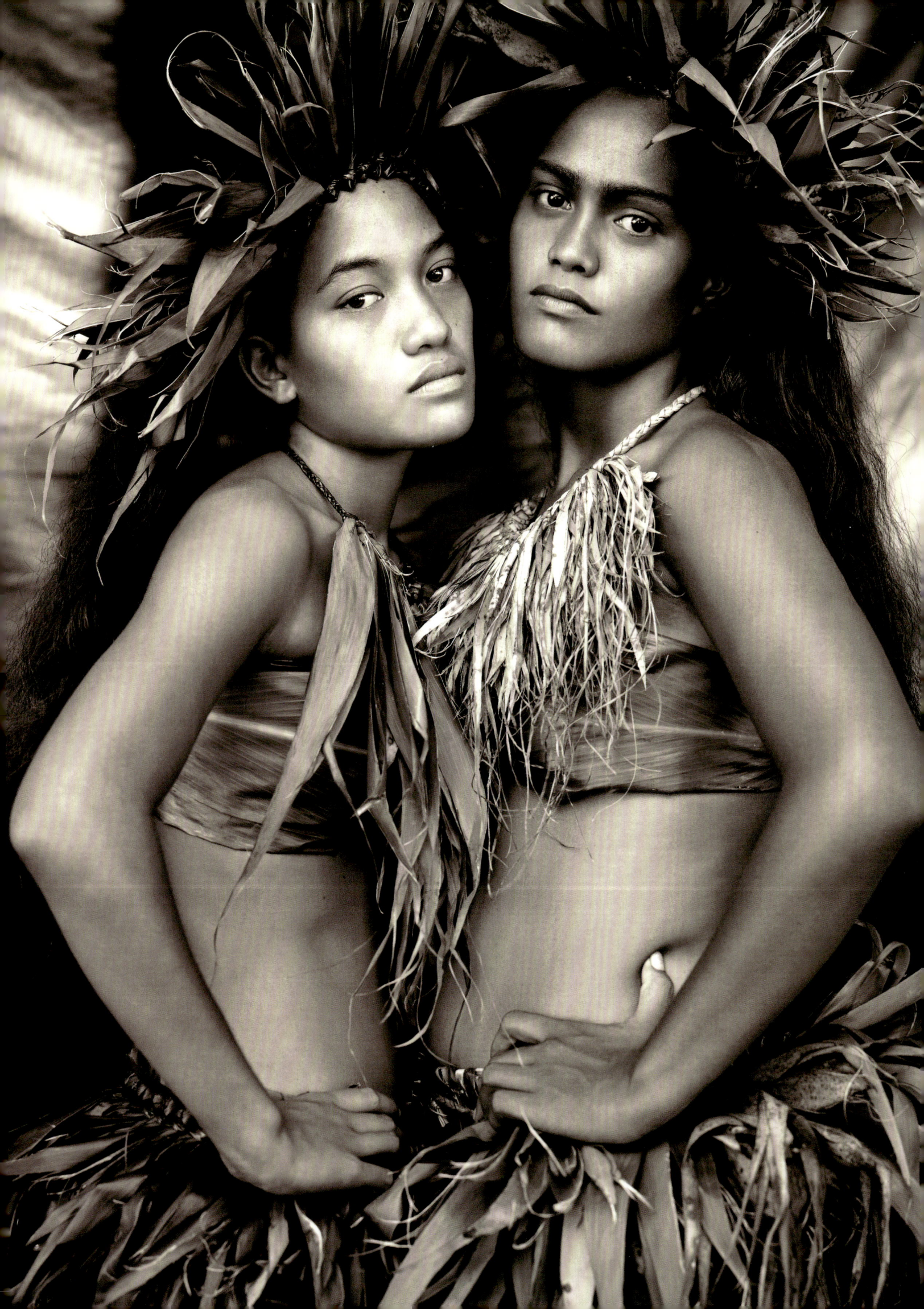

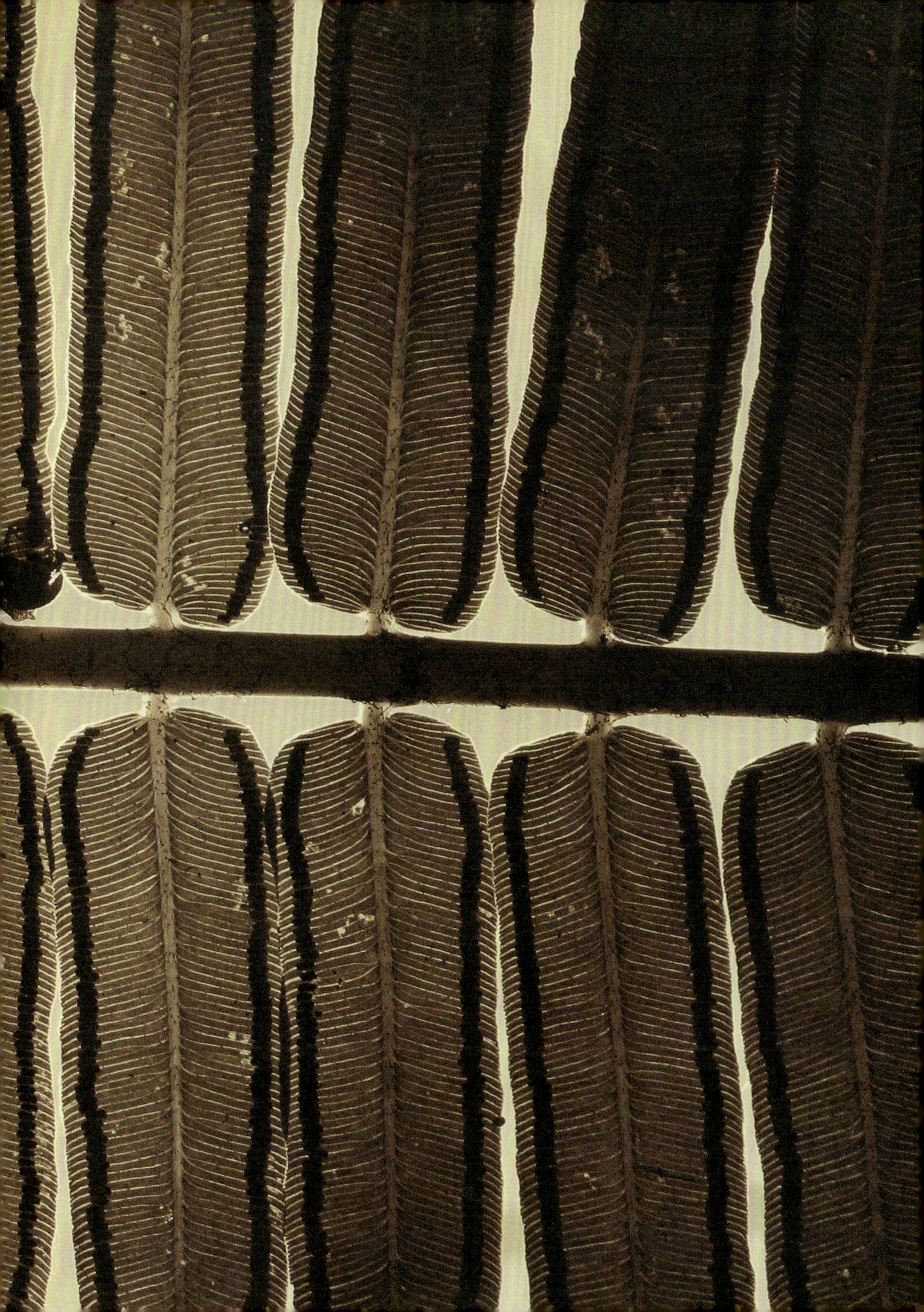

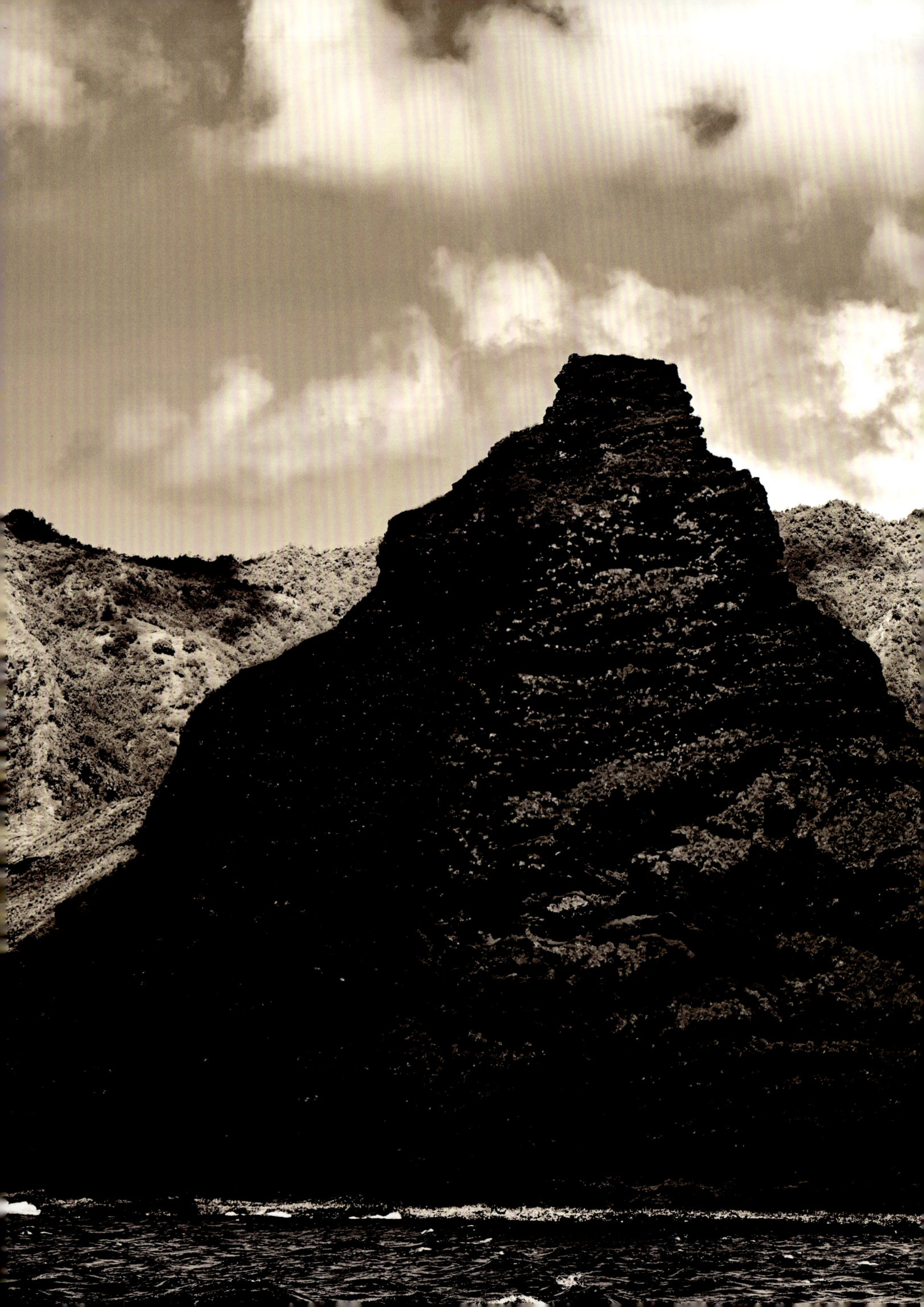

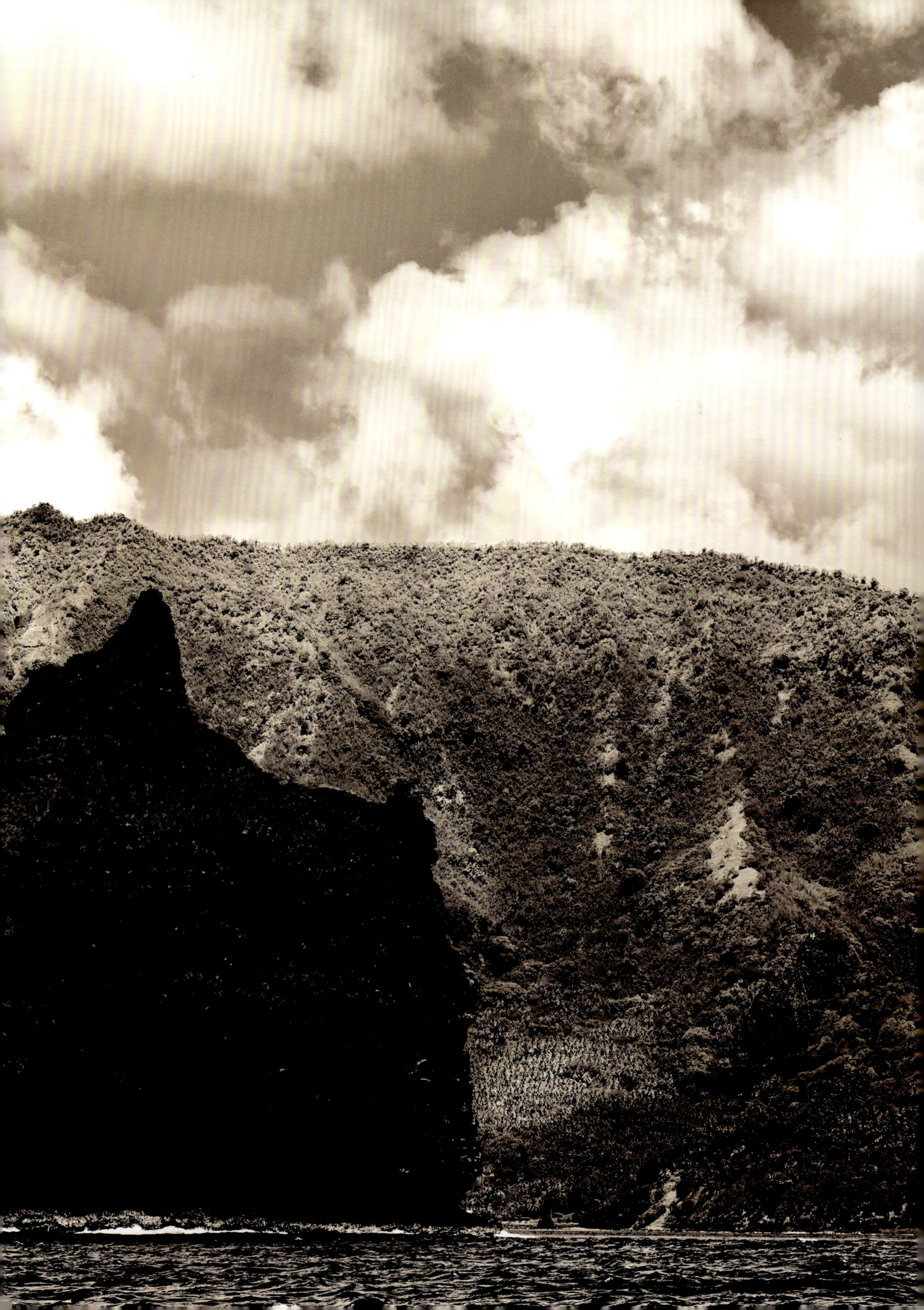

"FRANÇOIS'S TALENT, VISION, AND
UNIVERSE MAKE HIM COMPLETELY
UNIQUE; IT IS REALLY INSPIRING. HE IS
THE PERFECT EXAMPLE OF SOMEONE
WHO KNOWS HOW TO ALWAYS
REINVENT HIMSELF AND SURPRISE US.
I HAD THE CHANCE TO WORK WITH
HIM ON DIFFERENT PROJECTS FROM
EDITORIALS TO HIS BOOK *FAERY LANDS*.
IT'S ALWAYS EXCITING EVERY TIME WE
GET TO WORK TOGETHER."
– GIOVANNI BIANCO,
CREATIVE DIRECTOR

"¡ LOVE GIOVANNI BIANCO.
SO CREATIVE AND PASSIONATE, HE
ALWAYS HAS A THOUSAND IDEAS IN
HIS POCKET AND SO MUCH ENERGY.
I ADORE HIM, A GREAT FRIEND."
– FRANÇOIS NARS

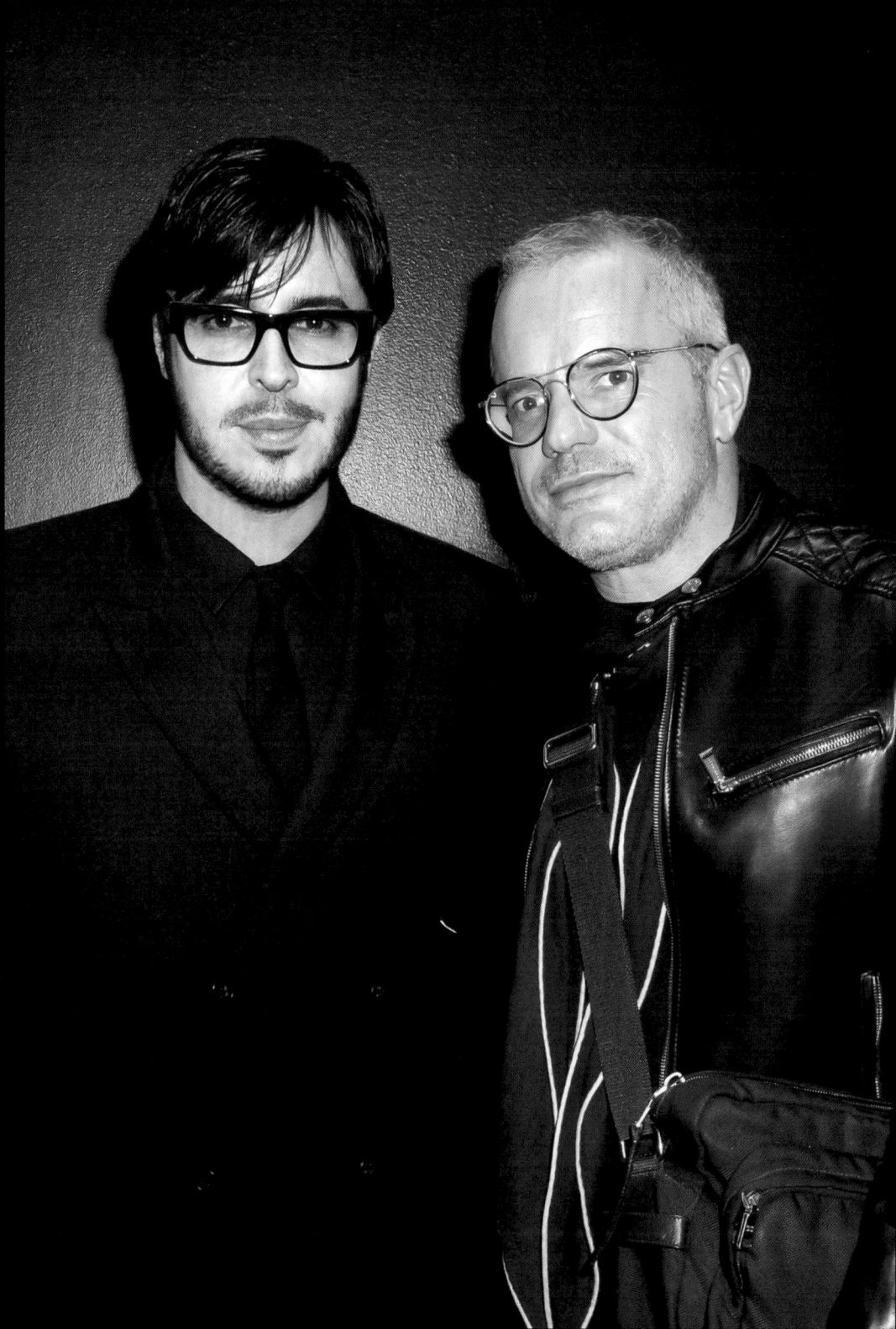

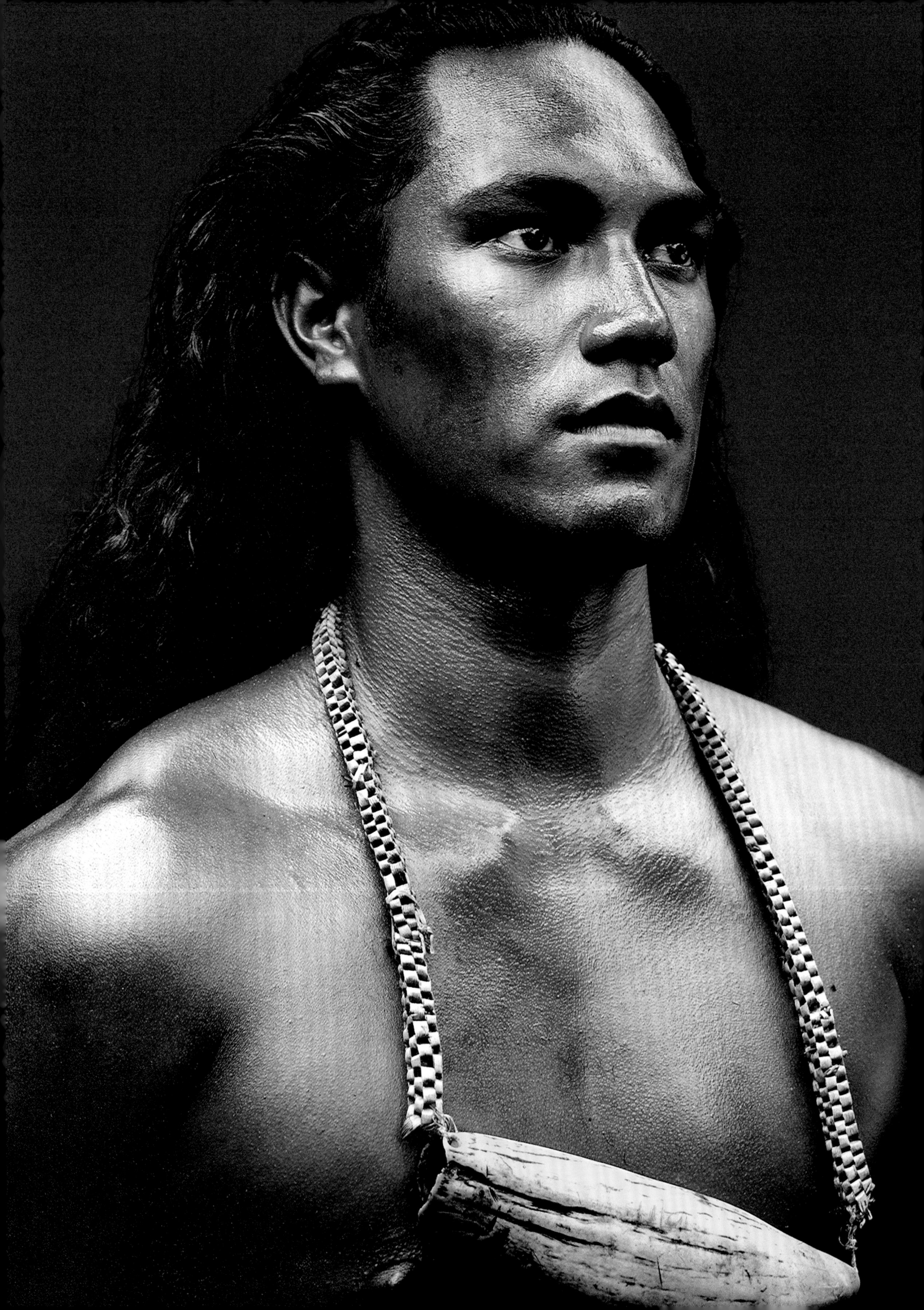

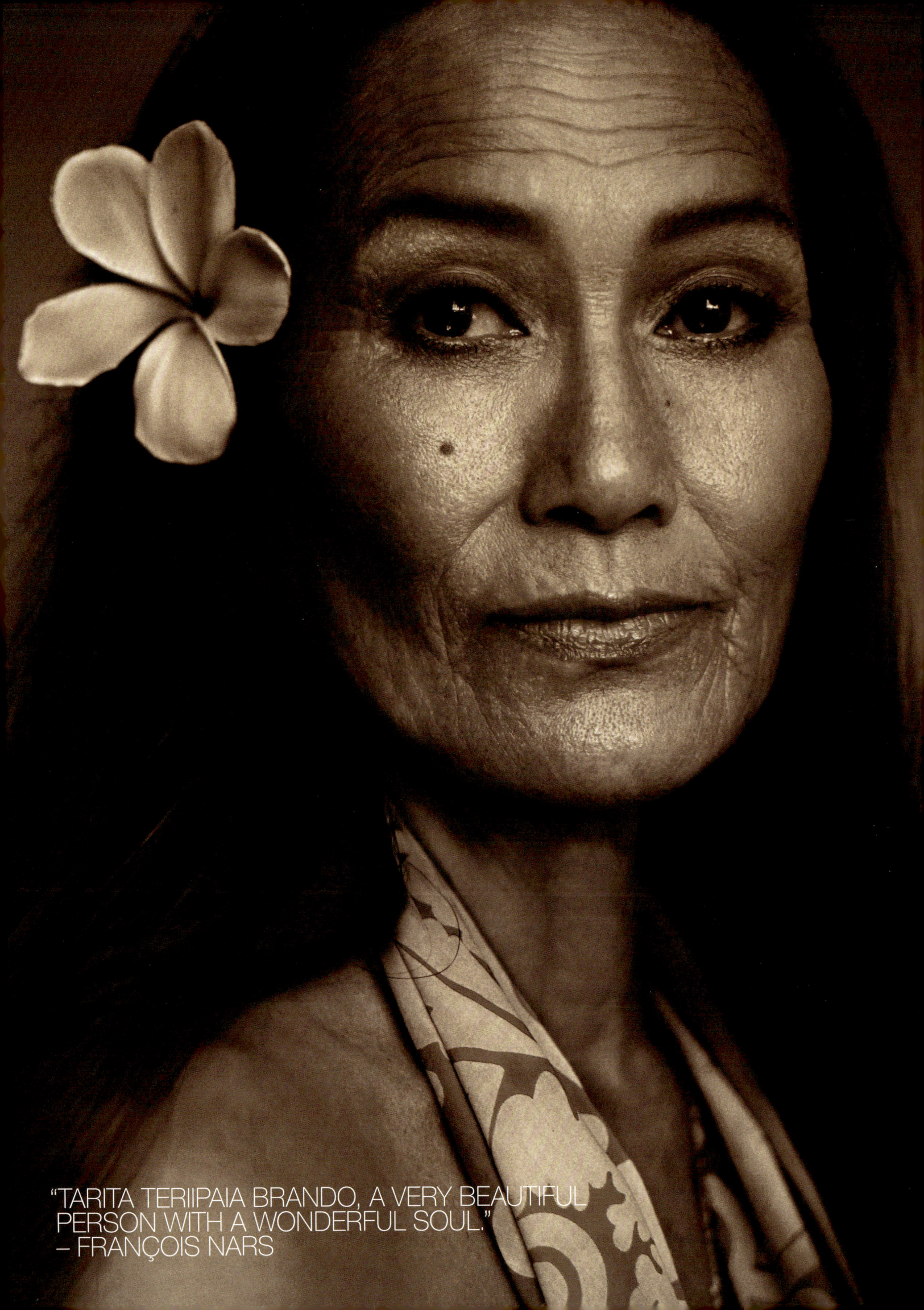

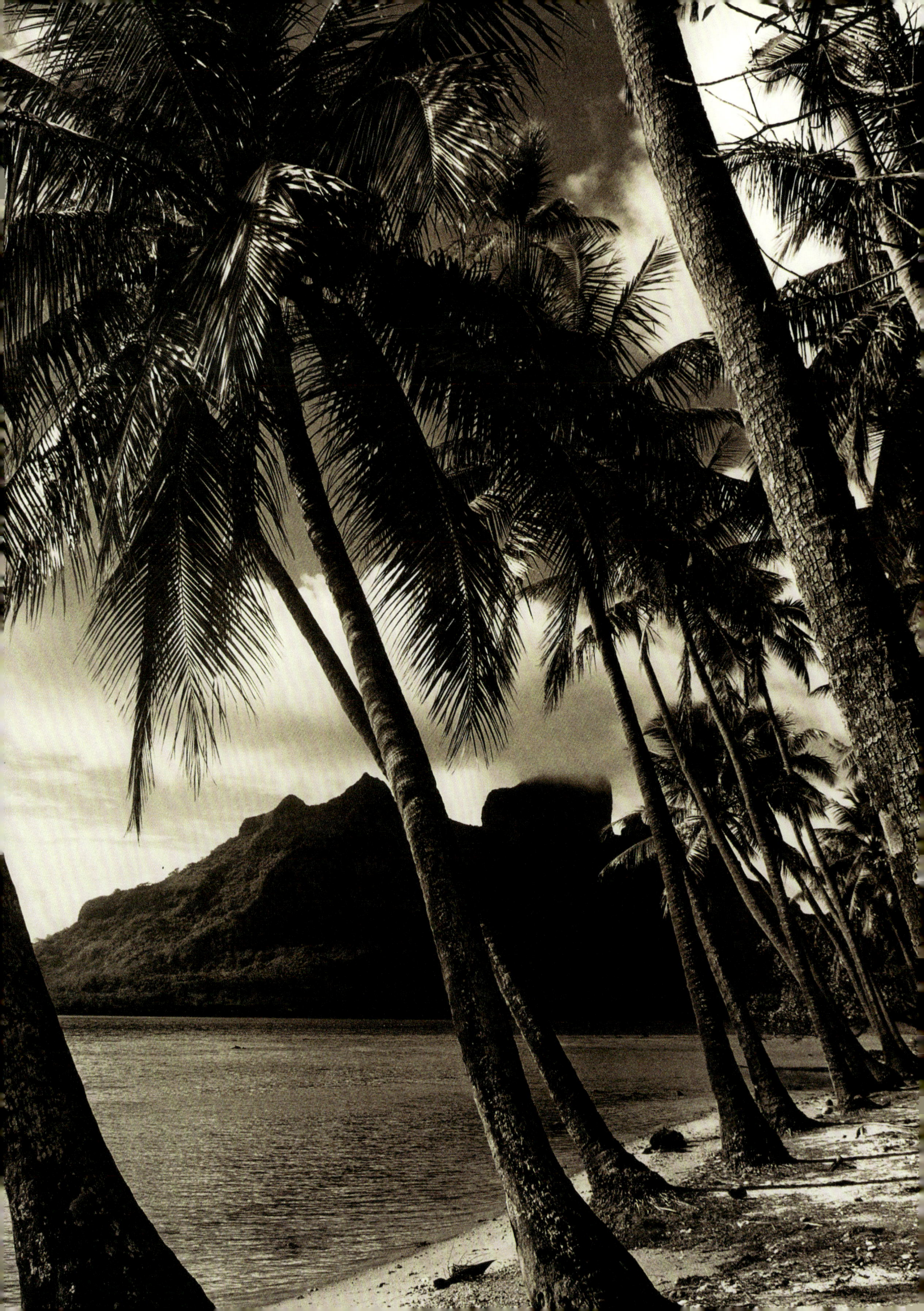

"I AM A FAMILY MAN.
I LOVE HAVING MY
FAMILY AROUND,
GOING ON HOLIDAYS
WITH THEM, AND
SPENDING A LOT OF
TIME TOGETHER."
– FRANÇOIS NARS

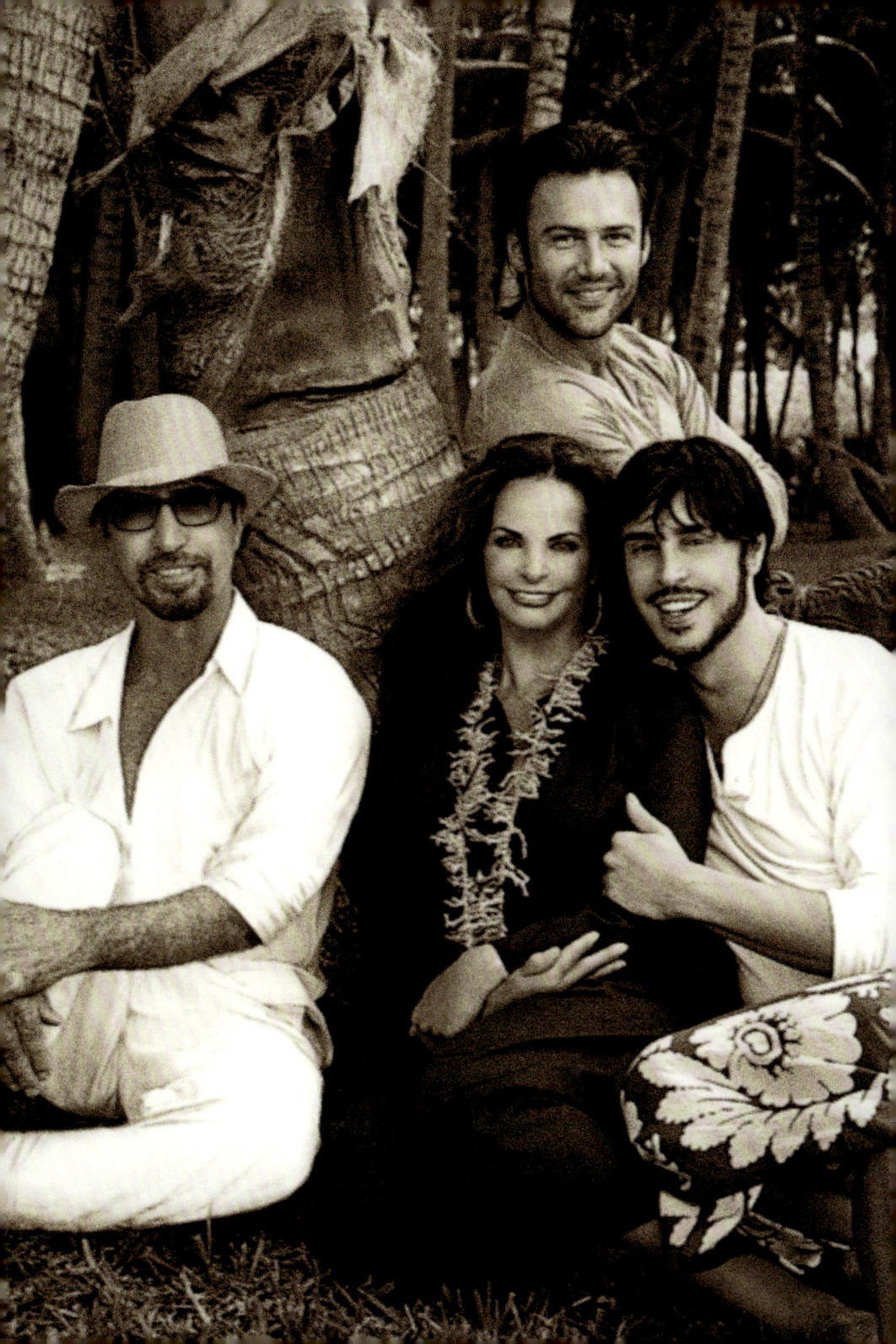

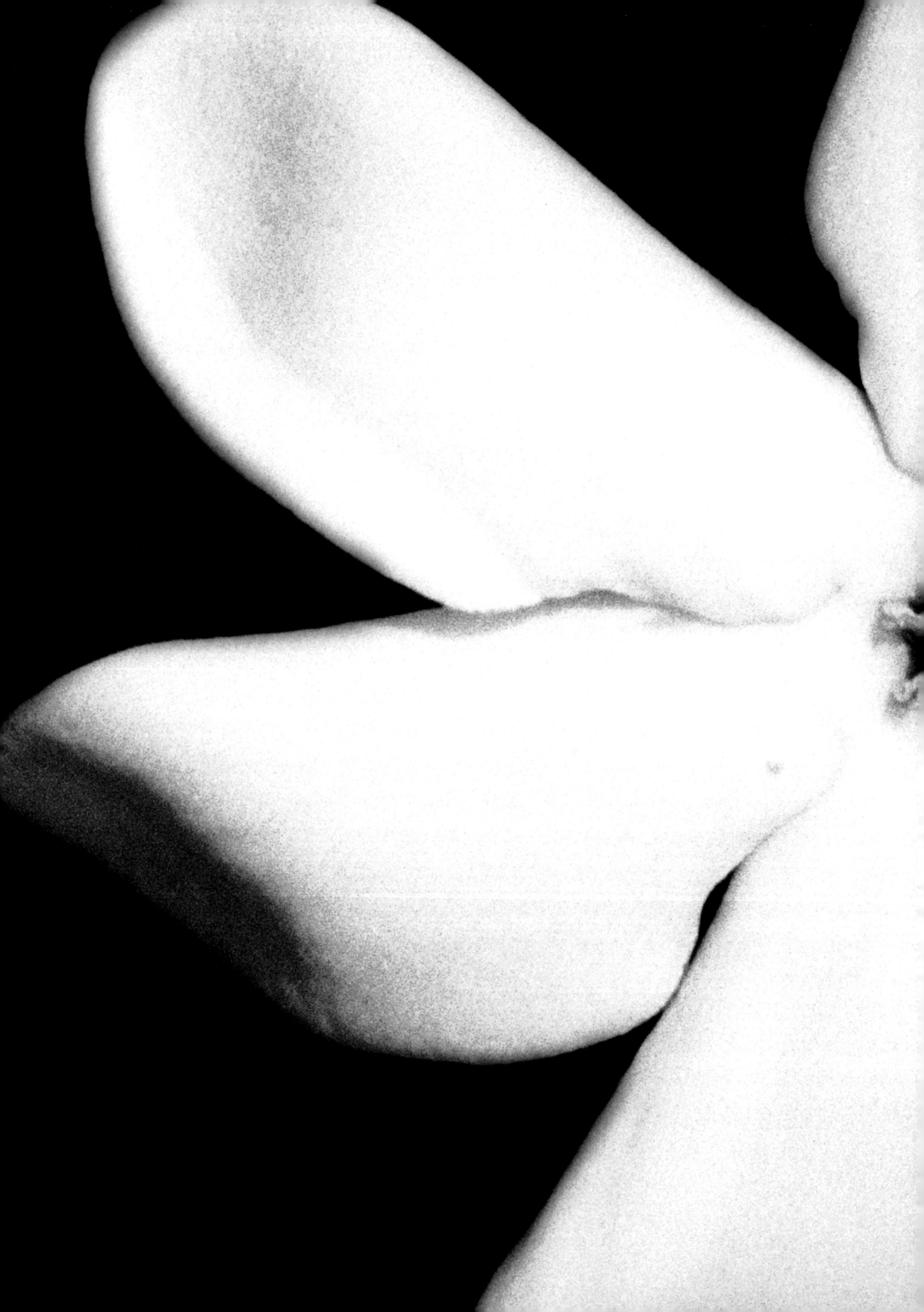

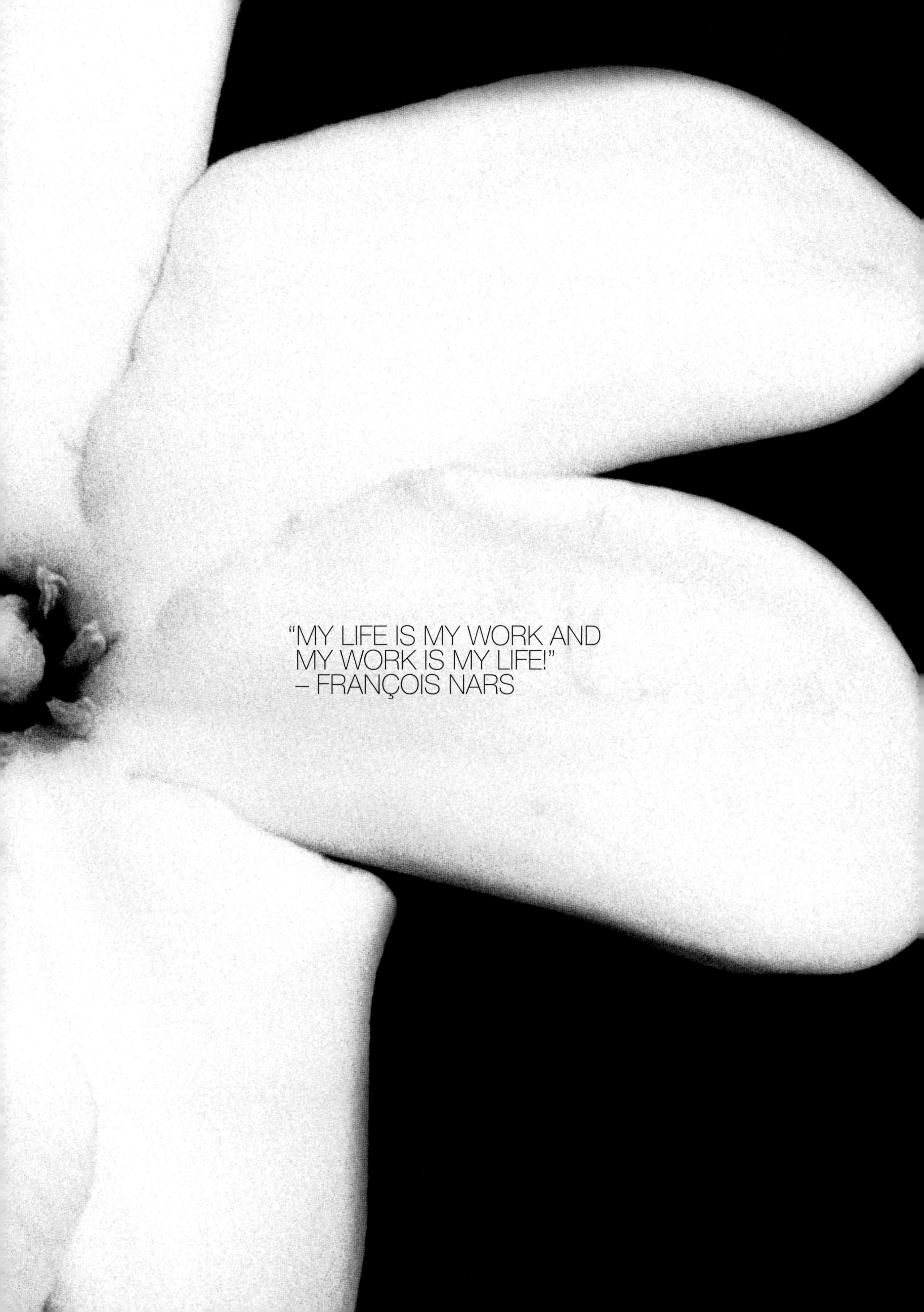

"MY LIFE IS MY WORK AND
MY WORK IS MY LIFE!"
– FRANÇOIS NARS

"NEVER BE SATISFIED WITH WHAT YOU HAVE DONE. ALWAYS TRY TO DO BETTER." – FRANÇOIS NARS

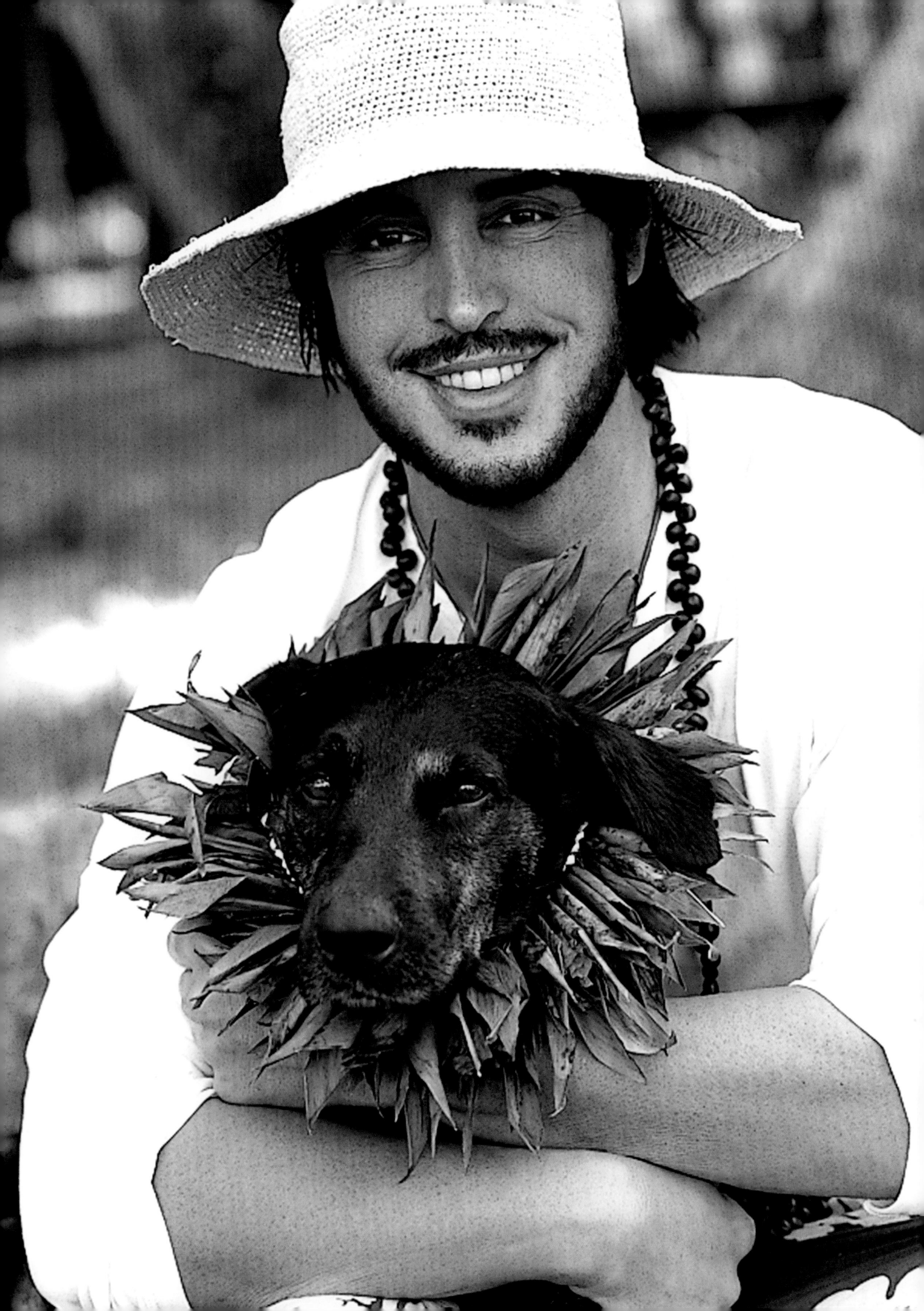

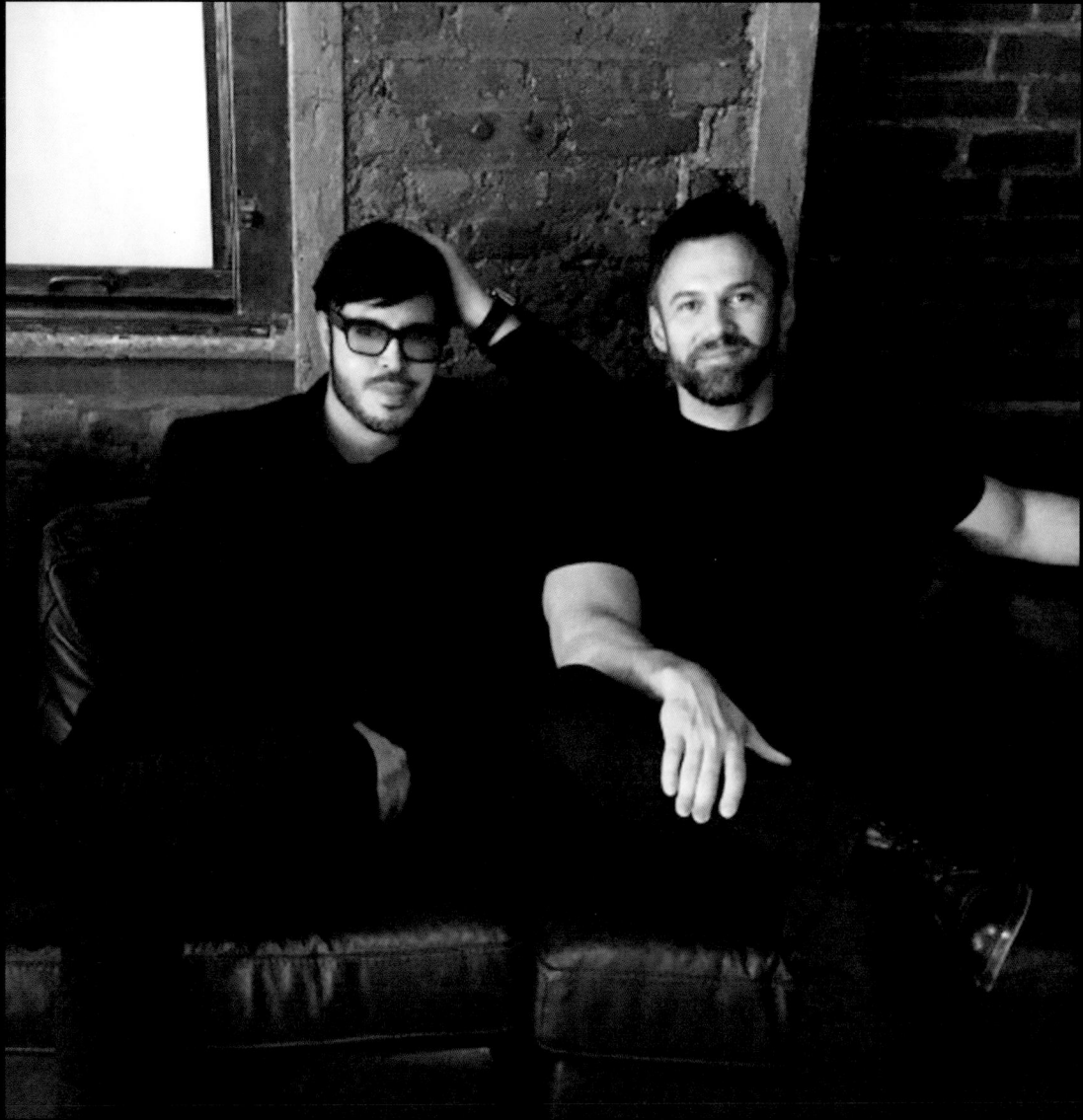

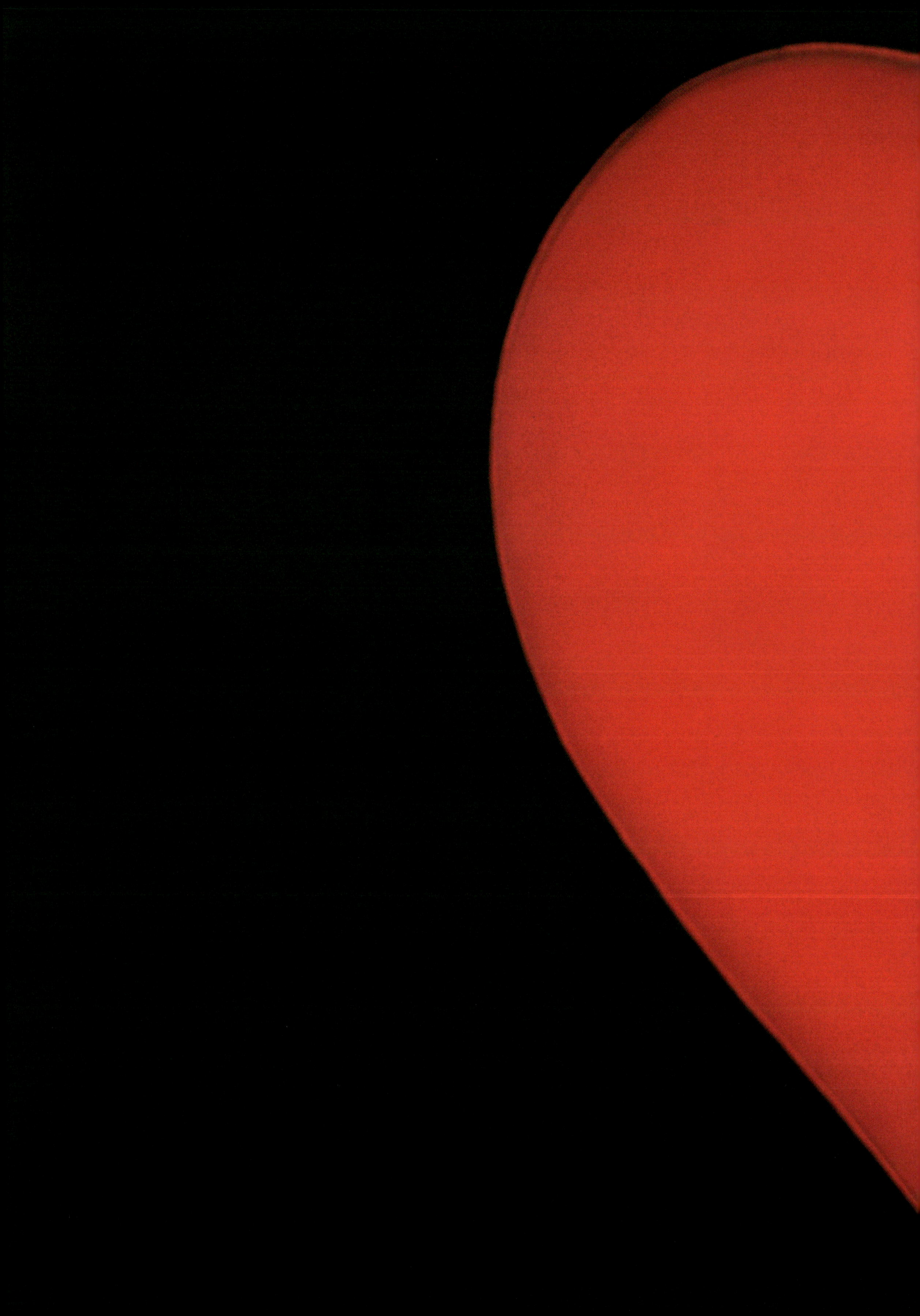

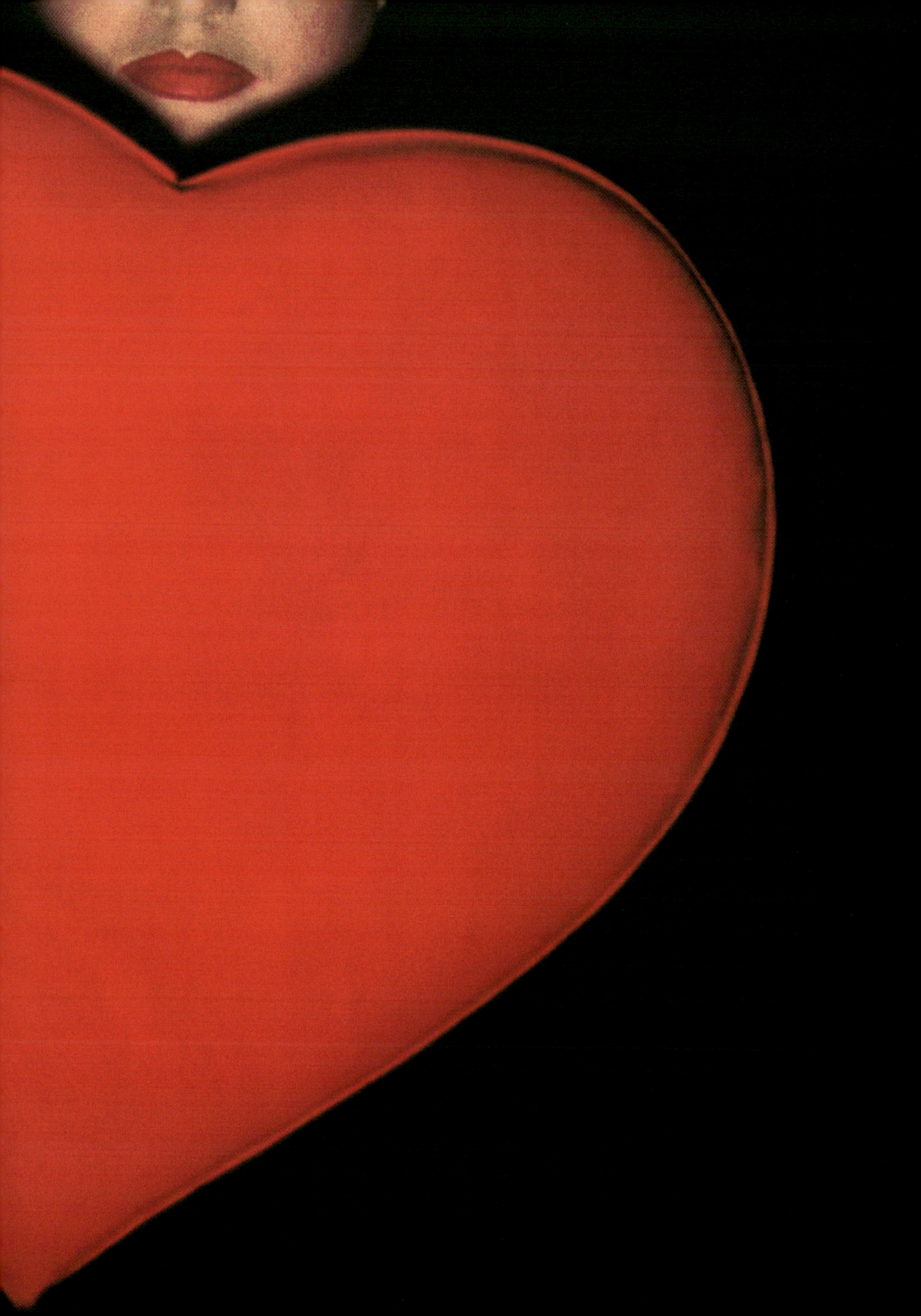

MY SINCEREST THANKS TO EVERYONE WHO WAS INVOLVED IN THE MAKING OF THE BOOK.

WITH VERY HEARTFELT GRATITUDE TO MY PARENTS, JEAN JACQUES AND CLAUDETTE NARS, TO CSABA, TO MARINA SCHIANO, AS WELL AS TO ALL MY FRIENDS, ARTISTS, AND MODELS INCLUDED IN THIS BOOK.

WITH TREMENDOUS GRATITUDE TO FABIEN BARON, YUKI IWASHIRO, THERESA GRILL, AND EVERYONE AT BARON & BARON.

THANK YOU TO ALL THE ARTISTS, INDIVIDUALS, AND ORGANIZATIONS WHO HAVE GIVEN RIGHTS OR CONTRIBUTED TO OBTAIN PERMISSION TO REPRODUCE THE IMAGES FEATURED IN THE BOOK.

TO ALL THE PHOTOGRAPHERS CREDITED IN THESE PAGES, TO ALL ARCHIVES, ESTATES, LICENSING AGENCIES, AND AGENTS—ANDRÉ WERTHER, ART + COMMERCE, ART PARTNER LICENSING, ARTISTS RIGHTS SOCIETY, CREATIVE EXCHANGE AGENCY, AUTHENTIC BRANDS GROUP, BARBARA RIX-SIEFF, THE RICHARD AVEDON FOUNDATION, THE HELMUT NEWTON FOUNDATION, THE JOHN KOBAL FOUNDATION, HULTON ARCHIVE, FONDATION PIERRE BERGÉ - YVES SAINT LAURENT, JEREMIAH NEWTON, THE ESTATE OF MARILYN MONROE LLC, THE ANDY WARHOL FOUNDATION FOR THE VISUAL ARTS, INC, THE CASATI ARCHIVES, THE HUMPHREY BOGART ESTATE. TO THE MODEL AND CELEBRITY AGENCIES - DNA MODELS, 42WEST, FORD MODELS, ID-PR, IMG MODELS, MAJOR MODEL MANAGEMENT, MARILYN MODEL AGENCY, MIKAS, NEXT MANAGEMENT, ONE MANAGEMENT, SOUL ARTIST MANAGEMENT, STORM MODEL MANAGEMENT, THE LIONS MODEL MANAGEMENT, TRUMP MODELS, UNITED TALENT AGENCY, VIVA MODEL MANAGEMENT, VOYEZ MON AGENT V.M.A, WILHELMINA MODELS, WOMEN MANAGEMENT. TO ALL OTHER ORGANIZATIONS AND COMPANIES—HEARST CORPORATION, LAGARDÈRE GROUP, CONDÉ NAST CORPORATION, BARNEYS NEW YORK, CALVIN KLEIN STUDIO LLC, CARITA SA, GIANNI VERSACE S.P.A. SPECIAL THANKS TO SARAH MOON, STEVEN KLEIN, AND KONSTANTIN KAKANIAS.

MANY THANKS TO BARBARA CALCAGNI, LOUIS DESAZARS, CHLOE WARNER, YANA CHERNOVA, MAGALIE PARKSUWAN, JULIA SLOAN, KELLY VIRTUE, GENEVIEVE LEON, GARY MOZER, GABRIELLE DE LESQUEN, AND EVERYONE AT NARS; KIM GENTILE, SASHA ERWITT, NORKIN DIGITAL, STEPHAN SAGMILLER, MILANI PRESS, MAXIME POIBLANC, ANTHONY PETRILLOSE AND THE RIZZOLI TEAM, AND EVERYONE WHO HAS BEEN DEDICATED TO THE CREATION OF THIS BOOK.

LAST BUT NOT LEAST, A SPECIAL THANKS TO ALL WHO HAVE WORKED WITH ME OVER THE COURSE OF ALL THESE YEARS: TO THE MAKEUP ARTISTS: LENA KORO, JAMES KALIARDOS, DIANE KENDAL, AYAKO YOSHIMURA, JAMES BOEHMER, FRANCELLE DALY, WILLIAM KAHN. TO THE HAIRSTYLISTS: PETER SAVIC, ORIBE, DIDIER MALIGE, FRANCO GOBBI, GARREN, LAURENT PHILLIPON, DUFFY, PETER GREY. TO THE STYLISTS: PATTI WILSON, TAYLOR KIM, LUDIVINE POIBLANC, LAETITIA DE L'ESCAILLE, ISABEL DUPRÉ, KARL TEMPLER. TO THE PHOTO ASSISTANTS: DAVID DIESING, JOHN ENGSTROM, LUCAS FLORES PIRAN, ROB KASSABIAN, MARKUS MAMOSER, QUINTON JONES, KEVIN VAST, JASON WALKER, DAVID SCHINMAN. TO OTHER CREATIVE AND PRODUCTION PARTNERS: SOPHIE THEALLET, STEFAN BECKMAN, ALESSANDRO ZOPPIS, EVERYONE AT MILK STUDIOS, AND ALL NAMES I HAVE NOT MENTIONED. — FRANÇOIS NARS.

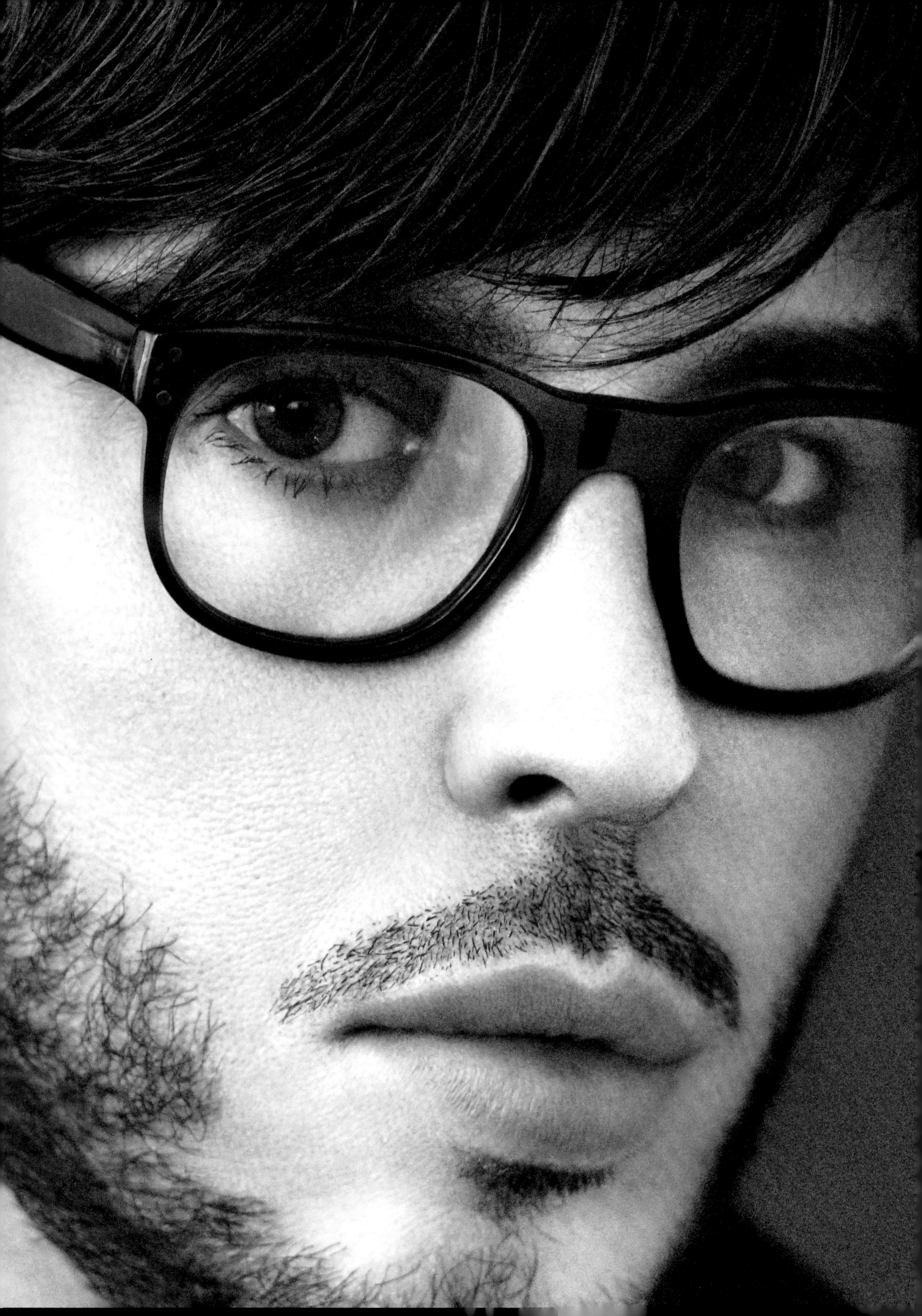

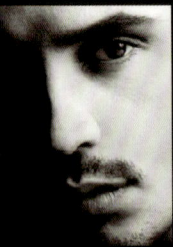

FRANÇOIS NARS, PHOTOGRAPH BY CHRIS MILITSCHER. © NARS COSMETICS.

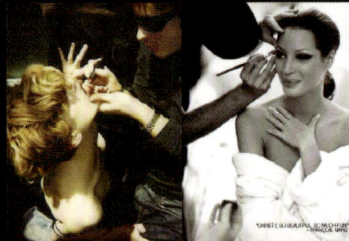

FRANÇOIS NARS DOING MAKEUP ON *LEFT:* KRISTEN MCMENAMY, CIRCA 1996. © NARS COSMETICS; *RIGHT:* CHRISTY TURLINGTON, PREVIOUSLY PUBLISHED IN *VOGUE* ITALIA, 1992. © WALTER CHIN/ TRUNK ARCHIVE.

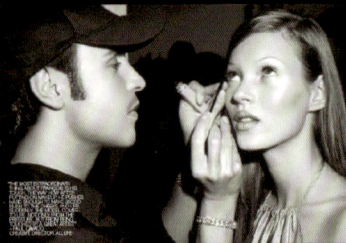

KATE MOSS AND FRANÇOIS NARS, 1992. © ROXANNE LOWIT.

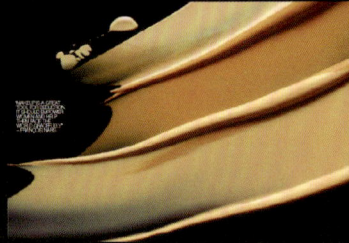

NARS PURE RADIANT TINTED MOISTURIZER PHOTOGRAPH BY MAXIME POIBLANC. © NARS COSMETICS.

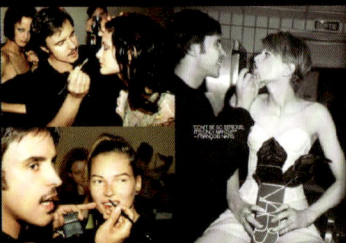

FRANÇOIS NARS DOING MAKEUP ON *LEFT:* SHALOM HARLOW (TOP), KATE MOSS (BOTTOM), CIRCA 1997. © NARS COSMETICS; *RIGHT:* KRISTEN MCMENAMY, 1995. © ROXANNE LOWIT.

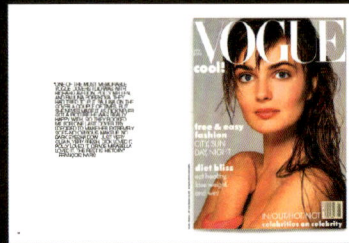

VOGUE, MAY 1986. PAULINA PORIZKOVA, PHOTOGRAPH BY RICHARD AVEDON, MAKEUP BY FRANÇOIS NARS. © THE RICHARD AVEDON FOUNDATION.

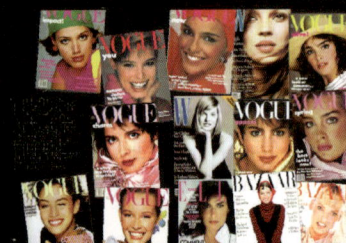

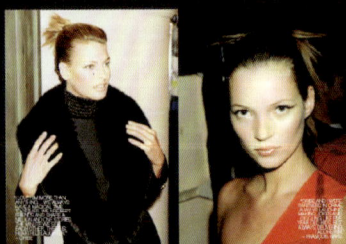

SELECTION OF U.S. MAGAZINE COVERS— ALL MAKEUP BY FRANÇOIS NARS. *FROM TOP LEFT TO BOTTOM RIGHT, BY TITLE: VOGUE:* MARCH 1984, APRIL 1984, JANUARY 1985, MAY 1984, JULY 1985, AUGUST 1985, FEBRUARY 1995, APRIL 1988, MAY 1988, ALL PHOTOGRAPHS BY RICHARD AVEDON. © THE RICHARD AVEDON FOUNDATION/CONDÉ NAST USA; *W:* JULY 1996, FEBRUARY 1994. © MICHAEL THOMSON/CONDÉ NAST USA; *ELLE:* SEPTEMBER 1983. © GILLES BENSIMON, COURTESY OF HACHETTE FILIPACCHI PRESSE, FRANCE; *HARPER'S BAZAAR:* NOVEMBER 1993, AUGUST 1994, ALL PHOTOGRAPHS BY PATRICK DEMARCHELIER. REPRINTED WITH THE PERMISSION OF HEARST COMMUNICATIONS, INC.

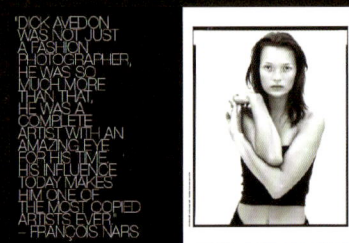

KATE MOSS IN CALVIN KLEIN'S CK BE CAMPAIGN, 1996, PHOTOGRAPH BY RICHARD AVEDON, MAKEUP BY FRANÇOIS NARS. © THE RICHARD AVEDON FOUNDATION.

LEFT AND RIGHT: STEPHANIE SEYMOUR WITH MARCUS SCHENKENBERG, VERSACE FALL 1993 CAMPAIGN, MAKEUP BY FRANÇOIS NARS. ALL PHOTOGRAPHS BY RICHARD AVEDON. © THE RICHARD AVEDON FOUNDATION.

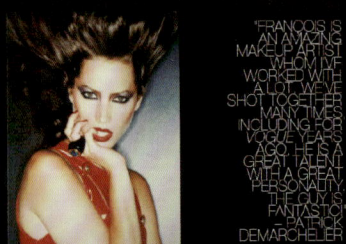

LEFT AND RIGHT: LINDA EVANGELISTA *(LEFT)* AND KATE MOSS *(RIGHT)* BACKSTAGE, NEW YORK, CIRCA 1995. © NARS COSMETICS.

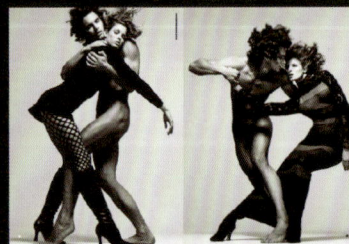

GIANNI VERSACE, DESIGNER, NOVEMBER 11 1981, PHOTOGRAPH BY RICHARD AVEDON. © THE RICHARD AVEDON FOUNDATION.

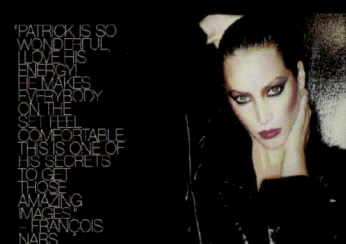

CHRISTY TURLINGTON BY PATRICK DEMARCHELIER. PREVIOUSLY PUBLISHED BY *HARPER'S BAZAAR*, AUGUST 1994. REPRINTED WITH THE PERMISSION OF HEARST COMMUNICATIONS, INC.

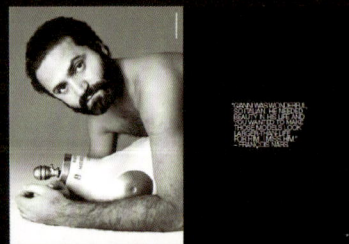

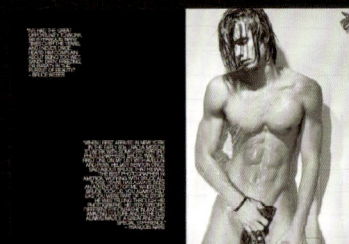

MARCUS SCHENKENBERG IN A CALVIN KLEIN JEANS CAMPAIGN, 1991, PHOTOGRAPH BY BRUCE WEBER, MAKEUP BY FRANÇOIS NARS. © BRUCE WEBER.

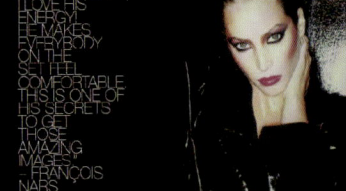

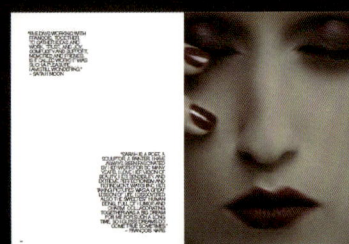

CHRISTY TURLINGTON BY PATRICK DEMARCHELIER. PREVIOUSLY PUBLISHED BY *HARPER'S BAZAAR*, AUGUST 1994. REPRINTED WITH THE PERMISSION OF HEARST COMMUNICATIONS, INC.

FROM THE NARS SARAH MOON HOLIDAY 2016 COLLECTION. © SARAH MOON.

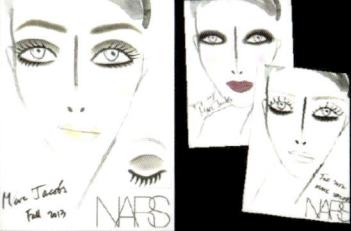

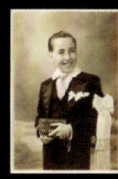

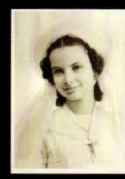

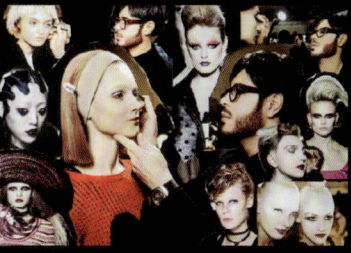

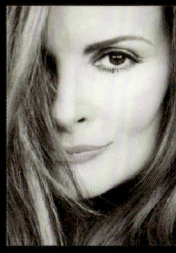

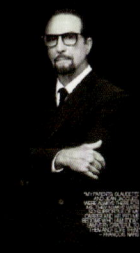

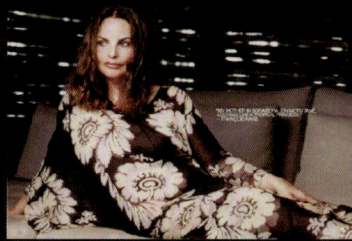

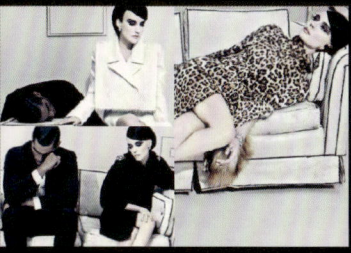

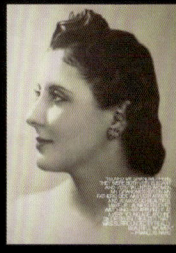

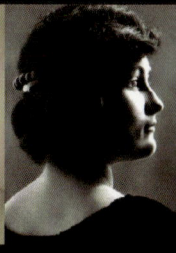

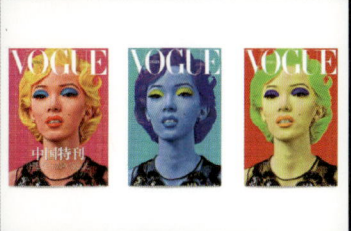

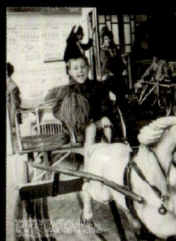

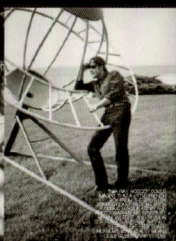

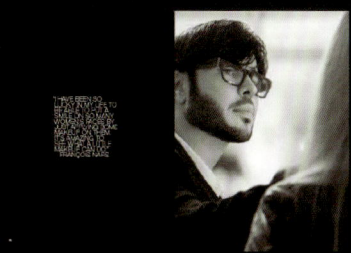

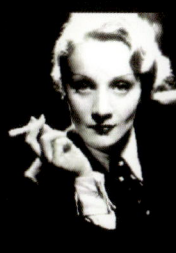

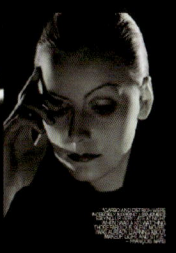

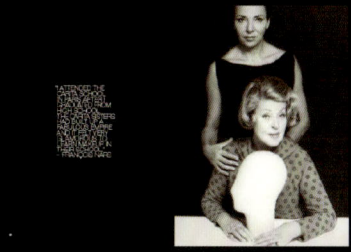

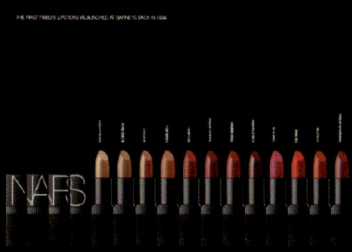

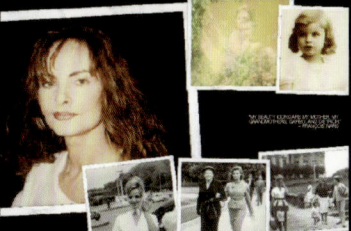

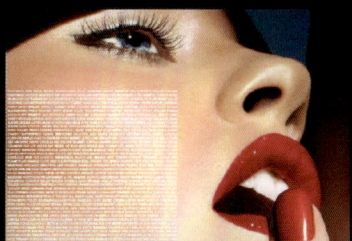

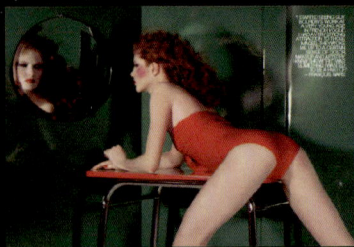

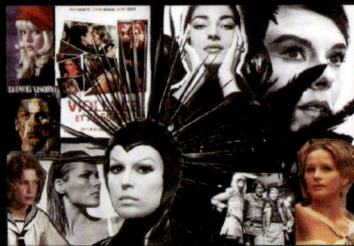

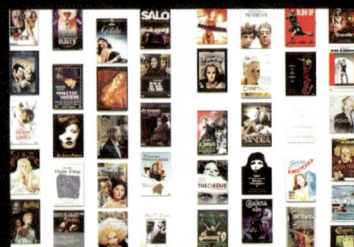

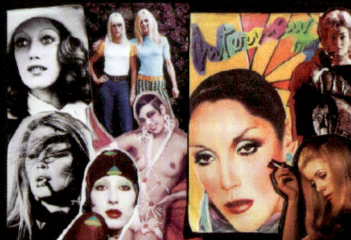

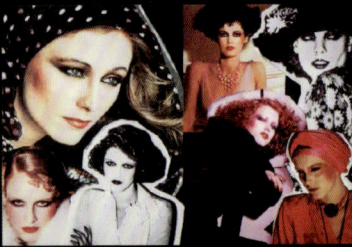

FRANÇOIS NARS'SS INSPIRATION COLLAGE OF MODELS FROM THE 1970S. *CLOCKWISE FROM TOP LEFT:* SUSAN MONCUR BY GIAN PAOLO BARBIERI. © GIAN PAOLO BARBIERI; DAYLE HADDON BY GUY BOURDIN. © ESTATE OF GUY BOURDIN/ART + COMMERCE; CHRISTIANA STEIDTEN BY GIAN PAOLO BARBIERI. © GIAN PAOLO BARBIERI; CARRIE NYGREN, BOTH PHOTOGRAPHS BY GUY BOURDIN. © ESTATE OF GUY BOURDIN/ ART + COMMERCE; CAROLE SINGLETON BY GIAN PAOLO BARBIERI. © GIAN PAOLO BARBIERI; GUNILLA LINDBLAD BY HANS FEURER. © HANS FEURER.

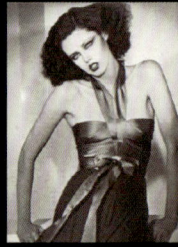

DAYLE HADDON, PHOTOGRAPH BY GUY BOURDIN, PREVIOUSLY PUBLISHED IN *VOGUE* PARIS, SEPTEMBER 1974. © ESTATE OF GUY BOURDIN/ ART + COMMERCE.

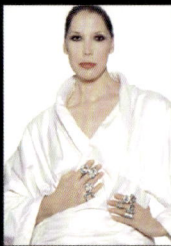

MARINA SCHIANO, PHOTOGRAPH BY FRANÇOIS NARS. © FRANÇOIS NARS.

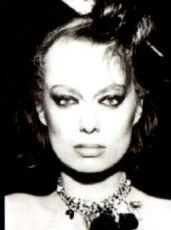

VIBEKE KNUDSEN, PHOTOGRAPH BY HANS FEURER, PREVIOUSLY PUBLISHED IN *VOGUE* PARIS JUNE/JULY 1976. © HANS FEURER.

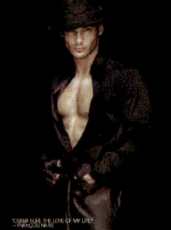

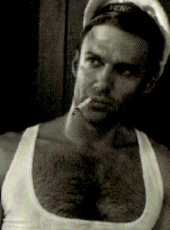

CSABA EGRI, PHOTOGRAPHS BY FRANÇOIS NARS. © FRANÇOIS NARS.

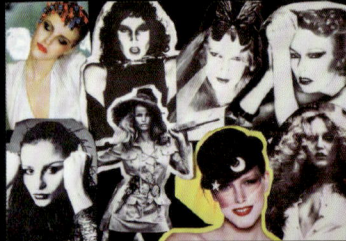

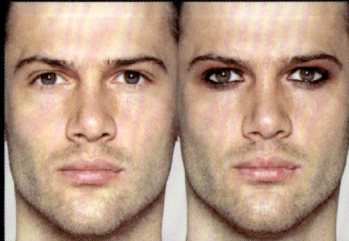

FRANÇOIS NARS'SS INSPIRATION COLLAGE OF MODELS FROM THE 1970S. *CLOCKWISE FROM TOP LEFT:* CAROLE SINGLETON, ANJELICA HUSTON, CARRIE NYGREN, AND UNKNOWN MODEL, ALL PHOTOGRAPHS BY GUY BOURDIN. © ESTATE OF GUY BOURDIN/ ART + COMMERCE; JERRY HALL; CARRIE NYGREN BY FOULI ELIA. © HACHETTE FILIPACCHI PRESSE, FRANCE; VERUSCHKA VON LEHNDORFF BY FRANCO RUBARTELLI. © CONDÉ NAST FRANCE; APPOLONIA VON RAVENSTEIN.

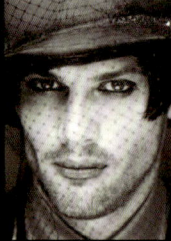

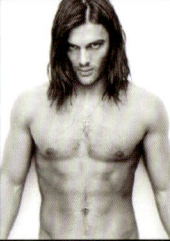

CSABA EGRI, PHOTOGRAPHS BY FRANÇOIS NARS. © FRANÇOIS NARS.

CSABA EGRI, PHOTOGRAPHS BY FRANÇOIS NARS, PREVIOUSLY PUBLISHED IN *NARS MAKEUP YOUR MIND,* 2001. © FRANÇOIS NARS.

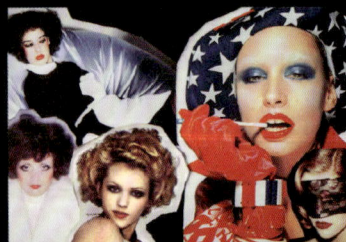

FRANÇOIS NARS'SS INSPIRATION COLLAGE OF MODELS FROM THE 1970S. *CLOCKWISE FROM TOP LEFT:* NICOLLE MEYER BY GUY BOURDIN, CHARLES JOURDAN FALL 1977 CAMPAIGN. © ESTATE OF GUY BOURDIN/ART + COMMERCE; DONNA JORDAN, CAROLE SINGLETON, BOTH PHOTOGRAPHS BY CHRIS VON WANGENHEIM. © ESTATE OF CHRIS VON WANGENHEIM/LICENSED BY VAGA, NEW YORK, NY; LOUISE DESPOINTES BY GUY BOURDIN © ESTATE OF GUY BOURDIN/ART + COMMERCE; TRACY WEED BY BARRY LATEGAN FOR *VOGUE* ITALIA, SEPTEMBER 1972. © BARRY LATEGAN, COURTESY OF *VOGUE* ITALIA.

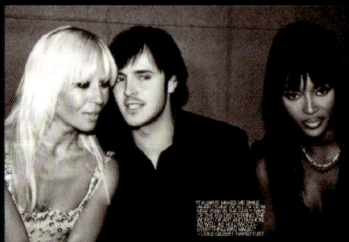

DONATELLA VERSACE, FRANÇOIS NARS, AND NAOMI CAMPBELL, 1995. © STEVE EICHNER/WIREIMAGE/GETTY IMAGES.

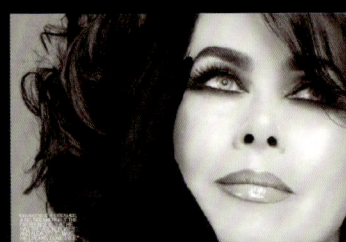

FROM LEFT TO RIGHT, BY ROW: FRANÇOIS NARS WITH CHRISTY TURLINGTON, 1992. © ROXANNE LOWIT; SHALOM HARLOW, 1994. © ROXANNE LOWIT; TONI GARRN, 2014. © WILL RAGOZZINO/BFANYC/SIPA USA; SERGE LUTENS, CHARLOTTE RAMPLING, ALL PHOTOGRAPHS BY DAVID DIESING, 2014. © FRANÇOIS NARS; MARINA SCHIANO, 2001. © NARS COSMETICS; CHRISTIAN LACROIX, PHOTOGRAPH BY DAVID DIESING, 2014. © FRANÇOIS NARS; LINDA EVANGELISTA BY LENA KORO. © FRANÇOIS NARS; SARAH MOON AND PATTI WILSON, 2015. © SARAH MOON; LIV TYLER, PHOTOGRAPH BY DAVID DIESING, 2013. © FRANÇOIS NARS; NAOMI CAMPBELL, 2009. © MIKE COPPOLA; JAMES KALIARDOS, PHOTOGRAPH BY DAVID DIESING, 2013. © FRANÇOIS NARS.

DAYLE HADDON, MODEL, PHOTOGRAPH BY FRANÇOIS NARS, 2009, PREVIOUSLY PUBLISHED IN *NARS 15X15.* © NARS COSMETICS.

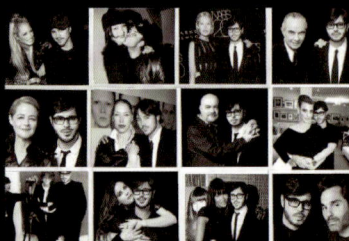

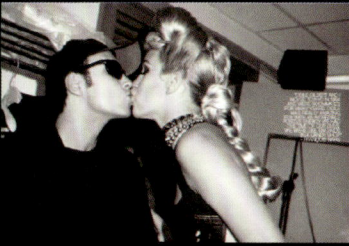

FRANÇOIS NARS WITH A MODEL, 1992.
© ROXANNE LOWIT.

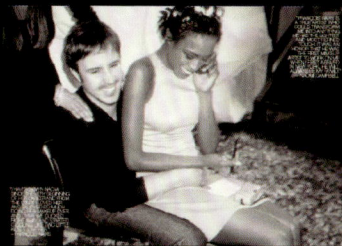

FRANÇOIS NARS AND NAOMI CAMPBELL,
PHOTOGRAPHER UNKNOWN.
© NARS COSMETICS.

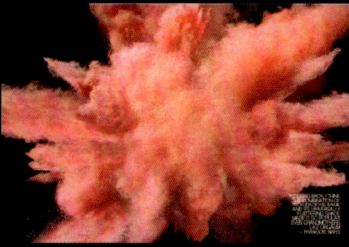

NARS ORGASM BLUSH, PHOTOGRAPH BY
BRENTON CARTER. © NARS COSMETICS.

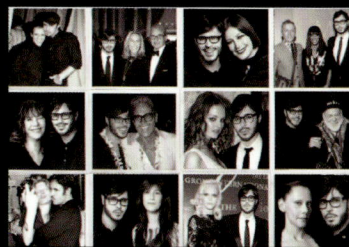

FROM LEFT TO RIGHT, BY ROW:
FRANÇOIS NARS WITH AZZEDINE ALAÏA,
1992. © ROXANNE LOWIT; CARLYNE
CERF DE DUDZEELE AND ORIBE, 2014.
© FRANÇOIS NARS; SUSAN MONCUR,
PHOTOGRAPH BY DAVID DIESING, 2015.
© FRANÇOIS NARS; SIMON DOONAN AND
PATTI WILSON, 2011. © DAVID X PRUTTING
& NEIL RASMUS/BFANYC/SIPA USA; JANE
BIRKIN, PHOTOGRAPH BY LUCAS FLORES
PIRAN, 2016. © FRANÇOIS NARS; ORIBE.
© FRANÇOIS NARS ARCHIVES; LYDIA
HEARST, 2007. © SHANE GRITZINGER/
FILMMAGIC/GETTY IMAGES; BRUCE
WEBER, PHOTOGRAPH BY DAVID
DIESING, 2015. © FRANÇOIS NARS;
KRISTEN MCMENAMY, CIRCA 1997.
© FRANÇOIS NARS ARCHIVES;
CHARLOTTE GAINSBOURG, PHOTOGRAPH
BY DAVID DIESING, 2014. © FRANÇOIS
NARS; GINTA LAPINA, 2011. © WILL
RAGOZZINO/BFANYC /SIPA USA; SUSANNE
BARTSCH, PHOTOGRAPH BY LUCAS
FLORES PIRAN, 2015. © FRANÇOIS NARS.

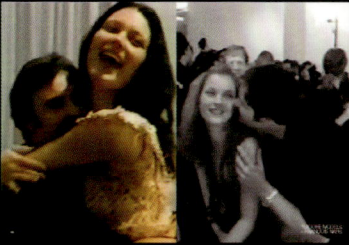

FRANÇOIS NARS WITH SHALOM HARLOW
(*LEFT*) AND KATE MOSS (*RIGHT*).
© NARS COSMETICS.

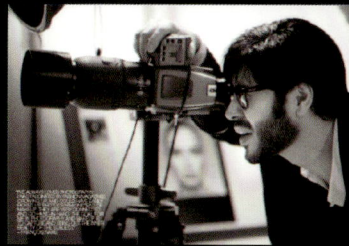

FROM LEFT TO RIGHT, BY ROW:
FRANÇOIS NARS WITH STEVEN KLEIN
AND STEPHANIE SEYMOUR, 2014.
© NEIL RASMUS/BFANYC/SIPA USA; TILDA
SWINTON BY ALESSANDRO ZOPPIS.
© FRANÇOIS NARS; BETTY CATROUX,
PHOTOGRAPH BY DAVID DIESING, 2013.
© FRANÇOIS NARS; DAYLE HADDON,
2007. © PATRICK MCMULLAN; TYSON
BALLOU, 2009. © JAMIE MCCARTHY/
GETTY IMAGES; ALICIA KEYS, 2015.
© NEIL RASMUS/BFANYC/SIPA USA;
GISELE BÜNDCHEN, PHOTOGRAPH BY
DAVID DIESING, 2015. © FRANÇOIS NARS;
LISA MARIE, 2009. © PATRICK MCMULLAN;
SYLVIE VARTAN, PHOTOGRAPH BY DAVID
DIESING, 2014. © FRANÇOIS NARS;
MARC JACOBS, OLIVIER THESKYENS,
AND LYDIA HEARST, ALL IN 2009. © JAMIE
MCCARTHY/GETTY IMAGES; GRACE
CODDINGTON, 2014. © NEIL RASMUS/
BFANYC/SIPA USA.

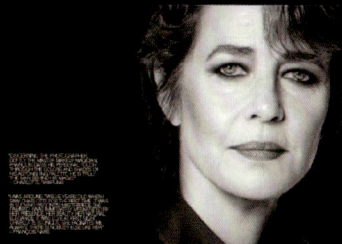

FRANÇOIS NARS SHOOTING FOR
*MAKEUP YOUR MIND EXPRESS
YOURSELF*, 2010. © NARS COSMETICS.

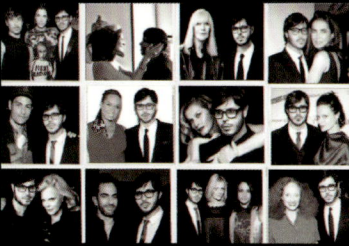

NARS AUDACIOUS LIPSTICK CAMPAIGN,
FALL 2014, CHARLOTTE RAMPLING,
ACTRESS, PHOTOGRAPH BY FRANÇOIS
NARS. © NARS COSMETICS.

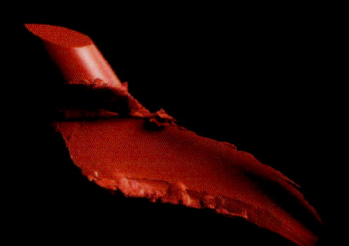

NARS HEAT WAVE LIPSTICK,
PHOTOGRAPH BY MAXIME POIBLANC.
© NARS COSMETICS.

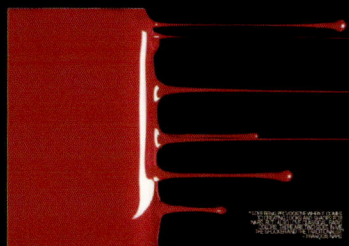

NARS SOUP CAN NAIL POLISH,
PHOTOGRAPH BY MAXIME POIBLANC.
© NARS COSMETICS.

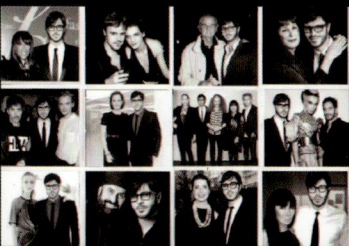

FROM LEFT TO RIGHT, BY ROW:
FRANÇOIS NARS WITH PATTI WILSON,
2011. © WILL RAGGOZINO/BFANYC/SIPA
USA; MICHELE HICKS, 1996. © ROXANNE
LOWIT; PATRICK DEMARCHELIER, 2010.
© PATRICK MCMULLAN; ANJELICA
HUSTON, PHOTOGRAPH BY DAVID DIESING,
2015. © FRANÇOIS NARS; STEVEN KLEIN
AND TAYLOR SCHILLING, SIGOURNEY
WEAVER, ALL IN 2014. © NEIL RASMUS/
BFANYC/SIPA USA; MARINA SCHIANO,
GRACE CODDINGTON, ANNA SUI, AND
CALVIN KLEIN, 2011. © DAVID X PRUTTING &
NEIL RASMUS/BFANYC/SIPA USA; DAPHNE
GUINNESS AND MARC JACOBS, 2009. ©
PATRICK MCMULLAN; DARIA STROKOUS,
2014. © NEIL RASMUS/BFANYC/SIPA USA;
PETER SAVIC, 2016. © FRANÇOIS NARS;
ISABELLA ROSSELLINI, 2010. © RABBANI
AND SOLIMENE/WIREIMAGE/GETTY IMAGES;
LENA KORO. © FRANÇOIS NARS ARCHIVES.

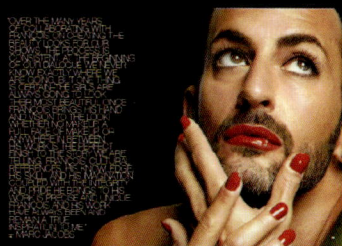

MARC JACOBS, DESIGNER,
PHOTOGRAPH BY FRANÇOIS NARS, 2009,
PREVIOUSLY PUBLISHED IN *NARS 15X15*.
© NARS COSMETICS.

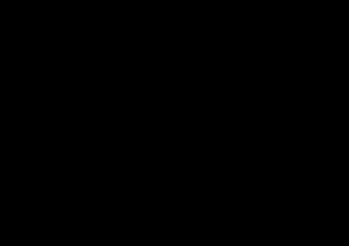

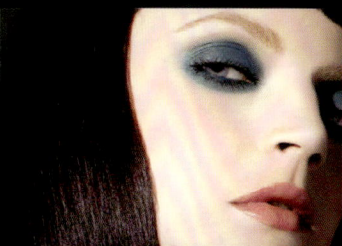

NARS SUMMER 2009 CAMPAIGN, MODEL
GUINEVERE VAN SEENUS, PHOTOGRAPH
BY FRANÇOIS NARS. © NARS COSMETICS.

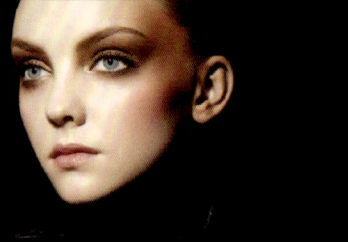

MODEL
HEATHER MARKS, PHOTOGRAPH BY
FRANÇOIS NARS. © NARS COSMETICS.

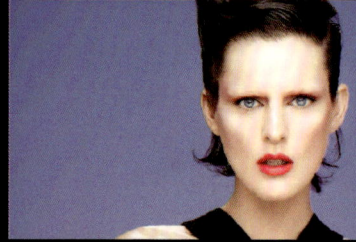

SPRING 2013, MODEL STELLA TENNANT,
PHOTOGRAPH BY FRANÇOIS NARS.
© NARS COSMETICS.

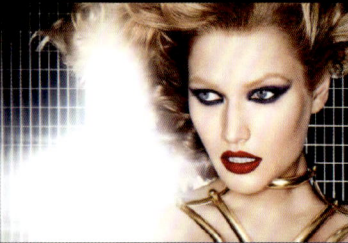

NARS FALL 2013 CAMPAIGN, MODEL TONI
GARRN, PHOTOGRAPH BY FRANÇOIS
NARS. © NARS COSMETICS.

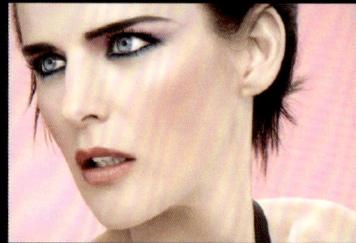

NARS SPRING 2013 CAMPAIGN, MODEL
STELLA TENNANT, PHOTOGRAPH BY
FRANÇOIS NARS. © NARS COSMETICS.

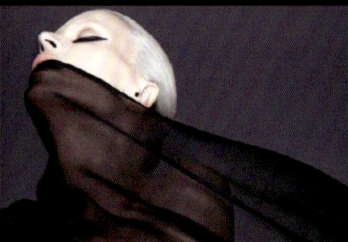

NARS FALL 2012 CAMPAIGN, MODEL
KRISTEN MCMENAMY, PHOTOGRAPH BY
FRANÇOIS NARS. © NARS COSMETICS.

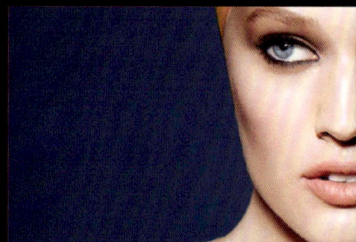

NARS MATTE MULTIPLE CAMPAIGN,
SPRING 2014, MODEL TONI GARRN,
PHOTOGRAPH BY FRANÇOIS NARS.
© NARS COSMETICS.

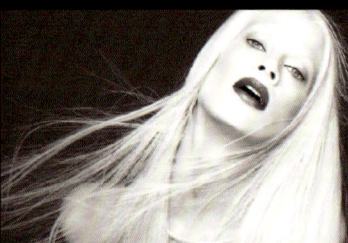

NARS FALL 2012 CAMPAIGN, MODEL
KRISTEN MCMENAMY, PHOTOGRAPH BY
FRANÇOIS NARS. © NARS COSMETICS.

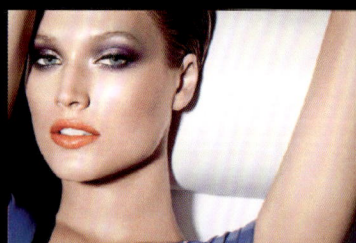

NARS SPRING 2014 CAMPAIGN, MODEL
TONI GARRN, PHOTOGRAPH BY
FRANÇOIS NARS. © NARS COSMETICS.

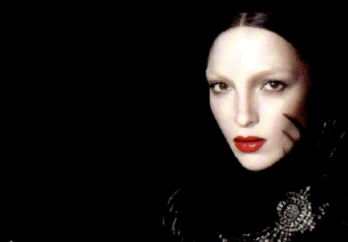

NARS LARGER THAN LIFE®
LIP GLOSS CAMPAIGN, HOLIDAY 2011,
MODEL MARIACARLA BOSCONO,
PHOTOGRAPH BY FRANÇOIS NARS.
© NARS COSMETICS.

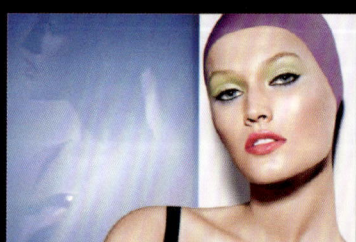

NARS SUMMER 2014 CAMPAIGN,
MODEL TONI GARRN, PHOTOGRAPH BY
FRANÇOIS NARS. © NARS COSMETICS.

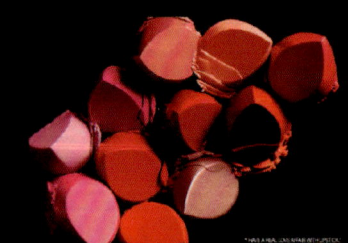

NARS LIPSTICK, PHOTOGRAPH BY
MAXIME POIBLANC. © NARS COSMETICS.

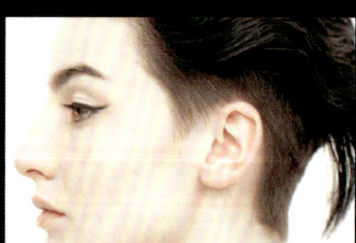

ERIN O'CONNOR, MODEL, PHOTOGRAPH
BY FRANÇOIS NARS, 1997, PREVIOUSLY
PUBLISHED IN X-RAY. © FRANÇOIS NARS.

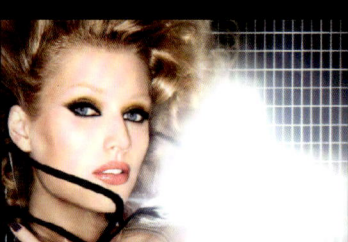

NARS EYE PAINT CAMPAIGN, FALL 2013,
MODEL TONI GARRN, PHOTOGRAPH BY
FRANÇOIS NARS. © NARS COSMETICS.

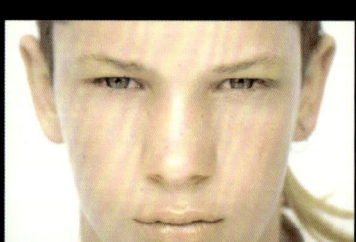

DAIN WILKERSON, MODEL, PHOTOGRAPH
BY FRANÇOIS NARS, 1997, PREVIOUSLY
PUBLISHED IN X-RAY. © FRANÇOIS NARS.

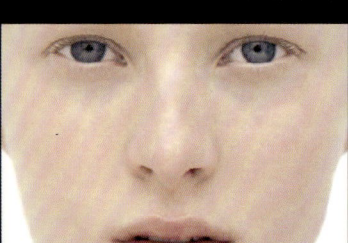

KAREN ELSON, MODEL, PHOTOGRAPH
BY FRANÇOIS NARS, 1997, PREVIOUSLY
PUBLISHED IN X-RAY. © FRANÇOIS NARS.

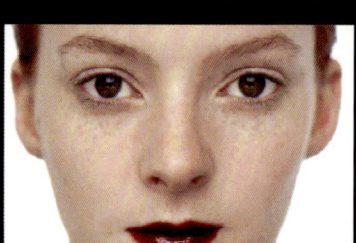

NARS SPRING 1999 CAMPAIGN, MODEL
SUNNIVA STORDHAL, PHOTOGRAPH BY
FRANÇOIS NARS. © NARS COSMETICS.

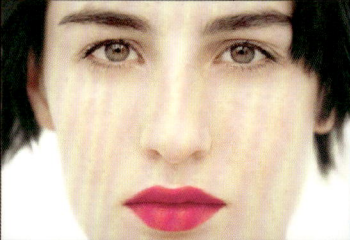

NARS SPRING 1998 CAMPAIGN, MODEL
ERIN O'CONNOR WITH SCHIAP LIPSTICK,
PHOTOGRAPH BY FRANÇOIS NARS.
© NARS COSMETICS.

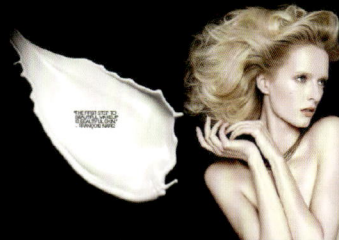

DARIA STROKOUS, PHOTOGRAPH BY
FRANÇOIS NARS. © NARS COSMETICS.

NARS AUDACIOUS LIPSTICK.
© ERIC MAILLET.

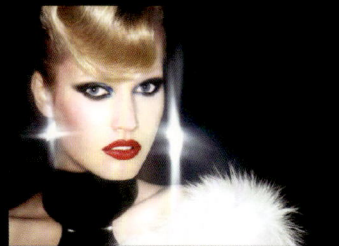

NARS HOLIDAY 2013 CAMPAIGN,
MODEL TONI GARRN, PHOTOGRAPH BY
FRANÇOIS NARS. © NARS COSMETICS.

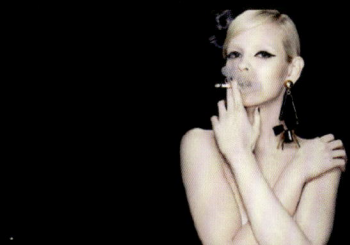

MODEL GINTA LAPINA, PHOTOGRAPH
BY FRANÇOIS NARS, PREVIOUSLY
PUBLISHED IN *VOGUE* JAPAN, APRIL 2011.
© FRANÇOIS NARS.

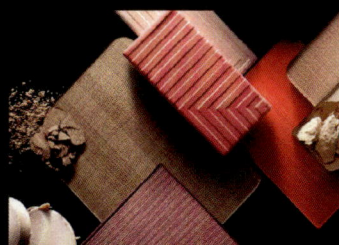

NARS DUAL INTENSITY BLUSH AND
BRONZER, PHOTOGRAPH BY BRENTON
CARTER. © NARS COSMETICS.

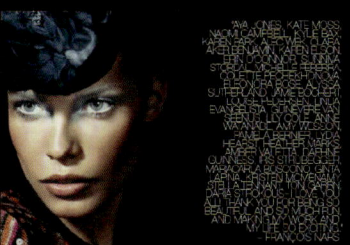

NARS FALL 2003 CAMPAIGN, MODEL
LOUISE PEDERSEN, PHOTOGRAPH BY
FRANÇOIS NARS. © NARS COSMETICS..

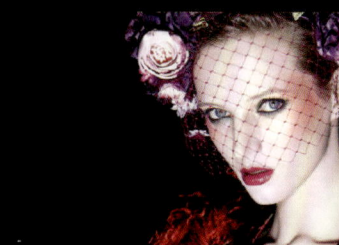

NARS HOLIDAY 2015 CAMPAIGN, MODEL
DARIA STROKOUS, PHOTOGRAPH BY
FRANÇOIS NARS. © NARS COSMETICS.

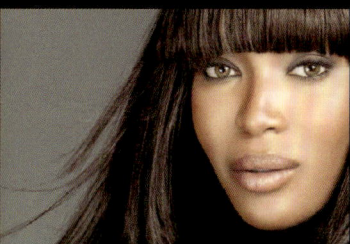

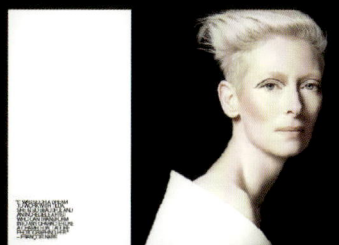

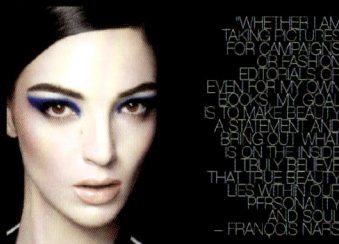

NAOMI CAMPBELL, MODEL,
PHOTOGRAPH BY FRANÇOIS NARS, 2009,
PREVIOUSLY PUBLISHED IN *NARS 15X15*.
© NARS COSMETICS.

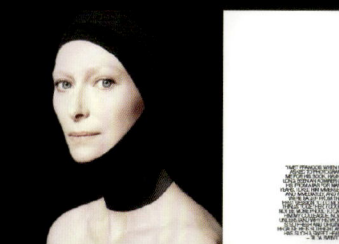

NARS ALL DAY LUMINOUS WEIGHTLESS
FOUNDATION CAMPAIGN, SPRING 2015,
TILDA SWINTON, ACTRESS, PHOTOGRAPH
BY FRANÇOIS NARS. © NARS COSMETICS.

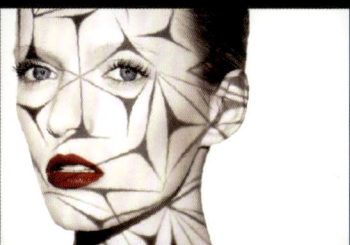

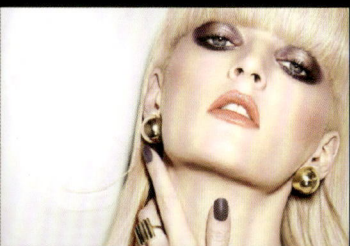

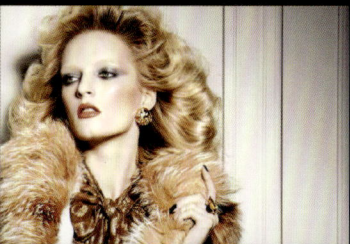

NARS HOLIDAY 2014 CAMPAIGN, MODEL
DARIA STROKOUS, PHOTOGRAPH BY
FRANÇOIS NARS. © NARS COSMETICS.

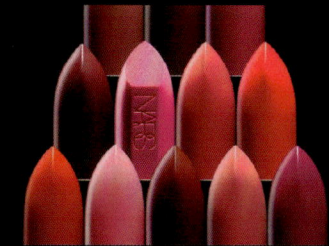

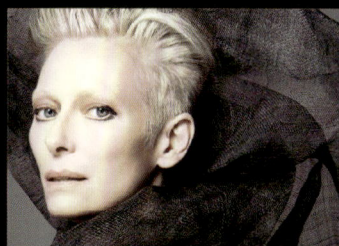

NARS DUAL INTENSITY BLUSH CAMPAIGN,
SPRING 2015, TILDA SWINTON, ACTRESS,
PHOTOGRAPH BY FRANÇOIS NARS.
© NARS COSMETICS.

NARS DUAL INTENSITY EYE SHADOW
CAMPAIGN, FALL 2014, MODEL DARIA
STROKOUS, PHOTOGRAPH BY FRANÇOIS
NARS. © NARS COSMETICS.

NARS SPRING 2015 CAMPAIGN, TILDA
SWINTON, ACTRESS, PHOTOGRAPH BY
FRANÇOIS NARS. © NARS COSMETICS.

NARS FALL 2014 CAMPAIGN, MODEL
DARIA STROKOUS, PHOTOGRAPH BY
FRANÇOIS NARS. © NARS COSMETICS.

NARS FALL 2011 CAMPAIGN, MODEL
MARIACARLA BOSCONO, PHOTOGRAPH
BY FRANÇOIS NARS. © NARS COSMETICS.

NARS HOLIDAY 2004 CAMPAIGN,
PHOTOGRAPH BY GUY BOURDIN.
© ESTATE OF GUY BOURDIN,
REPRODUCED WITH THE PERMISSION
OF ART + COMMERCE.

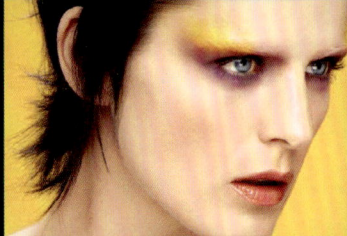

NARS SUMMER 2013 CAMPAIGN, MODEL
STELLA TENNANT, PHOTOGRAPH BY
FRANÇOIS NARS. © NARS COSMETICS.

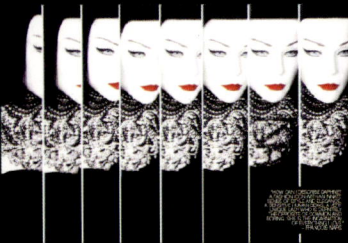

NARS FALL 2010 CAMPAIGN, ARTIST
DAPHNE GUINNESS, PHOTOGRAPH BY
FRANÇOIS NARS. © NARS COSMETICS.

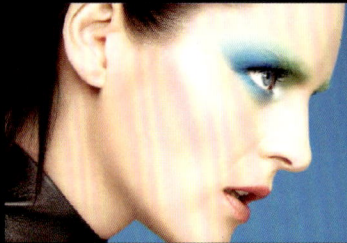

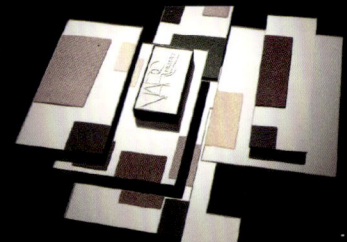

NARS SUMMER 2013 VISUAL, MODEL
STELLA TENNANT, PHOTOGRAPH BY
FRANÇOIS NARS. © NARS COSMETICS.

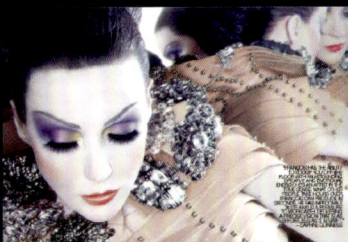

NARS HOLIDAY 2010 CAMPAIGN, ARTIST
DAPHNE GUINNESS, PHOTOGRAPH BY
FRANÇOIS NARS. © NARS COSMETICS.

NARSISSIST EYE PALETTE,
PHOTOGRAPH BY BRENTON CARTER.
© NARS COSMETICS.

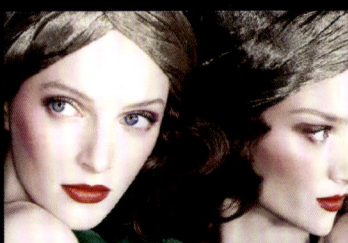

NARS FALL 2015 CAMPAIGN, MODEL
DARIA STROKOUS, PHOTOGRAPH BY
FRANÇOIS NARS. © NARS COSMETICS.

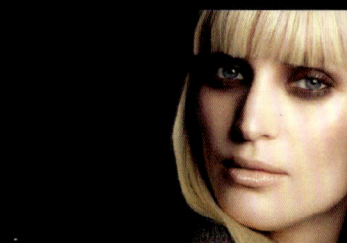

NARS HOLIDAY 2007 CAMPAIGN, MODEL
AMY WESSON, PHOTOGRAPH BY
FRANÇOIS NARS. © NARS COSMETICS.

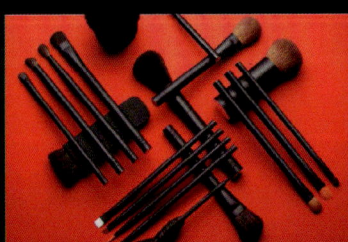

NARS ARTISTRY BRUSHES,
PHOTOGRAPH BY BRENTON CARTER.
© NARS COSMETICS.

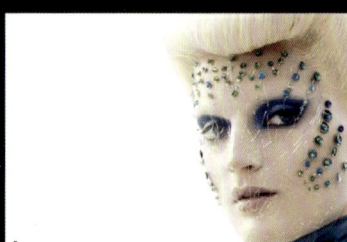

NARS HOLIDAY 2005 CAMPAIGN, MODEL
GUINEVERE VAN SEENUS, PHOTOGRAPH
BY FRANÇOIS NARS. © NARS COSMETICS

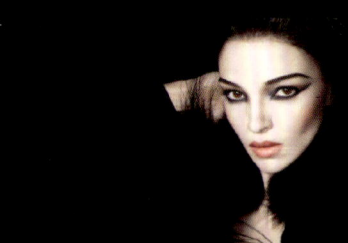

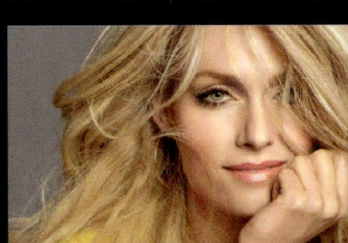

NARS LARGER THAN LIFE® LONGWEAR
EYELINER CAMPAIGN, FALL 2011, MODEL
MARIACARLA BOSCONO, PHOTOGRAPH BY
FRANÇOIS NARS. © NARS COSMETICS.

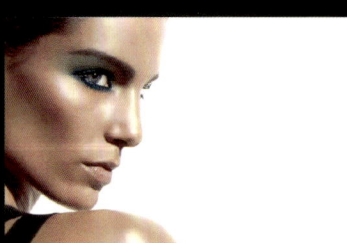

NARS SUMMER 2011 CAMPAIGN, MODEL
IRIS STRUBEGGER, PHOTOGRAPH BY
FRANÇOIS NARS. © NARS COSMETICS.

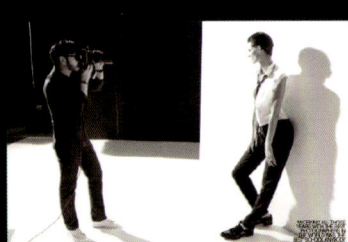

FRANÇOIS NARS AND MODEL IRIS
STRUBEGGER ON A SHOOT FOR
THE NARS SPRING 2011 CAMPAIGN.
© NARS COSMETICS.

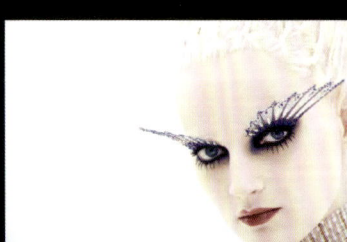

NARS FALL 2005 CAMPAIGN, MODEL
GUINEVERE VAN SEENUS, PHOTOGRAPH
BY FRANÇOIS NARS. © NARS COSMETICS

NARS SPRING 2010 CAMPAIGN, MODEL
AMBER VALLETTA, PHOTOGRAPH BY
FRANÇOIS NARS. © NARS COSMETICS.

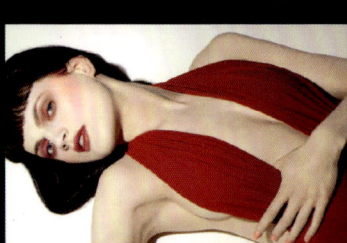

NARS SPRING 2009 CAMPAIGN, MODEL
GUINEVERE VAN SEENUS, PHOTOGRAPH
BY FRANÇOIS NARS. © NARS COSMETICS

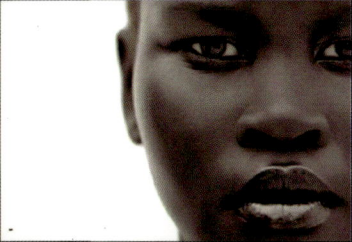

NARS 2006 CAMPAIGN, MODEL ALEC WECK, PHOTOGRAPH BY FRANÇOIS NARS. © NARS COSMETICS.

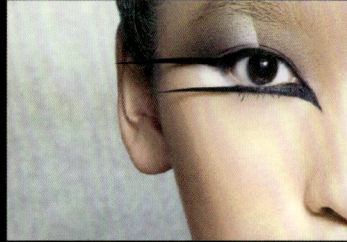

NARS 2006 CAMPAIGN, MODEL NAOMI CAMPBELL, PHOTOGRAPH BY FRANÇOIS NARS. © NARS COSMETICS.

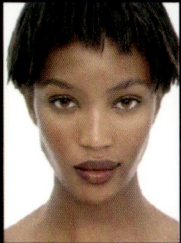

LEFT: CLARA AKER BENJAMIN, MODEL, PREVIOUSLY PUBLISHED IN *X-RAY*, 1997, PHOTOGRAPH BY FRANÇOIS NARS. © NARS COSMETICS. *RIGHT*: NARS FALL 1997 CAMPAIGN, MODEL KAREN ELSON, PHOTOGRAPH BY FRANÇOIS NARS. © NARS COSMETICS.

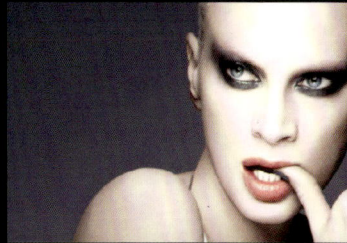

JASON FIDELE, MODEL/MUSICIAN, PREVIOUSLY PUBLISHED IN *X-RAY*, 1997, PHOTOGRAPH BY FRANÇOIS NARS. © FRANÇOIS NARS.

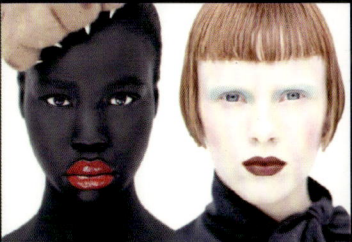

NARS 1996 CAMPAIGN, MODEL KAREN PARK GOUDE, PHOTOGRAPH BY FRANÇOIS NARS. © NARS COSMETICS.

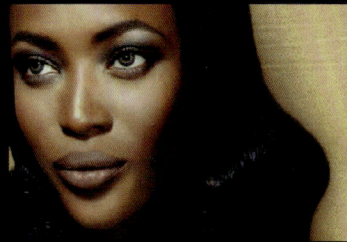

NARS 1997 CAMPAIGN, MODEL ELONORA JAGER, PHOTOGRAPH BY FRANÇOIS NARS. © NARS COSMETICS.

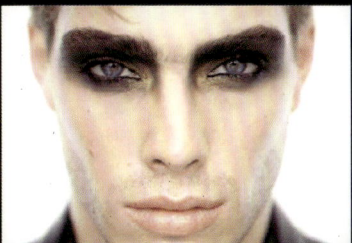

NARS EYE SHADOWS, PHOTOGRAPH BY MAXIME POIBLANC. © NARS COSMETICS.

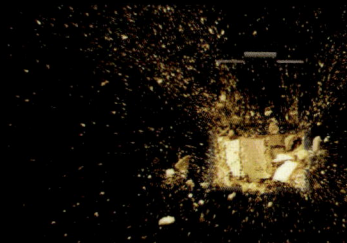

NARS HOLIDAY 2006 CAMPAIGN, MODEL ANNE WATANABE, PHOTOGRAPH BY FRANÇOIS NARS. © NARS COSMETICS.

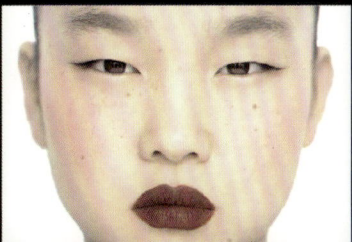

NARS FALL 2006 CAMPAIGN, MODEL ANNE WATANABE, PHOTOGRAPH BY FRANÇOIS NARS. © NARS COSMETICS.

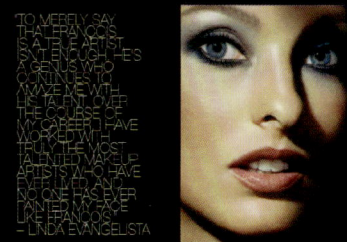

NARS FALL 2012 CAMPAIGN, MODEL KRISTEN MCMENAMY, PHOTOGRAPH BY FRANÇOIS NARS. © NARS COSMETICS.

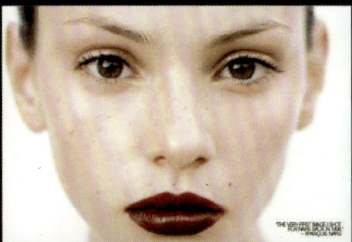

NARS FALL 2004 CAMPAIGN, MODEL NAOMI CAMPBELL, PHOTOGRAPH BY FRANÇOIS NARS. © NARS COSMETICS.

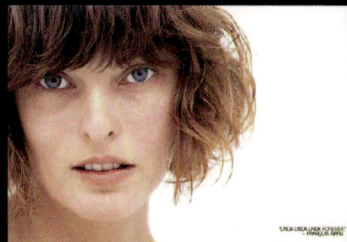

NARS GOLDFINGER EYE SHADOW. © NARS COSMETICS.

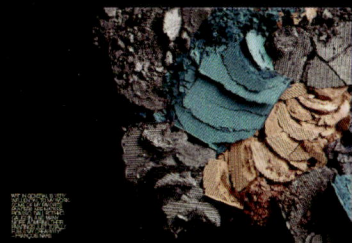

TO MERELY SAY THAT FRANÇOIS IS A GENIUS WHO CONTINUES TO AMAZE ME WITH HIS TALENT OVER MY CAREER? I HAVE WORKED WITH TRULY THE MOST TALENTED MAKEUP ARTISTS AND I HAVE NO ONE HAS EVER PAINTED MY FACE LIKE FRANÇOIS
— LINDA EVANGELISTA

NARS SPRING 2004 CAMPAIGN, MODEL LINDA EVANGELISTA, PHOTOGRAPH BY FRANÇOIS NARS. © NARS COSMETICS.

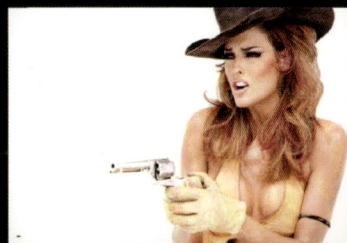

LINDA EVANGELISTA, PHOTOGRAPH BY FRANÇOIS NARS, 1997, PREVIOUSLY PUBLISHED IN *X-RAY*. © FRANÇOIS NARS.

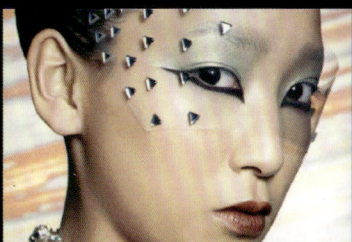

LINDA EVANGELISTA, PHOTOGRAPH BY FRANÇOIS NARS, 1997, PREVIOUSLY PUBLISHED IN *X-RAY*. © FRANÇOIS NARS.

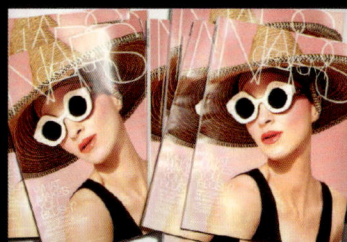

NARS ORGASM CAMPAIGN, SUMMER 2016, MODEL MARIACARLA BOSCONO, PHOTOGRAPH BY FRANÇOIS NARS. © NARS COSMETICS.

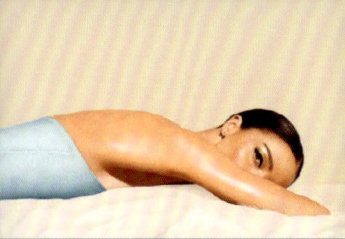

NARS BRONZING CAMPAIGN, SUMMER 2016, MODEL MARIACARLA BOSCONO, PHOTOGRAPH BY FRANÇOIS NARS. © NARS COSMETICS.

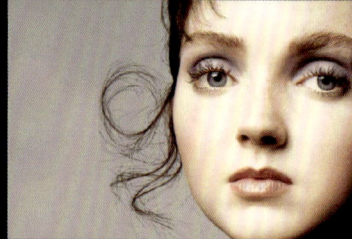

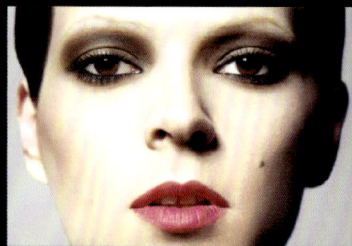

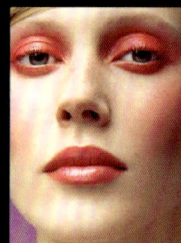

NARS SUMMER 2006 CAMPAIGN, MODEL LILY COLE, PHOTOGRAPH BY FRANÇOIS NARS. © NARS COSMETICS.

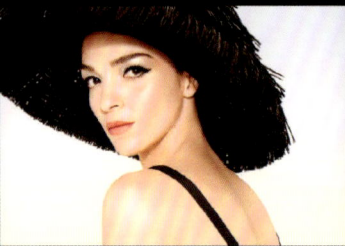

NARS SPRING 2016 CAMPAIGN, MODEL MARIACARLA BOSCONO, PHOTOGRAPH BY FRANÇOIS NARS. © NARS COSMETICS.

NARS FALL 2001 CAMPAIGN, MODEL ELEONORA (BIMBA) BOSE, PHOTOGRAPH BY FRANÇOIS NARS. © NARS COSMETICS

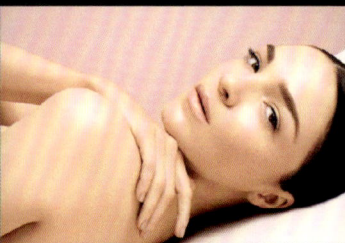

NARS VELVET MATTE SKIN TINT CAMPAIGN, SPRING 2016, MODEL MARIACARLA BOSCONO, PHOTOGRAPH BY FRANÇOIS NARS. © NARS COSMETICS.

NARS SPRING 2001 CAMPAIGN, MODEL COLETTE PECHEKHONOVA, PHOTOGRAPH BY FRANÇOIS NARS. © NARS COSMETICS.

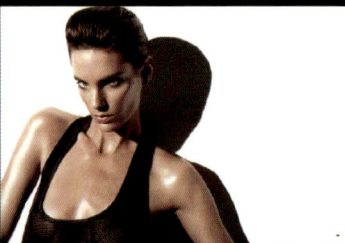

NARS ILLUMINATOR CAMPAIGN, SPRING 2011, MODEL IRIS STRUBEGGER, PHOTOGRAPH BY FRANÇOIS NARS. © NARS COSMETICS.

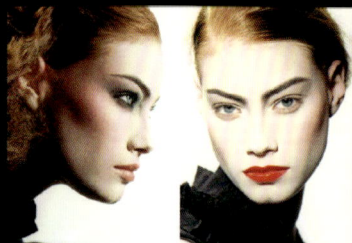

NARS SPRING 2002 CAMPAIGN, MODEL ALYSSA SUTHERLAND, PHOTOGRAPHS BY FRANÇOIS NARS. © NARS COSMETICS.

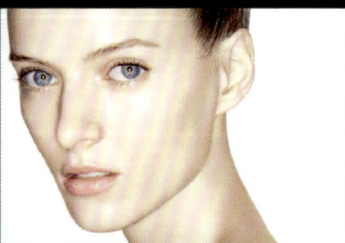

NARS SKIN CAMPAIGN, FALL 2015, MODEL DARIA STROKOUS, PHOTOGRAPH BY FRANÇOIS NARS. © NARS COSMETICS.

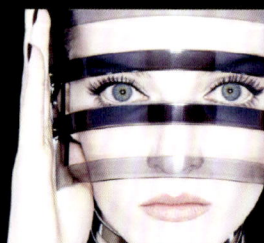

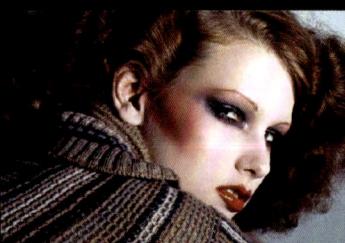

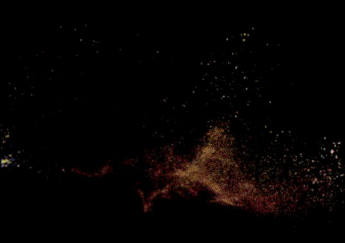

NARS AUDACIOUS MASCARA CAMPAIGN, FALL 2015, MODEL DARIA STROKOUS, PHOTOGRAPH BY FRANÇOIS NARS. © NARS COSMETICS.

NARS SUMMER 2005 CAMPAIGN, MODEL CARRIE NYGREN, PHOTOGRAPH BY GUY BOURDIN. © ESTATE OF GUY BOURDIN, REPRODUCED WITH THE PERMISSION OF ART + COMMERCE.

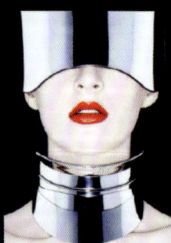

NARS AUDACIOUS LIPSTICK CAMPAIGN, FALL 2015, MODEL DARIA STROKOUS, PHOTOGRAPH BY FRANÇOIS NARS. © NARS COSMETICS.

NARS EYE SHADOWS, PHOTOGRAPH BY MAXIME POIBLANC. © NARS COSMETICS.

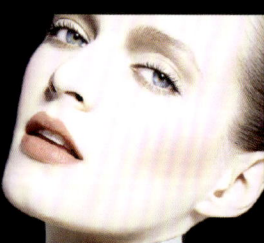

NARS HOT SAND CAMPAIGN, SPRING 2016, MODEL DARIA STROKOUS, PHOTOGRAPH BY FRANÇOIS NARS. © NARS COSMETICS.

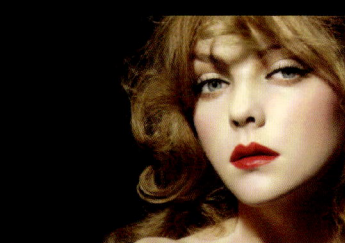

NARS PURE MATTE LIPSTICK CAMPAIGN, FALL 2009, MODEL HEATHER MARKS, PHOTOGRAPH BY FRANÇOIS NARS. © NARS COSMETICS.

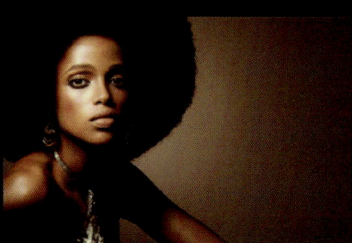

NARS AUDACIOUS CAMPAIGN, FALL 2016, MODEL AYA JONES, PHOTOGRAPH BY FRANÇOIS NARS. © NARS COSMETICS.

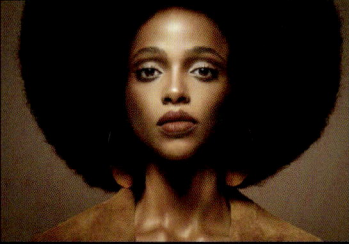

NARS... CAMPAIGN, MODEL AYA JONES, PHOTOGRAPH BY FRANÇOIS NARS. © NARS COSMETICS.

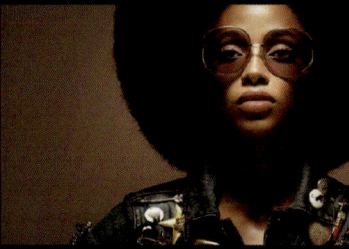

NARS VELVET LIP GLIDE CAMPAIGN, FALL 2016, MODEL AYA JONES, PHOTOGRAPH BY FRANÇOIS NARS. © NARS COSMETICS.

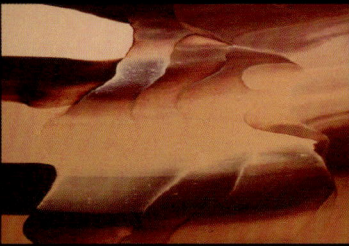

NARS FOUNDATIONS, PHOTOGRAPH BY MAXIME POIBLANC. © NARS COSMETICS.

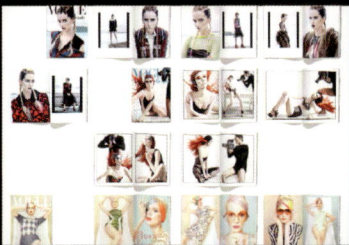

FRANÇOIS NARS'SS EDITORIALS FOR *VOGUE* JAPAN. *FROM TOP LEFT, BY ROW*: AUGUST 2013, *THE AVANT GARDE*, MODEL DARIA STROKOUS; JUNE 2010, *POOL PARTY*, MODEL TAO OKAMOTO; JUNE 2012, *THE RESORT TO BEAUTY*, MODEL DARIA STROKOUS. ALL PHOTOGRAPHS BY FRANÇOIS NARS. © FRANÇOIS NARS/2014 CONDÉ NAST JAPAN.

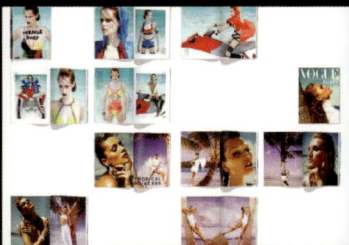

FRANÇOIS NARS'SS EDITORIALS FOR *VOGUE* JAPAN. *FROM TOP LEFT, BY ROW*: JULY 2014, *MIRACLE BODY*, MODEL THAIRINE GARCIA; AUGUST 2012, *TROPICAL PRINCESS*, MODEL TORI GARNN. ALL PHOTOGRAPHS BY FRANÇOIS NARS. © FRANÇOIS NARS/2014 CONDÉ NAST JAPAN.

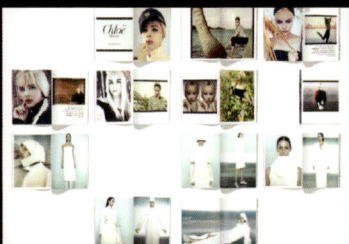

FRANÇOIS NARS'SS EDITORIALS FOR LEADING FASHION MAGAZINES. *FROM TOP LEFT, BY ROW: INSTYLE* SEPTEMBER 2012, *JOURNEY TO NARS*, MODEL CHLOE MORETZ; *VOGUE* JAPAN, *SHADES OF WHITE*. © 2016 CONDÉ NAST JAPAN. ALL PHOTOGRAPHS BY FRANÇOIS NARS. © FRANÇOIS NARS.

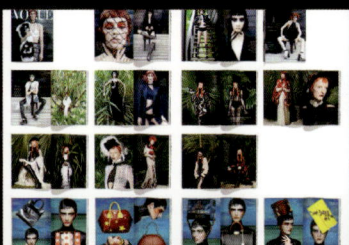

FRANÇOIS NARS'SS EDITORIALS FOR LEADING FASHION MAGAZINES. *FROM TOP LEFT, BY ROW*: *VOGUE* KOREA, JULY 2013, COVER AND FASHION EDITORIAL, MODEL KWAK JI YOUNG. © 2014 CONDÉ NAST KOREA; *MARIE CLAIRE* U.S., SEPTEMBER 2015, *IDYLL WILD*, MODEL DARIA STROKOUS; *V*, FALL 2014, *NARS ATTACKS*, MODEL DARIA STROKOUS. ALL PHOTOGRAPHS BY FRANÇOIS NARS. © FRANÇOIS NARS.

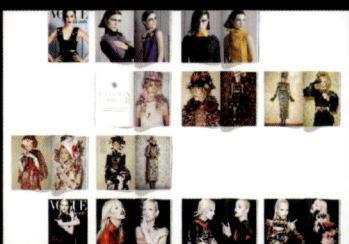

FRANÇOIS NARS'SS EDITORIALS FOR LEADING FASHION MAGAZINES. *FROM TOP LEFT, BY ROW*: *VOGUE* JAPAN, OCTOBER 2010, *NOUVELLE FEMME FATALE*, MODEL ANNA DE RIJK. © 2014 CONDÉ NAST JAPAN; *HARPER'S BAZAAR* AUSTRALIA, SEPTEMBER 2015, *PASSION FLOWER*, MODEL DARIA STROKOUS; *VOGUE* JAPAN, APRIL 2011, *THE CHINA SYNDROME*, MODEL GINTA LAPINA. © 2014 CONDÉ NAST JAPAN. ALL PHOTOGRAPHS BY FRANÇOIS NARS. © FRANÇOIS NARS.

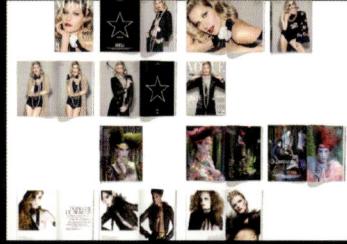

FRANÇOIS NARS'SS EDITORIALS FOR LEADING FASHION MAGAZINES. *FROM TOP LEFT, BY ROW: VOGUE* BRAZIL, DECEMBER 2015, *GISELE*, MODEL GISELE BÜNDCHEN. © EDIÇÕES GLOBO CONDÉ NAST; *VOGUE* RUSSIA, JANUARY 2011, MODEL IRIS STRUBEGGER. © CONDÉ NAST RUSSIA; *VOGUE* PARIS, OCTOBER 2009, *DÉBAUCHE DE PIGMENTS*. © CONDÉ NAST FRANCE. ALL PHOTOGRAPHS BY FRANÇOIS NARS. © FRANÇOIS NARS.

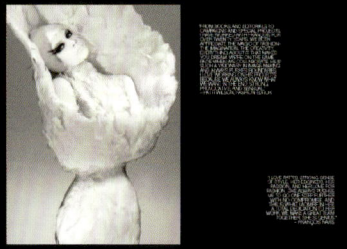

MUSE MAGAZINE, 2009–2010, MODEL NATASHA POLY, PHOTOGRAPH BY FRANÇOIS NARS. © FRANÇOIS NARS.

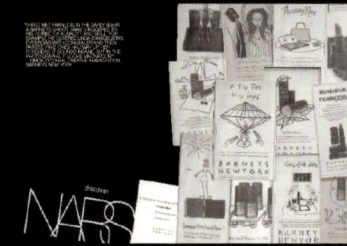

NARS'SS EARLY YEARS AT BARNEYS NEW YORK. *FROM LEFT TO RIGHT*: A BARNEYS NEW YORK INVITATION FOR THE NARS LAUNCH, 1994; NARS ADS IN *BARNEYS NEW YORK MAGAZINE*, 1994 TO 1997. ALL PHOTOGRAPHS © NARS COSMETICS/ BARNEYS INC.

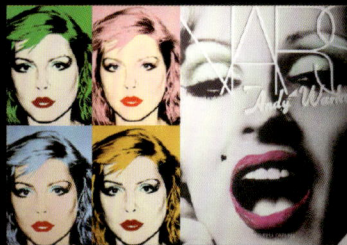

NARS ANDY WARHOL HOLIDAY 2012 COLLECTION. *FROM LEFT TO RIGHT*: DEBBIE HARRY; BEAUTIFUL DARLING. ALL PHOTOGRAPHS © 2015 THE ANDY WARHOL FOUNDATION FOR THE VISUAL ARTS, INC./ARTISTS RIGHT SOCIETY (ARS), NEW YORK/NARS COSMETICS.

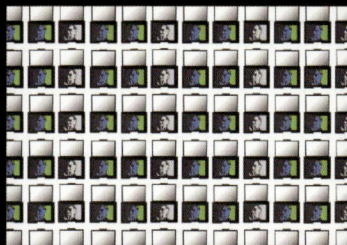

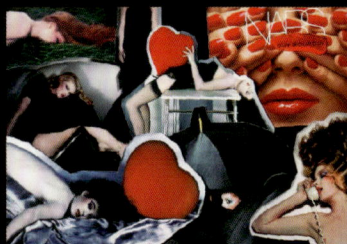

NARS ANDY WARHOL HOLIDAY 2012 COLLECTION. SELF PORTRAIT EYE SHADOW PALETTES. © 2015 THE ANDY WARHOL FOUNDATION FOR THE VISUAL ARTS, INC./ARTISTS RIGHT SOCIETY (ARS), NEW YORK/NARS COSMETICS.

NARS GUY BOURDIN HOLIDAY 2013 COLLECTION. ALL PHOTOGRAPHS BY GUY BOURDIN. © ESTATE OF GUY BOURDIN, REPRODUCED WITH THE PERMISSION OF ART + COMMERCE/ NARS COSMETICS.

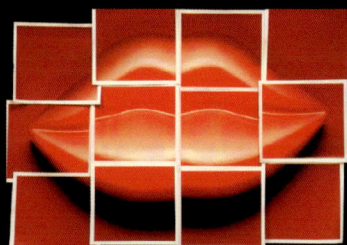

NARS GUY BOURDIN HOLIDAY 2013 GIFTING, LIP KEEPSAKE. © NARS COSMETICS.

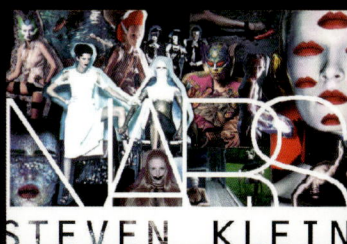

NARS STEVEN KLEIN HOLIDAY 2015 COLLECTION. ALL PHOTOGRAPHS BY STEVEN KLEIN. © STEVEN KLEIN/ NARS COSMETICS.

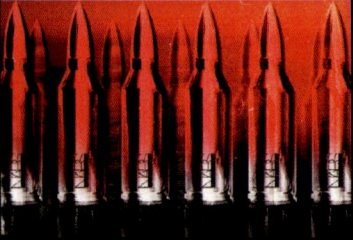

NARS STEVEN KLEIN HOLIDAY 2015
GIFTING, BULLET KEEPSAKE.
© NARS COSMETICS.

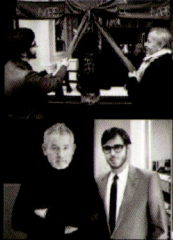

FRANÇOIS NARS AND FABIEN BARON
OPENING NARS'SS FIRST FLAGSHIP
BOUTIQUE, NEW YORK, 2011.
© DAVID X PRUTTING/BFA/SIPA USA.

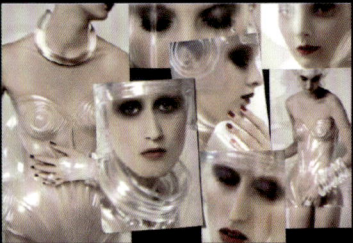

NARS SARAH MOON HOLIDAY 2016
COLLECTION. MODELS ANNA CLEVELAND
AND CODIE YOUNG. ALL PHOTOGRAPHS
BY SARAH MOON. © SARAH MOON/
NARS COSMETICS.

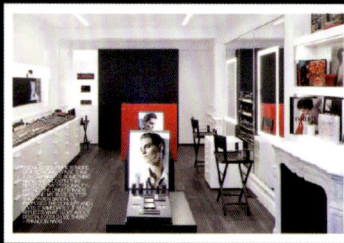

NARS'SS FIRST FLAGSHIP BOUTIQUE,
413 BLEECKER STREET, NEW YORK.
© DEAN KAUFMAN.

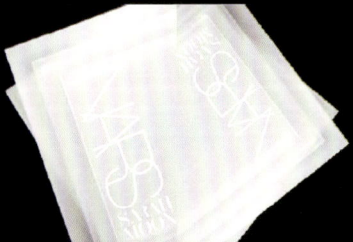

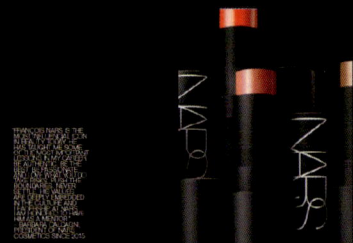

NARS SARAH MOON HOLIDAY 2016
GIFTING, KEEPSAKE.
© NARS COSMETICS.

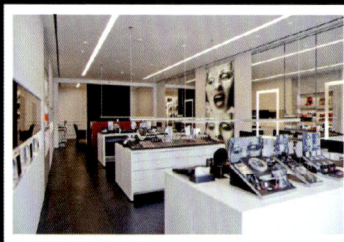

NARS'SS FLAGSHIP BOUTIQUE IN LOS
ANGELES, 8412 MELROSE AVENUE, WEST
HOLLYWOOD. © NARS COSMETICS.

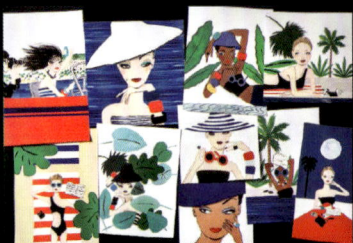

NARS SUMMER 2016 COLLECTION.
ALL ILLUSTRATIONS BY KONSTANTIN
KAKANIAS. © KONSTANTIN KAKANIAS/
NARS COSMETICS.

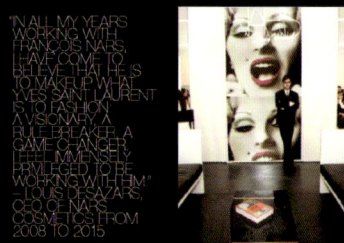

FRANÇOIS NARS IN THE NARS BOUTIQUE
FOR THE LAUNCH OF THE NARS ANDY
WARHOL HOLIDAY 2012 COLLECTION,
LOS ANGELES. © 2015 THE ANDY
WARHOL FOUNDATION FOR THE VISUAL
ARTS, INC./ARTISTS RIGHT SOCIETY (ARS
NEW YORK/NARS COSMETICS.

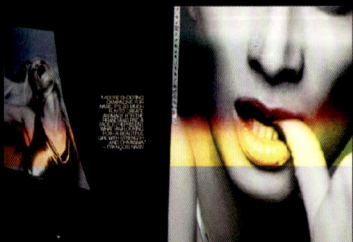

FILM STILLS FROM THE BEHIND-THE-
SCENES OF THE NARS FALL 2012 CAMPAIGN
SHOOT. © NARS COSMETICS.

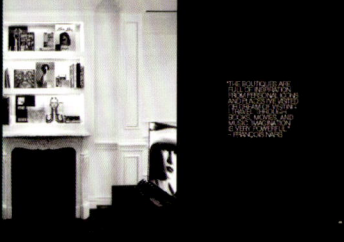

NARS'SS FIRST FLAGSHIP BOUTIQUE,
413 BLEECKER STREET, NEW YORK.
© DEAN KAUFMAN.

NARS MATTE MULTIPLE, PHOTOGRAPH BY
BRENTON CARTER. © NARS COSMETICS.

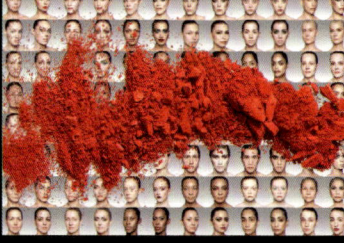

NARS BLUSH EXHIBIT A AND COLLAGE
OF PORTRAITS PHOTOGRAPHED
BY FRANÇOIS NARS, PREVIOUSLY
PUBLISHED IN MAKEUP YOUR MIND
EXPRESS YOURSELF, 2011.
© NARS COSMETICS.

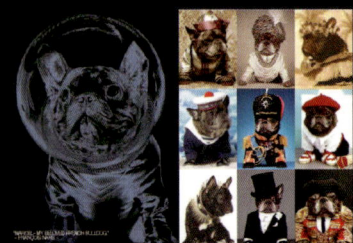

MARCEL, FRANÇOIS NARS'SS FRENCH
BULLDOG, THE FACE OF NARS HOLIDAY
CARDS FOR MORE THAN TEN YEARS
UNTIL 2012, ALL PHOTOGRAPHS BY
FRANÇOIS NARS. © FRANÇOIS NARS.

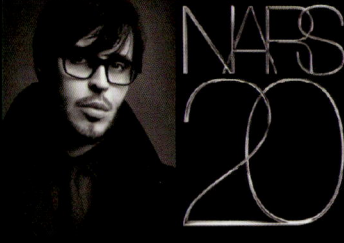

LEFT: FRANÇOIS NARS.
© PATRICK DEMARCHELIER. RIGHT:
NARS'SS TWENTIETH ANNIVERSARY
LOGO. © NARS COSMETICS.

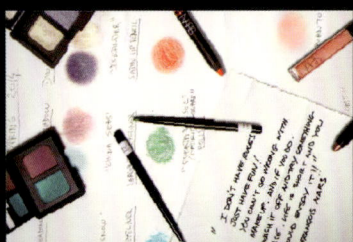

FRANÇOIS NARS DEVELOPING THE FALL
2014 COLOR COLLECTION.
© NARS COSMETICS.

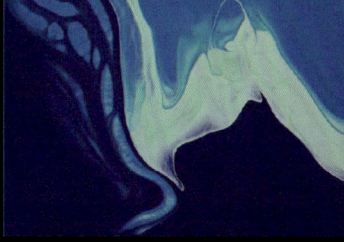

NARS STILL-LIFE, PHOTOGRAPH BY
MAXIME POIBLANC. © NARS COSMETICS.

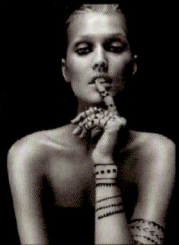

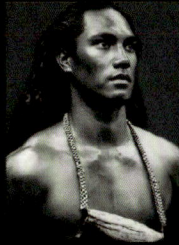

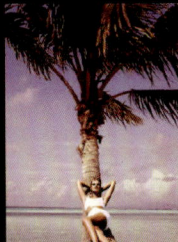

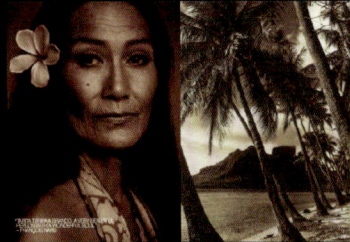

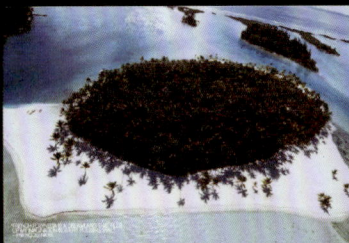

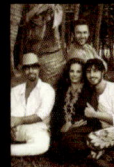

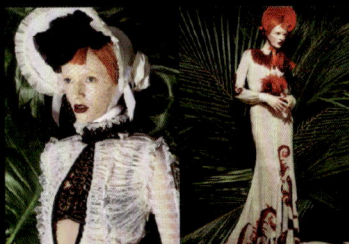

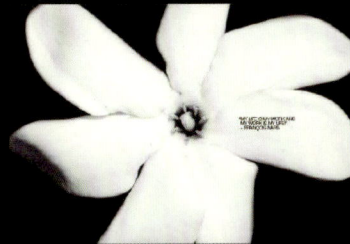

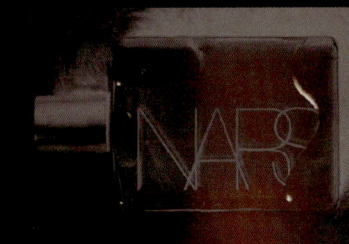

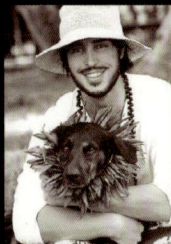

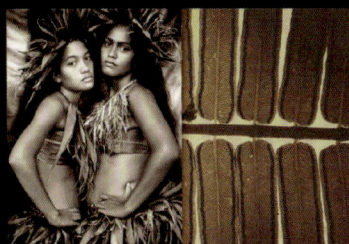

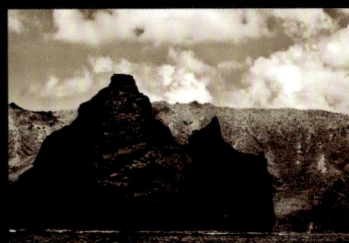

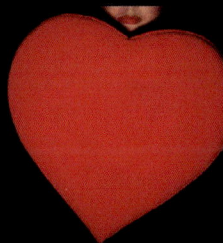

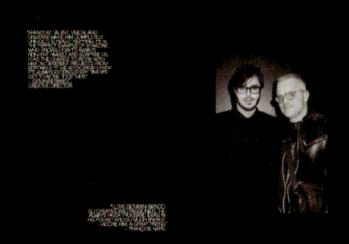

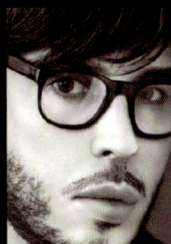

FIRST PUBLISHED IN THE UNITED STATES OF AMERICA IN 2016 BY
RIZZOLI INTERNATIONAL PUBLICATIONS INC.
300 PARK AVENUE SOUTH, NEW YORK, NY 10010
WWW.RIZZOLIUSA.COM

FRANÇOIS NARS
© 2016 NARS COSMETICS DIVISION OF SHISEIDO AMERICAS CORPORATION

BOOK AND COVER DESIGN: FABIEN BARON, BARON & BARON INC.
FOREWORD COPYRIGHT © FABIEN BARON

DISTRIBUTED IN THE U.S. TRADE BY RANDOM HOUSE, NEW YORK.

PRINTED IN ITALY.

ISBN: 978-0-8478-5821-7
LIBRARY OF CONGRESS CONTROL NUMBER: 2016935271

2016 2017 2018 2019 / 10 9 8 7 6 5 4 3 2 1